Inflammatory Bowel Disease: Clinical Gastroenterology

Inflammatory Bowel Disease: Clinical Gastroenterology

Edited by Remy Bowen

hayle
medical

New York

Hayle Medical,
750 Third Avenue, 9th Floor,
New York, NY 10017, USA

Visit us on the World Wide Web at:
www.haylemedical.com

ISBN: 978-1-63241-913-2

Cataloging-in-Publication Data

 Inflammatory bowel disease : clinical gastroenterology / edited by Remy Bowen.
    p. cm.
 Includes bibliographical references and index.
 ISBN 978-1-63241-913-2
 1. Inflammatory bowel diseases. 2. Gastroenterology. 3. Inflammatory bowel diseases--Treatment.
 4. Gastroenteritis. I. Bowen, Remy.

RC862.I53 I54 2020

616.344--dc23

Table of Contents

Preface

Every book is initially just a concept; it takes months of research and hard work to give it the final shape in which the readers receive it. In its early stages, this book also went through rigorous reviewing. The notable contributions made by experts from across the globe were first molded into patterned chapters and then arranged in a sensibly sequential manner to bring out the best results.

Inflammatory bowel disease (IBD) is a pathological condition of the colon and the small intestine. It is a complex multifactorial disease arising due to a genetic predisposition to the disease and interaction with environmental stimuli. Dietary patterns, alterations in the gut microbiome and loss of integrity of the intestinal epithelium can contribute to IBD. The common forms of inflammatory bowel disease are ulcerative colitis and Crohn's disease. Ulcerative colitis is restricted to the colon and rectum, whereas Crohn's disease affects any part of the gastrointestinal tract. Microscopically, the former extends only to the mucosa while the latter affects the full thickness of the bowel wall. Both these diseases have extra-intestinal manifestations such as arthritis, liver problems, eye problems, etc. Anemia is a common complication of both these diseases. This book explores all the important aspects of clinical gastroenterology in the present day scenario. It includes some of the vital pieces of work being conducted across the world, on inflammatory bowel disease. It is a resource guide for experts as well as students.

It has been my immense pleasure to be a part of this project and to contribute my years of learning in such a meaningful form. I would like to take this opportunity to thank all the people who have been associated with the completion of this book at any step.

Editor

Rate and Predictors of Mucosal Healing in Patients with Inflammatory Bowel Disease Treated with Anti-TNF-Alpha Antibodies

Florian Beigel[1]*, Matthias Deml[1], Fabian Schnitzler[1], Simone Breiteneicher[1], Burkhard Göke[1], Thomas Ochsenkühn[2], Stephan Brand[1]

1 Department of Medicine II, University Hospital Munich-Grosshadern, Ludwig-Maximilians-University, Munich, Germany, 2 Isarmedizin Zentrum, Munich, Germany

Abstract

Objective: Mucosal healing (MH) is an important treatment goal in patients with inflammatory bowel disease (IBD), but factors predicting MH under medical therapy are largely unknown. In this study, we aimed to characterize predictive factors for MH in anti-TNF-alpha antibody-treated IBD patients.

Methods: We retrospectively analyzed 248 IBD patients (61.3% CD, 38.7% UC) treated with anti-TNF-alpha antibodies (infliximab and/or adalimumab) for MH, defined as macroscopic absence of inflammatory lesions (Mayo endoscopy score 0 or SES-CD score 0) in colonoscopies which were analyzed before and after initiation of an anti-TNF-alpha antibody treatment.

Results: In patients treated with only one anti-TNF-alpha antibody ("TNF1 group", n = 202), 56 patients (27.7%) achieved complete MH at follow-up colonoscopy (median overall follow-up time: 63 months). In a second cohort (n = 46), which comprised patients who were consecutively treated with two anti-TNF-alpha antibodies ("TNF2 group"), 13 patients (28.3%) achieved complete MH (median overall follow-up time: 64.5 months). Compared to patients without MH, CRP values at follow-up colonoscopy were significantly lower in patients with MH (TNF1 group: $p = 8.35 \times 10^{-5}$; TNF2 group: $p = 0.002$). Multivariate analyses confirmed CRP at follow-up colonoscopy as predictor for MH in the TNF1 group ($p = 0.012$). Overall need for surgery was lower in patients with MH (TNF1 group: $p = 0.01$; TNF2 group: $p = 0.03$).

Conclusions: We identified low serum CRP level at follow-up colonoscopy as predictor for MH, while MH was an excellent negative predictor for the need for surgery.

Editor: Udai P. Singh, University of South Carolina School of Medicine, United States of America

Funding: F. Beigel is supported by grants from the Deutsche Forschungsgemeinschaft (DFG, BE 4490/2-1). S. Brand is supported by grants from the Deutsche Forschungsgemeinschaft (DFG, BR 1912/5-1), the Else Kröner-Fresenius-Stiftung (Else Kröner Exzellenzstipendium 2010; 2010_EKES.32). The funders had no role in study design, data collection and analysis, decision to publish, or preparation of the manuscript.

Competing Interests: F. Beigel, F. Schnitzler, T. Ochsenkühn and S. Brand received lecture fees, travel support and financial support for research from: Abbott, MSD.

* Email: florian.beigel@med.uni-muenchen.de

¶ These authors share senior authorship on this work.

Introduction

Treatment of patients with inflammatory bowel disease (IBD) has been focused but is also currently focused on symptomatic relief and clinical improvement. However, since the course of IBD may progress from an inflammatory to a stricturing and penetrating type of disease with a high rate of bowel surgery (up to 80% in Crohn's disease (CD)) [1,2], early and sufficient treatment strategies to protect the mucosal integrity and therefore prevent disease progression are warranted. Colonoscopy is the gold standard for diagnosing mucosal injury in IBD patients and to evaluate the efficacy of therapy. Various endoscopic scores (e.g. Mayo [3], Matts [4] and Lichtiger score [5] in ulcerative colitis; CDEIS [6] or SES-CD [7] in CD) are used in clinical practice and clinical studies to assess the mucosal status in IBD patients. Since routine surveillance colonoscopy in asymptomatic IBD patients

without dysplastic lesions depending on the severity and type of IBD are recommended only every 2–15 years, the mucosal status after initiation or maintenance of a new therapy often remains unclear in most of these patients. Moreover, willingness for control colonoscopy in asymptomatic patients is low.

There is growing evidence, that mucosal healing (MH) is associated with a better long-term outcome, lower need for surgeries and hospitalisation and improved quality of life in IBD patients [8,9,10]. Moreover, in a statement of the European Crohn's and Colitis Organization (ECCO) regarding the impact of MH on the course of IBD, the need for further studies was addressed [11].

Therefore, we aimed to analyze in this study the real-life prevalence and predictive factors of mucosal healing in IBD patients treated with anti-TNF-alpha antibodies in a large single center cohort.

Materials and Methods

Ethics statement

This was a retrospective study using medical records, and statistical analysis was anonymized. The ethics committee of the University of Munich was consulted (UE number 055-13) and a formal written waiver for the need of ethics approval was obtained. Written informed consent of the patients was not obtained, since patient records and relevant data were anonymized and de-identified prior to analysis.

Study cohorts

All patients, who received anti-TNF-alpha antibody treatment (infliximab or adalimumab) at our IBD center for the first time and during the time period from 2002 to 2013, were eligible for this study. Out of this cohort, patients with at least one colonoscopy before start of (baseline colonoscopy) and one during anti-TNF-alpha antibody treatment (follow-up colonoscopy) were included in this study (Figure 1). If more than one baseline or follow-up colonoscopy was available for analysis, the last colonoscopy before start of anti-TNF-alpha antibody treatment and the first colonoscopy after start of anti-TNF-alpha antibody treatment were used for analysis, respectively. Patients, who were treated with a second anti-TNF-alpha antibody after loss of response or intolerance to the first anti-TNF-alpha antibody between the time periods from baseline to follow-up colonoscopy, were assigned to the cohort "TNF2 group". All other patients were assigned to the cohort "TNF1 group". For further analyses, patients were divided according their disease entities (CD group and UC group).

Medical records were analyzed regarding the following parameters: demographics, C-reactive protein (CRP) value at baseline and follow-up colonoscopy, white blood cell count (WBC) at baseline and follow-up colonoscopy, age at first diagnosis, disease duration, type of anti-TNF-alpha antibody, concomitant medication, time to first anti-TNF-alpha antibody treatment, duration of anti-TNF-alpha antibody treatment, time between baseline and follow-up colonoscopy, smoking, BMI, extraintestinal manifestation, family history of IBD, reason for second (follow-up) endoscopy and hospitalization or surgery from baseline colonoscopy until last follow-up.

Medical treatment

Adalimumab was injected at doses of 160 mg loading dose, following 80 mg and then 40 mg subcutaneously every other week. Infliximab infusions were administered using a dose of 5 mg/kg body weight intravenously over 2 hours at weeks 0, 2, 6 (induction therapy) and thereafter every 8 weeks (maintenance therapy). Thiopurines were given at the full dose (mercaptopurine 1.0–1.5 mg/kg body weight, azathioprine 2.0–2.5 mg/kg body weight) from the beginning of therapy.

Endoscopy and histopathological analysis

Colonoscopy reports of baseline and follow-up colonoscopies were analyzed by two independent medical reviewers. The Mayo endoscopy score [3] was used for patients with UC and the SES-CD score [7] for patients with CD. Patients with macroscopic absence of IBD-defining markers and a Mayo endoscopy subscore of 0 (UC) or a SES-CD score of 0 (CD) were defined as patients with MH. All other patients were defined as patients without MH.

Statistical analysis

Comparison of demographic and clinical characteristics of the study populations was performed using the χ^2-test or Fisher's exact test for categorical variables and by using the Wilcoxon-Mann-Whitney test for continuous variables. Survival analyses techniques were used to model the time to surgery. All statistical analyses were performed using R (R.2.13.2). Hypotheses were tested at 5% level of significance (two-sided).

Results

Patients' characteristics

Data of 802 IBD patients were available for analysis (Figure 1). Out of these patients, 248 patients met the inclusion criteria and were eligible for the study. 152 patients (61.3%) had CD and 96 (38.7%) had UC.

In the TNF1 group (n = 202), 120 patients (59.4%) had CD and 82 patients (40.6%) had UC. One hundred and eight patients were female (52.5%); median of overall follow-up time for all patients was 63 months (range 3–127 months).

The TNF2 group consisted of 46 patients, 32 (69.6%) with CD and 14 (30.4%) with UC. Twenty patients were female (43.5%), median of follow-up time for the patients of the TNF2 group was 64.5 months (range 9–126). The demographic and clinical characteristics of the study cohorts are provided in table 1 and tables S1 and S6 (UC/CD subcohorts).

In the TNF2 group, 42 patients were switched from infliximab to adalimumab and 4 patients were switched from adalimumab to infliximab. Reasons for the switch from a first anti-TNF-alpha antibody to a second anti-TNF-alpha antibody in these patients were allergic reactions (n = 30; 65.2%), intolerance (n = 3; 6.5%) and loss of response (n = 13; 28.3%).

The most common reason for the second (follow-up) endoscopy was routine control colonoscopy (174 patients = 86.1% in the TNF1 group, and 40 patients = 87.0% in the TNF2 group). Only a minority of the patients had second (follow-up) endoscopy due to disease flares (28 = 13.9% in the TNF1 group, and 6 patients = 13.0% in the TNF2 group).

The median time from first anti-TNF-alpha antibody treatment to follow-up colonoscopy was 11 months in the TNF1 group and 25.5 months in the TNF2 group.

Mucosal healing at follow-up colonoscopy

In the TNF1 group, 56 patients (27.7%) had complete mucosal healing (as defined in the Methods section; Mayo endoscopy score 0 or SES-CD score 0) at follow-up colonoscopy, while 146 patients (72.3%) had no mucosal healing (Figure 2).

In the TNF2 group, 13 patients (28.3%) patients had complete mucosal healing at follow-up colonoscopy, while 33 patients (71.4%) had no mucosal healing at follow-up colonoscopy (Figure 2).

In the subanalysis of UC patients (n = 96), in the TNF1 group (n = 82) 23 patients (28.0%) patients had complete mucosal healing at follow-up colonoscopy, while 59 patients (72.0%) had no mucosal healing at follow-up colonoscopy (Table S2). In the TNF2 group (n = 14), 5 patients (35.7%) had complete mucosal healing at follow-up colonoscopy, while 9 patients (64.3%) had no mucosal healing at follow-up colonoscopy (Table S3).

In the subanalysis of CD patients (n = 152), in the TNF1 group (n = 120) 33 patients (27.5%) patients had complete mucosal healing at follow-up colonoscopy, while 87 patients (72.5%) had no mucosal healing at follow-up colonoscopy (Table S7). In the TNF2 group (n = 32), 8 patients (25.0%) patients had complete mucosal healing at follow-up colonoscopy, while 24 patients

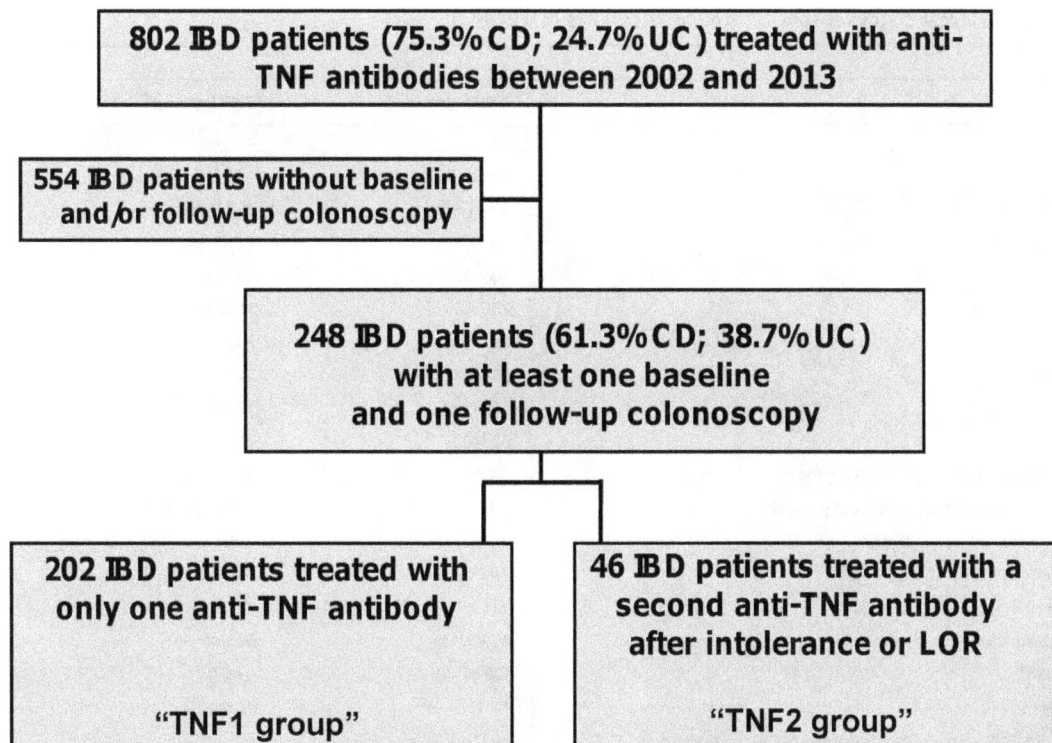

Figure 1. Study design. Data of 802 patients were available for analysis (75.3% patients with Crohn's disease and 24.7% patients with ulcerative colitis). In 554 IBD patients, there was no baseline and/or follow-up colonoscopy available. Accordingly, 248 patients were included in the analysis, while 202 patients were treated with one anti-TNF antibody between baseline and follow-up colonoscopy (TNF1 group) and 46 patients were treated with a second anti-TNF antibody after loss of response or intolerance to a first anti-TNF antibody (TNF2 group).

(75.0%) had no mucosal healing at follow-up colonoscopy (Table S8).

Univariate analyses reveals serum CRP levels as predictive factor for mucosal healing at follow-up colonoscopy

In patients with MH, CRP values of follow-up colonoscopy were significantly lower compared to CRP values at baseline colonoscopy (median 0.9 mg/dL at baseline vs. 0.3 mg/dL at follow-up; p = 0.002), while there was no significant difference of CRP values from baseline to follow-up colonoscopy in patients without MH (median 1.1 mg/dL at baseline vs. 0.55 mg/dL at follow-up; p = 0.07; Table 2). Interestingly, combination therapy with thiopurines and anti-TNF-alpha antibodies had no influence on mucosal healing status (10 patients with mucosal healing vs. 29 patients without mucosal healing; p = 1.0).

Similar to the TNF1 group, in the TNF2 group CRP values at follow-up colonoscopy were lower in patients with mucosal healing compared to baseline values, but not statistically significant (CRP median 0.6 mg/dL at baseline vs. 0.3 mg/dL at follow-up; p = 0.16). In patients without MH, CRP values at follow-up were not significantly different to CRP values at baseline colonoscopy (CRP median 0.7 mg/dL at baseline vs. 0.8 mg/dL at follow-up; p = 0.14, Table 3).

At baseline colonoscopy, CRP values were not significantly different in patients with or without MH in the TNF1 group (p = 0.95). However, CRP values were significantly lower at follow-up colonoscopy in patients with MH compared to patients without MH in the TNF1 group (p = 8.35E-05; Figure 3). Similar to the TNF1 group, baseline colonoscopy CRP values were not significantly different in patients with or without MH in the

TNF2 group (p = 0.06). In patients with MH of the TNF2 group, CRP values at follow-up colonoscopy were significantly lower compared to patients without MH (p = 0.002; Figure 4).

In the subanalysis of UC patients, CRP values in the TNF1 group at follow-up colonoscopy were significantly lower in patients with MH compared to patients without MH (CRP median 0.10 mg/dL (MH) vs. 0.50 mg/dL (no MH); p = 0.0002; Figure S1), while CRP values at baseline colonoscopy were not significantly different (CRP median 0.6 mg/dL (MH) vs. 1.0 mg/dL (no MH); p = 0.58). In patients with MH, CRP values of follow-up colonoscopy were significantly lower compared to CRP values at baseline colonoscopy (CRP median 0.6 mg/dL at baseline vs. 0.1 mg/dL at follow-up; p = 0.03), while there was no significant difference of CRP values from baseline to follow-up colonoscopy in patients without MH (CRP median 1.0 mg/dL at baseline vs. 0.5 mg/dL at follow-up; p = 0.10). In the TNF2 group, CRP values at follow-up colonoscopy were significantly lower in patients with mucosal healing compared to patients without MH (CRP median 0.20 mg/dL (MH) vs. 0.80 mg/dL (no MH); p = 0.03; Figure S2), while CRP values at baseline colonoscopy were not significantly different (CRP median 0.55 mg/dL (MH) vs. 0.6 mg/dL (no MH); p = 0.26). In patients with MH, CRP values of follow-up colonoscopy were significantly lower compared to CRP values at baseline colonoscopy (CRP median 0.55 mg/dL at baseline vs. 0.20 mg/dL at follow-up; p = 0.01); there was no significant difference of CRP values from baseline to follow-up colonoscopy in patients without MH (CRP median 0.6 mg/dL at baseline vs. 0.8 mg/dL at follow-up; p = 0.80).

Table 1. Demographic and clinical characteristics of the study cohorts (n = 248).

	TNF1 group	TNF2 group
Patients (n =)	202	46
Median age (yrs) [Range]	38 [18–72]	43.5 [17–73]
Median age at diagnosis (yrs) [Range]	25 [6–63]	26 [7–68]
Median disease duration (yrs) [Range]	10 [0–45]	9.5 [2–44]
Female sex (%)	106 (52.5)	20 (43.5)
Smoker (%)	73 (36.2)	14 (30.4)
Family history of IBD (%)	27 (13.4)	2 (4.3)
Extraintestinal manifestation (%)	80 (39.6)	24 (52.2)
Crohn's disease (%)	120 (59.4)	32 (69.6)
Ulcerative colitis (%)	82 (40.6)	14 (30.4)
Mean CRP-value at baseline colonoscopy (mg/dL) [Range]	2.409 [0.1–33.8]	2.425 [0.1–15.4]
Mean CRP-value at follow-up colonoscopy (mg/dL) [Range]	1.341 [0.1–23.1]	1.351 [0.1–10.1]
Mean WBC at baseline colonoscopy (G/L) [Range]	9.263 [2.3–23.1]	9.697 [4.4;23.9]
Mean WBC at follow-up colonoscopy (G/L) [Range]	7.493 [1.6;17.3]	8.389 [2.7;19.5]
Thiopurine treatment ever (%)	172 (85.1)	44 (95.7)
Median thiopurine treatment duration (months) [Range]	40 [0;211]	60.5 [43;237]
Infliximab treated patients (%)	188 (93.1)	4 (8.7)
Adalimumab treated patients (%)	14 (6.9)	42 (91.3)
Anti-TNF-alpha antibody and thiopurine treated patients at follow-up (%)	39 (19.3)	5 (10.9)
Median duration infliximab treatment (months) [Range]	11 [0–70]	18 [1–39]
Median duration adalimumab treatment (months) [Range]	6 [1–41]	10.5 [0–44]
Median time to first anti-TNF-alpha antibody treatment (years) [Range]	7 [0–42]	7 [0–39]
Median time from baseline to follow-up colonoscopy (months) [Range]	19 [0–123]	39.5 [1–104]
Median time from first to second anti-TNF-alpha antibody treatment (months) [Range]	n/a	7.5 [0–68]
Patients with surgery until follow-up (%)	34 (16.8)	10 (23.8)
Patients hospitalized until follow-up (%)	57 (28.2)	18 (39.1)
Median follow-up (months) [Range]	63 [3–127]	64.5 [9–126]

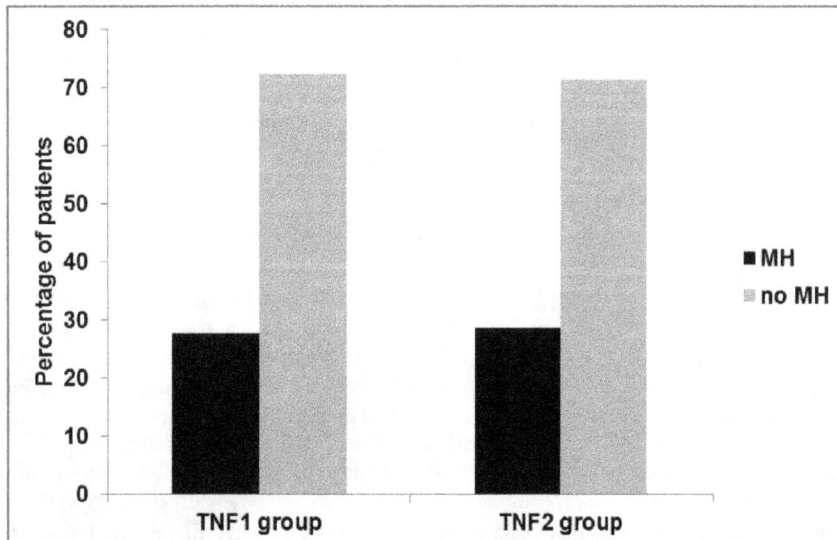

Figure 2. Rates of mucosal healing in both groups. In the TNF1 group, 146 patients (72.3%) had no MH, while 56 patients (27.7%) had MH. In the TNF2 group, 13 patients (28.6%) patients had MH, while 33 patients (71.4%) had no MH at follow-up colonoscopy.

Table 2. Demographic and clinical characteristics of the TNF1 group (n = 202) regarding MH.

	MH	No MH	p-value	OR [95%CI]
Patients (n =)	56 (27.7)	146 (72.3)	N/A	N/A
Median age (yrs) [Range]	38 [19;67]	37.5 [18;72]	0.961	1.001 [0.978;1.023]
Median age at diagnosis (yrs) [Range]	27.5 [14;48]	25 [6;63]	0.665	1.006 [0.980;1.033]
Median disease duration (yrs) [Range]	9.5 [0;33]	10 [0;45]	0.719	0.994 [0.961;1.027]
Female sex (%)	31 (55.4)	75 (51.4)	0.644	0.864 [0.465;1.605]
Smoker (%)	24 (42.9)	49 (33.6)	0.361	0.875 [0.658;1.165]
Family history of IBD (%)	3 (5.4)	24 (16.4)	0.048	3.556 [1.012;12.493]
Extraintestinal manifestation (%)	23 (41.1)	57 (39)	0.872	0.872 [0.428;1.778]
Diagnosis Crohn's disease/Ulcerative colitis	33/23	87/59	0.932	0.973 [0.520;1.821]
Mean (median) CRP-value at baseline colonoscopy (mg/dL) [Range]	2.441 (0.9) [0.1;14.8]	2.398 (1.1) [0.1;33.8]	0.948	0.997 [0.910;1.093]
Mean (median) CRP-value at follow-up colonoscopy (mg/dL) [Range]	0.583 (0.3) [0.1;4.3]	1.641 (0.550) [0.1;23.1]	0.040	1.705 [1.180;2.464]
Mean (median) WBC at baseline colonoscopy (G/L) [Range]	9.234 (8.5) [2.3;19.7]	9.274 (8.5) [3.5;23.1]	0.951	1.003 [0.916;1.098]
Mean (median) WBC at follow-up colonoscopy (G/L) [Range]	6.531(6.3) [1.6;14.6]	7.882 (7.700) [3.3;17.3]	0.02	1.250 [1.084;1.442]
Thiopurine treatment ever (%)	46 (82.1)	126 (86.3)	0.906	0.906 [0.176;4.649]
Median thiopurine treatment duration (months) [Range]	24 [4;104]	44.5 [0;211]	0.261	1.013 [0.990;1.037]
Infliximab treated patients (%)	53 (94.6)	135 (92.5)	0.7615	N/A
Adalimumab treated patients (%)	3 (5.4)	11 (7.5)	0.7615	N/A
Anti-TNF-alpha antibody and thiopurine treated patients at follow-up (%)	10 (17.9)	29 (19.9)	1.000	N/A
Median duration infliximab treatment (months) [Range]	12.5 [0;69]	10 [0;70]	0.4191	0.992 [0.971;1.012]
Median duration adalimumab treatment (months) [Range]	12 [0;69]	10 [0;70]	0.727	0.996 [0.975;1.018]
Median thiopurine treatment duration (months) [Range]	22.5 [1;41]	6 [1;25]	0.078	0.883 [0.769;1.014]
Median time to first anti-TNF-alpha antibody treatment (years) [Range]	6 [0;30]	7 [0;42]	0.835	0.996 [0.960;1.033]
Median time from baseline to follow-up colonoscopy (months) [Range]	19.5 [0;106]	19 [0;123]	0.853	0.999 [0.984;1.013]
Patients with surgery until follow-up (%)	3 (5.4)	31 (21.2)	0.006	N/A
Patients hospitalized until follow-up (%)	10 (17.9)	47 (32.2)	0.054	N/A
Median follow-up (months) [Range]	70 [22;127]	60 [3;125]	0.141	0.991 [0.980;1.003]

In the subanalysis of CD patients, CRP values in the TNF1 group at follow-up colonoscopy were significantly lower in patients with MH compared to patients without MH (CRP median 0.40 mg/dL (MH) vs. 0.60 mg/dL (no MH); p = 0.01; Figure S3), while CRP values at baseline colonoscopy were not significantly different (CRP median 1.5 mg/dL (MH) vs. 1.15 mg/dL (no MH); p = 0.57). In patients with MH, CRP values of follow-up colonoscopy were significantly lower compared to CRP values at baseline colonoscopy (median 1.5 mg/dL at baseline vs. 0.4 mg/dL at follow-up; p = 0.02), while there was no significant difference of CRP values from baseline to follow-up colonoscopy in patients without MH (median 1.15 mg/dL at baseline vs. 0.6 mg/dL at follow-up; p = 0.23). In the TNF2 group, CRP values at follow-up colonoscopy were significantly lower in patients with MH compared to patients without MH (CRP median 0.60 mg/dL (MH) vs. 0.70 mg/dL (no MH); p = 0.01; Figure S4), while CRP values at baseline colonoscopy were not significantly different

(CRP median 0.6 mg/dL (MH) vs. 2.3 mg/dL (no MH); p = 0.08). However, in patients with MH, CRP values of follow-up colonoscopy were not significantly lower compared to CRP values at baseline colonoscopy (median 0.6 mg/dL at baseline vs. 0.6 mg/dL at follow-up; p = 0.24); there was also no significant difference of CRP values from baseline to follow-up colonoscopy in patients without MH (median 2.3 mg/dL at baseline vs. 0.7 mg/dL at follow-up; p = 0.16).

Mulitvariate analyses reveals serum CRP levels as predictive factor for mucosal healing at follow-up colonoscopy

Multivariate analysis confirmed CRP at follow-up colonoscopy as predictive factor for MH (p = 0.01) in the TNF1 group, while CRP at follow-up colonoscopy was not predictive for MH in the TNF2 group (p = 0.11, Tables 4 and 5).

Table 3. Demographic and clinical characteristics of the TNF2 group (n = 46) regarding MH.

	MH	No MH	p-value	OR [95%CI]
Patients (n=)	13 (28.6)	33 (71.4)	N/A	N/A
Median age (yrs) [Range]	44 [26;73]	42 [17;69]	0.277	0.974 [0.929;1.021]
Median age at diagnosis (yrs) [Range]	33 [7;68]	25 [10;55]	0.142	0.965 [0.921;1.012]
Median disease duration (yrs) [Range]	8 [3;39]	12 [2;44]	0.607	1.018 [0.950;1.091]
Female sex (%)	7 (53.8)	13 (39.4)	0.376	0.557 [0.153;2.034]
Smoker (%)	4 (30.8)	10 (30.3)	0.530	0.763 [0.327;1.777]
Family history of IBD (%)	1 (7.7)	1 (3.0)	0.477	0.355 [0.02;6.172]
Extraintestinal manifestation (%)	3 (23.1)	21 (63.6)	0.035	5.091 [1.12;23.142]
Diagnosis Crohn's disease/Ulcerative colitis	8/5	24/9	0.460	0.60 [0.155;2.325]
Mean (median) CRP-value at baseline colonoscopy (mg/dL) [Range]	1.167 (0.6) [0.1;4.9]	2.902 (0.67) [0.1;15.4]	0.212	1.329 [0.850;2.079]
Mean (median) CRP-value at follow-up colonoscopy (mg/dL) [Range]	0.380 (0.300) [0.1;0.8]	1.645 (0.8) [0.1;10.1]	0.003	0.31 [0.144;0.661]
Mean (median) WBC at baseline colonoscopy (G/L) [Range]	9.144 (8.1) [6.8;12.6]	10.064 (9.1) [4.4;23.9]	0.581	1.075 [0.831;1.390]
Mean (median) WBC at follow-up colonoscopy (G/L) [Range]	8.265 (7.0) [4;19.3]	8.430 (7.70) [2.7;19.5]	0.904	1.011 [0.849;1.204]
Thiopurine treatment ever (%)	13 (100)	31 (93.9)	1.000	N/A
Median thiopurine treatment duration (months) [Range]	75 [75;75]	46 [43;237]	0.725	1.006 [0.971;1.043]
Infliximab after adalimumab treated patients (%)	1 (7.7)	3 (9.1)	1.000	N/A
Adalimumab after infliximab treated patients (%)	12 (92.3)	30 (91.9)	1.000	N/A
Anti-TNF-alpha antibody and thiopurine treated patients at follow-up (%)	1 (7.7)	4 (12.1)	1.000	N/A
Median duration infliximab treatment (months) [Range]	17 [9;95]	29 [0;68]	0.985	1.000 [0.969;1.032]
Median duration adalimumab treatment (months) [Range]	17 [17;17]	19 [1;39]	0.865	1.015 [0.855;1.205]
Median thiopurine treatment duration (months) [Range]	9.5 [2;44]	13 [0;42]	0.458	0.981 [0.931;1.033]
Median time to first anti-TNF-alpha antibody treatment (years) [Range]	5 [0;37]	8 [0;39]	0.625	1.017 [0.950;1.089]
Median time from baseline to follow-up colonoscopy (months) [Range]	45 [14;90]	33 [1;104]	0.332	0.988 [0.964;1.012]
Median time from first to second anti-TNF-alpha antibody treatment (months) [Range]	5 [1;68]	10 [0;56]	0.576	1.013 [0.968;1.06]
Patients with surgery until follow-up (%)	0 (0)	10 (30.3)	0.042	N/A
Patients hospitalized until follow-up (%)	2 (15.4)	16 (48.5)	0.049	N/A
Median follow-up (months) [Range]	77 [14;123]	58 [9;126]	0.461	0.993 [0.973;1.012]

In the subanalysis of UC patients, CRP at follow-up colonoscopy was not predictive for MH in the TNF1 group (p = 0.06) and the TNF2 group (p = 0.39) (Tables S4 and S5). In the subanalysis of CD patients, CRP at follow-up colonoscopy was also not predictive for MH in the TNF1 group (p = 0.08) and the TNF2 group (p = 0.28) (Tables S9 and S10).

Rate of hospitalization and surgery

Ten patients with MH and 47 patients without MH in the TNF1 group (p = 0.054) and 2 patients with MH and 16 patients without MH in the TNF2 group (p = 0.05) were hospitalized due to IBD (Tables 2 and 3).

Overall, 3 patients with MH and 31 patients without MH in the TNF1 group (p = 0.006) and no patient with MH and 10 patients without MH (p = 0.04) had surgery until follow-up in the TNF2 group (Tables 2 and 3). Accordingly, Kaplan-Mayer estimation revealed significantly lower need for surgery in patients with MH compared to patients without MH in both groups (Figures 5 and 6).

In the subanalysis of UC patients, 1 patients with MH and 21 patients without MH in the TNF1 group (p = 0.005) and no patient with MH and 5 patients without MH in the TNF2 group (p = 0.08) were hospitalized due to IBD. Overall, no patient with MH and 7 patients without MH in the TNF1 group (p = 0.18) and

Rate and Predictors of Mucosal Healing in Patients with Inflammatory Bowel Disease Treated with Anti-TNF-Alpha...

7

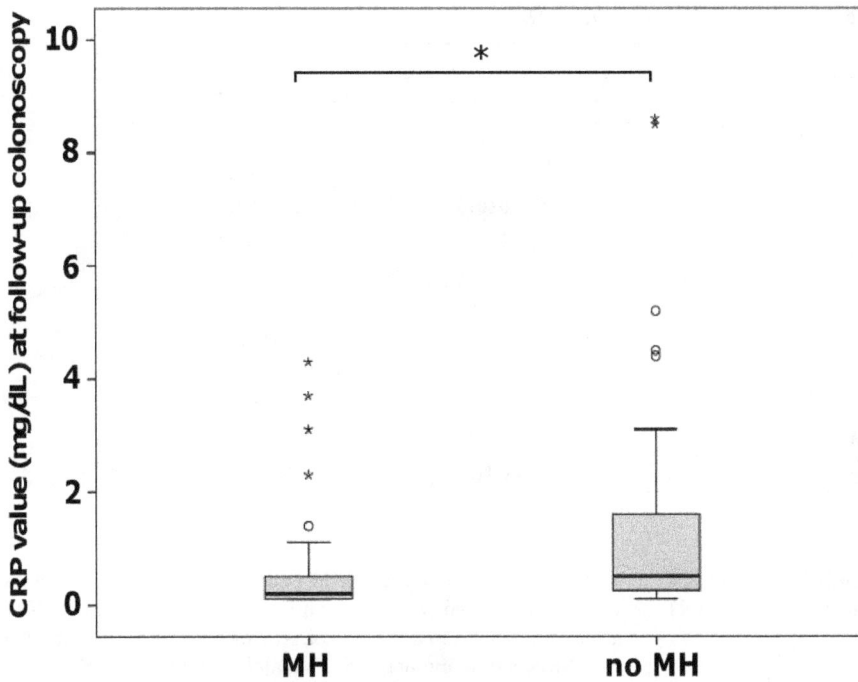

Figure 3. CRP values at follow-up colonoscopy (TNF1 group). At follow-up colonoscopy, CRP values were significantly lower in patients with MH compared to patients without MH (*p = 8.34E-05).

no patient with MH and 3 patients without MH (p = 0.25) had surgery until follow-up in the TNF2 group (Tables S2 and S3).

In the subanalysis of CD patients, 9 patients with MH and 26 patients without MH in the TNF1 group (p = 0.82) and 2 patients with MH and 11 patients without MH in the TNF2 group (p = 0.42) were hospitalized due to IBD. Overall, 3 patients with MH and 24 patients without MH in the TNF1 group (p = 0.049) and no patient with MH and 7 patients without MH (p = 0.14) had surgery until follow-up in the TNF2 group (Tables S7 and S8).

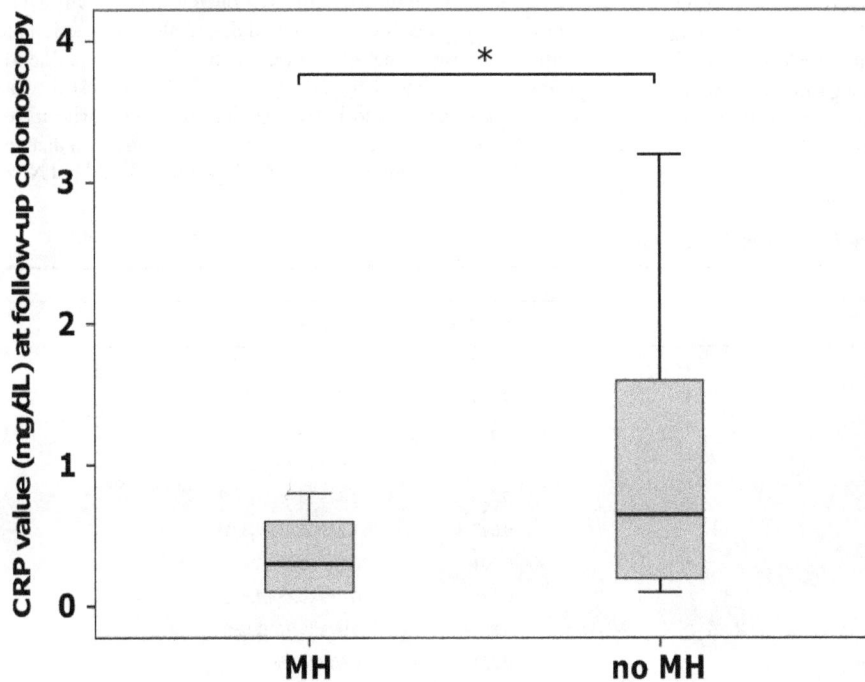

Figure 4. CRP values at follow-up colonoscopy (TNF2 group). At follow-up colonoscopy, there was a trend for lower CRP in patients with MH compared to patients without MH (*p = 0.002).

Table 4. Multivariate analysis for outcome MH in the TNF1 group (n = 202).

	p-value	OR [95%CI]
CRP-value at baseline colonoscopy	0.398	1.080 [0.904;1.290]
CRP-value at follow-up colonoscopy	0.012	1.687 [1.124;2.533]
WBC at baseline colonoscopy	0.685	0.976 [0.870;1.096]
WBC at follow-up colonoscopy	0.026	1.187 [1.021;1.380]
Age at diagnosis	0.869	0.901 [0.262;3.098]
Age	0.854	1.123 [0.326;3.865]
Gender	0.174	0.602 [0.289;1.251]
Smoker	0.428	0.871 [0.620;1.225]
Duration anti-TNF-alpha antibody treatment	0.691	0.992 [0.951;1.034]
Time to first anti-TNF-alpha antibody treatment	0.102	1.176 [0.968;1.429]
Time from baseline to follow-up colonoscopy	0.893	1.002 [0.967;1.039]

Kaplan-Mayer estimation revealed significantly lower need for surgery in patients with MH compared to patients without MH only in the TNF1 group of CD patients (Figures S5, S6, S7, S8).

Discussion

Mucosal healing (MH) in patients with IBD is an important treatment goal, leading to better long-term remission rates, better quality of life, lower need for hospitalisation and surgeries, and lower rates of colorectal cancer [9,12,13,14]. MH can be achieved with various treatment strategies including immunosuppressive therapies such as methotrexate or thiopurines and anti-TNF-alpha antibodies [8,15,16,17,18]. Former studies have demonstrated that corticosteroids are not suitable for maintenance of mucosal healing [19], and combination therapy with thiopurines and anti-TNF-alpha antibodies is superior compared to thiopurine monotherapy in CD regarding remission rates and MH [20]. Emerging data indicate that early use of anti-TNF-alpha antibodies lead to better long-term outcome in IBD patients by preventing mucosal damage [8,10,13,21]. However, results from prospective large-scale studies are still very limited.

In our study, we found a MH prevalence of 27.7% in patients who were treated with one anti-TNF-alpha antibody (TNF1 group) and 28.3% in a second cohort which included patients who were switched to another anti-TNF-alpha antibody (TNF2 group) due to intolerance or loss of response. The MH rates in our cohort were somewhat lower than that of previously published studies which is related to the strict definition of MH in our study which required complete endoscopic MH (Mayo endoscopic subscore 0 for UC patients or SES-CD score 0 for CD patients, respectively). Of note, our study comprises a large cohort with a long follow-up time (median overall follow-up time: TNF1 group 63 months, TNF2 group 64.5 months) compared to most other clinical studies which have much shorter follow-up times. Another new finding of our study is that switch from a first anti-TNF-alpha antibody to a second anti-TNF-alpha antibody had no significant impact on MH rates, independently from the reason for switch. However, since most of our patients were switched due to allergic reaction or intolerance, MH rates might be lower when switch is done due to loss of response. Similar to recent studies, which demonstrated a lower need for surgeries and hospitalization in patients who have MH [9,14], we confirmed these findings. Regarding predictive factors for MH, CRP values in the TNF1 group and in the TNF2

Table 5. Multivariate analysis for outcome MH in the TNF2 group (n = 46).

	p-value	OR [95%CI]
CRP-value at baseline colonoscopy	0.197	1.976 [0.702;5.561]
CRP-value at follow-up colonoscopy	0.106	3.640 [0.761;17.415]
WBC at baseline colonoscopy	0.350	1.149 [0.859;1.538]
WBC at follow-up colonoscopy	0.719	0.957 [0.753;1.252]
Age at diagnosis	0.556	0.825 [0.436;1.563]
Age	0.527	1.228 [0.650;2.321]
Gender	0.201	0.137 [0.007;2.877]
Smoker	0.135	0.419 [0.134;1.312]
Duration anti-TNF-alpha antibody treatment	0.857	0.993 [0.924;1.068]
Time to first anti-TNF-alpha antibody treatment	0.231	0.600 [0.259;1.386]
Time from baseline to follow-up colonoscopy	0.201	1.098 [0.951;1.267]
Time from first to second anti-TNF-alpha antibody treatment	0.639	0.973 [0.866;1.092]

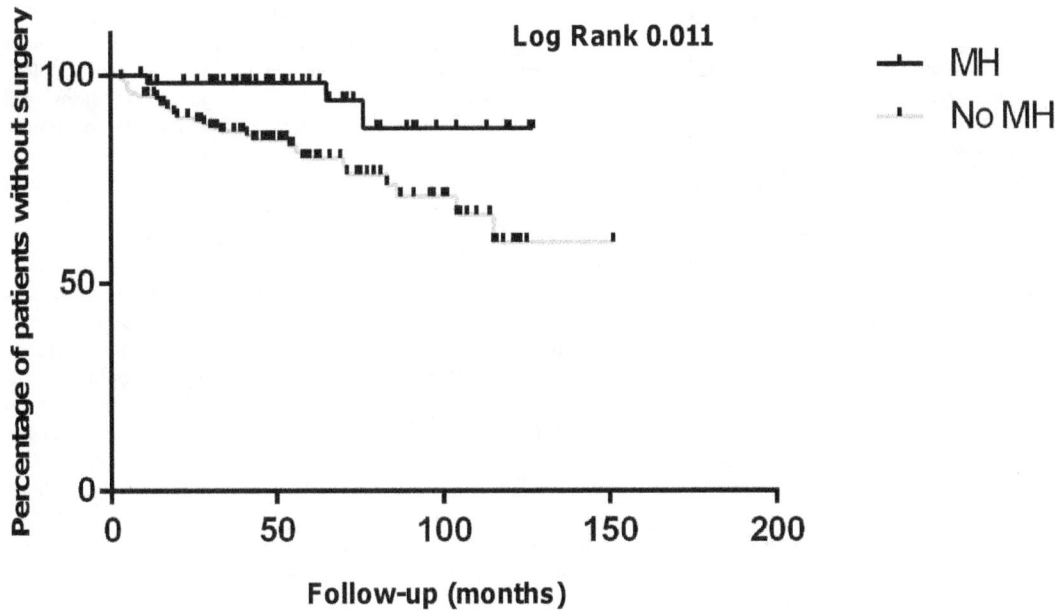

Figure 5. Kaplan-Mayer estimate for surgery-free time intervals in the TNF1 group over the follow-up time. During the follow-up time, 3 patients with MH underwent surgery as compared to 31 patients without MH patients (logrank p = 0.01).

group at follow-up colonoscopy were significantly lower in patients with MH, when compared to patients without MH. Multivariate analysis confirmed CRP as a predictive marker in the TNF1 group, while smoking was negatively associated with MH in this group.

When dividing our patient cohort regarding their disease entity (CD and UC), the MH rates remain similar to the overall cohorts (CD: TNF1 group 27.5%, TNF2 group 25.0%; UC: TNF1 group 28.0%, TNF2 group 35.7%). In univariate analyses, both in CD and UC patients, low CRP levels at follow-up were associated with MH. However, multivariate analyses could not confirm CRP at

follow-up as a predictive marker in both groups. This might be explained by the relative small sample size, especially in the TNF2 groups.

Interestingly, a recent study also demonstrated normalisation of CRP as a strong predictor of efficacy and mucosal healing during the first year of adalimumab therapy in CD [18]. In this study, logistic regression analysis revealed normalisation of CRP (defined as CRP<10 mg/L) at week 12 after initiation of adalimumab therapy as a predictive factor for MH (p<0.001). Another study also showed that CRP correlated with MH (p = 0.033) in CD patients treated with infliximab [22].

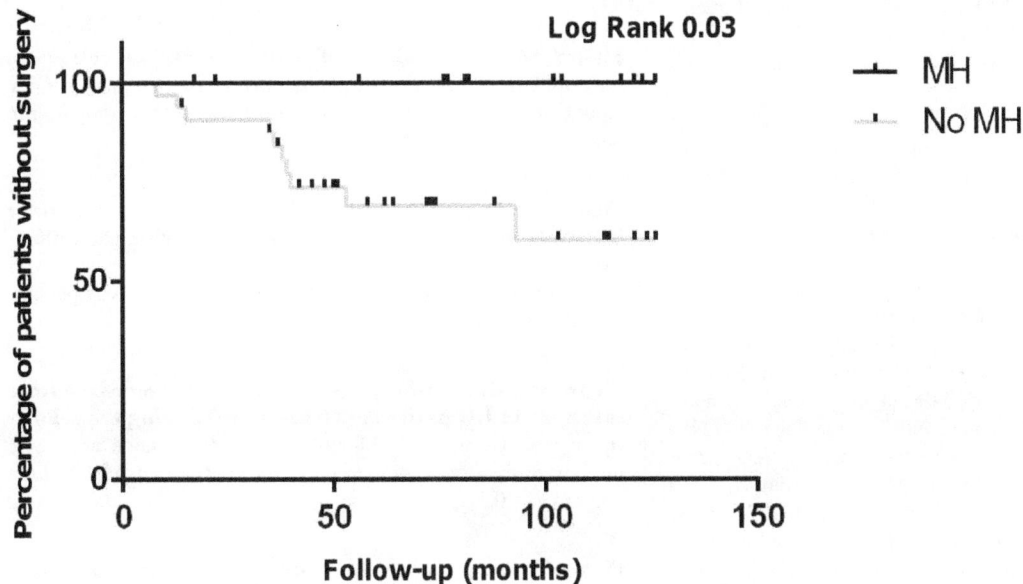

Figure 6. Kaplan-Mayer estimate for surgery-free time intervals in the TNF2 group over the follow-up time. During the follow-up time, no patient with MH underwent surgery as compared to 10 patients without MH (logrank p = 0.03).

The anti-TNF-alpha antibodies infliximab and adalimumab have the potential to induce and maintain MH in IBD [13,17,23]. Moreover, there is evidence that early infliximab-induced MH is associated with a better long-term outcome and a lower need for major abdominal surgeries in CD and UC [8,9,24]. A recent retrospective analysis demonstrated that infliximab induced MH in 45% of CD patients 3 months after start of inflixmab which was highly predictive for MH after 12 months [25]. One possible mechanism by which infliximab induces mucosal healing in UC is down-regulation of basic fibroblast growth factor/syndecan 1 [26]. Another study revealed a significant induction of regulatory macrophages in patients with mucosal healing after treatment with infliximab which was more pronounced in patients receiving infliximab/azathioprine combination treatment [27]. This might be an explanation for the better outcome of this combination treatment regime in clinical practice and as demonstrated in the SONIC trial [20]. However, in our study combination therapy with anti-TNF-alpha antibody and thiopurines was not associated with a higher rate of MH. Other important mechanisms by which anti-TNF-alpha antibodies may promote MH are downregulation of proinflammatory cytokines/chemokines [28], matrix-metallo-proteinases, tissue inhibitors of metalloproteinases [29] and apoptosis/necroptosis [30].

One may speculate if early start of anti-TNF-alpha antibody treatment could have improved the rates of MH in our study cohort, since most of the patients in our study underwent step-up strategies and were treated with an anti-TNF-alpha antibody only 7 years (median) after the first diagnosis of IBD. In the large anti-TNF-alpha antibody landmark trials, MH rates are varying with the different time points of assessment. In CD patients, infliximab induced MH rates ranging from 29% to 45% [20,31] and 27% with adalimumab [32]. In studies with UC patients, MH rates are higher and ranged from 47% with adalimumab [23] and 60% with infliximab [24]. However, in contrast to these anti-TNF-alpha antibody studies, in which patients have routine colonoscopy after a defined time point after initiation of anti-TNF-alpha antibody treatment, in clinical practice patients without clinical symptoms are often not willing to undergo colonoscopy. Accordingly, data from these patients are missing and in a real life situation there might be higher rates of MH in anti-TNF-alpha antibody-treated patients who have no colonoscopy after start of anti-TNF-alpha antibody therapy, since clinical activity was obviously low and there was no need for routine diagnostic colonoscopy.

There are some limitations of our study, mostly due to its retrospective nature: first, there were limited data on clinical scores like CDAI/CAI. However, there is evidence that CDAI and CAI as subjective scoring systems are not suitable to determine MH [33]. Moreover, only in a few patients neutrophil-derived fecal stool markers like calprotectin were available to be correlated with MH. Second, time periods between baseline and follow-up colonoscopy were varying (see table 1). However, there was no significant difference in the time interval between baseline and follow-up colonoscopy among patients with and without MH. In the majority of our patients (88%), the main reason for second (follow-up) colonoscopy was routine control of ongoing anti-TNF-alpha antibody therapy, and only few colonoscopies were performed due to flare of the disease (12%). Accordingly, CRP values at baseline colonoscopy were not significantly different in both groups, which suggest similar clinical disease activity.

As noted above, colonoscopy as an invasive procedure has a low acceptance rate in asymptomatic IBD patients. Other non-invasive diagnostic modalities for the assessment of MH like fecal calprotectin [34,35], lactoferrin [35] or combination of fecal calprotectin and clinical activity scores (e.g. Harvey-Bradshaw index) [36] and radiological techniques (e.g. MR enteroclysis [37]) may serve as additional or alternative markers of MH in the near future. However, despite the presence of complete MH, histological findings which predict disease relapse like basal plasma cell infiltration in UC patients [38], are valuable markers and should be additionally taken into account when monitoring IBD patients.

In summary, in nearly 30% of IBD patients treated with anti-TNF-alpha antibodies we observed complete MH. Switch from one anti-TNF-alpha antibody to a second anti-TNF-alpha antibody had no significant impact on MH rates in our study. We confirmed former findings that the need for surgeries and hospitalisation was lower in patients with MH than in patients without MH. After initiation of an anti-TNF-alpha antibody therapy, low CRP values at follow-up colonoscopy compared to a baseline colonoscopy were associated with MH. Therefore, in clinical practice the CRP value seems to be an easy-to-use marker for MH in IBD patients. Further prospective studies comparing step-up versus early interventional top-down strategies and defined colonoscopy intervals after the start of anti-TNF-alpha antibody treatment are warranted to assess their value for complete MH and long term outcome of these patients.

Supporting Information

Figure S1   CRP values of UC patients at follow-up colonoscopy (TNF1 group). At follow-up colonoscopy, CRP values were significantly lower in patients with MH compared to patients without MH (*p = 0.0002).

Figure S2   CRP values of UC patients at follow-up colonoscopy (TNF2 group). At follow-up colonoscopy, CRP values were significantly lower in patients with MH compared to patients without MH (*p = 0.03).

Figure S3   CRP values of CD patients at follow-up colonoscopy (TNF1 group). At follow-up colonoscopy, CRP values were significantly lower in patients with MH compared to patients without MH (*p = 0.01).

Figure S4   CRP values of CD patients at follow-up colonoscopy (TNF2 group). At follow-up colonoscopy, CRP values were significantly lower in patients with MH compared to patients without MH (*p = 0.01).

Figure S5   Kaplan-Mayer estimate for surgery-free time intervals in UC patients (TNF1 group) during the follow-up time. During the follow-up time, no patient with MH underwent surgery as compared to 7 patients without MH patients (logrank p = 0.09).

Figure S6   Kaplan-Mayer estimate for surgery-free time intervals in UC patients (TNF2 group) during the follow-up time. During the follow-up time, no patient with MH underwent surgery as compared to 3 patients without MH patients (logrank p = 0.17).

Figure S7   Kaplan-Mayer estimate for surgery-free time intervals in CD patients (TNF1 group) during the follow-up time. During the follow-up time, 3 patients with MH underwent surgery as compared to 24 patients without MH patients (logrank p = 0.04).

Figure S8 Kaplan-Mayer estimate for surgery-free time intervals in CD patients (TNF2 group) during the follow-up time. During the follow-up time, no patient with MH underwent surgery as compared to 7 patients without MH patients (logrank p = 0.09).

Table S1 Demographic and clinical characteristics of the UC study cohort (n = 96).

Table S2 Demographic and clinical characteristics of the UC TNF1 group (n = 82) regarding MH.

Table S3 Demographic and clinical characteristics of the UC TNF2 group (n = 14) regarding MH.

Table S4 Multivariate analysis for outcome MH in the UC TNF1 group.

Table S5 Multivariate analysis for outcome MH in the UC TNF2 group.

Table S6 Demographic and clinical characteristics of the CD study cohort (n = 152).

Table S7 Demographic and clinical characteristics of the CD TNF1 group (n = 120) regarding MH.

Table S8 Demographic and clinical characteristics of the CD TNF2 group (n = 32) regarding MH.

Table S9 Multivariate analysis for outcome MH in the MC TNF1 group.

Table S10 Multivariate analysis for outcome MH in the MC TNF2 group.

Author Contributions

Conceived and designed the experiments: FB MD BG TO S. Brand. Performed the experiments: FB MD FS. Analyzed the data: FB MD S. Breiteneicher. Contributed reagents/materials/analysis tools: BG. Wrote the paper: FB S. Brand.

References

1. Cosnes J, Gower-Rousseau C, Seksik P, Cortot A (2011) Epidemiology and natural history of inflammatory bowel diseases. Gastroenterology 140: 1785–1794.
2. Cosnes J, Cattan S, Blain A, Beaugerie L, Carbonnel F, et al. (2002) Long-term evolution of disease behavior of Crohn's disease. Inflamm Bowel Dis 8: 244–250.
3. Schroeder KW, Tremaine WJ, Ilstrup DM (1987) Coated oral 5-aminosalicylic acid therapy for mildly to moderately active ulcerative colitis. A randomized study. N Engl J Med 317: 1625–1629.
4. Matts SG (1961) The value of rectal biopsy in the diagnosis of ulcerative colitis. Q J Med 30: 393–407.
5. Lichtiger S, Present DH, Kornbluth A, Gelernt I, Bauer J, et al. (1994) Cyclosporine in severe ulcerative colitis refractory to steroid therapy. N Engl J Med 330: 1841–1845.
6. Mary JY, Modigliani R (1989) Development and validation of an endoscopic index of the severity for Crohn's disease: a prospective multicentre study. Groupe d'Etudes Therapeutiques des Affections Inflammatoires du Tube Digestif (GETAID). Gut 30: 983–989.
7. Daperno M, D'Haens G, Van Assche G, Baert F, Bulois P, et al. (2004) Development and validation of a new, simplified endoscopic activity score for Crohn's disease: the SES-CD. Gastrointest Endosc 60: 505–512.
8. Colombel JF, Rutgeerts P, Reinisch W, Esser D, Wang Y, et al (2011). Early mucosal healing with infliximab is associated with improved long-term clinical outcomes in ulcerative colitis. Gastroenterology 141: 1194–1201.
9. Schnitzler F, Fidder H, Ferrante M, Noman M, Arijs I, et al. (2009) Mucosal healing predicts long-term outcome of maintenance therapy with infliximab in Crohn's disease. Inflamm Bowel Dis 15: 1295–1301.
10. Baert F, Moortgat L, Van Assche G, Caenepeel P, Vergauwe P, et al. (2009) Mucosal healing predicts sustained clinical remission in patients with early-stage Crohn's disease. Gastroenterology 138: 463–468; quiz e410–461.
11. Peyrin-Biroulet L, Ferrante M, Magro F, Campbell S, Franchimont D, et al (2011). Results from the 2nd Scientific Workshop of the ECCO. I: Impact of mucosal healing on the course of inflammatory bowel disease. J Crohns Colitis 5: 477–483.
12. Dave M, Loftus EV Jr. (2012) Mucosal healing in inflammatory bowel disease-a true paradigm of success? Gastroenterol Hepatol (N Y) 8: 29–38.
13. Rutgeerts P, Van Assche G, Sandborn WJ, Wolf DC, Geboes K, et al. (2012). Adalimumab induces and maintains mucosal healing in patients with Crohn's disease: data from the EXTEND trial. Gastroenterology 142: 1102–1111 e1102.
14. Pineton de Chambrun G, Peyrin-Biroulet L, Lemann M, Colombel JF (2010) Clinical implications of mucosal healing for the management of IBD. Nat Rev Gastroenterol Hepatol 7: 15–29.
15. Kozarek RA, Patterson DJ, Gelfand MD, Botoman VA, Ball TJ, et al. (1989) Methotrexate induces clinical and histologic remission in patients with refractory inflammatory bowel disease. Ann Intern Med 110: 353–356.
16. D'Haens G, Geboes K, Rutgeerts P (1999) Endoscopic and histologic healing of Crohn's (ileo-) colitis with azathioprine. Gastrointest Endosc 50: 667–671.
17. D'Haens G, Van Deventer S, Van Hogezand R, Chalmers D, Kothe C, et al. (1999) Endoscopic and histological healing with infliximab anti-tumor necrosis factor antibodies in Crohn's disease: A European multicenter trial. Gastroenterology 116: 1029–1034.
18. Kiss LS, Szamosi T, Molnar T, Miheller P, Lakatos L, et al. (2011) Early clinical remission and normalisation of CRP are the strongest predictors of efficacy, mucosal healing and dose escalation during the first year of adalimumab therapy in Crohn's disease. Aliment Pharmacol Ther 34: 911–922.
19. Olaison G, Sjodahl R, Tagesson C (1990) Glucocorticoid treatment in ileal Crohn's disease: relief of symptoms but not of endoscopically viewed inflammation. Gut 31: 325–328.
20. Colombel JF, Sandborn WJ, Reinisch W, Mantzaris GJ, Kornbluth A, et al. (2010) Infliximab, azathioprine, or combination therapy for Crohn's disease. N Engl J Med 362: 1383–1395.
21. Ordas I, Feagan BG, Sandborn WJ (2011) Early use of immunosuppressives or TNF antagonists for the treatment of Crohn's disease: time for a change. Gut 60: 1754–1763.
22. Jurgens M, Mahachie John JM, Cleynen I, Schnitzler F, Fidder H, et al. (2011) Levels of C-reactive protein are associated with response to infliximab therapy in patients with Crohn's disease. Clin Gastroenterol Hepatol 9: 421–427 e421.
23. Sandborn WJ, van Assche G, Reinisch W, Colombel JF, D'Haens G, et al. (2012) Adalimumab induces and maintains clinical remission in patients with moderate-to-severe ulcerative colitis. Gastroenterology 142: 257–265 e251–253.
24. Colombel JF, Rutgeerts P, Reinisch W, Esser D, Wang Y, et al. (2011) Early Mucosal Healing With Infliximab Is Associated With Improved Long-term Clinical Outcomes in Ulcerative Colitis. Gastroenterology 141: 1194–1201.
25. af Bjorkesten CG, Nieminen U, Turunen U, Arkkila PE, Sipponen T, et al. (2011) Endoscopic monitoring of infliximab therapy in Crohn's disease. Inflamm Bowel Dis 17: 947–953.
26. Ierardi E, Giorgio F, Zotti M, Rosania R, Principi M, et al (2011). Infliximab therapy downregulation of basic fibroblast growth factor/syndecan 1 link: a possible molecular pathway of mucosal healing in ulcerative colitis. J Clin Pathol 64: 968–972.
27. Vos AC, Wildenberg ME, Arijs I, Duijvestein M, Verhaar AP, et al. (2011) Regulatory macrophages induced by infliximab are involved in healing in vivo and in vitro. Inflamm Bowel Dis 18: 401–408.
28. van Assche G, Vermeire S, Rutgeerts P (2010) Mucosal healing and anti TNFs in IBD. Curr Drug Targets 11: 227–233.
29. de Bruyn M, Machiels K, Vandooren J, Lemmens B, Van Lommel L, et al. (2013) Infliximab Restores the Dysfunctional Matrix Remodeling Protein and Growth Factor Gene Expression in Patients with Inflammatory Bowel Disease. Inflamm Bowel Dis.
30. Gunther C, Martini E, Wittkopf N, Amann K, Weigmann B, et al. (2011) Caspase-8 regulates TNF-alpha-induced epithelial necroptosis and terminal ileitis. Nature 477: 335–339.
31. Hanauer SB, Feagan BG, Lichtenstein GR, Mayer LF, Schreiber S, et al. (2002) Maintenance infliximab for Crohn's disease: the ACCENT I randomised trial. Lancet 359: 1541–1549.
32. Rutgeerts P, Van Assche G, Sandborn WJ, Wolf DC, Geboes K, et al. (2012) Adalimumab Induces and Maintains Mucosal Healing in Patients With Crohn's Disease: Data From the EXTEND Trial. Gastroenterology.
33. af Bjorkesten CG, Nieminen U, Turunen U, Arkkila P, Sipponen T, et al. (2012) Surrogate markers and clinical indices, alone or combined, as indicators for

endoscopic remission in anti-TNF-treated luminal Crohn's disease. Scand J Gastroenterol 47: 528–537.

34. D'Haens G, Ferrante M, Vermeire S, Baert F, Noman M, et al (2012). Fecal calprotectin is a surrogate marker for endoscopic lesions in inflammatory bowel disease. Inflamm Bowel Dis 18:2218–2224.

35. Sipponen T, Karkkainen P, Savilahti E, Kolho KL, Nuutinen H, et al. (2008) Correlation of faecal calprotectin and lactoferrin with an endoscopic score for Crohn's disease and histological findings. Aliment Pharmacol Ther 28: 1221–1229.

36. Af Bjorkesten CG, Nieminen U, Turunen U, Arkkila P, Sipponen T, et al (2012). Surrogate markers and clinical indices, alone or combined, as indicators for endoscopic remission in anti-TNF-treated luminal Crohn's disease. Scand J Gastroenterol 47: 528–537.

37. Ordas I, Rimola J, Rodriguez S, Paredes JM, Martinez-Perez MJ, et al. (2013) Accuracy of Magnetic Resonance Enterography in Assessing Response to Therapy and Mucosal Healing in Patients With Crohn's Disease. Gastroenterology 146: 374–382.

38. Bessissow T, Lemmens B, Ferrante M, Bisschops R, Van Steen K, et al. (2012) Prognostic value of serologic and histologic markers on clinical relapse in ulcerative colitis patients with mucosal healing. Am J Gastroenterol 107: 1684–1692.

2

Association between the Pro12Ala Polymorphism of Peroxisome Proliferator-Activated Receptor Gamma 2 and Inflammatory Bowel Disease

Zhi-Feng Zhang[1]*[9], **Ning Yang**[2][9], **Gang Zhao**[1], **Lei Zhu**[1], **Li-Xia Wang**[1]

1 Department of Gastroenterology, The First Affiliated Hospital of Dalian Medical University, Dalian, China, 2 Department of Nephrology, The First Affiliated Hospital of Dalian Medical University, Dalian, China

Abstract

Background: Peroxisome proliferator-activated receptor gamma (PPARγ), a nuclear receptor, has been implicated playing a role in the development of inflammatory bowel disease (IBD). However, previous studies evaluating the association between the PPARγ2 Pro12Ala polymorphism and IBD are inconsistent. We performed a meta-analysis to determine whether the PPARγ2 Pro12Ala mutation was associated with the presence of IBD.

Methods and Findings: Electronic databases were searched for case-control studies evaluating the association between the Pro12Ala mutation and the presence of IBD. Effects were summarized with the methods recommended by the Cochrane Collaboration. A total of 7 studies including 1002 ulcerative colitis (UC) cases, 1090 Crohǹs disease (CD) cases and 1983 controls were involved in this meta-analysis. In the overall analysis, no significant association of this polymorphism with UC or CD was found. In the subgroup analyses in different populations, AlaAla genotype seemed to protect the European Caucasian population against the development of CD (Pro vs Ala: OR = 1.135, 95%CI = 0.951–1.354, P = 0.162, Bon = 1.000; ProPro vs ProAla: OR = 1.042, 95%CI = 0.852–1.273, P = 0.690, Bon = 1.000; ProPro vs AlaAla: OR = 2.379, 95%CI = 1.110–5.100, P = 0.026, Bon = 0.156; ProAla vs AlaAla: OR = 2.315, 95%CI = 1.064–5.037, P = 0.034, Bon = 0.204; Pro homozygotes vs Ala positives: OR = 1.094, 95%CI = 0.899–1.330, P = 0.371, Bon = 1.000; Pro positives vs Ala homozygotes: OR = 2.360, 95%CI = 1.103–5.053, P = 0.027, Bon = 0.162; heterozygotes vs all homozygotes: OR = 0.976, 95%CI = 0.799–1.192, P = 0.809, Bon = 1.000). There was no significant association of this polymorphism with UC or CD in the East Asian population and the Turkish population.

Conclusion: AlaAla genotype may be a protective factor in the European Caucasian population against the development of CD in a recessive way.

Editor: Tatjana Adamovic, Karolinska Institutet, Sweden

Funding: The authors have no support or funding to report.

Competing Interests: The authors have declared that no competing interests exist.

* E-mail: zhifeng_zhang@tom.com

[9] These authors contributed equally to this work.

Introduction

Inflammatory bowel disease (IBD) clinically classified into ulcerative colitis (UC) and Crohǹs disease (CD) is a non specific chronic intestinal inflammatory disorder with the characteristics of relapses and remissions. When diagnosed, patients with UC or CD need lifelong medications. Moreover, strictures, abscesses, fistulas, extra intestinal involvements and even carcinomas would complicate IBD and eventually affect the progression of IBD. In the last three decades, we have witnessed a time trend increase of the prevalence of IBD especially of CD both in developed and developing regions [1].

Although the treatment of IBD has advanced considerably and guidelines have just been revised, IBD is still incurable [2]. Clarifying the etiology of IBD may help us to find optimal therapies. To date, it is believed that the inappropriate response of the intestinal mucosal immune system to indigenous intestinal flora

and other antigens is crucial in IBD development [3]. The mechanism of the inappropriate response is different in UC and CD. The deficiency of the innate immune system which permits intestinal pathogens to break through the intestinal barrier and activate the adaptive immune system may be responsible for the uncontrolled inflammation in CD, while UC is probably caused by the primarily upregulated response of the intestinal mucosal immune system [4].

Peroxisome proliferator-activated receptor gamma (PPARγ), a nuclear receptor, has been implicated as playing some role in the development of UC and CD [5,6]. One experimental study even showed the beneficial effect of a PPARγ agonist on UC [7]. The CCA-to-GCA (Pro-to-Ala) mutation in codon 12 of exon B of the PPARγ2 is a common single nucleotide polymorphism (SNP) [8]. The Pro12Ala mutation may affect the activity of PPARγ in epithelial cells and immunocytes, and consequently interfere with the susceptibility of a host to develop IBD. In order to elucidate the association between the Pro12Ala mutation and the development of IBD, some molecular epidemiological researches were conducted worldwide. One case-control study conducted in Japan indicated that the Pro12Ala mutation was more frequently found in UC patients [9]. Another study showed a significant association between this mutation and the development of CD [10]. However, a research conducted in China and Holland failed to confirm the association between the Pro12Ala polymorphism and IBD [11]. One reason of the inconsistent results of previous studies may be the sample size not large enough in some studies. Meta-analysis is a well-established method combining all available published data to increase the statistical power of the analysis. Hence we performed this meta-analysis to determine whether the Pro12Ala mutation was associated with the development of IBD.

Methods

Searching strategies

PubMed (1966 to June 2011) and Scopus (1966 to June 2011) were searched using the combinations of text words and medical subject headings (MeSH) including "inflammatory bowel disease", "ulcerative colitis", "Crohn's disease", "IBD", "UC", "CD", "peroxisome proliferator-activated receptor", "PPAR", "polymorphism", "polymorphisms", "single nucleotide", "allele" and "genotype". Chinese medical databases including Wanfang database (1982 to June 2011), China National Knowledge Infrastructure (CNKI, 1994 to June 2011) and Chinese Biomedical Literature Database (CBM, 1978 to June 2011) were also searched for relevant articles. We searched reference lists, relevant meta-analyses and reviews in order to get additional articles.

Study selection criteria

The following selection criteria were employed in this meta-analysis: 1) Case-control studies evaluating the association between the PPARγ2 Pro12Ala mutation and the presence of IBD. 2) Diagnosis of IBD according to clinical manifestations, radiological changes, endoscopic manifestations, and histological evaluations comprehensively. 3) Hardy-Weinberg equilibrium fulfilled in the control arm of each research. 4) Articles with a full text not just an abstract. 5) Articles providing raw data or Odds ratio (OR) and its 95% confidence interval (CI) for each comparison. Exclusion criteria were as the follows: 1) Repetitive publications. 2) Family based case-control studies.

Data extraction

Two reviewers screened the titles and abstracts of potentially relevant articles. And the full texts of highly relevant articles would be thoroughly read by two reviewers. When a discrepancy was encountered, a third reviewer would be referred to and the decision would be made through discussions. Publication year, region the study was conducted in, ethnicity, available allele and genotype frequencies in each arm and the method of polymorphism assessment of each study were exacted.

Assessment of the risks of bias

We also assessed the potential risks of bias with the items including 1) Selection bias (differential selections of cases and controls; selections based on UC or CD severity), 2) Information bias (quality control measures in the genotyping process, blinding of laboratory personnel or researchers and phenotype misclassification) and 3) confounding factors (cases and controls matching).

Data analysis

Hardy-Weinberg equilibrium was assessed using the $\chi2$ test. Paired combinations of genotypes were employed to determine the hereditary models: 1) an allelic analysis (Pro vs Ala); 2) a genotypic analysis (ProPro vs AlaAla, ProPro vs ProAla, ProAla vs AlaAla) and 3) another genotypic analysis comparing each genotype with the other two (Pro homozygotes vs Ala positives, Pro positives vs Ala homozygotes, heterozygotes vs all homozygotes). If the comparisons of ProPro vs AlaAla, ProPro vs ProAla and Pro homozygotes vs Ala positives were statistically significant, the Ala allele would be a dominant allele. If the comparisons of ProPro vs AlaAla, ProAla vs AlaAla and Pro positives vs Ala homozygotes were statistically significant, the Ala allele would be a recessive allele. OR and its 95% CI were calculated with the methods recommended by the Cochrane Collaboration, and a fixed value of 0.5 was added to all cells of study results tables where no events were observed in one or both groups [12]. The Cochrane Q $\chi2$ test and the CI overlapping status of each selected study were used to detect the heterogeneity among studies. The I^2 statistics was also used to evaluate the risks of heterogeneity among studies: 0%–40% represented no risk of heterogeneity, 30%–60% represented a low risk of heterogeneity, 50%–90% represented substantial heterogeneity and 75%–100% represented considerable heterogeneity [12]. If the P value was more than 0.1, the I^2 statistics indicating no or a low risk of heterogeneity and the CI of each study overlapped, a fixed model was employed and the Mantel-Haenszel method was implemented to synthesize data. If the P value was less than 0.1, the I^2 statistics indicating substantial or considerable heterogeneity or the CI of each study did not overlapped, a random model was employed and the DerSimonian-Laird method was applied to synthesize data. Funnel plots were used to examine bias in the results of the meta-analyses [13,14]. The step down Bonferroni method was used for the multiple comparison adjustments [15]. Stata 11.0 software (StataCorp LP, College Station, Texas, USA) was used for meta-analyses and Hardy-Weinberg equilibrium tests. R 2.13.0 software (The R Foundation for Statistical Computing, http://cran.csdb.cn/) was used for the step down Bonferroni adjustments (Bon). Values of $P<0.05$ were considered statistically significant. All the above methods had been used for pooling data in two previous published genetic association meta-analyses [16.17].

Results

Characteristics of selected studies

91 articles were identified during premature searches with our searching strategy of the five databases (PubMed: 30; Scopus: 56; Wanfang database: 2; CNKI: 1; CBM: 2). 59 articles were retrieved after excluding overlapping studies. After excluding reviews, animal studies, comments, letters and studies not evaluating IBD, 16 studies assessing the association between the PPARγ polymorphism and IBD were found. Among the remaining 16 articles, 8 studies did not evaluate the Pro12Ala mutation and one republication was identified. Only 7 articles met our selection criteria. After searching reference lists, relevant meta-analyses and reviews, we did not find additional studies. The selection process is illustrated in Figure 1. These 7 studies including 1002 UC cases, 1090 CD cases and 1983 controls were involved in this meta-analysis [9–11,18–21]. Among the selected researches, 3 studies were conducted in the European Caucasian population, 3 studies were conducted in the East Asian population and one study was conducted in the Turkish population. The control arm of each study conformed to the Hardy-Weinberg equilibrium. The characteristics of selected studies are illustrated

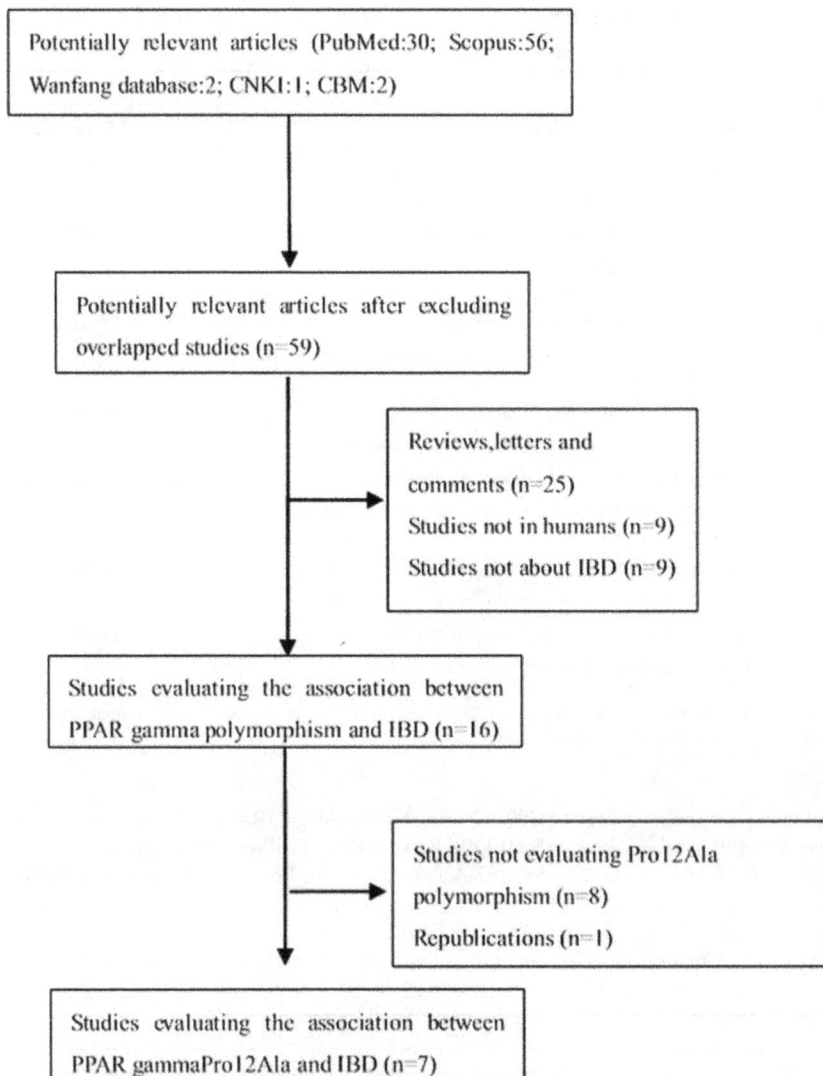

Figure 1. Flow diagram of the study selection process.

in Table 1 and Table 2. The PRISMA Checklist is shown in Text S1. The detailed searching process of Scopus is demonstrated in Text S2.

Assessment of the risks of bias

Selection bias: Cases were selected from diagnosed UC and CD patients in medical institutions in all the included studies. 3 studies recruited healthy blood donors as controls [10,20,21]. One study recruited healthy medical staff as controls [11]. While the other 3 studies only described healthy subjects as controls. Only one study used colonoscopy to exclude IBD in the controls [9]. Only one study described the severity of cases, which was mild to moderate [20].

Information bias: 3 studies used polymerase chain reaction-restriction fragment length polymorphism (PCR-RFLP) as the single nucleotide polymorphism (SNP) detection method [11,19, 20]. Mutagenically separated polymerase chain reaction (MS-PCR) was employed by one study to detect SNP [18]. Two studies used Taqman SNP genotyping assays (Taqman) to detect SNP [10,21]. One study detected SNP with real time polymerase chain reaction (RT-PCR) [9]. Investigators were blinded to data in two studies [19,21]. Negative and positive controls were processed with

each batch of samples and all experiments were repeated twice to ensure consistency for quality control purposes in one study [11]. One study genotyped 10% of the samples again to confirm reproducibility [21]. No phenotype misclassification was reported in the selected studies.

Confounding factors: Age and gender distribution were comparable among arms in most studies, while controls were slightly older as compared to CD patients in one study [20]. Regarding the possible influence of the Pro12Ala polymorphism in PPARγ2 gene on the risk of development of the type 2 diabetes mellitus, one study excluded diabetics from the study and control groups [18].

Meta-analysis

The CI overlapping status, Cochrane Q $\chi2$ tests, I^2 statistics and the detailed meta-analysis results are shown in Figure 2 and Figure 3.

Meta-analysis in the overall population

The association between the PPARγ Pro12Ala polymorphism and UC was investigated in 6 studies with 1002 UC cases and

Table 1. Characteristics of included studies evaluating the association between the PPARγ Pro12Ala mutation and the presence of IBD.

Author	Year	Location	Ethnicity	Case and control selection	SNP method
Atug O [18]	2008	Turkey	Turkish	Case: patients diagnosed in medical institutions	MS-PCR
				Control: healthy volunteers matched for age and gender	
Wang F [19]	2008	Japan	East Asian	Case: patients diagnosed in medical institutions	PCR-RFLP
				Control: healthy control subjects without detailed descriptions of matching methods	
Ferreira P [20]	2010	Portugal	European Caucasian	Case: patients diagnosed in medical institutions	PCR-RFLP
				Control: healthy blood donors without detailed descriptions of matching methods	
Shrestha UK [11]	2010	China	East Asian	Case: patients diagnosed in medical institutions	PCR-RFLP
				Control: healthy controls matched for age and gender	
Andersen V [21]	2011	Denmark	European Caucasian	Case: patients diagnosed in medical institutions	Taqman
				Control: healthy blood donors without detailed descriptions of matching methods	
Aoyagi Y [9]	2010	Japan	East Asia	Case: patients diagnosed in medical institutions	RT-PCR
				Control: healthy controls matched for age and gender	
Poliska S [10]	2011	Hungary	European Caucasian	Case: patients diagnosed in medical institutions	Taqman
				Control: healthy controls matched for age and gender	

SNP: single nucleotide polymorphism; MS-PCR: mutagenically separated polymerase chain reaction; PCR-RFLP: polymerase chain reaction-restriction fragment length polymorphism; Taqman: Taqman SNP genotyping assays; RT-PCR: real time polymerase chain reaction.

1867 controls [9–11,18,19,21]. There was no significant association between this polymorphism and UC in the overall population (Pro vs Ala: OR = 0.884, 95%CI = 0.625–1.251, P = 0.486, Bon = 1.000; ProPro vs ProAla: OR = 1.088, 95%CI = 0.883–1.340, P = 0.429, Bon = 1.000; ProPro vs AlaAla: OR = 0.644, 95%CI = 0.347–1.197, P = 0.165, Bon = 1.000; ProAla vs AlaAla:

Table 2. Allele and genotype frequencies of the arms of included studies evaluating the association between the PPARγ Pro12Ala mutation and the presence of IBD.

Author	Arms	Pro	Ala	Pro/Pro	Pro/Ala	Ala/Ala	HWE test
Atug O [18]	UC (n = 45)	83	7	38	7	0	
	CD (n = 69)	127	11	58	11	0	
	Control (n = 100)	187	13	87	13	0	P = 0.487
Wang F [19]	UC (n = 118)	231	5	113	5	0	
	Control (n = 142)	277	7	135	7	0	P = 0.763
Ferreira P [20]	CD (n = 90)	163	17	74	15	1	
	Control (n = 116)	209	23	95	19	2	P = 0.371
Shrestha UK [11]	UC (n = 212)	400	24	189	22	1	
	CD (n = 32)	61	3	29	3	0	
	Control(n = 220)	416	24	198	20	2	P = 0.079
Andersen V [21]	UC (n = 495)	844	146	364	116	15	
	CD (n = 327)	564	90	240	84	3	
	Control (n = 779)	1315	243	549	217	13	P = 0.105
Aoyagi Y [9]	UC (n = 29)	52	6	25	2	2	
	CD (n = 10)	20	0	10	0	0	
	Control (n = 134)	264	4	130	4	0	P = 0.861
Poliska S [10]	UC (n = 103)	178	28	77	24	2	
	CD (n = 562)	990	134	433	124	5	
	Control (n = 492)	854	130	375	104	13	P = 0.083

UC: ulcerative colitis; CD: Crohn's disease; HWE test: Hardy-Weinberg equilibrium test.

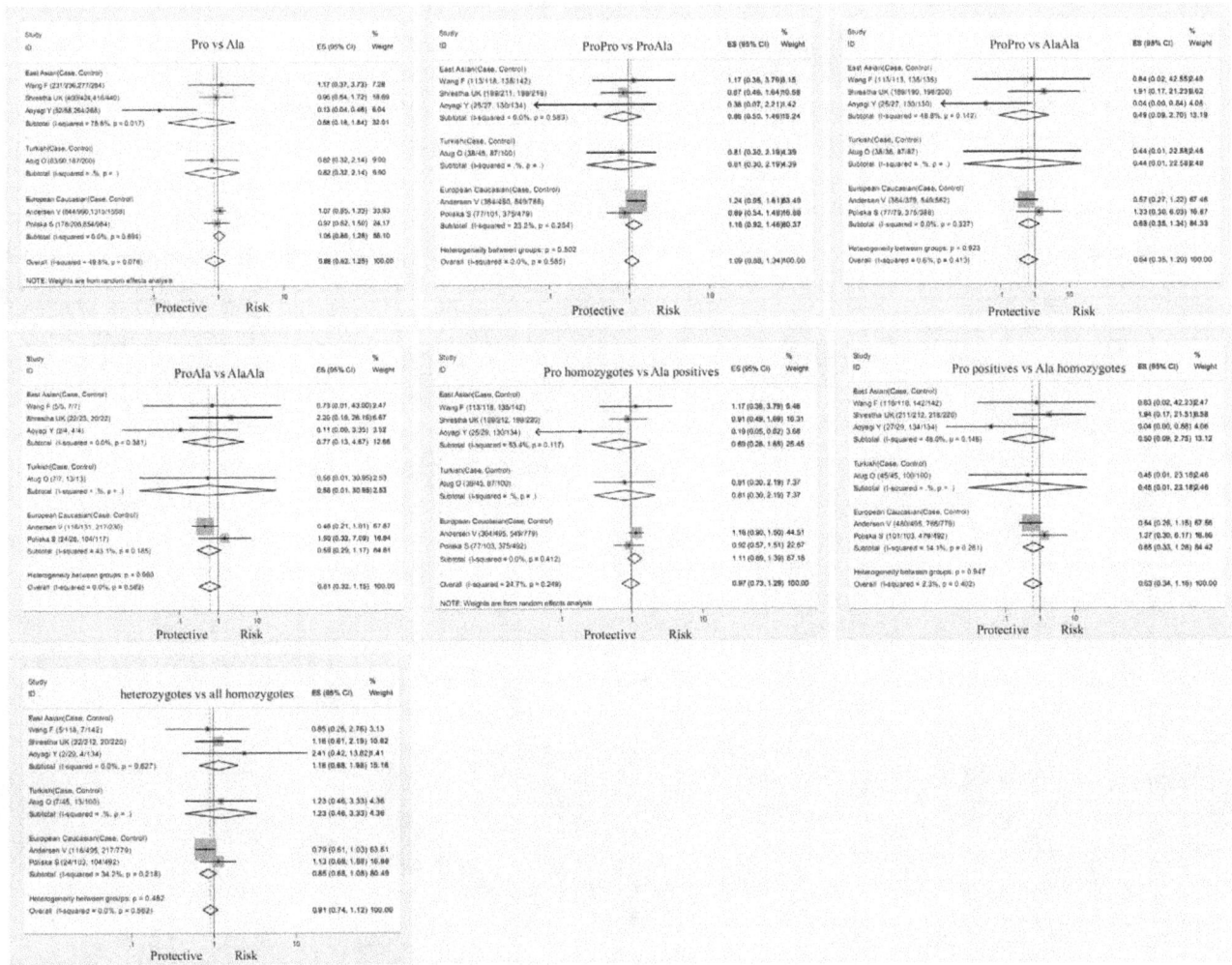

Figure 2. Forest plots for meta-analyses of the association between the PPARγ Pro12Ala mutation and the presence of UC.

OR = 0.606, 95%CI = 0.320–1.149, *P* = 0.125, Bon = 0.875; Pro homozygotes vs Ala positives: OR = 0.968, 95%CI = 0.727–1.289, *P* = 0.823, Bon = 1.000; Pro positives vs Ala homozygotes: OR = 0.625, 95%CI = 0.337–1.159, *P* = 0.136, Bon = 0.952; heterozygotes vs all homozygotes: OR = 0.910, 95%CI = 0.739–1.120, *P* = 0.372, Bon = 1.000). Between-study heterogeneity was detected in the contrasts of Pro vs Ala and Pro homozygotes vs Ala positives. The association between the PPARγ Pro12Ala polymorphism and CD was investigated in 6 studies with 1090 CD cases and 1841 controls [9–11,18,20,21]. No significant association between this polymorphism and CD in the overall population was found either (Pro vs Ala: OR = 1.117, 95%CI = 0.941–1.325, *P* = 0.204, Bon = 1.000; ProPro vs Pro-Ala: OR = 1.024, 95%CI = 0.845–1.242, *P* = 0.807, Bon = 1.000; ProPro vs AlaAla: OR = 1.918, 95%CI = 0.938–3.922, *P* = 0.074, Bon = 0.518; ProAla vs AlaAla: OR = 1.986, 95%CI = 0.953–4.139, *P* = 0.067, Bon = 0.469; Pro homozygotes vs Ala positives: OR = 1.075, 95%CI = 0.890–1.297, *P* = 0.454, Bon = 1.000; Pro positives vs Ala homozygotes: OR = 1.906, 95%CI = 0.933–3.893, *P* = 0.077, Bon = 0.539; heterozygotes vs all homozygotes: OR = 0.991, 95%CI = 0.818–1.201, *P* = 0.927, Bon = 1.000). Between-study heterogeneity was not detected in all the contrasts.

Analysis in the European Caucasian population

The association between the PPARγ Pro12Ala polymorphism and UC in the European Caucasian population was investigated in 2 studies with 598 UC cases and 1271 controls [10,21]. There was no significant association between the Pro12Ala polymorphism and UC in the European Caucasian population (Pro vs Ala: OR = 1.047, 95%CI = 0.858–1.277, *P* = 0.651, Bon = 1.000; Pro-Pro vs ProAla: OR = 1.157, 95%CI = 0.917–1.459, *P* = 0.219, Bon = 1.000; ProPro vs AlaAla: OR = 0.680, 95%CI = 0.346–1.335, *P* = 0.263, Bon = 1.000; ProAla vs AlaAla: OR = 0.586, 95%CI = 0.293–1.173, *P* = 0.131, Bon = 0.917; Pro homozygotes vs Ala positives: OR = 1.109, 95%CI = 0.886–1.388, *P* = 0.365, Bon = 1.000; Pro positives vs Ala homozygotes: OR = 0.653, 95%CI = 0.334–1.280, *P* = 0.215, Bon = 1.000; heterozygotes vs all homozygotes: OR = 0.854, 95%CI = 0.678–1.077, *P* = 0.183, Bon = 1.000). Between-study heterogeneity was not detected in all the contrasts. The association between the PPARγ Pro12Ala polymorphism and CD in the European Caucasian population was investigated in 3 studies with 979 CD cases and 1387 controls [10,20,21]. The AlaAla genotype seemed to protect the European Caucasian population against the development of CD in a recessive way(Pro vs Ala: OR = 1.135, 95%CI = 0.951–1.354, *P* = 0.162, Bon = 1.000; ProPro vs ProAla: OR = 1.042,

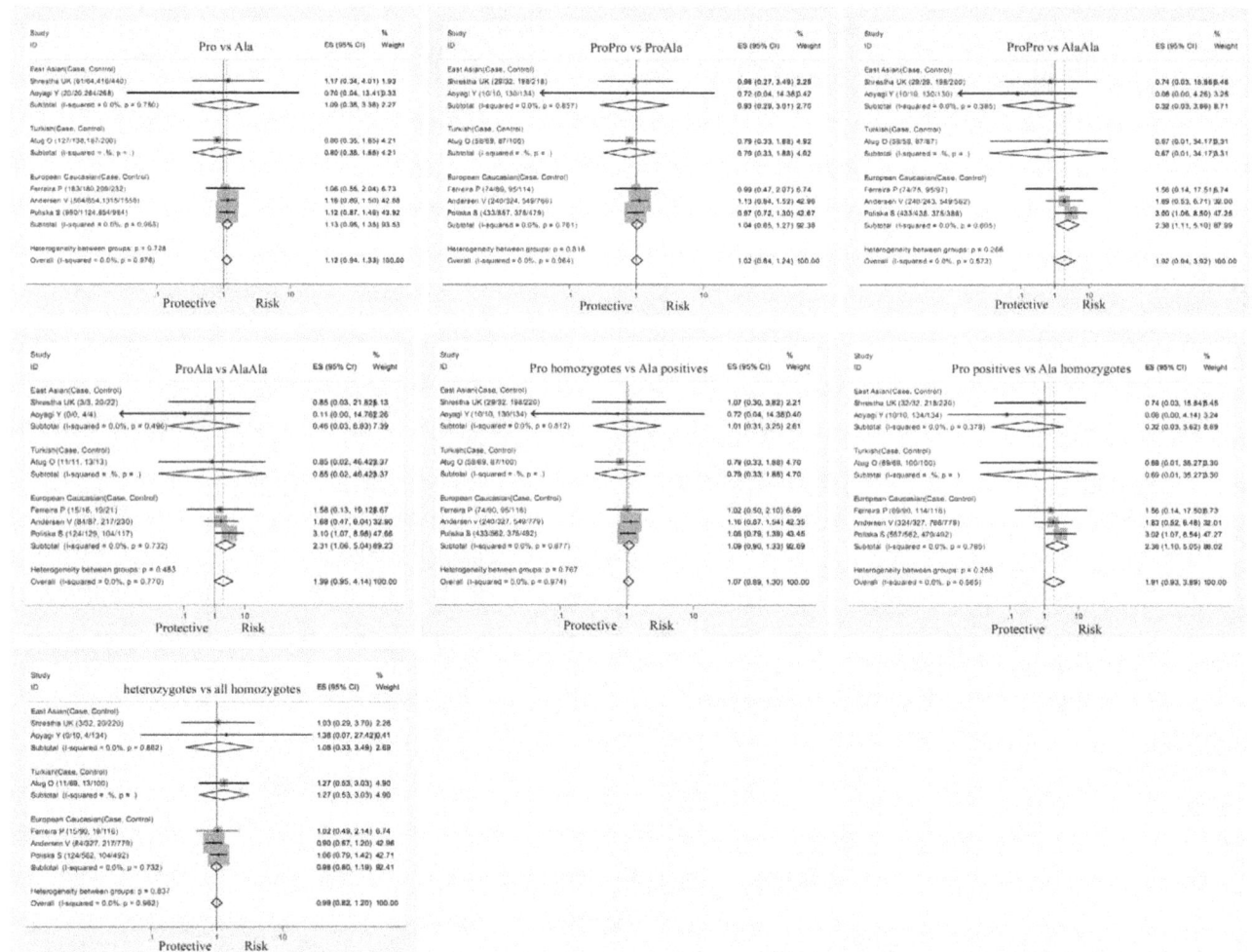

Figure 3. Forest plots for meta-analyses of the association between the PPARγ Pro12Ala mutation and the presence of CD.

95%CI = 0.852–1.273, P = 0.690, Bon = 1.000; ProPro vs AlaAla: OR = 2.379, 95%CI = 1.110–5.100, P = 0.026, Bon = 0.156; ProAla vs AlaAla: OR = 2.315, 95%CI = 1.064–5.037, P = 0.034, Bon = 0.204; Pro homozygotes vs Ala positives: OR = 1.094, 95%CI = 0.899–1.330, P = 0.371, Bon = 1.000; Pro positives vs Ala homozygotes: OR = 2.360, 95%CI = 1.103–5.053, P = 0.027, Bon = 0.162; heterozygotes vs all homozygotes: OR = 0.976, 95%CI = 0.799–1.192, P = 0.809, Bon = 1.000). Between-study heterogeneity was not detected in all the contrasts.

Analysis in the East Asian population

The association between the PPARγ Pro12Ala polymorphism and UC in the East Asian population was investigated in 3 studies with 359 UC cases and 496 controls [9,11,19]. There was no significant association between this polymorphism and UC in the East Asian population (Pro vs Ala: OR = 0.576, 95%CI = 0.180–1.844, P = 0.353, Bon = 1.000; ProPro vs ProAla: OR = 0.856, 95%CI = 0.502–1.460, P = 0.568, Bon = 1.000; ProPro vs AlaAla: OR = 0.490, 95%CI = 0.089–2.700, P = 0.413, Bon = 1.000; ProAla vs AlaAla: OR = 0.774, 95%CI = 0.128–4.669, P = 0.780, Bon = 1.000; Pro homozygotes vs Ala positives: OR = 0.686, 95%CI = 0.284–1.654, P = 0.401, Bon = 1.000; Pro positives vs Ala homozygotes: OR = 0.500, 95%CI = 0.091–2.750, P = 0.425, Bon = 1.000; heterozygotes vs all homozygotes: OR = 1.164, 95%CI = 0.683–

1.984, P = 0.577, Bon = 1.000). Between-study heterogeneity was detected in the contrasts of Pro vs Ala and Pro homozygotes vs Ala positives. The association between the PPARγ Pro12Ala polymorphism and CD in the East Asian population was investigated in 2 studies with 42 CD cases and 354 controls [9,11].There was no significant association between this polymorphism and CD in the East Asian population (Pro vs Ala: OR = 1.086, 95%CI = 0.349–3.382, P = 0.886, Bon = 1.000; ProPro vs ProAla: OR = 0.933, 95%CI = 0.289–3.012, P = 0.907, Bon = 1.000; ProPro vs AlaAla: OR = 0.324, 95%CI = 0.029–3.663, P = 0.363, Bon = 1.000; ProAla vs AlaAla: OR = 0.458, 95%CI = 0.031–6.825, P = 0.571, Bon = 1.000; Pro homozygotes vs Ala positives: OR = 1.011, 95%CI = 0.315–3.249, P = 0.985, Bon = 1.000; Pro positives vs Ala homozygotes: OR = 0.321, 95%CI = 0.028–3.623, P = 0.358, Bon = 1.000; heterozygotes vs all homozygotes: OR = 1.082, 95%CI = 0.335–3.493, P = 0.896, Bon = 1.000). Between-study heterogeneity was not detected in all the contrasts.

Analysis in the Turkish population

The association between the PPARγ Pro12Ala polymorphism and IBD in the Turkish population was investigated in 1 study with 45 UC cases, 69 CD cases and 100 controls [18]. And this study showed no significant association between this polymorphism and UC or CD in the Turkish population.

Moreover, the conclusions of our meta-analysis did not change when we used a fixed model and a random model to perform our meta-analysis respectively.

Evaluation of reporting bias

Obvious asymmetry was revealed by the shapes of the Begg funnel plots in the overall UC analysis and the overall CD analysis. The study with the smallest sample size reported by Aoyagi was a clear outlier which might be suggestive of a small-study effect. The Begg funnel plots corresponding to the allelic analysis are shown in Figure 4.

Discussion

The core pathophysiological process of UC is the uncontrolled inflammation mainly affecting the colon. Environmental factors including commensal flora and other antigens and host factors including genetic dispositions are all involved in the UC development [3,4]. The primarily upregulated response of the intestinal mucosal immune system is probably responsible for the uncontrolled inflammation of UC [4].

Firstly, dysfunction of the cellular and immune intestinal barrier which separates the microbial flora from host tissues renders a host susceptible to invasive factors [22]. Secondly, environmental factors including the dietary factor and microbia activate the Toll-like receptors (TLRs), which then activate NF-κB and cause the expression of pro-inflammatory genes consequently [23]. In the inflammation regulation networks, activation of PPARγ could suppress the activation of NFκB and TLRs [24,25], therefore inhibit the cascades of inflammation. Decreased PPARγ expression in epithelial cells was also found in UC patients in one study [26]. Moreover, a randomized placebo-controlled trial suggested that a PPARγ agonist was efficacious in the treatment of mild to moderately active UC [27]. All of these indicate normal expression of PPARγ as a protecting factor against the development of UC. Pro12Ala mutation is a common mutation, which downregulates the activity of PPARγ as indicated in one study [28]. Therefore the Pro12Ala mutation may be a risk factor for UC. However, our meta-analysis did not find a significant association between this mutation and the development of UC in the overall, European Caucasian and East Asian population. Our explanation is that the Pro12Ala mutation only affects the function of PPARγ2, and the function of PPARγ1 which makes up a large portion of PPARγ in intestines is intact. So the effect of the Pro12Ala mutation on the whole PPARγ function is limited, which would attenuate the effect of the Pro12Ala mutation on UC.

The mechanism of the uncontrolled inflammation in CD is different from that in UC. The deficiency of the innate immune system which permits intestinal pathogens to break through the intestinal barrier and activates the adaptive immune system may be responsible for the uncontrolled inflammation in CD [4]. The impaired function of macrophages may be the central process in the innate immune system deficiency [4,29,30], which causes granulomas in CD consequently. Nod proteins and PPARγ are all involved in the maintenance of normal innate immune system [6,31]. Gene mutations of the elements constituting the innate immune system may contribute to the CD development. Genetics play more important roles in the development of CD than in the development of UC [32,33]. NOD2/CARD15 polymorphism is the first confirmed risk factor for CD in Caucasian populations [34]. This encourages researchers to find other CD susceptible gene polymorphisms. A recent meta-analysis of genome-wide association scans identified *PTPN2, IL18RAP, TAGAP,* and *PUS10* loci as new CD risk factors [35], which widened our understanding of the gene background of CD. The PPARγ Pro12Ala mutation would decrease the function of PPARγ [28], and consequently abate its suppression on the activation of NFκB and TLRs [24,25], which would enhance the function of the innate immune system and protect a host against the development of CD.

Our meta-analysis supports this hypothesis. The AlaAla genotype seemed to protect the European Caucasian population against the development of CD. The Pro12Ala mutation only affects the function of PPARγ2, which supports PPARγ2 as a modulator in the innate immune system maintenance. However, we did not find an association between this polymorphism and CD in the East Asian population. This is in consistence with the observation of NOD2/CARD15 polymorphism on CD in the non Caucasian populations [36,37]. We deduce that the PPARγ Pro12Ala mutation, the NOD2/CARD15 polymorphism and other unknown gene polymorphisms mainly occurred in the Caucasian population may function synergistically in the CD development. Further these polymorphisms may constitute the gene background of the Caucasian population in turn.

However, the conclusions of this meta-analysis should be interpreted cautiously. This meta-analysis has some limitations. Firstly, only one study used colonoscopy to exclude IBD in the controls [9]. Only one study described the severity of cases, which was mild to moderate [20]. All of the above could cause selection

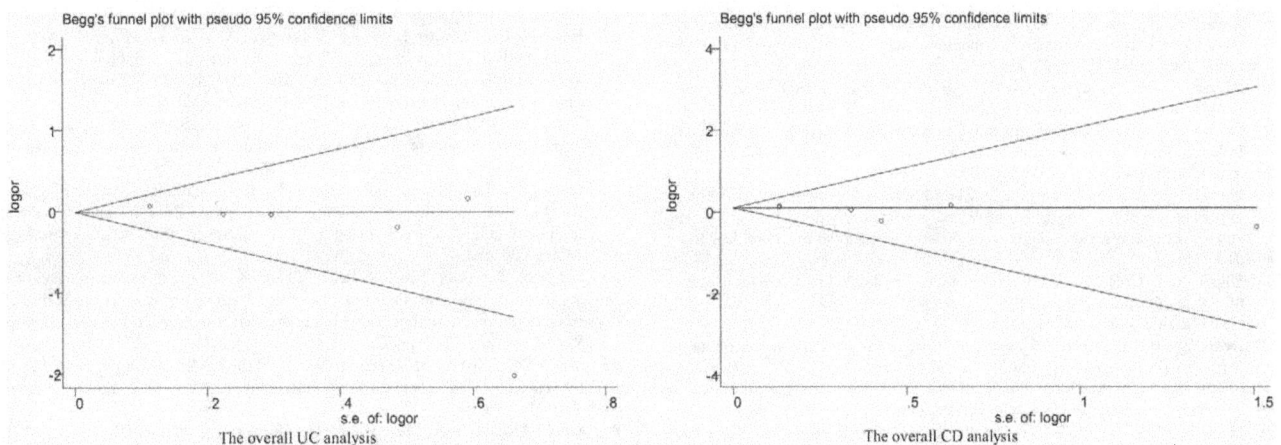

Figure 4. Begg funnel plots of the overall UC analysis and the overall CD analysis.

bias in some studies. Secondly, only two studies described the measures for genotyping quality control [11,21], and two studies used blindness measures [19,21]. Information bias could not be excluded completely. Thirdly, the controls were slightly older as compared to CD patients in one study [20], which would affect the comparability between arms in this study. Fourthly, the number of included studies was not large enough although we endeavored to collect relevant full text published studies. Fifthly, Obvious asymmetry was revealed by the shapes of the Begg funnel plots in the overall UC analysis and the overall CD analysis. The study with the smallest sample size reported by Aoyagi was a clear outlier, which might be suggestive of a small-study effect. Thus a reporting bias cannot be excluded. More high quality and large sample studies evaluating the association between the Pro12Ala mutation and the presence of IBD are still needed. An update of our meta-analysis is necessary in the future. Furthermore, only one study evaluated the interaction between diets and the Pro12Ala polymorphism which showed that a high intake of saturated and mono-unsaturated fat was associated with a more active CD only in wild type carriers [20]. The combined effect of diets and this polymorphism still needs to be elucidated. Studies investigating the interaction between the PPARγ Pro12Ala mutation and the NOD2/CARD15 polymorphism in the CD development in the Caucasian population are also wanted.

In conclusion, based on published full text case-control studies, our meta-analysis demonstrates that the AlaAla genotype may be a protecting factor in the European Caucasian population against the development of CD in a recessive way.

Acknowledgments

The authors thank two anonymous reviewers for questions and comments, which substantially improved the paper.

Author Contributions

Conceived and designed the experiments: Z-FZ NY. Performed the experiments: Z-FZ NY. Analyzed the data: Z-FZ NY GZ LZ L-XW. Contributed reagents/materials/analysis tools: Z-FZ NY GZ LZ L-XW. Wrote the paper: Z-FZ.

References

1. Cosnes J, Gower-Rousseau C, Seksik P, Cortot A (2011) Epidemiology and natural history of inflammatory bowel diseases. Gastroenterology 140(6): 1785–1794.
2. Mowat C, Cole A, Windsor A, Ahmad T, Arnott I, et al. (2011) Guidelines for the management of inflammatory bowel disease in adults. Gut 60(5): 571–607.
3. Baumgart DC, Carding SR (2007) Inflammatory bowel disease: cause and immunobiology. Lancet 369(9573): 1627–1640.
4. Marks DJ (2011) Defective innate immunity in inflammatory bowel disease: a Crohn's disease exclusivity? Curr Opin Gastroenterol 27(4): 328–334.
5. Yamamoto-Furusho JK, Peñaloza-Coronel A, Sánchez-Muñoz F, Barreto-Zuñiga R, Dominguez-Lopez A (2011) Peroxisome proliferator-activated receptor-gamma (PPAR-γ) expression is downregulated in patients with active ulcerative colitis. Inflamm Bowel Dis 17(2): 680–681.
6. Peyrin-Biroulet L, Beisner J, Wang G, Nuding S, Oommen ST, et al. (2010) Peroxisome proliferator-activated receptor gamma activation is required for maintenance of innate antimicrobial immunity in the colon. Proc Natl Acad Sci U S A 107(19): 8772–8777.
7. Celinski K, Dworzanski T, Korolczuk A, Slomka M, Radej S, et al. (2011) Activated and inactivated PPARs-γ modulate experimentally induced colitis in rats. Med Sci Monit 17(4): BR116–124.
8. Yen CJ, Beamer BA, Negri C, Silver K, Brown KA, et al. (1997) Molecular scanning of the human peroxisome proliferator activated receptor gamma (hPPAR gamma) gene in diabetic Caucasians: identification of a Pro12Ala PPAR gamma 2 missense mutation. Biochem Biophys Res Commun 241: 270–274.
9. Aoyagi Y, Nagata S, Kudo T, Fujii T, Wada M, et al. (2010) Peroxisome proliferator-activated receptor γ 2 mutation may cause a subset of ulcerative colitis. Pediatr Int 52(5): 729–734.
10. Poliska S, Penyige A, Lakatos PL, and the Hungarian IBD Study Group, Papp M, et al. (2011) Association of peroxisome proliferator-activated receptor gamma polymorphisms with inflammatory bowel disease in a hungarian cohort. Inflamm Bowel Dis. Available: http://onlinelibrary.wiley.com/doi/10.1002/ibd.21798/pdf. Accessed 2011 June 30.
11. Shrestha UK, Karimi O, Crusius JB, Zhou F, Wang Z, et al. (2010) Distribution of peroxisome proliferator-activated receptor-gamma polymorphisms in Chinese and Dutch patients with inflammatory bowel disease. Inflamm Bowel Dis 16(2): 312–319.
12. Higgins JPT, Green S, eds (2011) Cochrane Handbook for Systematic Reviews of Interventions Version 5.1.0 [updated March 2011]. The Cochrane Collaboration. Accessed 2011 June 30.
13. Dear K, Begg C (1992) An approach to assessing publication bias prior to performing a meta-analysis. Stat Sci 7: 237–245.
14. Sterne JA, Egger M (2001) Funnel plots for detecting bias in meta-analysis: guidelines on choice of axis. J Clin Epidemiol 54: 1046–1055.
15. Holm S (1979) A Simple Sequentially Rejective Bonferroni Test Procedure. Scand J Stat 6: 65–70.
16. Xin XY, Ding JQ, Chen SD (2010) Apolipoprotein E promoter polymorphisms and risk of Alzheimer's disease: evidence from meta-analysis. J Alzheimers Dis 19(4): 1283–1294.
17. Lehmann DJ, Cortina-Borja M, Warden DR, Smith AD, Sleegers K, et al. (2005) Large meta-analysis establishes the ACE insertion-deletion polymorphism as a marker of Alzheimer's disease. Am J Epidemiol 162: 305–317.
18. Atug O, Tahan V, Eren F, Tiftikci A, Imeryuz N, et al. (2008) Pro12Ala polymorphism in the peroxisome proliferator-activated receptor-gamma (PPARgamma) gene in inflammatory bowel disease. J Gastrointestin Liver Dis 17(4): 433–437.
19. Wang F, Tahara T, Arisawa T, Sakata M, Takahama K, et al. (2008) Polymorphism of peroxisome proliferator-activated receptor gamma is not associated to Japanese ulcerative colitis. Hepatogastroenterology 55(81): 73–75.
20. Ferreira P, Cravo M, Guerreiro CS, Tavares L, Santos PM, et al. (2010) Fat intake interacts with polymorphisms of Caspase9, FasLigand and PPARgamma apoptotic genes in modulating Crohn's disease activity. Clin Nutr 29(6): 819–823.
21. Andersen V, Christensen J, Ernst A, Jacobsen BA, Tjønneland A, et al. (2011) Polymorphisms in NF-κB, PXR, LXR, PPARγ and risk of inflammatory bowel disease. World J Gastroenterol 17(2): 197–206.
22. Salim SY, Söderholm JD (2011) Importance of disrupted intestinal barrier in inflammatory bowel diseases. Inflamm Bowel Dis 17(1): 362–381.
23. Becker CE, O'Neill LA (2007) Inflammasomes in inflammatory disorders: the role of TLRs and their interactions with NLRs. Semin Immunopatho 29: 239–248.
24. Genolet R, Wahli W, Michalik L (2004) PPARs as drug targets to modulate inflammatory responses? Curr Drug Targets Inflamm Allergy 3: 361–375.
25. Reynolds CM, Draper E, Keogh B, Rahman A, Moloney AP, et al. (2009) A conjugated linoleic acid-enriched beef diet attenuates lipopolysaccharide-induced inflammation in mice in part through PPARgamma-mediated suppression of toll-like receptor 4. J Nutr 139(12): 2351–2357.
26. Dubuquoy L, Jansson EA, Deeb S, Rakotobe S, Karoui M, et al. (2003) Impaired expression of peroxisome proliferator-activated receptor gamma in ulcerative colitis. Gastroenterology 124: 1265–1276.
27. Lewis JD, Lichtenstein GR, Deren JJ, Sands BE, Hanauer SB (2008) Rosiglitazone for Ulcerative Colitis Study Group. Rosiglitazone for active ulcerative colitis: a randomized placebo-controlled trial. Gastroenterology 134(3): 688–695.
28. Masugi J, Tamori Y, Mori H, Koike T, Kasuga M (2000) Inhibitory effect of a proline-to-alanine substitution at codon 12 of peroxisome proliferator-activated receptor-gamma 2 on thiazolidinedione-induced adipogenesis. Biochem Biophys Res Commun 268: 178–182.
29. Marks DJ, Harbord MW, MacAllister R, Rahman FZ, Young J, et al. (2006) Defective acute inflammation in Crohn's disease: a clinical investigation. Lancet 367: 668–678.
30. Smith AM, Rahman FZ, Hayee B, Graham SJ, Marks DJ, et al. (2009) Disordered macrophage cytokine secretion underlies impaired acute inflammation and bacterial clearance in Crohn's disease. J Exp Med 206: 1883–1897.
31. Magalhaes JG, Sorbara MT, Girardin SE, Philpott DJ (2011) What is new with Nods? Curr Opin Immunol 23: 29–34.

32. Vind I, Jespersgaard C, Hougs L, Riis L, Dinesen L, et al. (2005) Genetic and environmental factors in monozygotic twins with Crohn's disease and their first-degree relatives: a case report. Digestion 1: 262–265.

33. Jess T, Riis L, Jespersgaard C, Hougs L, Andersen PS, et al. (2005) Disease concordance, zygosity, and NOD2/CARD15 status: follow-up of a population-based cohort of Danish twins with inflammatory bowel disease. Am J Gastroenterol 100: 2486–2492.

34. Torok HP, Glas J, Lohse P, Folwaczny C (2003) Alterations of the CARD15/NOD2 gene and the impact on management and treatment of Crohn's disease patients. Dig Dis 21: 339–345.

35. Franke A, McGovern DP, Barrett JC, Wang K, Radford-Smith GL, et al. (2010) Genome-wide meta-analysis increases to 71 the number of confirmed Crohn's disease susceptibility loci. Nat Genet 42: 1118–1125.

36. Leong RW, Armuzzi A, Ahmad T, Wong ML, Tse P, et al. (2003) NOD2/CARD15 gene polymorphisms and Crohn's disease in the Chinese population. Aliment Pharmacol Ther 1: 1465–1470.

37. Inoue N, Tamura K, Kinouchi Y, Fukuda Y, Takahashi S, et al. (2002) Lack of common NOD2 variants in Japanese patients with Crohn's disease. Gastroenterology 123: 86–91.

3

Serological Markers for Inflammatory Bowel Disease in AIDS Patients with Evidence of Microbial Translocation

Anupa Kamat[1], **Petronela Ancuta**[2], **Richard S. Blumberg**[3], **Dana Gabuzda**[1]*

1 Department of Cancer Immunology and AIDS, Dana Farber Cancer Institute, Harvard Medical School, Boston, Massachusetts, United States of America, 2 Departement de Microbiologie et Immunologie, Centre de Recherche du Centre Hospitalier de l'Universite de Montreal (CRCHUM) Universite de Montreal and INSERM Unit 743, Montreal, Quebec, Canada, 3 Department of Medicine, Brigham and Women's Hospital, Harvard Medical School, Boston, Massachusetts, United States of America

Abstract

Background: Breakdown of the gut mucosal barrier during chronic HIV infection allows translocation of bacterial products such as lipopolysaccharides (LPS) from the gut into the circulation. Microbial translocation also occurs in inflammatory bowel disease (IBD). IBD serological markers are useful in the diagnosis of IBD and to differentiate between Crohn's disease (CD) and ulcerative colitis (UC). Here, we evaluate detection of IBD serological markers in HIV-infected patients with advanced disease and their relationship to HIV disease markers.

Methods: IBD serological markers (ASCA, pANCA, anti-OmpC, and anti-CBir1) were measured by ELISA in plasma from AIDS patients (n = 26) with low CD4 counts (<300 cells/μl) and high plasma LPS levels, and results correlated with clinical data. For meta-analysis, relevant data were abstracted from 20 articles.

Results: IBD serological markers were detected in approximately 65% of AIDS patients with evidence of microbial translocation. An antibody pattern consistent with IBD was detected in 46%; of these, 75% had a CD-like pattern. Meta-analysis of data from 20 published studies on IBD serological markers in CD, UC, and non-IBD control subjects indicated that IBD serological markers are detected more frequently in AIDS patients than in non-IBD disease controls and healthy controls, but less frequently than in CD patients. There was no association between IBD serological markers and HIV disease markers (plasma viral load and CD4 counts) in the study cohort.

Conclusions: IBD serological markers may provide a non-invasive approach to monitor HIV-related inflammatory gut disease. Further studies to investigate their clinical significance in HIV-infected individuals are warranted.

Editor: Derya Unutmaz, New York University, United States of America

Funding: This work was supported by NIH DA26322 and MH083588. R.B. was supported by NIH DK44319, DK51362, DK53056, and the Harvard Digestive Diseases Center. P.A. was supported by New Investigator Awards from Fonds de la Recherche en Santé Québec (FRSQ) and INSERM. Core facilities were supported by the Harvard Center for AIDS Research and DFCI/Harvard Center for Cancer Research grants. NNTC sites were supported by MH59745, NS38841, MH59656, NS54591, and MH59724. The funders had no role in study design, data collection and analysis, decision to publish, or preparation of the manuscript.

Competing Interests: The authors have declared that no competing interests exist.

* E-mail: dana_gabuzda@dfci.harvard.edu

Introduction

CD4 T-cells in gut-associated lymphoid tissue (GALT) are primary target cells of HIV, and GALT is an important site for HIV replication and pathogenesis [1–4]. Significant CD4 T cell loss occurs in the gastrointestinal tract within the first few weeks of infection [5–7]. Later on, during chronic HIV infection, loss of GALT integrity and breaching of the gut mucosal barrier leads to microbial translocation [8–10], which is evidenced by the release of microbial products such as bacterial endotoxins (lipopolysaccharides (LPS), a component of gram negative bacteria) into the circulation (endotoxemia) [11]. Microbial translocation from a leaky gut may contribute to immune activation during chronic HIV infection [11–15]. Elevated levels of plasma LPS and bacterial 16S rDNA have been used to measure translocation of microbial products from the gastrointestinal tract [11,16].

Microbial translocation is also a noted feature in inflammatory bowel disease (IBD) [17–20]. IBD comprises a group of intestinal diseases characterized by chronic inflammation of the bowel;

Crohn's disease (CD) and ulcerative colitis (UC) are the common clinical subtypes of IBD. The intestinal bacterial flora triggers and drives an aberrant immune response in a genetically susceptible host, resulting in chronic inflammation of the gut [21,22]. Low level endotoxemia has pathogenic significance in IBD; it occurs in 31%–48% of CD patients and 17%–28% of UC patients [18,23], with a higher incidence in patients with active IBD (94% in CD, 88% in UC) [19].

The role of enteric microflora in IBD pathophysiology is highlighted by the presence of antibody reactivity to microbial antigens. These serological markers can be helpful to distinguish between CD and UC as well as aiding in the diagnosis of IBD along with clinical history, endoscopy, and physical examination [24]. The currently available IBD serological markers are: ASCA (anti-*Saccharomyces cerevisiae* antibody) [25–31], pANCA (perinuclear anti-neutrophil antibody) [25–30,32], and anti-OmpC (antibody against outer membrane porin C of *E.coli*) [28,33–37]. ASCA, which is directed against a mannose epitope in the phosphopepti-domannan of the *Saccharomyces cerevisiae* cell wall [30–32], is associated with CD [25–27,37–41]. The sensitivity and specificity for detection of ASCA antibodies in CD are 50%–70% and 80%–90%, respectively [25,27,29,30,32,37,42,43]. pANCA is an antibody directed against cytoplasmic constituents of neutrophils with a perinuclear staining pattern [25,44,45]. pANCA is detected in 40%–80% of UC patients, but also in 6%–20% of CD patients who can be classified as having a UC-like phenotype [30,32,37,46,47], with sensitivity and specificity between 55%–70% and 80%–95% in UC patients [27,29,30,32,37,43,45–47]. Anti-OmpC antibodies are detected in 40%–55% of CD patients [25,48–51], with sensitivity and specificity ranging between 20%–55% and 75%–95%, respectively [25,34,37,50,52]. Anti-CBir1 (antibodies against bacterial flagellin) is a new serological marker associated with IBD [28,35,53–58]. CBir1 flagellin is an immuno-dominant and colitogenic antigen of enteric microbial flora [58]. Anti-CBir1 is detected in approximately 50% of CD patients [28,35,53,55–58], and is independently associated with compli-cated CD [25,33,35,59].

A number of parallels are observed between HIV and IBD in terms of gut disease [60–62]. Small intestinal villous atrophy and enterocyte defects have been described in HIV-infected patients. Because these defects usually occur in the absence of enteric pathogens, the term HIV enteropathy has been used [60,62,63]. Characteristic features of HIV enteropathy are diarrhea, gastro-intestinal inflammation, increased intestinal permeability, and decreased mucosal repair and regeneration [1,2,60,64]. Previous studies reported infrequent cases of IBD in HIV-infected patients [61,65–67]. To our knowledge, however, no reports have examined the prevalence of ASCA, OmpC, and CBir1 antibodies in HIV infection.

We previously demonstrated that elevated circulating LPS levels correlate with monocyte activation during HIV infection, and may thereby contribute to chronic immune activation [12]. In the present study, we evaluated detection of IBD serological markers in AIDS patients with low CD4 counts (<300 cells/µl) and high plasma LPS levels. We detected IBD serological antibodies in approximately 65% of subjects. A serological pattern consistent with IBD was detected in 46% of AIDS patients; of these, 75% showed a CD-like pattern, while 25% had a UC pattern. IBD serological markers may provide a non-invasive approach to monitor HIV-related gut disease. Further studies to determine their prognostic significance in HIV-infected individuals are warranted.

Methods

Subjects

AIDS patients with CD4 counts <300 cells/µl were recruited at the Lemuel Shattuck Hospital (n = 20), or at 3 sites in the National NeuroAIDS Tissue Consortium (NNTC) (Manhattan HIV Brain Bank, National Neurological AIDS Bank, Texas NeuroAIDS Research Center) (n = 6) with written informed consent and IRB approval at each study site. Patients with active bacterial or opportunistic infections were excluded. There was no available radiographic, endoscopic, or histopathologic data for the gut. All plasma samples were stored at −80°C until analyzed.

Laboratory assays

Frozen plasma samples were shipped on dry ice to Prometheus Laboratories (San Diego, CA) and analyzed in a blinded fashion; Prometheus staff did not have access to clinical information except for HIV/HCV status. Prometheus IBD Serology 7 is the most comprehensive IBD test available, utilizing several proprietary markers and incorporating computer-based Smart Diagnostic

Algorithm pattern recognition technology to aid in the diagnosis of IBD as well as differentiate between CD and UC. Prometheus IBD Serology 7 tests include the following assays: ASCA IgA and IgG, anti-OmpC IgA antibodies, IgG anti-CBir1, and pANCA autoantibody by ELISA, and immunofluorescence assay (IFA) to determine the perinuclear pattern of neutrophils and DNAse sensitivity. The reference cut-off for each assay was defined by Prometheus laboratories (ASCA IgA <20 EU/ml, ASCA IgG <40 EU/ml, anti-OmpC <16.5 EU/ml, anti-CBir1 <21 EU/ml, and pANCA autoantibody <12.1 EU/ml). Positive samples showing patterns consistent with IBD were reported based on analysis by Prometheus Smart Diagnostic Algorithm Technology.

Quantification of cytokines and chemokines

A multiplex immunoassay (Bio-source 25-plex Human Cytokine Assay; Invitrogen., CA, USA), consisting of fluorescent micro-spheres conjugated with a monoclonal antibody specific for a target protein, was used according to the manufacturer's instructions to measure levels of the following cytokines IL-1β, IL-2, IL-4, IL-5, IL-6, IL-7, IL-8, IL-10, IL-12, IL-13, IL-17, IFN-α, IFNγ, TNF-α granulocyte-monocyte colony stimulating factor (GM-CSF), monocyte chemoattractive protein (MCP-1/CCL2), macrophage inflammatory protein (MIP-1β/MIP-1α), IP-10, MIG, Eotaxin and RANTES. Briefly, plasma was diluted 1:2 and incubated with antibody-coupled beads. Complexes were washed and then incubated with biotinylated detection antibody followed by streptavidin-phycoerythrin prior to assessing titers of cytokine concentration. Recombinant cytokines were used to establish standard curves. Cytokine levels were determined using a multiplex array reader from Luminex^{TM} Instrumentation System (Bio-Plex Workstation from Bio-Rad Laboratories, USA). Analyte concentration was calculated using Bioplex Manager Software.

Statistical analysis

Data were analyzed using the Mann-Whitney U test and Spearman rank correlation coefficient. Differences were consid-ered significant at p<0.05.

Results

IBD serological markers in AIDS

To investigate the frequency and pattern of IBD serological markers in AIDS patients, we used the Prometheus IBD Serology 7 test to detect IBD serological markers in plasma samples. Subjects were selected from a larger cohort of 119 AIDS subjects with CD4 counts <300 cells/µl described in a previous study [12] on the basis of high plasma LPS above the median value for AIDS patients in the study cohort (>80 pg/ml) levels; LPS levels were determined in the previous study using the Diazo-coupled *Limulus* amebocyte lysate (LAL) assay. The study cohort consisted of 26 AIDS patients with relatively high plasma viral loads (median 10,935 copies/ml, range <50–2,210,000) and low CD4 counts (median 80 cells/µl, range 3–261), together with a high frequency of intravenous drug abuse (IVDU) (65%), HCV co-infection (50%), and HIV-associated dementia (HAD) (50%). Eleven subjects were both IVDU and HCV positive. Demographic and clinical characteristics of the study cohort are shown in Table 1. All subjects were on HAART, but only 23% were virologically suppressed (<400 plasma HIV RNA copies/ml).

In the study cohort (n = 26), ASCA IgA, pANCA, and anti-OmpC were detected in 31% (8/26), while ASCA IgG and anti-CBir1 were detected in 15% (4/26) (Table 2). Prometheus laboratories classified subjects as having a CD- or UC-like pattern according to Smart Diagnostic Algorithm Technology. According

Table 1. Demographic and clinical characteristics of HIV patients in the study cohort (n = 26).

Age (years)	
Median (range)	45 (32–63)
Gender	
Male	19 (73%)
Female	7 (27%)
Race/ethnicity	
African American	6 (23%)
Caucasian	12 (46%)
Hispanic	8 (31%)
Plasma HIV RNA (copies/ml)	
Mean ± SD	215,718±590,409
Median (range)	10,935 (<50–2,210,000)
>400 copies/ml	18 (69%)
<400 copies/ml	6 (23%)
Unknown	2 (8%)
CD4 T Cell Count (cells/μl)	
Mean ± SD	98.6±84.4
Median (range)	80 (3–261)
Plasma LPS (pg/ml)	
Mean± SD	128.07±56.18
Median (range)	109 (82.5–279.6)
HCV Co-infection	
Negative	7 (27%)
Positive	13 (50%)
Unknown	6 (23%)
Substance abuse	
No IVDU	9 (35%)
Heroin IVDU	8 (31%)
Heroin and Cocaine IVDU	5 (19%)
Cocaine IVDU	4 (15%)

to this classification, 46% (12/26) of the subjects showed a pattern consistent with IBD, with 75% (9/12) having a CD-like pattern and 25% (3/12) having a UC-like pattern. In subjects with a positive IBD pattern, ASCA IgA and IgG antibodies were detected in 50% and 33%, while anti-OmpC, anti-CBir1, and pANCA were detected in 67%, 33%, and 42%, respectively (Table 2). Three patients with a pANCA (+) anti-OmpC (+) pattern and 1 with a pANCA (+) anti-CBir1 (+) pattern (n = 1) could also be classified as having a pattern consistent with UC-like CD [25,29,48,68,69,70]. Thus, IBD serological markers were detected in approximately 65% of AIDS patients with high plasma LPS levels, with 46% having an IBD-like pattern and the majority of these having a CD-like pattern.

IBD serological markers in subgroups with IV heroin use, HCV co-infection, or HIV-associated dementia (HAD)

Previous studies reported that AIDS patients with heroin IVDU, HCV co-infection or HAD have higher plasma LPS levels compared to respective control groups [12,71]. Furthermore, substance abuse and HCV co-infection are associated with an increased incidence of bacterial infections [72]. We therefore

examined the pattern of ASCA, pANCA, anti-OmpC, and anti-CBir1 in AIDS patients classified according to these subgroups (Table 2 and data not shown). There was no significant difference in the frequency or magnitude of IBD serological markers between IVDU heroin users compared to patients with no substance abuse, HCV-positive compared to HCV-negative subjects, or HAD compared to non-HAD subjects (Table 2 and data not shown). Thus, there was no difference in magnitude or frequency of IBD serological markers in these clinical subgroups.

Higher ASCA IgG, anti-OmpC, and anti-CBir1 levels but similar plasma viral load and CD4 counts in AIDS patients with IBD-like serological pattern

Higher levels of ASCA IgG (median 31.4 EU/ml, range 12–120 compared to 12 EU/ml, 12–27.9, p = 0.027), anti-OmpC (25.9 EU/ml, 4.7–111, compared to 7.1 EU/ml, 1–15.3, p = 0.005), and anti-CBir1 (18.6 EU/ml, 8–37.7, compared to 9.1 EU/ml, 5.5–15.6, p = 0.001) were detected in subjects with a positive IBD pattern as compared to those with a negative pattern (Table 3 and Figure S1). In contrast, there was no significant difference in ASCA IgA and pANCA antibody levels between these two groups (p = 0.135 and p = 0.540). We then investigated the relationship of IBD serological markers to HIV disease markers, plasma LPS, and EndoCAb levels. HIV RNA levels, CD4 cell counts, plasma sCD14, plasma LPS, and IgM EndoCAb levels were similar in the 2 groups (Table 3). Furthermore, there were no significant correlations (Spearman correlation) between levels of individual IBD serological markers and HIV RNA levels, CD4 cell counts, plasma sCD14, or plasma LPS levels (data not shown). Thus, we found no association between IBD serological markers and HIV disease markers or plasma LPS levels in the study cohort.

No association of IBD serological markers with plasma cytokines and chemokines in AIDS patients

In IBD, the dysregulated inflammatory response is associated with upregulation of mucosal and systemic levels of cytokines (i.e., IL-1, IL-6, IL-8, IL-12, and TNF) [73]. We used a multiplex assay to measure levels of 25 cytokines and chemokines in plasma samples from 20 AIDS patients in the study cohort and explore their relationship to individual IBD serological markers. We detected higher levels of IL-2R, CXCL9, CXCL10, CCL2, and IL-6 (p = 0.001, 0.0003, 0.0002, 0.017, and 0.0005, respectively) in plasma of AIDS patients compared to healthy uninfected controls (data not shown). No significant differences in cytokine/chemokine levels were seen when AIDS subjects were grouped according to positive (n = 9) versus negative IBD (n = 11) pattern (data not shown). Only IL-10 showed a trend towards significance (median 7.26 (range 0–41.94 pg/ml) versus 2.14 (0–8 pg/ml) respectively, p = 0.087, data not shown), with higher levels in patients with a positive IBD pattern. We then examined the association of individual IBD serological markers with levels of IL-1β, IL-2R, IL-6, IL-10, IL-17, IP-10, IFNγ, TNF, MIP-1α, MIP-1β, and MCP-1, and found a positive correlation only between anti-CBir1 antibody and IL-6 (r = 0.447, p = 0.048, Figure S2). Together with previous studies demonstrating that CBir1 antigen can induce IL-6 and other proinflammatory cytokines [56,58], this finding raises the possibility that translocation of flagellin into the circulation may be a factor that contributes to immune activation in AIDS.

Magnitude of IBD serological antibody response in AIDS

Previous data suggested that the magnitude of antibody responses to microbial antigens is associated with increased risk

Table 2. Profile of inflammatory bowel disease (IBD) serological markers in AIDS subjects.

	HIV positive subjects n = 26 n (%)	Smart Algorithm positive subjects n = 12 n (%)	Heroin IVDU subjects n = 13 n (%)	HCV positive subjects n = 13 n (%)
ASCA IgA	8 (31)	6 (50)	4 (31)	5 (38)
ASCA IgG	4 (15)	4 (33)	2 (15)	2 (15)
Anti-OmpC IgA	8 (31)	8 (67)	4 (31)	3 (23)
Anti-CBir1	4 (15)	4 (33)	2 (15)	2 (15)
NSNA (IBD Specific pANCA)				
pANCA Autoantibody	8 (31)	5 (42)	5 (38)	2 (15)
IFA Perinuclear Pattern	5 (19)	4 (33)	2 (15)	2 (15)
DNAse Sensitivity	5 (19)	4 (33)	2 (15)	2 (15)
Crohn's- like pattern*	9 (35)	9 (75)	5 (38)	4 (31)
UC-like pattern*	3 (11)	3 (25)	1(7.6)	1 (7.6)
UC-like Crohn's pattern				
ANCA (+) OmpC (+)**	3 (11)	3 (11)	1 (7.6)	1 (7.6)
ANCA (+) CBir (+)***	1 (3.8)	1 (3.8)	1 (7.6)	0 (0)

Abbreviations: Heroin IVDU - Intravenous drug users using heroin, or heroin and cocaine; ASCA IgA/Ig - Anti-Saccharomyces cerevisiae antibodies; Anti-OmpC IgA- Anti-Outer membrane porin C on E.coli; Anti-CBir1- recognizes bacterial flagellin antigen associated with IBD; pANCA autontibody - IBD- specific pANCA autoantibody (NSNA, Neutrophil-specific nuclear autoantibody);
*Based on Prometheus Smart Algorithm;
**patients with UC-like pattern according to Smart Algorithm also classified as having a UC-like CD pattern;
***One patient with CD-like pattern according to Prometheus Smart Algorithm also classified as having UC-like CD pattern.

of complicated CD [25,42,59]. We tested this hypothesis with respect to HIV disease progression by counting the number of positive antibodies (ASCA, pANCA, anti-OmpC, and anti-CBir1) and scoring these from 0–3 (Table 4). None of the subjects showed a positive response for all 4 antibodies; 26.9% (7/26) had a score of 1, 30.7% (8/26) had a score of 2, 7.6% (2/26) had a score of 3, and 34.6% (9/26) had a score of zero. Forty-two percent (6/14) of subjects with CD4 T - cell counts <100 cells/μl versus 27% (3/11) with >100

cells/μl had antibody responses to 2 antigens, but this difference did not reach statistical significance (p = 0.676). Subjects grouped according to HIV RNA levels >10,000 versus <10,000 copies/ml, heroin use versus no heroin use, HAD versus non-HAD, or LPS > median value of 109 pg/ml versus <109 pg/ml had no difference in the magnitude of antibody response. Thus, the magnitude of IBD serological antibody responses was not associated with HIV disease markers, high LPS levels, or clinical subgroups in the study cohort.

Table 3. Clinical and serological profile in AIDS subjects having a serological pattern consistent with IBD versus not consistent with IBD.

	Pattern consistent with IBD** (n = 12)	Pattern not consistent with IBD** (n = 14)	p-value
Age (years)	45	44	0.149
Plasma HIV RNA (copies/ml)	9,725	10,935	0.665
CD4 cell count (cells/μl)	84	66	0.956
Plasma sCD14 (μg/ml)	2.5	2.6	0.897
Plasma LPS (pg/ml)	121	105	0.207
Plasma EndoCAb (MMU/ml)	57	75	0.738
ASCA IgA (EU/ml)	19.7	12	0.135
ASCA IgG (EU/ml)	31.4	12	0.027*
Anti-OmpC IgA (EU/ml)	25.9	7.1	0.005*
Anti- CBir1 (EU/ml)	18.6	9.1	0.001*
pANCA AutoAb (EU/ml)	12.1	12.1	0.540

Abbreviations: IBD - Inflammatory bowel disease;
**numbers represent median values; Statistical analysis was performed using Mann-Whitney test,
*p<0.05 statistically significant; ASCA IgA/IgG- Anti-Saccharomyces cerevisiae antibodies; Anti-OmpC IgA- Anti-Outer membrane porin C on E.coli; Anti-CBir1- recognizes bacterial flagellin antigen associated with IBD; pANCA autoantibody-IBD-specific pANCA autoantibody (NSNA, Neutrophil-specific nuclear autoantibody).

Table 4. Clinical characteristics of AIDS patients in relation to the magnitude of IBD serological antibody response.

Subjects	Number of IBD serological antibodies n (%)			
	0	1	2	3
AIDS patients (n = 26)	9 (34.6)	7 (26.9)	8 (30.7)	2 (7.6)
CD4 <100 cells/µl (n = 14)	4 (28.5)	3 (21.4)	6 (42.8)	1 (7.1)
Plasma HIV RNA >10,000 HIV RNA copies/ml (n = 12)	3 (25.0)	3 (25.0)	5 (41.6)	1 (8.3)
LPS >109 pg/ml* (n = 13)	4 (30.7)	4 (30.7)	4 (30.7)	1 (7.6)
Heroin IVDU (n = 13)	3 (23.0)	6 (46.1)	3 (23.0)	1 (7.6)
HAD (n = 13)	4 (30.7)	4 (30.7)	4 (30.7)	1 (7.6)

Abbreviations used: HAD- HIV-associated dementia; Heroin IVDU- heroin intravenous drug users; LPS- Lipopolysaccharide; Antibodies tested- ASCA IgA/IgG- Anti-Saccharomyces cerevisiae antibodies; Anti-OmpC IgA- Anti-Outer membrane porin C on E.coli; Anti-CBir1- recognizes bacterial flagellin antigen associated with IBD; pANCA autoantiody- IBD-specific pANCA autoantibody (NSNA, Neutrophil-specific nuclear autoantibody);
*represents cut-off above the median value for the study cohort.

Discussion

In this study, we examined IBD serological markers in AIDS patients with high plasma LPS levels and detected an IBD-like serological pattern in 46%. Among subjects with a positive IBD pattern, 75% had a CD-like pattern and 25% had a UC-like pattern. The association of pANCA with CD markers has been described as a UC-like Crohn's pattern [25,29,43,69,70]. Based on this classification, 15% of the study cohort had a UC-like CD pattern. These findings are consistent with the frequent occurrence of HIV-related gut disease involving the small and large intestine in AIDS patients [1,2,3,4]. Antibodies to microbial antigens (ASCA IgG, anti-OmpC, and anti-CBir1) were detected at higher levels in AIDS patients with compared to those without an IBD serological pattern. These findings together with the detection IBD serological markers in approximately 65% of AIDS patients with high plasma LPS suggest that IBD markers, in particular ASCA, anti-OmpC, and anti-CBir1, may provide a non-invasive approach to monitor HIV-related inflammatory gut disease, and possibly therapeutic responses.

Our original hypothesis was that high plasma LPS levels or HIV disease markers would be associated with detection of IBD serological markers. However, we found no difference in LPS levels between AIDS subjects with versus without an IBD-like serological pattern, and no association between the frequency or magnitude of IBD serological markers and HIV RNA levels, CD4 cell counts, plasma sCD14 or LPS levels. We found a higher magnitude of antibody responses to 2 antigens in AIDS patients with low CD4 counts or high viral loads as compared to other clinical subgroups, but this difference did not reach statistical significance. pANCA antibodies were previously detected in 18% to 41.9% of patients with symptomatic HIV infection [74,75,76], and in 20% of heroin users with systemic complications irrespective of HIV infection [77]. Consistent with these findings, we detected pANCA in 31% of AIDS patients and 38% of heroin users. Nonetheless, detection or levels of pANCA did not discriminate between subgroups classified according to positive IBD pattern, HIV disease markers, or IV heroin use. Together, these unexpected findings could reflect differences in gut commensalism, other host factors that affect gut homeostasis, or limitations of our study such as the small sample size, cross-sectional design, or selection of subjects with high LPS levels. Alternatively, the severity of HIV- related gut disease may not be detected by serological measurements of IBD markers or HIV

disease biomarkers. We also cannot exclude the possibility that the absence of antibody responses to microbial antigens in 35% (9/26) of AIDS patients with high LPS levels reflects weakened humoral immune responses. Another limitation of our study is the lack of endoscopy or gut pathology data for the study cohort. Viazis et al [66] examined IBD outcomes in HIV-infected subjects who had an IBD diagnosis and found that these patients have a better disease course with lower probability of IBD relapse as compared to HIV-negative IBD patients. This was attributed to lower CD4 T-cell counts in HIV-infected individuals suppressing disease activity in CD. If true, low CD4 counts in our study cohort might influence relationships between HIV disease markers or LPS levels and IBD serological antibodies. The Th17 subset of CD4+ T-cells play an important role in the pathogenesis of IBD; HIV preferentially infects and depletes these cells in GALT, which may also help to explain the better disease course observed in patients with an IBD diagnosis who are HIV-positive compared to those who are HIV-negative. Larger prospective studies are needed to determine the clinical significance of IBD serological markers in HIV-infected patients and their relationship to HIV-related gut disease.

To assess the diagnostic precision of IBD serological antibodies and their ability to distinguish between CD, UC, inflammatory and non-inflammatory non-IBD disease subjects, and healthy controls, we performed meta-analysis of serological data from 20 published studies [25,27–30,33–35,37,42,49,52,53,55,57,58,78–81]. Extensive meta-analysis was previously reported for ASCA and pANCA antibodies [43]. To our knowledge, however, the present study is the first meta-analysis for all available IBD serological markers. Consistent with previous reports [25,27,29,30,34,37,79,81], our meta-analysis demonstrated that the prevalence of ASCA IgA/IgG was 45% in CD subjects as compared to 7.9% and 3.7% in non-IBD and healthy controls, respectively, and pANCA was prevalent in 42.4% of UC subjects (Table 5) [26,27,29,32,37,44,82]. Anti-OmpC and anti-CBir1 were prevalent in 29.4% and 55.2% of CD subjects, respectively, compared to 17.6% and 25.5% in non-IBD disease controls, and 10.7% and 6.3% in healthy controls. A separate meta-analysis of 10 published studies that used Prometheus Laboratories IBD Serological Markers (Table S1) demonstrated similar findings, with ASCA, anti-OmpC, and anti-CBir1 more prevalent in CD (48.5%, 32.2%, and 55.8%, respectively), pANCA more prevalent in UC (67.9%), and ASCA, pANCA, and anti-OmpC prevalent in

Table 5. Meta-analysis of 20 studies using IBD serological markers.

Marker	Number of studies				Number of subjects				Positive for antibodies n (%)			
	CD	UC	Disease ontrols	Healthy ontrols	CD	UC	Disease controls	Healthy ontrols	CD	UC	Disease Controls	Healthy Controls
ASCA IgA/IgG*	15	9	6	6	4893	1026	455	1071	2206 (45)	110 (10.7)	36 (7.9)	40 (3.7)
ANCA	10	8	6	6	2424	826	381	871	352 (14)	351 (42.4)	54 (16)	23 (2.6)
Anti-OmpC	10	4	2	3	4116	448	176	401	1211 (29.4)	90 (20)	31 (17.6)	43 (10.7)
Anti-CBir1	6	2	2	2	2261	100	43	80	1249 (55.2)	11 (11)	11 (25.5)	5 (6.3)

CD- Crohn's Disease; UC- Ulcerative colitis;
*- any one of the antibodies present; Disease controls include inflammatory and non-inflammatory non-IBD disease controls (n = 633), including 264 non-IBD inflammatory gut diseases (i.e., colitis, gastroenteritis, celiac disease, etc); 193 non-inflammatory gut diseases (i.e., abdominal pain, diarrhea, lactose intolerance, etc); 90 rheumatologic disorders, and 86 other (i.e., constipation, nausea, rectal bleeding, etc).
The meta-analysis includes 19 studies with CD patients [25,27,28,29,30,33,34,35,37,42,49,52,53,55,57,58,78,79,81], 12 with UC patients [25,27,29,30,34,37,42,52,57,58,78,79,81], 10 with non-IBD disease controls [25,29,30,37,52,57,58,78,79,80,81], and 8 with healthy controls [25,27,29,30,34,42,57,58,81].

1.6%–6.3% of non-IBD disease controls and 3.9%–9.9% of healthy controls (Table S1). We detected ASCA, anti-OmpC, and anti-CBir1 in 15%–31% of AIDS patients with high LPS levels compared to 29.4%–55.2% in CD, 7.9%–25.5% in non-IBD disease controls, and 3.7%–0.7% in healthy controls. Thus, IBD serological markers were detected more frequently in AIDS patients than in non-IBD disease controls or healthy subjects, but less frequently than in CD patients.

IBD serological markers alone are not recommended for diagnosis and monitoring of IBD because they are not robust enough for routine use [50,83]. Moreover, prediction of IBD using Smart Diagnostic Algorithm Technology has not been published in peer-reviewed journals and test validation was done using only healthy controls [83]. To our knowledge, there are no published prospective studies on IBD serological markers in predicting disease course in UC or CD. As such, prospective studies are needed to determine their prognostic significance. Nonetheless, our meta-analysis highlights the utility of IBD serological markers in discriminating between CD, UC, non-IBD controls, and healthy controls, and their potential use for further studies of gut disease in HIV infection.

Several cytokines with proinflammatory activities (IL-1, IL-6, IL-8, IL-12, and TNF-α) are upregulated in IBD, and are likely to play an important role in clinical and immunopathological manifestations of the disease [56,73]. Plasma IL-10 concentrations are elevated in subjects with active CD and UC [84] or with UC [85]. Similarly, higher levels of IL-10 in AIDS patients with compared to those without an IBD-like pattern were suggested by a trend towards significance in the present study. Higher levels of IL-6 [56,73] and negative correlation between IL-6 and anti-CBir1 were previously reported in CD subjects [56]. In contrast, we found a positive correlation between IL-6 and anti-CBir1 in AIDS patients. These findings suggest complex relationships between antibody responses to CBir1 antigen and IL-6 induction, and raise the possibility that translocation of flagellin from the gut into the circulation, or associated pathogenic processes, might contribute to immune activation in chronic HIV infection.

Limitations of this study are its cross-sectional design and small sample size, which may have decreased the power to detect significant associations between IBD serological markers and HIV disease markers. Another limitation is the narrow selection criteria used to define the study cohort, limited to AIDS subjects with CD4 counts <300 cells/µl and high plasma LPS levels. These narrow selection criteria may in part explain our inability to detect a significant difference in HIV disease markers, plasma LPS levels, or plasma cytokine/chemokine levels between patients with and without an IBD-like pattern. In view of these limitations, we recognize the need for further studies to examine the detection of IBD serological markers and frequency of an IBD-like pattern in patients with acute or chronic HIV infection before progression to AIDS and in relation to gut disease documented by endoscopic or pathologic exam. Despite these limitations, this study opens the door for new opportunities to explore and validate the detection of IBD serological markers in peripheral blood samples as novel markers of gut disease in HIV infection.

In summary, we detected at least one IBD serological marker in approximately 65% of AIDS patients with high LPS levels, and an IBD-like serological pattern in 46%. Detection of these markers, particularly ASCA, anti-OmpC, and anti-CBir1, could provide a potential non-invasive approach to monitor HIV-related gut disease. Further studies are warranted to understand the clinical significance of IBD serological markers in HIV infection and their utility as tools for studies of HIV-related gut disease and monitoring therapeutic responses.

Supporting Information

Figure S1 Differences in levels of IBD serological markers (A- ASCA IgA, B- ASCA IgG, C - Anti-OmpC and D- Anti-CBir1) in subjects with versus without IBD pattern are shown. Lines indicate median levels for each group. Mann Whitney test was used to assess the difference in antibody levels between the two groups, *p<0.05 was considered statistically significant. (EPS)

Figure S2 IL-6 levels correlated positively with levels of anti-CBir1 (n = 20 AIDS patients, Spearman correlation). (EPS)

Table S1 Meta-analysis of 10 studies using Prometheus laboratories IBD Serology 7 (DOC)

Acknowledgments

We thank investigators at NNTC sites and Dr. David Stone (Shattuck Hospital) for providing plasma samples from AIDS patients and clinical data.

Author Contributions

Conceived and designed the experiments: AK RB DG. Performed the experiments: AK PA. Analyzed the data: AK RB DG. Wrote the paper: AK DG.

References

1. Brenchley JM, Douek DC (2008) HIV infection and the gastrointestinal immune system. Mucosal Immunol 1: 23–30.
2. Dandekar S (2007) Pathogenesis of HIV in the gastrointestinal tract. Curr HIV/AIDS Rep 4: 10–15.
3. Kotler DP (2005) HIV infection and the gastrointestinal tract. Aids 19: 107–117.
4. Lackner AA, Mohan M, Veazey RS (2009) The gastrointestinal tract and AIDS pathogenesis. Gastroenterology 136: 1965–1978.
5. Brenchley JM, Schacker TW, Ruff LE, Price DA, Taylor JH, et al. (2004) CD4+ T cell depletion during all stages of HIV disease occurs predominantly in the gastrointestinal tract. J Exp Med 200: 749–759.
6. Chase A, Zhou Y, Siliciano RF (2006) HIV-1-induced depletion of CD4+ T cells in the gut: mechanism and therapeutic implications. Trends Pharmacol Sci 27: 4–7.
7. Guadalupe M, Reay E, Sankaran S, Prindiville T, Flamm J, et al. (2003) Severe CD4+ T-cell depletion in gut lymphoid tissue during primary human immunodeficiency virus type 1 infection and substantial delay in restoration following highly active antiretroviral therapy. J Virol 77: 11708–11717.
8. Brenchley JM, Price DA, Douek DC (2006) HIV disease: fallout from a mucosal catastrophe? Nat Immunol 7: 235–239.
9. Haynes BF (2006) Gut microbes out of control in HIV infection. Nat Med 12: 1351–1352.
10. Paiardini M, Frank I, Pandrea I, Apetrei C, Silvestri G (2008) Mucosal immune dysfunction in AIDS pathogenesis. AIDS Rev 10: 36–46.
11. Brenchley JM, Price DA, Schacker TW, Asher TE, Silvestri G, et al. (2006) Microbial translocation is a cause of systemic immune activation in chronic HIV infection. Nat Med 12: 1365–1371.
12. Ancuta P, Kamat A, Kunstman KJ, Kim EY, Autissier P, et al. (2008) Microbial translocation is associated with increased monocyte activation and dementia in AIDS patients. PLoS One 3: e2516.
13. Hofer U, Speck RF (2009) Disturbance of the gut-associated lymphoid tissue is associated with disease progression in chronic HIV infection. Semin Immunopathol.
14. Hunt PW, Brenchley J, Sinclair E, McCune JM, Roland M, et al. (2008) Relationship between T cell activation and CD4+ T cell count in HIV-seropositive individuals with undetectable plasma HIV RNA levels in the absence of therapy. J Infect Dis 197: 126–133.
15. Marchetti G, Bellistri GM, Borghi E, Tincati C, Ferramosca S, et al. (2008) Microbial translocation is associated with sustained failure in CD4+ T-cell reconstitution in HIV-infected patients on long-term highly active antiretroviral therapy. Aids 22: 2035–2038.
16. Jiang W, Lederman MM, Hunt P, Sieg SF, Haley K, et al. (2009) Plasma levels of bacterial DNA correlate with immune activation and the magnitude of immune restoration in persons with antiretroviral-treated HIV infection. J Infect Dis 199: 1177–1185.
17. Caradonna L, Amati L, Magrone T, Pellegrino NM, Jirillo E, et al. (2000) Enteric bacteria, lipopolysaccharides and related cytokines in inflammatory bowel disease: biological and clinical significance. J Endotoxin Res 6: 205–214.
18. Pastor Rojo O, Lopez San Roman A, Albeniz Arbizu E, de la Hera Martinez A, Ripoll Sevillano E, et al. (2007) Serum lipopolysaccharide-binding protein in endotoxemic patients with inflammatory bowel disease. Inflamm Bowel Dis 13: 269–277.
19. Gardiner KR, Halliday MI, Barclay GR, Milne L, Brown D, et al. (1995) Significance of systemic endotoxaemia in inflammatory bowel disease. Gut 36: 897–901.
20. McGuckin MA, Eri R, Simms LA, Florin TH, Radford-Smith G (2009) Intestinal barrier dysfunction in inflammatory bowel diseases. Inflamm Bowel Dis 15: 100–113.
21. Murphy SJ, Ullman TA, Abreu MT (2008) Gut microbes in Crohn's disease: getting to know you better? Am J Gastroenterol 103: 397–398.
22. Macpherson AJ, Harris NL (2004) Interactions between commensal intestinal bacteria and the immune system. Nat Rev Immunol 4: 478–485.
23. Caradonna L, Amati L, Lella P, Jirillo E, Caccavo D (2000) Phagocytosis, killing, lymphocyte-mediated antibacterial activity, serum autoantibodies, and plasma endotoxins in inflammatory bowel disease. Am J Gastroenterol 95: 1495–1502.
24. Austin GL, Shaheen NJ, Sandler RS (2006) Positive and negative predictive values: use of inflammatory bowel disease serologic markers. Am J Gastroenterol 101: 413–416.
25. Ferrante M, Henckaerts L, Joossens M, Pierik M, Joossens S, et al. (2007) New serological markers in inflammatory bowel disease are associated with complicated disease behaviour. Gut 56: 1394–1403.
26. Israeli E, Grotto I, Gilburd B, Balicer RD, Goldin E, et al. (2005) Anti-Saccharomyces cerevisiae and antineutrophil cytoplasmic antibodies as predictors of inflammatory bowel disease. Gut 54: 1232–1236.
27. Koutroubakis IE, Petinaki E, Mouzas IA, Vlachonikolis IG, Anagnostopoulou E, et al. (2001) Anti-Saccharomyces cerevisiae mannan antibodies and antineutrophil cytoplasmic autoantibodies in Greek patients with inflammatory bowel disease. Am J Gastroenterol 96: 449–454.
28. Markowitz J, Kugathasan S, Dubinsky M, Mei L, Crandall W, et al. (2009) Age of diagnosis influences serologic responses in children with Crohn's disease: a possible clue to etiology? Inflamm Bowel Dis 15: 714–719.
29. Peeters M, Joossens S, Vermeire S, Vlietinck R, Bossuyt X, et al. (2001) Diagnostic value of anti-Saccharomyces cerevisiae and antineutrophil cytoplasmic autoantibodies in inflammatory bowel disease. Am J Gastroenterol 96: 730–734.
30. Quinton JF, Sendid B, Reumaux D, Duthilleul P, Cortot A, et al. (1998) Anti-Saccharomyces cerevisiae mannan antibodies combined with antineutrophil cytoplasmic autoantibodies in inflammatory bowel disease: prevalence and diagnostic role. Gut 42: 788–791.
31. Seibold F (2005) ASCA: genetic marker, predictor of disease, or marker of a response to an environmental antigen? Gut 54: 1212–1213.
32. Targan SR (1999) The utility of ANCA and ASCA in inflammatory bowel disease. Inflamm Bowel Dis 5: 61–63; discussion 66-67.
33. Arnott ID, Landers CJ, Nimmo EJ, Drummond HE, Smith BK, et al. (2004) Sero-reactivity to microbial components in Crohn's disease is associated with disease severity and progression, but not NOD2/CARD15 genotype. Am J Gastroenterol 99: 2376–2384.
34. Davis MK, Andres JM, Jolley CD, Novak DA, Haafiz AB, et al. (2007) Antibodies to Escherichia coli outer membrane porin C in the absence of anti-Saccharomyces cerevisiae antibodies and anti-neutrophil cytoplasmic antibodies are an unreliable marker of Crohn disease and ulcerative colitis. J Pediatr Gastroenterol Nutr 45: 409–413.
35. Dubinsky MC, Lin YC, Dutridge D, Picornell Y, Landers CJ, et al. (2006) Serum immune responses predict rapid disease progression among children with Crohn's disease: immune responses predict disease progression. Am J Gastroenterol 101: 360–367.
36. Mei L, Targan SR, Landers CJ, Dutridge D, Ippoliti A, et al. (2006) Familial expression of anti-Escherichia coli outer membrane porin C in relatives of patients with Crohn's disease. Gastroenterology 130: 1078–1085.
37. Zholudev A, Zurakowski D, Young W, Leichtner A, Bousvaros A (2004) Serologic testing with ANCA, ASCA, and anti-OmpC in children and young adults with Crohn's disease and ulcerative colitis: diagnostic value and correlation with disease phenotype. Am J Gastroenterol 99: 2235–2241.
38. Adams RJ, Heazlewood SP, Gilshenan KS, O'Brien M, McGuckin MA, et al. (2008) IgG antibodies against common gut bacteria are more diagnostic for Crohn's disease than IgG against mannan or flagellin. Am J Gastroenterol 103: 386–396.
39. Buckland MS, Mylonaki M, Rampton D, Longhurst HJ (2005) Serological markers (anti-Saccharomyces cerevisiae mannan antibodies and antineutrophil cytoplasmic antibodies) in inflammatory bowel disease: diagnostic utility and phenotypic correlation. Clin Diagn Lab Immunol 12: 1328–1330.
40. Desir B, Amre DK, Lu SE, Ohman-Strickland P, Dubinsky M, et al. (2004) Utility of serum antibodies in determining clinical course in pediatric Crohn's disease. Clin Gastroenterol Hepatol 2: 139–146.
41. Vermeire S, Peeters M, Vlietinck R, Joossens S, Den Hond E, et al. (2001) Anti-Saccharomyces cerevisiae antibodies (ASCA), phenotypes of IBD, and intestinal permeability: a study in IBD families. Inflamm Bowel Dis 7: 8–15.
42. Papp M, Altorjay I, Dotan N, Palatka K, Foldi I, et al. (2008) New serological markers for inflammatory bowel disease are associated with earlier age at onset, complicated disease behavior, risk for surgery, and NOD2/CARD15 genotype in a Hungarian IBD cohort. Am J Gastroenterol 103: 665–681.
43. Reese GE, Constantinides VA, Simillis C, Darzi AW, Orchard TR, et al. (2006) Diagnostic precision of anti-Saccharomyces cerevisiae antibodies and perinuclear antineutrophil cytoplasmic antibodies in inflammatory bowel disease. Am J Gastroenterol 101: 2410–2422.
44. Duerr RH, Targan SR, Landers CJ, Sutherland LR, Shanahan F (1991) Antineutrophil cytoplasmic antibodies in ulcerative colitis. Comparison with other colitides/diarrheal illnesses. Gastroenterology 100: 1590–1596.
45. Fleshner PR, Vasiliauskas EA, Kam LY, Fleshner NE, Gaiennie J, et al. (2001) High level perinuclear antineutrophil cytoplasmic antibody (pANCA) in ulcerative colitis patients before colectomy predicts the development of chronic pouchitis after ileal pouch-anal anastomosis. Gut 49: 671–677.
46. Sandborn WJ, Loftus EV, Jr., Colombel JF, Fleming KA, Seibold F, et al. (2001) Evaluation of serologic disease markers in a population-based cohort of patients with ulcerative colitis and Crohn's disease. Inflamm Bowel Dis 7: 192–201.
47. Winter HS, Landers CJ, Winkelstein A, Vidrich A, Targan SR (1994) Antineutrophil cytoplasmic antibodies in children with ulcerative colitis. J Pediatr 125: 707–711.
48. Bossuyt X (2006) Serologic markers in inflammatory bowel disease. Clin Chem 52: 171–181.
49. Landers CJ, Cohavy O, Misra R, Yang H, Lin YC, et al. (2002) Selected loss of tolerance evidenced by Crohn's disease-associated immune responses to auto- and microbial antigens. Gastroenterology 123: 689–699.
50. Peyrin-Biroulet L, Standaert-Vitse A, Branche J, Chamaillard M (2007) IBD serological panels: facts and perspectives. Inflamm Bowel Dis 13: 1561–1566.
51. Shih DQ, Targan SR, McGovern D (2008) Recent advances in IBD pathogenesis: genetics and immunobiology. Curr Gastroenterol Rep 10: 568–575.
52. Sabery N, Bass D (2007) Use of serologic markers as a screening tool in inflammatory bowel disease compared with elevated erythrocyte sedimentation rate and anemia. Pediatrics 119: e193–199.
53. Devlin SM, Yang H, Ippoliti A, Taylor KD, Landers CJ, et al. (2007) NOD2 variants and antibody response to microbial antigens in Crohn's disease patients and their unaffected relatives. Gastroenterology 132: 576–586.

54. Fleshner P, Ippoliti A, Dubinsky M, Vasiliauskas E, Mei L, et al. (2008) Both preoperative perinuclear antineutrophil cytoplasmic antibody and anti-CBir1 expression in ulcerative colitis patients influence pouchitis development after ileal pouch-anal anastomosis. Clin Gastroenterol Hepatol 6: 561–568.

55. Papadakis KA, Yang H, Ippoliti A, Mei L, Elson CO, et al. (2007) Anti-flagellin (CBir1) phenotypic and genetic Crohn's disease associations. Inflamm Bowel Dis 13: 524–530.

56. Shen C, Landers CJ, Derkowski C, Elson CO, Targan SR (2008) Enhanced CBir1-specific innate and adaptive immune responses in Crohn's disease. Inflamm Bowel Dis 14: 1641–1651.

57. Targan SR, Landers CJ, Yang H, Lodes MJ, Cong Y, et al. (2005) Antibodies to CBir1 flagellin define a unique response that is associated independently with complicated Crohn's disease. Gastroenterology 128: 2020–2028.

58. Lodes MJ, Cong Y, Elson CO, Mohamath R, Landers CJ, et al. (2004) Bacterial flagellin is a dominant antigen in Crohn disease. J Clin Invest 113: 1296–1306.

59. Mow WS, Vasiliauskas EA, Lin YC, Fleshner PR, Papadakis KA, et al. (2004) Association of antibody responses to microbial antigens and complications of small bowel Crohn's disease. Gastroenterology 126: 414–424.

60. Sharpstone D, Neild P, Crane R, Taylor C, Hodgson C, et al. (1999) Small intestinal transit, absorption, and permeability in patients with AIDS with and without diarrhoea. Gut 45: 70–76.

61. Sharpstone DR, Duggal A, Gazzard BG (1996) Inflammatory bowel disease in individuals seropositive for the human immunodeficiency virus. Eur J Gastroenterol Hepatol 8: 575–578.

62. Olsson J, Poles M, Spetz AL, Elliott J, Hultin L, et al. (2000) Human immunodeficiency virus type 1 infection is associated with significant mucosal inflammation characterized by increased expression of CCR5, CXCR4, and beta-chemokines. J Infect Dis 182: 1625–1635.

63. Kewenig S, Schneider T, Hohloch K, Lampe-Dreyer K, Ullrich R, et al. (1999) Rapid mucosal CD4(+) T-cell depletion and enteropathy in simian immunodeficiency virus-infected rhesus macaques. Gastroenterology 116: 1115–1123.

64. Bjarnason I, Sharpstone DR, Francis N, Marker A, Taylor C, et al. (1996) Intestinal inflammation, ileal structure and function in HIV. Aids 10: 1385–1391.

65. Lautenbach E, Lichtenstein GR (1997) Human immunodeficiency virus infection and Crohn's disease: the role of the CD4 cell in inflammatory bowel disease. J Clin Gastroenterol 25: 456–459.

66. Viazis N, Vlachogiannakos J, Georgiou O, Rodias M, Georgiadis D, et al. (2009) Course of inflammatory bowel disease in patients infected with human immunodeficiency virus. Inflamm Bowel Dis.

67. Yoshida EM, Chan NH, Herrick RA, Amar JN, Sestak PM, et al. (1996) Human immunodeficiency virus infection, the acquired immunodeficiency syndrome, and inflammatory bowel disease. J Clin Gastroenterol 23: 24–28.

68. Rutgeerts P, Vermeire S (2000) Serological diagnosis of inflammatory bowel disease. Lancet 356: 2117–2118.

69. Dubinsky M (2009) What is the role of serological markers in IBD? Pediatric and adult data. Dig Dis 27: 259–268.

70. Dubinsky MC (2008) What is the role of serological markers in the diagnosis of IBD? Inflamm Bowel Dis 14 Suppl 2: S185–186.

71. Balagopal A, Philp FH, Astemborski J, Block TM, Mehta A, et al. (2008) Human immunodeficiency virus-related microbial translocation and progression of hepatitis C. Gastroenterology 135: 226–233.

72. Friedman H, Newton C, Klein TW (2003) Microbial infections, immunomodulation, and drugs of abuse. Clin Microbiol Rev 16: 209–219.

73. Papadakis KA, Targan SR (2000) Role of cytokines in the pathogenesis of inflammatory bowel disease. Annu Rev Med 51: 289–298.

74. Cornely OA, Hauschild S, Weise C, Csernok E, Gross WL, et al. (1999) Seroprevalence and disease association of antineutrophil cytoplasmic autoantibodies and antigens in HIV infection. Infection 27: 92–96.

75. Klaassen RJ, Goldschmeding R, Dolman KM, Vlekke AB, Weigel HM, et al. (1992) Anti-neutrophil cytoplasmic autoantibodies in patients with symptomatic HIV infection. Clin Exp Immunol 87: 24–30.

76. Savige JA, Chang L, Crowe SM (1993) Anti-neutrophil cytoplasm antibodies in HIV infection. Adv Exp Med Biol 336: 349–352.

77. Nikolova M, Liubomirova M, Iliev A, Krasteva R, Andreev E, et al. (2002) Clinical significance of antinuclear antibodies, anti-neutrophil cytoplasmic antibodies and anticardiolipin antibodies in heroin abusers. Isr Med Assoc J 4: 908–910.

78. Dubinsky MC, Ofman JJ, Urman M, Targan SR, Seidman EG (2001) Clinical utility of serodiagnostic testing in suspected pediatric inflammatory bowel disease. Am J Gastroenterol 96: 758–765.

79. Mainardi E, Villanacci V, Bassotti G, Liserre B, Rossi E, et al. (2007) Diagnostic value of serological assays in pediatric inflammatory bowel disorders. Digestion 75: 210–214.

80. Mustila A, Paimela L, Leirisalo-Repo M, Huhtala H, Miettinen A (2000) Antineutrophil cytoplasmic antibodies in patients with early rheumatoid arthritis: an early marker of progressive erosive disease. Arthritis Rheum 43: 1371–1377.

81. Vermeire S, Joossens S, Peeters M, Monsuur F, Marien G, et al. (2001) Comparative study of ASCA (Anti-Saccharomyces cerevisiae antibody) assays in inflammatory bowel disease. Gastroenterology 120: 827–833.

82. Linskens RK, Mallant-Hent RC, Groothuismink ZM, Bakker-Jonges LE, van de Merwe JP, et al. (2002) Evaluation of serological markers to differentiate between ulcerative colitis and Crohn's disease: pANCA, ASCA and agglutinating antibodies to anaerobic coccoid rods. Eur J Gastroenterol Hepatol 14: 1013–1018.

83. Austin GL, Herfarth HH, Sandler RS (2007) A critical evaluation of serologic markers for inflammatory bowel disease. Clin Gastroenterol Hepatol 5: 545–547.

84. Kucharzik T, Stoll R, Lugering N, Domschke W (1995) Circulating antiinflammatory cytokine IL-10 in patients with inflammatory bowel disease (IBD). Clin Exp Immunol 100: 452–456.

85. Mitsuyama K, Tomiyasu N, Takaki K, Masuda J, Yamasaki H, et al. (2006) Interleukin-10 in the pathophysiology of inflammatory bowel disease: increased serum concentrations during the recovery phase. Mediators Inflamm 2006: 26875.

4

Functional Studies on the IBD Susceptibility Gene IL23R Implicate Reduced Receptor Function in the Protective Genetic Variant R381Q

Svetlana Pidasheva[1,2]*, Sara Trifari[2¤b], Anne Phillips[1¤c], Jason A. Hackney[1], Yan Ma[1], Ashley Smith[4], Sue J. Sohn[2], Hergen Spits[2¤a], Randall D. Little[6], Timothy W. Behrens[3], Lee Honigberg[4], Nico Ghilardi[2,5], Hilary F. Clark[1,2]*

1 Department of Bioinformatics and Computational Biology, Genentech Inc, South San Francisco, California, United States of America, 2 Department of Immunology, Genentech Inc, South San Francisco, California, United States of America, 3 ITGR Biomarker Discovery Group, Genentech Inc, South San Francisco, California, United States of America, 4 ITGR Early Development, Genentech Inc, South San Francisco, California, United States of America, 5 Department of Molecular Biology, Genentech Inc, South San Francisco, California, United States of America, 6 Genizon BioSciences, Inc., St. Laurent, Quebec, Canada

Abstract

Genome-wide association studies (GWAS) in several populations have demonstrated significant association of the *IL23R* gene with IBD (Crohn's disease (CD) and ulcerative colitis (UC)) and psoriasis, suggesting that perturbation of the IL-23 signaling pathway is relevant to the pathophysiology of these diseases. One particular variant, R381Q (rs11209026), confers strong protection against development of CD. We investigated the effects of this variant in primary T cells from healthy donors carrying IL23R^{R381} and IL23R^{Q381} haplotypes. Using a proprietary anti-IL23R antibody, ELISA, flow cytometry, phosphoflow and real-time RT-PCR methods, we examined IL23R expression and STAT3 phosphorylation and activation in response to IL-23. IL23R^{Q381} was associated with reduced STAT3 phosphorylation upon stimulation with IL-23 and decreased number of IL-23 responsive T-cells. We also observed slightly reduced levels of proinflammatory cytokine secretion in IL23R^{Q381} positive donors. Our study shows conclusively that IL23R^{Q381} is a loss-of-function allele, further strengthening the implication from GWAS results that the IL-23 pathway is pathogenic in human disease. This data provides an explanation for the protective role of R381Q in CD and may lead to the development of improved therapeutics for autoimmune disorders like CD.

Editor: Sunil K. Ahuja, South Texas Veterans Health Care System, United States of America

Funding: The funders (Genentech and Genizon) did have a role in study design, data collection and analysis, decision to publish, or preparation of the manuscript, since the authors are employees of these companies.

Competing Interests: The authors are employees of Genentech Inc., (www.gene.com) and Genizon Biosciences.

* E-mail: svetlana.pidasheva@gmail.com (SP); clark.hilary@gene.com (HFC)

¤a Current address: Academic Medical Center, University of Amsterdam, Amsterdam, The Netherlands
¤b Current address: La Jolla Institute for Allergy and Immunology, La Jolla, California, United States of America
¤c Current address: Gastrointestinal Unit, University of Edinburgh, Edinburgh, United Kingdom

Introduction

The inflammatory bowel diseases (IBD), Crohn's disease (CD) and ulcerative colitis (UC), have long been recognized as having a genetic element to disease susceptibility [1,2]. Following the discovery of NOD2 as a CD susceptibility gene, there have been over seventy susceptibility genes and loci implicated in IBD [3], especially with the advent of genome-wide association studies. These newly discovered genetic associations have shed light on the biological pathways involved in disease initiation and pathogenesis.

Several genes in the Th17 pathway have been linked with IBD susceptibility, including IL23R, TNFSF15, STAT3, IL12B, CCR6 and JAK2 [3]. Of all the Th17 pathway genes, the interleukin 23 receptor (*IL23R*) gene (GenBank accession: NM_144701, GeneID: 149233) on chromosome 1p31 confers the highest odds-ratio (OR) for disease development/lowest OR for disease protection [4,5,6,7,8,9,10,11,12], as well as being implicated in other chronic inflammatory diseases including psoriasis [13] and ankylosing spondylitis [14]. R381Q (rs11209026), the only coding IL23R variant identified by GWAS, confers an OR of 0.45 for Crohn's disease development (MAF 1.9% in CD, 7% in controls) [4], and an OR of 0.55 for UC development (MAF 3.7% in UC, 7% in controls) [15], implying a protective effect.

IL23R is most highly expressed on activated T cells, particularly of the Th17 subtype, natural killer (NK) cells and at lower levels on monocytes, macrophages and dendritic cells [16].

IL23R pairs with IL12RB1 to confer IL-23 responsiveness on cells expressing both receptor subunits [16,17]. Upon activation by IL-23, IL23R signals through the JAK/STAT pathway. IL23R associates constitutively with JAK2 and, in a ligand-dependent manner, with STAT3, STAT1, STAT4 and STAT5 can also be activated by IL-23 [16]. On ligand binding, JAK2 phosphorylates IL23R at Tyr705, recruiting STAT3 to the receptor complex, where it is further phosphorylated by JAK2. Phosphorylated

STAT3 homodimerizes and translocates to the nucleus where it triggers downstream expression of cytokines, including IL-17A, IL-17F, IL-22 and IL-21 in Th17 cells (reviewed in [18,19]).

As well as functioning as a mediator of cytokine production in Th17 pathway cells, several studies also suggest that IL23R is a key player in the proliferation and survival of Th17 cells [17,20,21]. Studies in intestinal tissue have shown that IL-17F and IL-22 mRNA expression (induced via IL-23 signaling) are significantly increased in inflamed colonic lesions in CD compared to uninflamed biopsies, and that IL-22 is associated with a higher expression of inflammatory mediators [22,23].

Because of its role in T cell biology and the compelling genetic evidence, we hypothesized that IL23R^{Q381} could potentially influence the response of the IL23R-expressing cells such as Th17 cells in the host. Indeed, a recent study by Di Meglio and colleagues [24] suggests that IL23R^{Q381} exerts its protective effects through attenuation of IL-23 induced Th17 function.

We investigated this possibility using primary T cells from healthy donors carrying IL23R^{R381} and IL23R^{Q381} haplotypes.

Results

Arginine 381 is absolutely conserved across different species

The R381Q polymorphism is located between the transmembrane domain and the putative JAK2 binding site in the cytoplasmic portion of IL23R protein, and is absolutely conserved across different species (Fig. 1 A, B). By virtue of its location, this polymorphism could potentially interfere with either surface localization of the IL23R [25] or signal transduction [26]; it is unlikely to interfere with ligand binding.

Untransformed polyclonal IL23R^{Q381} positive T cell lines have decreased number of IL23R positive cells and reduced IL-23 responsiveness compared to IL23R^{R381} T cell lines

To study the effects of the R381Q polymorphism we used untransformed polyclonal T cell lines from donors carrying either IL23R^{R381} or IL23R^{Q381}. IL23R positive cells were detected using proprietary monoclonal antibody against human IL23R (Fig. 1S). We genotyped 138 healthy donors and identified eighteen

IL23R^{Q381} heterozygous individuals and one homozygous individual. The calculated allele frequency of 7.1% of R381Q is consistent with the published estimates (7.0% [4] 7.3% [27]; 6.0% [28]). We generated T cell lines from five IL23R^{R381}, four IL23R^{Q381} heterozygous, and one IL23R^{Q381} homozygous donors. All donors were Caucasian of ages 25 to 65.

We observed no obvious differences in viability and proliferation rates between these T cell lines during *in vitro* expansion (Fig. S2A, B). However, flow cytometry analysis performed after six days of *in vitro* stimulation with feeder mixture (see Methods), revealed significantly diminished population of IL23R positive T cell from IL23R^{Q381} positive donors compared to their IL23R^{R381} counterparts (Fig. 2A, B). Consistently, when stimulated with IL-23 we observed fewer pSTAT3 positive cells in IL23R^{Q381} samples (Fig. 2C–D). In addition, the median fluorescence intensity (MFI) of IL-23 stimulated pSTAT3 positive cells was reduced (Fig. 2E), suggesting that not only was there a specific reduction of IL-23–responsive T-cells generated from IL23R^{Q381} positive individuals but also the strength of the IL-23 response for any given cell was decreased by the R381Q polymorphism. By comparison, IL-6-elicited STAT3 phosphorylation was unaffected by the IL23R genotype, demonstrating that IL23R^{Q381} positive cells are intrinsically capable of full STAT3 activation (Fig. 2C, D).

Untransformed polyclonal IL23R^{Q381} positive T cell have decreased IL-23-induced pSTAT1 and pSTAT5 compared to IL23R^{R381} T cell lines

To further characterize this phenomenon, we examined IL-23-induced STAT1 and STAT5 phosphorylation. To reduce background levels of STAT5 phosphorylation elicited by endogenously produced IL-2, we added a neutralizing monoclonal anti-human IL-2 antibody to the cultures during IL-23 stimulation. We observed significantly decreased levels of both STAT5 (Fig. 3A, C) and STAT1 phosphorylation (Fig. 3B, C) in IL23R^{Q381} bearing T cells compared to the IL-23R^{R381} positive lines. The MFI of pSTAT5 positive cells was slightly decreased and pSTAT1 positive cells significantly decreased after IL-23 stimulation, in agreement with the defect observed in STAT3 phosphorylation. On the other hand, when stimulated with IL-2, pSTAT5 levels were equivalent between IL23R^{R381} and IL23R^{Q381} cell lines (Fig. 3A, C).

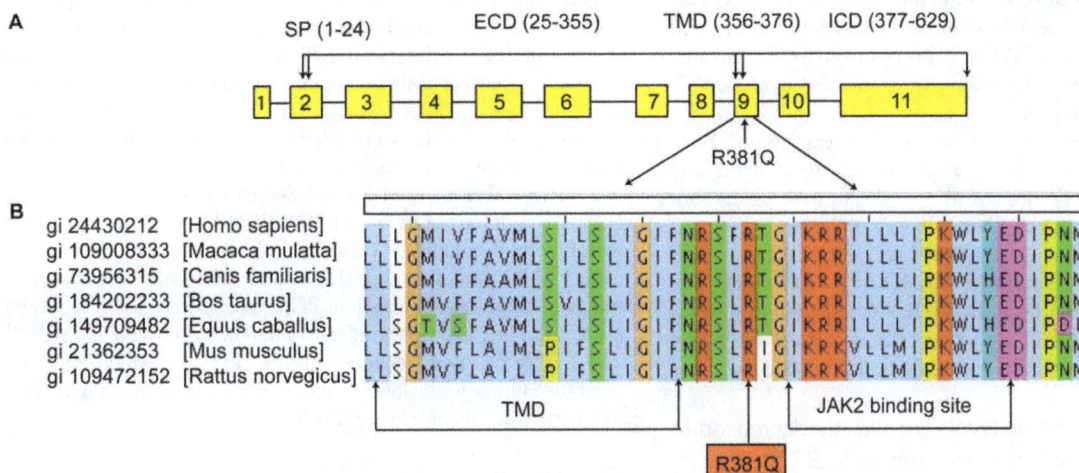

Figure 1. The arginine at position 381 of the IL23R is absolutely conserved across different species. (**A**) Map of the IL23R gene. (**B**) Sequence alignment of IL23R protein sequences from different species.

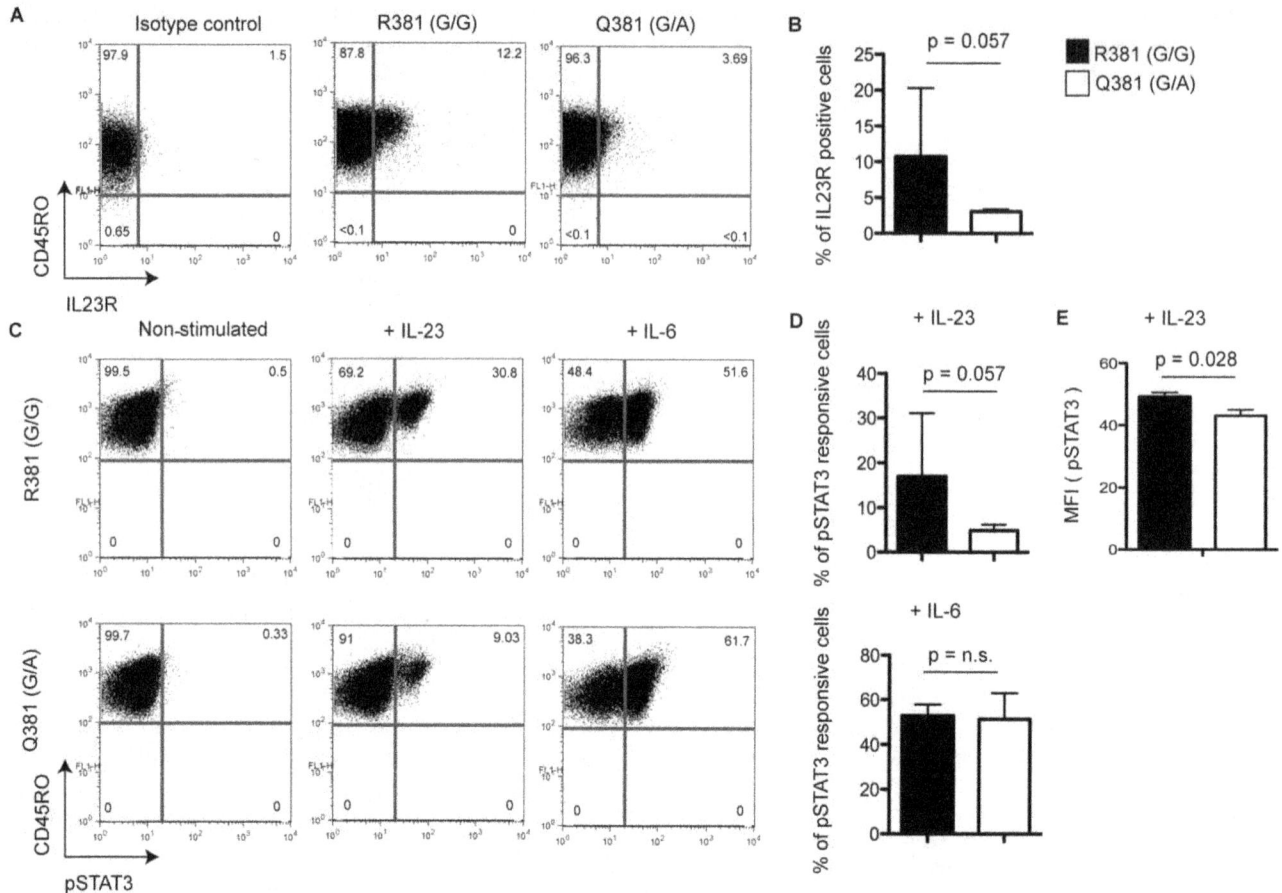

Figure 2. Untransformed polyclonal IL23R^{Q381} positive T cell lines have a decreased number of IL23R positive cells and reduced IL-23 responsiveness compared to IL23R^{R381} T cell lines. Flow cytometric analyses of T cell lines from IL23R^{R381} and IL23R^{Q381} donors is shown. Numbers in the quadrants indicate percent cells in that quadrant. (**A**) IL23R cell surface expression on non-permeabilized T cells of representative donors and (**B**) the mean percent (n = 4) of IL23R positive cells is shown. The error bars indicate standard deviation (SD). IL-23 and IL-6 induced STAT3 phosphorylation in (**C**) representative donors and (**D**) 4 donors per group. (**E**) The MFI pSTAT3 signal in the pSTAT3 positive population (n = 4). Data are representative examples of at least three independent experiments. The Mann-Whitney test was used to calculate the p value.

In addition to T cell lines generated from IL23R^{R381} and IL23R^{Q381} donors, we analyzed freshly isolated peripheral blood mononuclear cells (PBMCs) from the same donors. IL23R expression is known to be activation dependent [29], and indeed we could not detect any IL23R expression on freshly isolated PBMC (data not shown). Therefore, we stimulated total PBMCs with agonist antibodies directed against CD3 and CD28 for 72 hours and then analyzed IL23R surface expression. After stimulation, we clearly observed IL23R expression on the IL23R^{R381} T cells, while the IL23R^{Q381} T cells had slightly, but not significantly decreased number of IL23R positive cells (Fig. 4A, B). We also observed decreased numbers of pSTAT3 positive IL23R^{Q381} CD4$^+$ cells, compared to IL23R^{R381} CD4$^+$ cells when we stimulated whole blood with IL-23. IL-6 stimulation resulted in similar numbers of pSTAT3 positive cells, regardless of IL23R genotype (Fig. 4C, D), confirming our data from T cell lines.

Peripheral blood cytokine levels are slightly decreased in IL23R^{Q381} positive donors compared to IL23R^{R381}

To investigate the functional impact of the IL23R^{R381Q} in terms of cytokine secretion, we used stimulated T cell lines from IL23R^{R381} and IL23R^{Q381} donors to measure the production of cytokines by intracellular staining (Fig. 5A–C). We observed

slightly, but not significantly decreased levels of IL-17A, IL-22 and IFN-g in IL23R^{Q381} positive donors. Similar results were observed when fresh PBMCs from IL23R^{R381} and IL23R^{Q381} positive donors were stimulated (Fig. S3A–C). Interestingly, a recent study [30] using primary T cells from IL23R^{R381} (n = 27) and IL23R^{Q381} (n = 13) positive donors showed that IL23R^{Q381} donors have decreased IL-23–dependent IL-17 and IL-22 production. Serum IL-22 levels were determined using enzyme-linked immunosorbent assay (ELISA), and we again observed a slight, but not significant, trend toward decreased IL-22 production in IL23R^{Q381} donors compared to IL23R^{R381} donors, in agreement with previously published data [31]. We also extracted RNA from fresh PBMCs and analyzed IL23R and RORC (a Th17 marker) mRNA expression by real-time PCR. We observed heterogeneity among donors, but no significant differences between IL23R^{R381} and IL23R^{Q381} positive donor groups (Fig. 5F), which could be attributed either to the low number of donors or the possibility that this variant is has no effect on mRNA processing.

Discussion

In the past several years, GWAS have lead to major breakthroughs in our understanding of the genetics of CD. However, there have been relatively few published studies

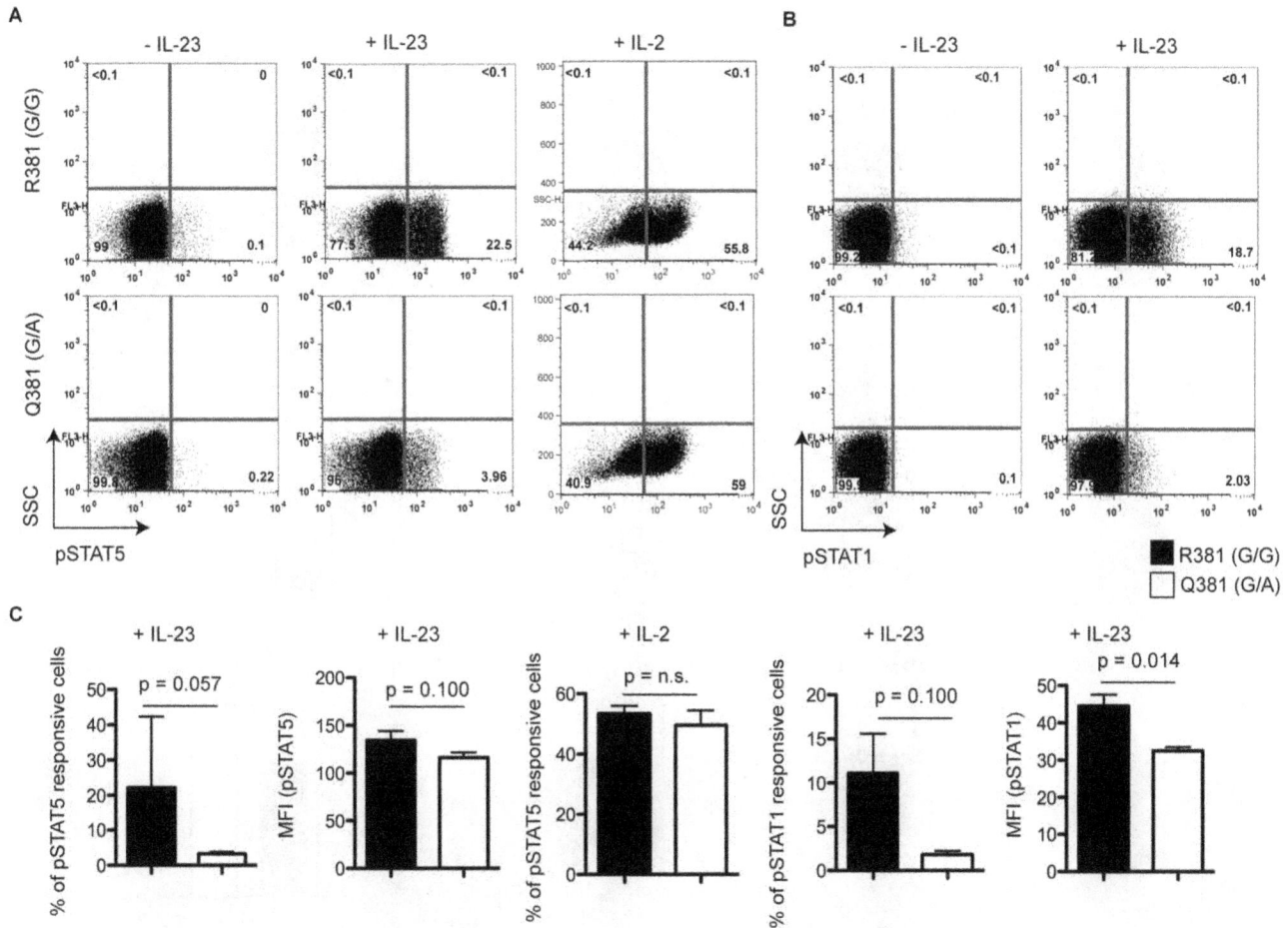

Figure 3. Untransformed polyclonal IL23R^{Q381} positive T cell have decreased IL-23 induced pSTAT1 and pSTAT5 compared to IL23R^{R381} T cell lines. (A) IL-23 and IL-2 induced pSTAT5 and (B) IL-23 induced pSTAT1 response in representative donors and (C) the mean of the percent positive from and MFI of pSTAT1 and pSTAT5 (n = 4). Data are representative examples of at least two independent experiments. The Mann-Whitney test was used to calculate the p value.

functionally validating disease-associated variants so far [24,30, 32,33]. We chose several relevant *in vitro* systems to demonstrate conclusively that the R381Q variant results in decreased population of IL-23 responsive cells, as well as an attenuation of signaling via the IL23R, manifesting in diminished IL-23 dependent activation of all STATs known to be associated with IL-23 signaling. Supporting our results, a recent study [24] using *in vitro* polarized Th17 cell from IL23R^{R381} (n = 22) and IL23R^{Q381} (n = 19) positive donors demonstrated that the cells from L23R^{Q381} positive donors had impaired IL-23-mediated IL-17A production and STAT3 phosphorylation.

Several mechanisms might contribute to this observation, including reduced capacity of IL23R^{Q381} to activate STAT proteins due to impaired association of JAK2 proteins with the cytoplasmic tail of the receptor. Arginine 381 is located near the JAK2 putative binding site (Fig. 1). However, in order to determine whether R381Q is truly a causative variant and not a tagging single nucleotide polymorphism (SNP), which tags a protective IL23R haplotype associated with decrease population of IL23R positive/responsive cells, further studies such as generation of a R381Q knock-in mouse model would have to be conducted.

One of the major advantages of our study was the availability of healthy donors willing to donate blood repeatedly for our primary T cells studies. It should be noted that, while we used T cells in our analysis, the protective effect of IL23R^{Q381} is likely to be co-mediated by other IL-23 responsive cell types (e.g. dendritic cells [16]) *in vivo*). We observed decreases in cytokine levels in IL23R^{Q381} positive donors compared to IL23R^{R381} donors in peripheral blood. However, the difference was not significant, potentially because of the small number of available samples.

For future studies it will be important to analyze a much larger cohort of donors. In addition, it will be interesting to conduct deep sequencing studies to identify additional genetic variants harbored in IL23R. Indeed, recent study by Monozawa and colleagues [34] reported a number of low frequency IL23R variants identified by resequencing of positional candidates.

It is important to note that despite the R381 risk variant having an allelic frequency of greater than 90% in Caucasian populations, the prevalence of CD in North American populations is only approximately 0.2% [35] [36]. This underlies the polygenic nature of CD susceptibility and the importance of other genes (e.g. *NOD2*, *ATG16L1*) as well as environmental influences (e.g. smoking, diet and possibly bacteria) on the risk of CD development.

IL23R is a key player in the proliferation and survival of Th17 cells, which are critical for host defense against bacterial, fungal and viral infections at mucosal surfaces [37]. Negative evolutionary selection to insure an appropriate defense response may

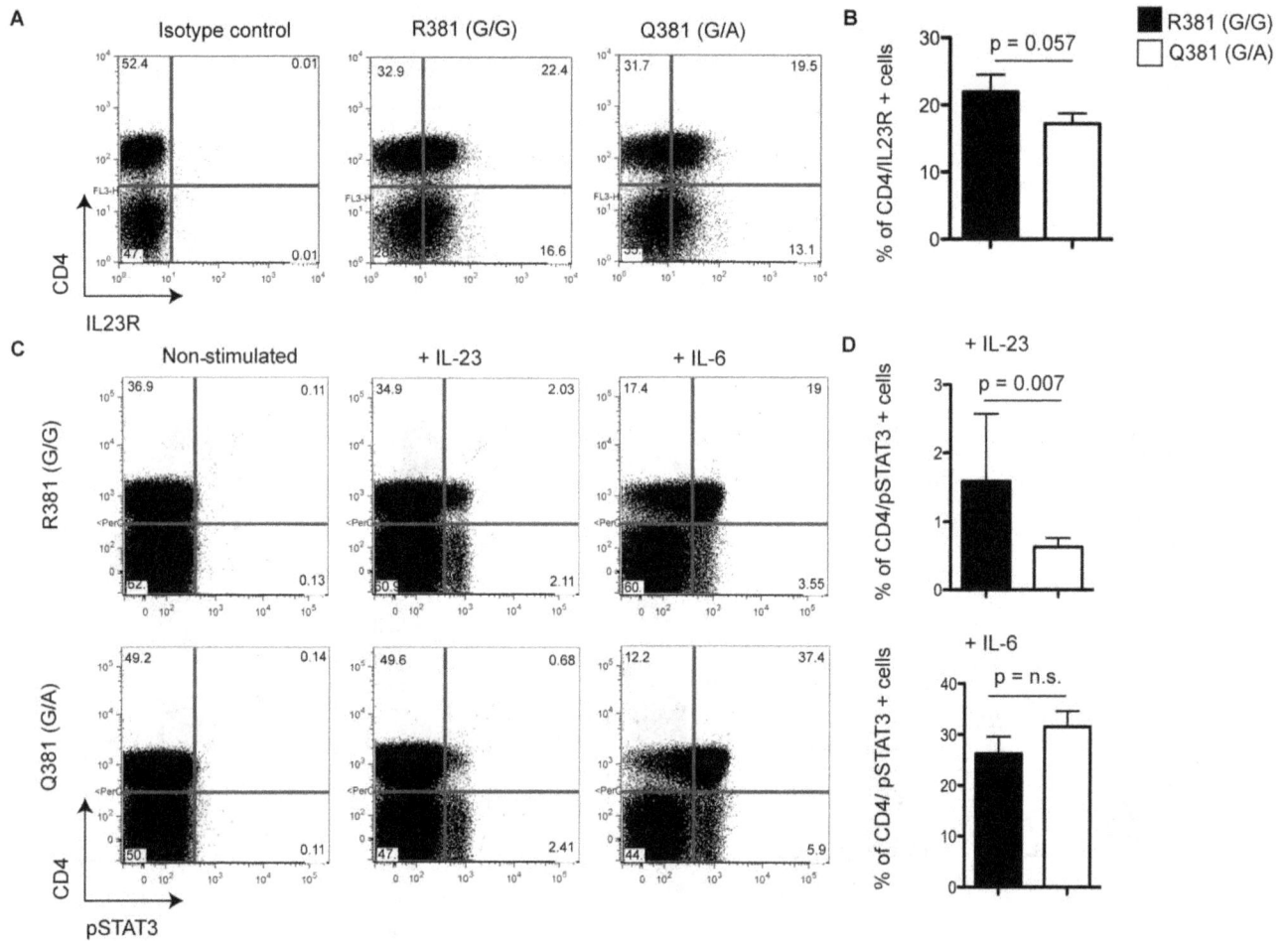

Figure 4. PBMCs from IL23R^{Q381} positive donors have decreased IL23R surface expression and reduced IL-23 responsiveness compared to IL23R^{R381}. Flow cytometric analyses of PBMCs from IL23R^{R381} and IL23R^{Q381} donors is shown. Numbers in the quadrants indicate percent cells in each. (**A**) IL23R expression on non-permeabilized PBMCs stimulated with anti-CD3 and anti-CD28 antibodies for 72 hours of representative donors and (**B**) the mean of the percent positive from 4 donors per group is shown. The error bars indicate SD. IL-23 and IL-6 induced STAT3 phosphorylatin in whole blood from (**C**) representative donors and (**D**) 4 donors per group. Data are representative examples of at least three independent experiments. The Mann-Whitney test was used to calculate the p value.

explain why only a small percentage of the population have this variant.

In summary, our data indicate that IL23R^{Q381} is a hypomorphic IL23R allele that results in a decreased population of IL-23 responsive cells, leading to diminished IL-23-induced STAT3 phosphorylation. This provides an explanation for the protective role of R381Q in CD and other autoimmune disorders (Fig. 6) and further supports the hypothesis that blocking the IL-23 pathway may lead to improved therapeutics for autoimmune disorders like CD [38] and psoriasis [39].

Materials and Methods

Antibodies and ELISA

Information for all antibodies used in this study is summarized in Table S1. A monoclonal antibody against human IL23R (clone 20G3.4) was generated by immunizing mice with a hIL23R-Ig fusion protein (Fig. 1S).

Biotinylated and FITC-conjugated versions of this antibody were used in this study. Serum IL-22 levels of human genotype specific healthy donors were measured using the IL-22 ELISA

MAX Set Deluxe kit (BioLegend, Inc) according to the manufacturer's instructions. Human IL-17A levels were measured in supernatants from PBMCs isolated from genotype specific healthy donors and stimulated with anti-CD3 (2.5 ug/ml) and anti-CD28 (1 ug/ml) antibodies+/−IL-23 (5 ng/ml) for 2 days. Supernatants were harvested and analyzed using hIL-17A ELISA (eBioscience) according to the manufacturer's instructions.

IL23R construct

Gateway recombination cloning technology (Invitrogen) was used to create all constructs. Full-length wild-type *IL23R* coding sequence was PCR amplified using following primers: forward 5′ GG**ACAAGTTTGTACAAAAAAGCAGGCT**TCACC*ATGAAT-CAGGTCACTATT* - 3′ (bold - attB1 site; underlined - kozak; italics - Il23R nucleotides 1–18). Reverse 5′ – GGGG**ACCACTTTG-TACAAGAAAGCTGGGTC**CTA*CTTTTCCAAGAGTGA* - 3′ (bold - attB1 site; underlined - stop; italics - Il23R nucleotides 1872–1886). PCR product was cloned into the pDONR221 donor vector (Invitrogen, Carlsbad, CA). Construct encoding IL23R^{R381} was subsequently transferred into a gateway adapted pMSCVpuro

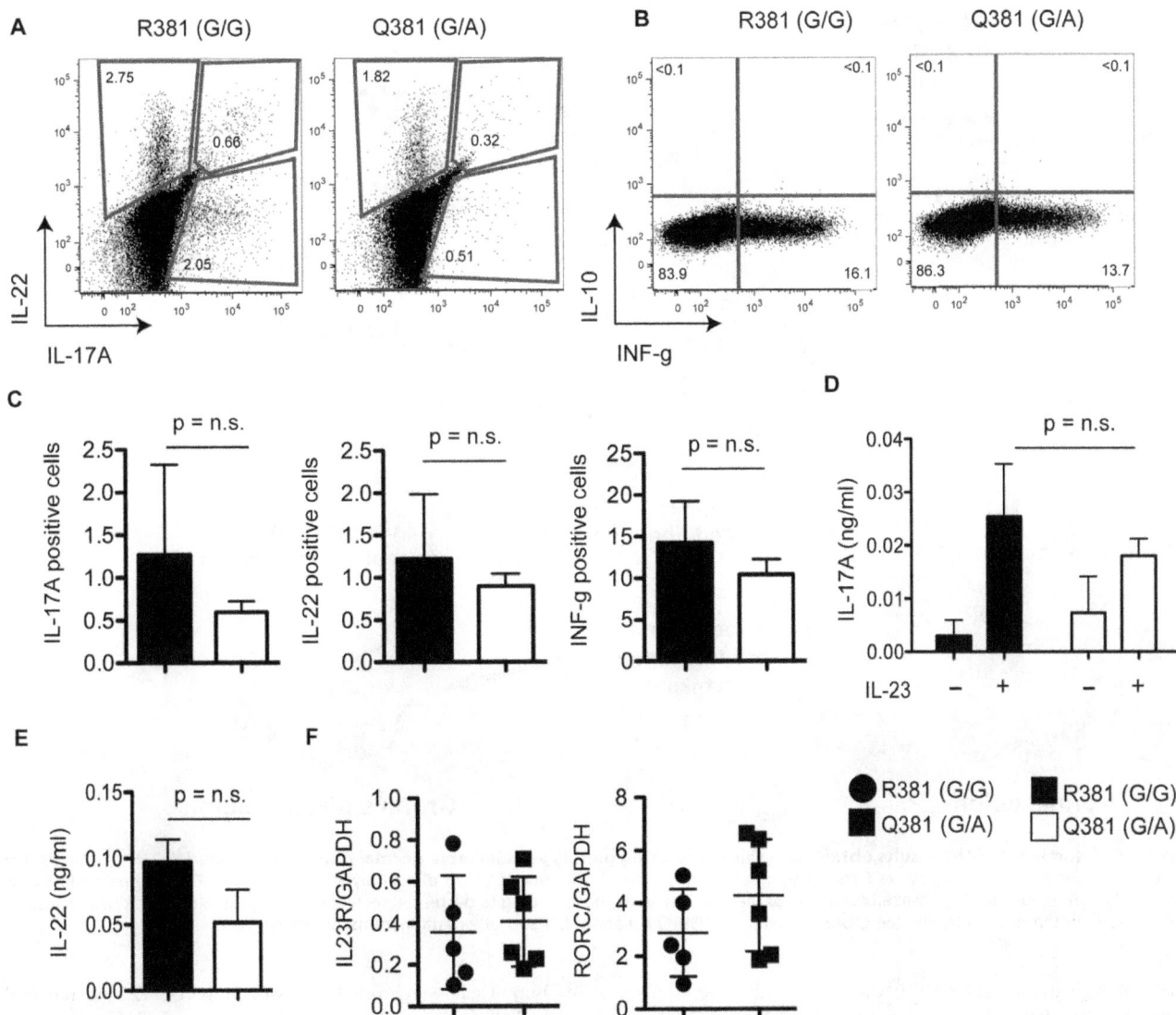

Figure 5. Peripheral blood cytokine levels are comparable in IL23R^Q381 and IL23R^R381 positive donors. ICS of cytokine production by T cell lines stimulated with anti-CD3/ CD28 dynabeads (**A**) representative donors for IL-22 and IL-17 and (**B**) IL-10 and INF-g (**C**) Frequency of cytokine positive cells (n = 4/per group). (**D**) Cytokine production by PBMCs stimulated with anti-CD3 and anti-CD28 antibodies+/−IL-23 and measured by ELISA (3 donors per group) (**E**) Serum IL-22 levels in IL23R^Q381 and IL23R^R381 positive donors (5 donors per group) measured by ELISA. (**F**) Real-time PCR analysis for IL23R and RORC mRNA expression, presented (in arbitrary units (AU)) relative to GAPDH expression (used as an internal "housekeeping" control). mRNA collected from PBMCs of IL23R^R381 (5 donors) and IL23R^Q381 (6 donors). Each symbol represents a donor. Data are representative examples of at least two independent experiments. The Mann-Whitney test was used to calculate the p value.

plasmid using LR Clonase, and final destination construct was sequence verified.

BaF3 cell culture and transduction

BaF3 cells [40] were maintained in RPMI supplemented with 10% bovine calf serum, L-Glutamine and Penicillin-Streptomycin (Invitrogen, Carlsbad, CA). Conditioned medium from WEHI-3B cells was used as a source of IL-3 and added to the culture at 2% final concentration. A pMSCV- based plasmid encoding hIL-12RB1 was introduced by electroporation, and positive single cell clones were identified and sorted by FACS into individual wells of 96-well plates. Human IL23R^R381 cDNA, cloned in the pMSCVpuro retroviral expression vector, was introduced into the same hIL-12RB1 containing BaF3 subclones by standard retroviral transduction. 293T cells in combination with the

retroviral packaging vector pCL-Eco (Imgenex) were used as a packaging system. Twenty-four hours after transduction, BaF3 cells were put in 1 μg/ml puromycin (Clontech) medium to select transduced cells. Relative IL23R and IL12RB1 mRNA abundances were verified by qPCR.

To detect IL23R cell surface expression BaF3 cells were stained with biotinylated IL23R antibody 20G3.4 in combination with streptavidin-PE (eBioscience). Isotype control antibodies were used as negative controls (BD biosciences).

Genotyping

Blood samples were obtained from healthy donors after written informed consent was provided. Ethical approval for the use of this material was obtained from the Western Institutional Review Board. Genomic DNA was isolated from 138 healthy donors, and

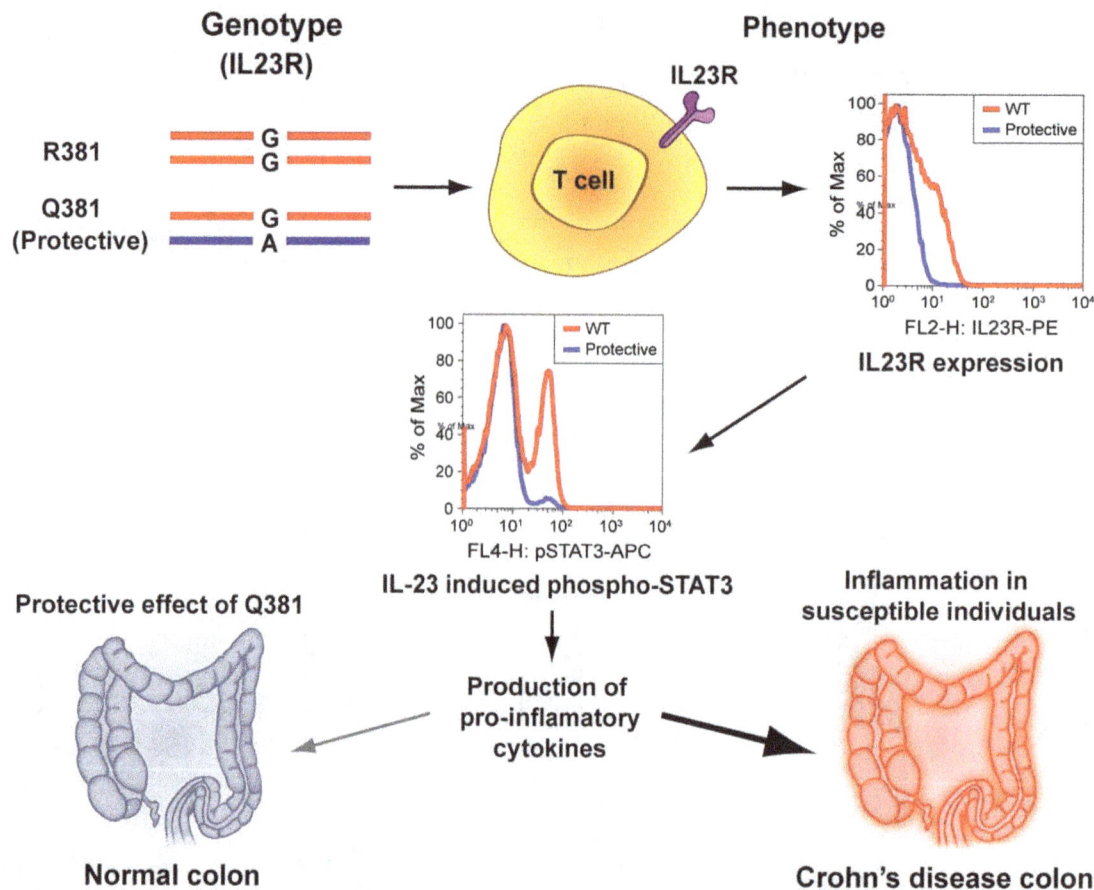

Figure 6. A summary of the results obtained in this study using genotype-selectable normal donors is depicted. IL23R^{Q381} donors had a significant decrease in IL23R positive T cells, leading to the decreased IL-23 induced STAT3 phosphorylation. Decreased STAT3 signaling in T cells like TH17 might modulate the extent and duration of the response in the host, leading to decreased secretion of proinflamatory cytokines such as IL-17 and IL-22 in the gut, explaining the protective effect of R381Q variant in CD and other autoimmune disorders.

the R381Q variant (rs11209026) was genotyped using Applied Biosystems TaqMan SNP genotyping assay (assay ID: C_1272298_10). Eighteen donors were identified as being IL23R^{Q381} heterozygous (GA) and 1 homozygous (AA).

T cell lines

T cell lines were generated as previously described [41,42,43]. Briefly, CD4$^+$ T cells were sorted from whole blood of IL23R^{R381} and IL23R^{Q381} positive donors using a human whole blood CD4 selection kit (RoboSep; StemCell Technologies) according to the manufacturer's instructions (purity of the CD4+ cells after enrichment was >95%). Cells were seeded at 5×10^5 cells/ml and stimulated with a feeder mixture containing 1×10^6/ml irradiated (6,000 rad) allogenic PBMC and 1×10^5/ml irradiated (10,000 rad) JY cells, 1 μg/ml phytohemagglutinin (Sigma), and 200 IU/ml recombinant human IL-2 (Roche). Cells were cultured in Yssel's medium (Gemini Bio-Products) supplemented with 1% human serum. T cells were restimulated with the feeder mixture every 2 weeks. Cell surface expression of IL23R was analyzed by flow cytometry 6 days after stimulation.

T cell culture

PBMCs were isolated from whole blood of IL23R^{R381} and IL23R^{Q381} positive donors using UNI-SEP (U-10, Accurate Chemical) pre-filled tubes containing a solution of 5.6% polysucrose and 9.6% sodium metrizoate (density 1.077 g/ml, osmolality 280 mOsm). Cells were stimulated with anti-CD3 (2.5 ug/ml) and anti-CD28 (1 ug/ml) antibodies for 72 hours. IL23R cell surface cell surface expression was analyzed by flow cytometry using biotinylated IL23R antibody in combination with streptavidin-PE (eBioscience).

Cell viability Assay

T cells were plated in 96-well plates in triplicates at 5×10^5 cells per well. IL-23 was added to a final concentration of 100 nM and a 1:4 dilution series was established. After 72 h of stimulation cells were analyzed by the CellTiter-Glow Luminescent Cell Viability Assay according to the instructions of the manufacturer (Promega Corp). All experiments were performed in triplicate wells.

Proliferation Assay

T cells were plated in 96-well plates in triplicates at 5×10^5 cells per well. IL-23 was added to a final concentration of 100 nM and a 1:2 dilution series was established. After 72 h of stimulation cells were analyzed by a 16-h pulse with 1 μCi/well [^{3}H] thymidine (Amersham Biosciences) followed by harvesting using a 96-well plate harvester and counting by liquid scintillation. All experiments were performed in triplicate wells.

Flow cytometry

All data were collected on FacsCalibur and LSR II instruments (BD Biosciences) and analyzed using FlowJo software (Tree Star).

A summary of all antibodies used in this study is provided in Table S1, and antibodies were used according to the instructions of the manufacturer unless otherwise indicated.

IL23R cell surface expression

T cells were stained with biotinylated IL23R antibody 20G3.4 in combination with streptavidin-PE (eBioscience). Isotype control antibodies were used as negative controls (BD biosciences).

STAT phosphorylation

Flow cytometric analyses of STAT phosphorylation were performed as previously described [43,44]. Briefly, T cells were starved overnight in Yssel's medium supplemented with mono-clonal anti-human IL-2 antibody to neutralize IL-2. Cells were stimulated with 10 ng/ml of rhIL-23 or 10 ng/ml of rhIL-6 or 1000 IU/ml of IL-2 and incubated at 37°C for 15 min. Cells were fixed, permeabilized and stained with phospho-STAT3, phospho-STAT1 and phospho-STAT5 specific antibodies to detect activated STAT3, STAT1 and STAT5, respectively.

Whole blood was stimulated with 10 ng/ml of IL-23 or 10 ng/ml of rhIL-6 and incubated at 37°C for 15 min, fixed and lysed to halt signaling and lyse red blood cells. Cells were permeabilized and stained with phospho-STAT3 specific antibodies to detect activated STAT3.

Intracellular cytokine staining (ICS)

Intracellular staining was done as previously described [45]. Briefly, T cells were stimulated either with Dynabeads CD3/CD28 T Cell Expander (Invitrogen) (bead:cell ratio = 1:10) or with 10 ng/ml PMA plus 500 ng/ml ionomycin (Sigma). After 3 hrs, BD Golgi Plug with brefeldin A (BD Biosciences) was added to block secretion. After an additional 3 hrs, T cells were stained with green live/dead dye (Invitrogen). Cells were fixed in 3% paraformaldehyde and permeabilized with Perm/Wash buffer (BD Biosciences). Permeabilized T cells were stained with anti-hIFN-g, anti-hIL-17, anti-hIL-10, anti-hIL-22 or isotype control antibodies (BD Biosciences).

Real-time quantitative RT-PCR

Total RNA was extracted from freshly isolated PBMCs of IL23R^{R381} and IL23R^{Q381} positive donors using RNeasy Micro kit (Qiagen). High-Capacity cDNA Archive kit (Applied Biosystems) was used for cDNA synthesis. Transcripts were quantified by real-time quantitative PCR on an ABI PRISM 7900 sequence detector (Applied Biosystems) with Applied Biosystems predesigned TaqMan Gene Expression Assays. The following probes were used: RORC (Hs01076112) and IL23R (Hs00332759). For each sample, mRNA abundance was normalized to the amount of GAPDH or RPL19 transcripts.

Sequence alignment by CLUSTAL W

IL23R protein sequences from all the species available in Genbank were aligned with Clustal W in FASTA format (http://www.ebi.ac.uk/clustalw/).

Statistical analyses

Statistical analyses were performed by the Mann-Whitney test using R and Graph Pad Prism software was used to calculate standard deviation. $P<0.05$ considered statistically significant.

Supporting Information

Figure S1 The specificity of anti-IL23R antibody is demonstrated using BaF3 cells retrovirally transduced with IL23R^{R381}. Representative analysis by flow cytometry show IL23R surface expression on non-permeabilized transduced BaF3 cells. Isotype control is indicated by gray shading, non-transformed BaF3 cells by a red line and IL23R^{R381} by a blue line.

Figure S2 Untransformed polyclonal IL23R^{Q381} positive T cell have comparable cell viability and proliferation rates to IL23R^{R381} cells. The mean percent (n = 4) of representative donors (**A**) cell viability and (**B**) proliferation rates after stimulation with IL-23 for 72 h. Data are representative examples of at least three independent experiments.

Figure S3 Cytokine levels are comparable in IL23R^{Q381} and IL23R^{R381} positive donors. ICS of cytokine production by PBMCs stimulated with anti-CD3/ CD28 dynabeads (**A**) representative donors for IL-22 and IL-17 and (**B**) IL-10 and INF-g (**C**) four donors per group is shown. Data are representative examples of at least three independent experiments. The Mann-Whitney test was used to calculate the p value.

Table S1 List of anti-human antibodies used in this study.

Acknowledgments

We thank W. Ouyang, J. Arron, N. Crellin, C. Kaplan, A. Abbas, D. Thibault, J. Tan and B. Lo for discussions; Genentech Bioinformatic and Computational Biology and Immunology departments and ITGR Biomarker Discovery Group for support; A. Bruce for artwork; J. Cupp, L. Gilmour, A. Paler Martinez, R. Neupane, C. Poon and W. Tombo from the Genentech flow cytometry lab for assistance in cell sorting and Luminex assays; and the Genentech Blood Donor Program for blood samples.

Author Contributions

Conceived and designed the experiments: SP HFC. Performed the experiments: SP ST AS SS. Analyzed the data: SP ST AS SS HFC NG. Contributed reagents/materials/analysis tools: NG. Wrote the paper: SP ST HFC JAH. Provided intellectual input: AP JAH YM HS RDL TWB LH.

References

1. Tysk C, Lindberg E, Jarnerot G, Floderus-Myrhed B (1988) Ulcerative colitis and Crohn's disease in an unselected population of monozygotic and dizygotic twins. A study of heritability and the influence of smoking. Gut 29: 990–996.

2. Thompson NP, Driscoll R, Pounder RE, Wakefield AJ (1996) Genetics versus environment in inflammatory bowel disease: results of a British twin study. Bmj 312: 95–96.

3. Franke A, McGovern DP, Barrett JC, Wang K, Radford-Smith GL, et al. (2010) Genome-wide meta-analysis increases to 71 the number of confirmed Crohn's disease susceptibility loci. Nat Genet 42: 1118–1125.

4. Duerr RH, Taylor KD, Brant SR, Rioux JD, Silverberg MS, et al. (2006) A genome-wide association study identifies IL23R as an inflammatory bowel disease gene. Science 314: 1461–1463.

5. Yamazaki K, McGovern D, Ragoussis J, Paolucci M, Butler H, et al. (2005) Single nucleotide polymorphisms in TNFSF15 confer susceptibility to Crohn's disease. Hum Mol Genet 14: 3499–3506.

6. Rioux JD, Xavier RJ, Taylor KD, Silverberg MS, Goyette P, et al. (2007) Genome-wide association study identifies new susceptibility loci for Crohn disease and implicates autophagy in disease pathogenesis. Nat Genet 39: 596–604.

7. Hampe J, Franke A, Rosenstiel P, Till A, Teuber M, et al. (2007) A genome-wide association scan of nonsynonymous SNPs identifies a susceptibility variant for Crohn disease in ATG16L1. Nat Genet 39: 207–211.

8. Libioulle C, Louis E, Hansoul S, Sandor C, Farnir F, et al. (2007) Novel Crohn disease locus identified by genome-wide association maps to a gene desert on 5p13.1 and modulates expression of PTGER4. PLoS Genet 3: e58.

9. Franke A, Hampe J, Rosenstiel P, Becker C, Wagner F, et al. (2007) Systematic association mapping identifies NELL1 as a novel IBD disease gene. PLoS One 2: e691.

10. Wellcome Trust Case Control Consortium (2007) Genome-wide association study of 14,000 cases of seven common diseases and 3,000 shared controls. Nature 447: 661–678.

11. Parkes M, Barrett JC, Prescott NJ, Tremelling M, Anderson CA, et al. (2007) Sequence variants in the autophagy gene IRGM and multiple other replicating loci contribute to Crohn's disease susceptibility. Nat Genet 39: 830–832.

12. Raelson JV, Little RD, Ruether A, Fournier H, Paquin B, et al. (2007) Genome-wide association study for Crohn's disease in the Quebec Founder Population identifies multiple validated disease loci. Proc Natl Acad Sci U S A 104: 14747–14752.

13. Capon F, Di Meglio P, Szaub J, Prescott NJ, Dunster C, et al. (2007) Sequence variants in the genes for the interleukin-23 receptor (IL23R) and its ligand (IL12B) confer protection against psoriasis. Hum Genet 122: 201–206.

14. Rueda B, Orozco G, Raya E, Fernandez-Sueiro JL, Mulero J, et al. (2008) The IL23R Arg381Gln non-synonymous polymorphism confers susceptibility to ankylosing spondylitis. Ann Rheum Dis 67: 1451–1454.

15. Silverberg MS, Cho JH, Rioux JD, McGovern DP, Wu J, et al. (2009) Ulcerative colitis-risk loci on chromosomes 1p36 and 12q15 found by genome-wide association study. Nat Genet 41: 216–220.

16. Parham C, Chirica M, Timans J, Vaisberg E, Travis M, et al. (2002) A receptor for the heterodimeric cytokine IL-23 is composed of IL-12Rbeta1 and a novel cytokine receptor subunit, IL-23R. J Immunol 168: 5699–5708.

17. Oppmann B, Lesley R, Blom B, Timans JC, Xu Y, et al. (2000) Novel p19 protein engages IL-12p40 to form a cytokine, IL-23, with biological activities similar as well as distinct from IL-12. Immunity 13: 715–725.

18. Ouyang W, Kolls JK, Zheng Y (2008) The biological functions of T helper 17 cell effector cytokines in inflammation. Immunity 28: 454–467.

19. Altshuler D, Daly MJ, Lander ES (2008) Genetic mapping in human disease. Science 322: 881–888.

20. Harrington LE, Hatton RD, Mangan PR, Turner H, Murphy TL, et al. (2005) Interleukin 17-producing CD4+ effector T cells develop via a lineage distinct from the T helper type 1 and 2 lineages. Nat Immunol 6: 1123–1132.

21. Aggarwal S, Ghilardi N, Xie MH, de Sauvage FJ, Gurney AL (2003) Interleukin-23 promotes a distinct CD4 T cell activation state characterized by the production of interleukin-17. J Biol Chem 278: 1910–1914.

22. Seiderer J, Elben I, Diegelmann J, Glas J, Stallhofer J, et al. (2008) Role of the novel Th17 cytokine IL-17F in inflammatory bowel disease (IBD): upregulated colonic IL-17F expression in active Crohn's disease and analysis of the IL17F p.His161Arg polymorphism in IBD. Inflamm Bowel Dis 14: 437–445.

23. Brand S, Beigel F, Olszak T, Zitzmann K, Eichhorst ST, et al. (2006) IL-22 is increased in active Crohn's disease and promotes proinflammatory gene expression and intestinal epithelial cell migration. Am J Physiol Gastrointest Liver Physiol 290: G827–838.

24. Di Meglio P, Di Cesare A, Laggner U, Chu CC, Napolitano L, et al. (2011) The IL23R R381Q Gene Variant Protects against Immune-Mediated Diseases by Impairing IL-23-Induced Th17 Effector Response in Humans. PLoS One 6: e17160.

25. Lerch-Bader M, Lundin C, Kim H, Nilsson I, von Heijne G (2008) Contribution of positively charged flanking residues to the insertion of transmembrane helices into the endoplasmic reticulum. Proc Natl Acad Sci U S A 105: 4127–4132.

26. Chaligne R, Tonetti C, Besancenot R, Roy L, Marty C, et al. (2008) New mutations of MPL in primitive myelofibrosis: only the MPL W515 mutations promote a G1/S-phase transition. Leukemia 22: 1557–1566.

27. Roberts RL, Gearry RB, Hollis-Moffatt JE, Miller AL, Reid J, et al. (2007) IL23R R381Q and ATG16L1 T300A are strongly associated with Crohn's disease in a study of New Zealand Caucasians with inflammatory bowel disease. Am J Gastroenterol 102: 2754–2761.

28. Newman WG, Zhang Q, Liu X, Amos CI, Siminovitch KA (2009) Genetic variants in IL-23R and ATG16L1 independently predispose to increased susceptibility to Crohn's disease in a Canadian population. J Clin Gastroenterol 43: 444–447.

29. Wilson NJ, Boniface K, Chan JR, McKenzie BS, Blumenschein WM, et al. (2007) Development, cytokine profile and function of human interleukin 17-producing helper T cells. Nat Immunol 8: 950–957.

30. Sarin R, Wu X, Abraham C (2011) Inflammatory disease protective R381Q IL23 receptor polymorphism results in decreased primary CD4+ and CD8+ human T-cell functional responses. Proc Natl Acad Sci U S A 108: 9560–9565.

31. Schmechel S, Konrad A, Diegelmann J, Glas J, Wetzke M, et al. (2008) Linking genetic susceptibility to Crohn's disease with Th17 cell function: IL-22 serum levels are increased in Crohn's disease and correlate with disease activity and IL23R genotype status. Inflamm Bowel Dis 14: 204–212.

32. Abraham C, Cho JH (2006) Functional consequences of NOD2 (CARD15) mutations. Inflamm Bowel Dis 12: 641–650.

33. Kuballa P, Huett A, Rioux JD, Daly MJ, Xavier RJ (2008) Impaired autophagy of an intracellular pathogen induced by a Crohn's disease associated ATG16L1 variant. PLoS One 3: e3391.

34. Momozawa Y, Mni M, Nakamura K, Coppieters W, Almer S, et al. (2011) Resequencing of positional candidates identifies low frequency IL23R coding variants protecting against inflammatory bowel disease. Nat Genet 43: 43–47.

35. Loftus CG, Loftus EV, Jr., Harmsen WS, Zinsmeister AR, Tremaine WJ, et al. (2007) Update on the incidence and prevalence of Crohn's disease and ulcerative colitis in Olmsted County, Minnesota, 1940–2000. Inflamm Bowel Dis 13: 254–261.

36. Bernstein CN, Wajda A, Svenson LW, MacKenzie A, Koehoorn M, et al. (2006) The epidemiology of inflammatory bowel disease in Canada: a population-based study. Am J Gastroenterol 101: 1559–1568.

37. Khader SA, Gaffen SL, Kolls JK (2009) Th17 cells at the crossroads of innate and adaptive immunity against infectious diseases at the mucosa. Mucosal Immunol 2: 403–411.

38. Sandborn WJ, Feagan BG, Fedorak RN, Scherl E, Fleisher MR, et al. (2008) A randomized trial of Ustekinumab, a human interleukin-12/23 monoclonal antibody, in patients with moderate-to-severe Crohn's disease. Gastroenterology 135: 1130–1141.

39. Malefyt RdW (2008) Future of psoriasis: an industry perspective on research. Expert Rev Dermatol 3: S13–S17.

40. Palacios R, Steinmetz M (1985) Il-3-dependent mouse clones that express B-220 surface antigen, contain Ig genes in germ-line configuration, and generate B lymphocytes in vivo. Cell 41: 727–734.

41. Trifari S, Sitia G, Aiuti A, Scaramuzza S, Marangoni F, et al. (2006) Defective Th1 cytokine gene transcription in CD4+ and CD8+ T cells from Wiskott-Aldrich syndrome patients. J Immunol 177: 7451–7461.

42. Yssel H, Spits H (2002) Generation and maintenance of cloned human T cell lines. Curr Protoc Immunol Chapter 7: Unit 7 19.

43. Crellin NK, Garcia RV, Levings MK (2007) Flow cytometry-based methods for studying signaling in human CD4+CD25+FOXP3+ T regulatory cells. J Immunol Methods 324: 92–104.

44. Schulz KR, Danna EA, Krutzik PO, Nolan GP (2007) Single-cell phospho-protein analysis by flow cytometry. Curr Protoc Immunol Chapter 8: Unit 8 17.

45. Trifari S, Kaplan CD, Tran EH, Crellin NK, Spits H (2009) Identification of a human helper T cell population that has abundant production of interleukin 22 and is distinct from T(H)-17, T(H)1 and T(H)2 cells. Nat Immunol 10: 864–871.

5

Host Genes Related to Paneth Cells and Xenobiotic Metabolism are Associated with Shifts in Human Ileum-Associated Microbial Composition

Tianyi Zhang[1,2], **Robert A. DeSimone**[2], **Xiangmin Jiao**[1], **F. James Rohlf**[3], **Wei Zhu**[1], **Qing Qing Gong**[4], **Steven R. Hunt**[5], **Themistocles Dassopoulos**[4], **Rodney D. Newberry**[4], **Erica Sodergren**[6], **George Weinstock**[6], **Charles E. Robertson**[7], **Daniel N. Frank**[8], **Ellen Li**[2,4]∗

1 Department of Applied Mathematics and Statistics, Stony Brook University, Stony Brook, New York, United States of America, **2** Department of Medicine, Stony Brook University, Stony Brook, New York, United States of America, **3** Department of Ecology and Evolution, Stony Brook University, Stony Brook, New York, United States of America, **4** Department of Medicine, Washington University-St. Louis School of Medicine, Saint Louis, Missouri, United States of America, **5** Department of Surgery, Washington University-St. Louis School of Medicine, Saint Louis, Missouri, United States of America, **6** The Genome Institute, Washington University-St. Louis School of Medicine, Saint Louis, Missouri, United States of America, **7** Department of Molecular, Cellular and Developmental Biology, University of Colorado, Boulder, Colorado, United States of America, **8** Department of Medicine, University of Colorado, Aurora, Colorado, United States of America

Abstract

The aim of this study was to integrate human clinical, genotype, mRNA microarray and 16 S rRNA sequence data collected on 84 subjects with ileal Crohn's disease, ulcerative colitis or control patients without inflammatory bowel diseases in order to interrogate how host-microbial interactions are perturbed in inflammatory bowel diseases (IBD). Ex-vivo ileal mucosal biopsies were collected from the disease unaffected proximal margin of the ileum resected from patients who were undergoing initial intestinal surgery. Both RNA and DNA were extracted from the mucosal biopsy samples. Patients were genotyped for the three major NOD2 variants (Leufs1007, R702W, and G908R) and the ATG16L1T300A variant. Whole human genome mRNA expression profiles were generated using Agilent microarrays. Microbial composition profiles were determined by 454 pyrosequencing of the V3–V5 hypervariable region of the bacterial 16 S rRNA gene. The results of permutation based multivariate analysis of variance and covariance (MANCOVA) support the hypothesis that host mucosal Paneth cell and xenobiotic metabolism genes play an important role in host microbial interactions.

Editor: Markus M. Heimesaat, Charité, Campus Benjamin Franklin, Germany

Funding: This work was supported partially by National Institutes of Health (NIH) UH2DK083994, the Crohn's and Colitis Foundation of America, the Simons Foundation and by the Leona M. and Harry B. Helmsley charitable trust through the Sinai-Helmsley Alliance for Research Excellence (SHARE) Network and NIH R21HG005964. The authors acknowledge use of the Washington University Digestive Diseases Research Core Center Tissue Procurement Facility (P30 DK52574). No additional external funding was received for this study. The funders had no role in study design, data collection and analysis, decision to publish, or preparation of the manuscript.

Competing Interests: The authors have declared that no competing interests exist.

* E-mail: Ellen.Li@stonybrook.edu

Introduction

Inflammatory bowel diseases are complex genetic disorders resulting from the interplay of genetic and environmental factors [1–3]. Crohn's diseases (CD) and ulcerative colitis (UC) represent the two major inflammatory bowel diseases (IBD) phenotypes and are distinguished by different patterns of disease location. The inflammation in CD patients may be located anywhere along the gastrointestinal tract, but in the majority (80%) of CD patients, the terminal ileum is involved. In UC, the inflammation is confined to the colon. Because there is evidence that isolated Crohn's colitis are associated with genetic factors that are distinct from ileal CD, and the overlap between genetic factors associated with UC and isolated Crohn's colitis, we have focused our attention on the ileal CD subphenotype as a relatively homogenous category that is distinct from isolated colitis (CD or UC) and non-IBD controls [4–6].

Single nucleotide polymorphisms in the NOD2 gene and the ATG16L1 gene have been linked to alterations in innate host immunity, particularly Paneth cell function and with ileal CD phenotype [7–14]. We previously reported that increased *CD3D* mRNA expression in disease affected ileum resected from 18 ileal CD patients was associated with NOD2 genotype [15]. We also observed alterations in mRNA gene expression in the disease unaffected proximal margin of resected ileum from 19 ileal CD patients compared to 9 control non-IBD patients, regardless of NOD2 genotype [15]. The microarray dataset has recently been further expanded to include 47 ileal CD, 27 UC and 25 non-IBD control subjects (total = 99).

Culture-independent microbiological technologies coupled with high-throughput DNAsequencing have uncovered alterations in human intestine-associated microbial compositions ("dysbiosis") in IBD patients compared with controls [16–25]. Ileal CD phenotype has been also associated with shifts in intestinal and fecal microbial composition, particularly reduced relative frequency of *Faecalibacterium prausnitzii* [19], [20], [23]. In addition to disease phenotype, exploratory analyses have also associated NOD2 genotype to intestinal associated microbial composition [22]. We have recently completed 16 S rRNA sequence analysis on an independent set of disease-unaffected ileal biopsies collected of 52 ileal CD, 58 colitis and 60 control patients without IBD undergoing initial surgical resection [24]. Of the 170 subjects with microbial composition data and 99 subjects with mRNA expression profiles, 84 subjects had paired microarray and microbial datasets. We report here the results of permutation based MANCOVA of these paired mRNA expression and microbial profiles in 34 ileal CD, 27 UC and 23 non-IBD control patients.

Results

Patient Characteristics

As shown in Table 1, 35% of ileal CD patients harbored at least one NOD2 risk allele (NOD2R) compared to 13% of nonIBD control patients, consistent with previous studies [1–3]. Only one ileal CD patient was homozygous for the ATG16L1 nonrisk allele. The patients were predominantly Caucasian. The median age of surgery was lower in ileal CD patients than nonIBD control patients. Thirty percent of colitis patients had a concomitant *C. difficile* infection, consistent with the increased incidence of this infection noted previously in IBD patients [26], [27]. Thirty to fifty percent of IBD patients and none of the non-IBD control patients were treated with 5-aminosalicylic acid (5-ASA), steroids, immunomodulators or an anti-TNFα agent. All of the subjects received intravenous antibiotics within one hour of incision [28].

Comparison of Ileal Mucosal Expression Profiles between Ileal CD, UC and non-IBD Control Subjects

Normalization and pre-processing of the data to filter out undetectable gene-probes resulted in a total of 26,765 gene-probes. Because this number of variables still greatly exceeded the sample size, we sought to further reduce the number of input microarray variables. We reasoned that genes that were differentially expressed between the three disease phenotypes were most likely to be involved in altering host-microbial interactions. Two-class unpaired SAM analysis was used to identify genes differentially expressed (fold change >1.5, FDR <0.05) between ileal CD and Control samples, between UC and Control samples, and between CD and UC samples [29]. The results indicate significant differences in gene expression patterns between all three disease phenotypes (see Table S1) [30], [31]. By taking the union of the candidate genes identified by the three two-class comparisons, the dimensions of the normalized microarray data was reduced from 26,765 to a 2,979 gene-probe set (see Fig. 1).

Hierarchical clustering of the 2,979 gene-probe set was then carried out by using 1-correlation dissimilarities and Ward linkage as previously described [32], [33]. The number of clusters was chosen to be 43, based on inspection of the R2 plot (see Table S2). Hierarchical clustering of the original 26,765 gene-probe set was also carried out using the same algorithms to 265 clusters. This number of clusters was again chosen based on inspection of the R2 plot. In all but four (clusters #14, 20, 31, 36) of the 43 clusters, greater than 40% of the gene-probes were concentrated in two of the 265 clusters obtained by clustering the original 26,765 gene-probe set, indicating that using SAM to reduce the number of

Table 1. Distribution of NOD2 composite and ATG16L1 genotype and clinical characteristics of ileal CD, colitis and control non-IBD patients.

Variables	Ileal CD (n = 34)	UC (n = 27)	Control (n = 23)	P-value	FDR
NOD2 genotype				0.11	0.15
NOD2R (R/R + R/NR)	35%	19%	13%		
NOD2NR (NR/NR)	65%	81%	87%		
ATG16L1 genotype				0.23	0.28
ATG16L1R/R	41%	41%	43%		
ATG16L1R/NR	56%	41%	35%		
ATG16L1NR/NR	3%	18%	22%		
Gender (male)	38%	59%	30%	0.095	0.14
Race (Caucasian)	94%	96%	96%	0.92	0.92
Median age (range) y	36 (21–59)	43 (17–64)	55 (32–84)	<0.001	<0.001
Current smoker	38%	11%	22%	0.048	0.08
Positive fecal C. difficile toxin	0%	30%	0%	<0.001	<0.001
Median BMI (range) kg/m²	25 (16–38)	24(18–43)	28(20–38)	0.43	0.47
5-ASA	52%	70%	0%	<0.001	<0.001
Steroids	55%	74%	0%	<0.001	<0.001
Immunomodulators	50%	52%	0%	<0.001	<0.001
Anti-TNFα biologics				0.003	0.006
Current (≤8 weeks)	35%	41%	0%		
Past (>8 weeks)	9%	7%	0%		
Never	56%	52%	100%		

The variables shown below are included in the subsequent MANCOVA analyses for 84 patients. Chi-square test for contingency table was used for categorical data and Kruskal-Wallis test was used for age and BMI. Variables that differed significantly (FDR ≤0.05) are **bolded**.

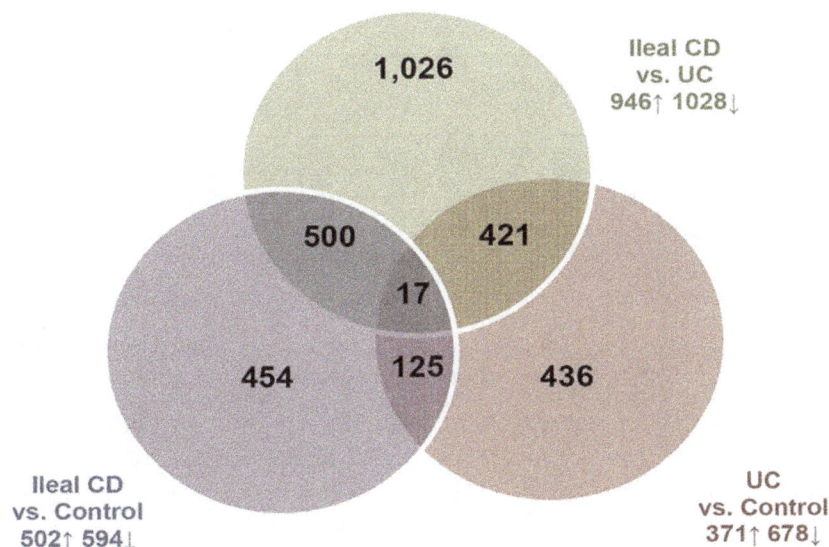

Figure 1. Venn diagram of the union of the gene-probes identified by SAM. Two-class unpaired SAM analyses of ileal CD vs Control samples, UC vs. Control Samples and ileal CD vs. UC samples have been conducted. The number of gene-probes that overlapped between the three separate analyses is shown within the Venn diagram. The total numbers of upregulated and downregulated gene-probes for each individual analysis are shown on the side.

probes did not appear to bias clustering. We reasoned that genes, which were highly correlated with each other, would be linked by common biological pathways. Ingenuity Pathway Analysis (IPA) canonical pathways were associated (P<0.01 and at least 4 gene probes) in 12 of 43 clusters (see Table S3). In addition, direct inspection of cluster #24 revealed that this cluster included a number of genes expressed in Paneth cells, such as the α-defensins.

Permutational based MANCOVA with Stepwise Variable Selection and Gene Cluster Centroids as Independent Variables

For 84 of 99 ileal mucosal samples with microarray profiles, 454 pyrosequencing of the V3, V4, and V5 (V3–V5) hypervariable regions of the 16 S rRNA gene was completed using primers adopted by the Human Microbiome Project [34], [35]. A vector consisting of the relative frequencies of six phyla/subphyla categories (excluding the seventh "other Taxa" category):1.) Actinobacteria, 2.) Bacteroidetes, 3.) Firmicutes. Clostridium Group IV, 4.) Firmicutes. Clostridium Group XIVa, 5.) Firmicutes. Bacilli, 6.) Proteobacteria, was used as the dependent variables. The 43 microarray cluster medians were used as cluster centroids [36], [37], in addition to disease phenotype and the other 12 input variables in the analysis. Using the stepwise variable selection method, permutation based MANCOVA selected disease phenotype, a Paneth cell gene enriched cluster, two xenobiotic metabolism gene enriched clusters, and NOD2 genotype as the independent variable set (see Table 2). Gene-probes included in these three clusters are listed in Table 3. We obtained similar results using the cluster mean or first principle component [36], [38] as the cluster centroids (data not shown). We also obtained similar results when parallel Sanger and 454 V1–V3 16 S sequence datasets were used (data not shown).

To examine correlations between gene transcripts and bacterial taxa at a more granular level, we selected individual gene transcripts within these microarray clusters and individual bacterial genera. The selected transcripts included the alpha

defensins, (*DEFA5* and *DEFA6*), which have exhibited altered regulation in ileal Crohn's disease [10], [39], [40], and included cellular detoxification genes, which have exhibited altered

Table 2. Selected variables associated (P≤0.05) with shifts in ileum associated microbial composition.

Selected Variables	Df	R²	P value
Phenotype	2	0.0460	0.037
Paneth cell cluster (Cluster 24)	1	0.0576	0.002
Xenobiotic cluster A (Cluster 13)	1	0.0319	0.024
Xenobiotic cluster B (Cluster 2)	1	0.0291	0.041
NOD2 genotype	1	0.0414	0.011

regulation in ulcerative colitis [41]. The bacteria genera selected included the Faecalibacterium and Shigella/Escherichia genera, because the relative frequency of *Faecalibacterium prausnizii* has been reported to be reduced and that of *Escherichia coli* have been reported to be increased in patients with ileal CD. Bacterial genera, previously selected as ulcerative colitis related were also included in this analysis [42].

As shown in Figure 2, a positive correlation (P<0.05) between the relative frequency of the Faecalibacterium genus (Firmicutes Phylum, Clostridium GroupIV) and mRNA expression levels of Paneth cell genes, including *DEFA5* and *DEFA6*, was observed in ileal CD patients but not in non-IBD controls or UC patients. Negative correlations (P<0.05) were observed between the relative frequency of the Bacteroidetes genus and Parabacteroides genus (Bacteroidetes phylum) and mRNA expression levels of the *REG* genes in ileal CD patients, but not in UC or non-IBD control patients. Furthermore, negative correlations (P<0.05) were observed between the relative frequency of the Parabacteroides genus (Bacteroidetes phylum) and mRNA expression levels of

Table 3. Gene list for the Paneth cell gene enriched cluster and the xenobiotic metabolism gene enriched clusters A and B.

Cluster Function	Gene list
Paneth Cell (cluster 24)	ENPP7, **DEFA5**, TM4SF20, RGN, MDK, **REG3A**, BCMO1, BAI2, GPR172B, CA9, ANGPTL4, ASAH2, CEL, NPC1L1, SERPINB5, SERPINA1, NPNT, VNN1, DDO, PRSS2, **PLA2G2A**, PRSS1, SLC2A12, CCK, CDKN1C, UNC5CL, FBXO2, KLK12, SIGLEC15, CLCA1, RHBG, CCL25, AZGP1, LCT, **DEFA6**, GCNT1, SLC16A4, UNC93A, LOC100128979, WNT11, VNN1, PEAR1, LOC643201, **ITLN2**, **REG4**, LOC100240735, LOC100240735, **REG3G**, PRSS2
Xenobiotic Metabolism Cluster A (cluster 13)	CPO, PRSS7, AATK, HEBP1, **ABCG5**, **CYP2C9**, GATM, SLC5A12, **GSTA1**, MS4A8B, SULT1E1, PTGR1, CYP2C19, CYP2C19, **ABCC2**, NR0B2, ABCA4, APOC3, CYBRD1, MME, MTTP, GSTA2, UNC93A, SST, ACE2, GSTA3, SOAT2, FBP1, TM4SF5, SLC23A3, EDN2, **NR1I3**, PDIA2, ENPEP, UGT2B4, C17ORF78, SLC5A11, ANO6, KCNH6, C19ORF77, C21ORF129, MGAM, ABCC2, PDZK1, CYP2C18, CPS1, NQO2, DNASE1, DHDH, OSR2, BST1, PIK3C2G, MEP1B, APOB, RBP2, AADAC, PEPD, MAOB, MAOB, APOA4, REEP6, MEP1A, GSTA5, PHYHIPL, OAT, MEP1A, **SULT2A1**, MGAT3, MME, GSTA2, TIAM2, LOC285733, EMB, SLC16A10, SLC6A4, EMB, LOC149703, TMEM229A, C19ORF69
Xenobiotic Metabolism Cluster B (cluster 2)	NELL2, ACOX2, CYP2J2, **SULT1A2**, PRR15L, GUCA2A, LGALS2, PCK2, DDC, RNF128, FMO1, FAM82A2, ABAT, SAT2, NAT8, AGXT2, BTNL3, MYO1A, MTHFS, SMPD3, CBS, VIL1, EDN3, ABCG2, MOSC2, G6PC, CDK20, CYP4F3, VIL1, ABHD6, HSD17B11, TRPM6, C9ORF24, KLKB1, TM4SF4, EFNA1, CBR1, ANKRD43, SLC9A3R1, SUSD2, SLC1A7, LINCR, CHP2, SLC17A4, MAF, FAM151A, OAZ1, KAZALD1, APOM, C9ORF40, ANXA13, GUCA2B, GLRX, C6ORF123, EPHX2, CTU2, CES2, PBX1, KAZALD, SP8, SULT1A4, TRPM6, VPS35, NAT8B, CSNK1D, STAU2, PTPRF, PGRMC2, AGPHD1, AGXT2, APOM, IYD, LRAT, LAMA1, ADI1

The genes selected for further correlation analyses are **bolded**.
See Table S3 for the complete list of all clusters.

cellular detoxification genes in non-IBD control and ileal CD patients but not in UC patients. The highest correlation (out of >500 comparisons) was observed between Faecalibacterium and *DEFA6* (r = 0.59, P = 0.00024, FDR = 0.057) in ileal CD patients.

Discussion

In this exploratory study, we report the results of the analysis integrating human ileal mucosal microarray expression profiles with microbiota profiles. Since the number of genes and bacterial taxa greatly exceed the number of samples, we sought to shrink these high dimensional datasets by grouping the bacteria taxa into broad phyla/subphyla categories, and by selecting potentially disease relevant transcripts by SAM followed by clustering using 1-correlation dissimilarity measure. We were gratified to observe that a number of the resulting clusters could be linked to canonical pathways by IPA. Furthermore inspection of one of the clusters revealed that it included a number of genes that were expressed in

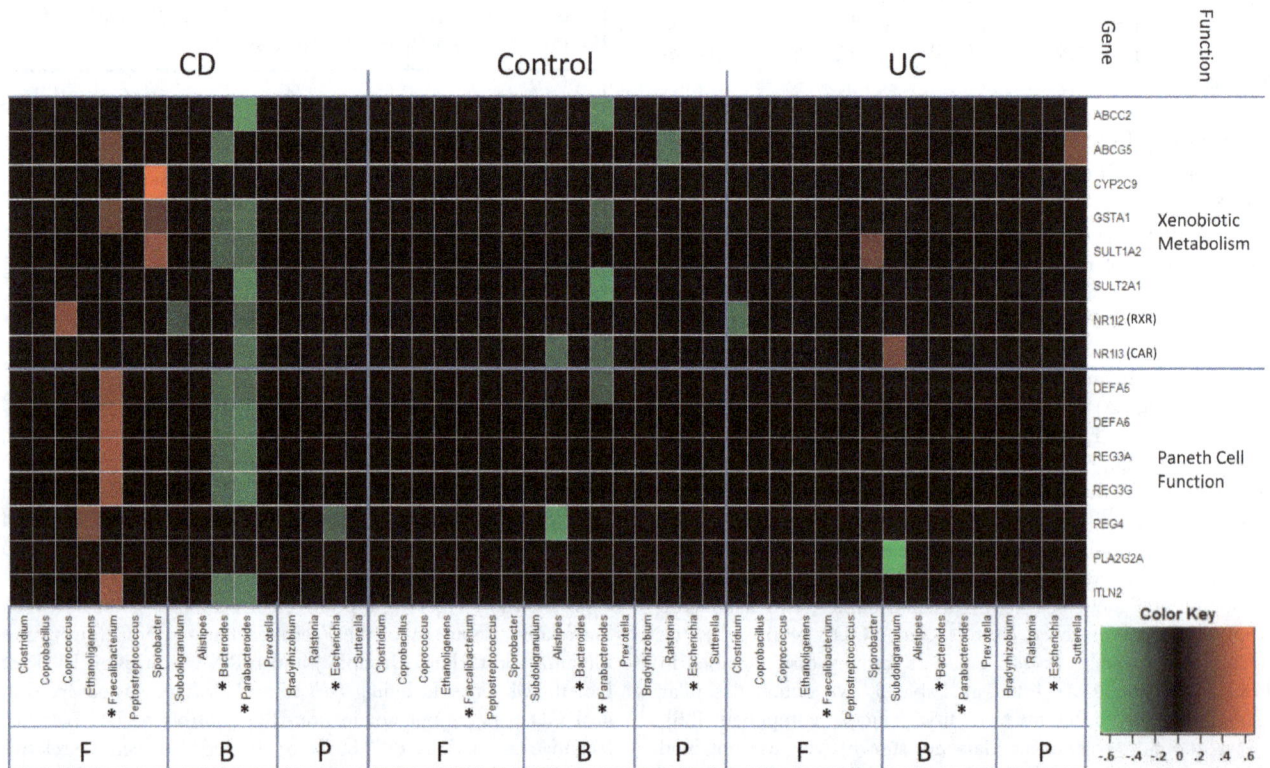

Figure 2. Correlations between selected mRNA transcripts and bacterial genera. Selected transcripts from the Paneth cell and xenobiotic metabolism microarray clusters are listed with their public reference along the vertical axis (see text). Selected bacterial genera are classified by phyla. CD, ileal CD phenotype; Control, non-IBD control phenotype; UC, UC phenotype; F, Firmicutes; B, Bacteroidetes; P, Proteobacteria. *Red squares* represent positive correlations (P<0.05), and *green squares* represent negative correlations (P<0.05).

Paneth cells. We therefore selected gene transcripts within these three microarray clusters for further analysis. These genes included the alpha defensins and members of the regenerating gene (REG) family. The alpha defensins are antimicrobial peptides that are secreted by Paneth cells. Manipulation of alpha defensin expression in experimental animals has been shown to alter gut microbial composition [43]. On the other hand, monoassociation of a Bacteroidetes species with germ free animals was shown to alter regulation of Paneth cell gene expression [44]. Altered expression of alpha defensins have been associated with the ileal Crohn's disease phenotype. The *REG* genes belong to the calcium (C-type) dependent lectin superfamily and have been noted to be upregulated in CD and UC intestinal tissues [45], [46]. Expression levels of cellular detoxification genes, which are target genes for the transcription factor pregnane X receptor (PXR and also termed NR1I2), have been previously noted to be down-regulated in the colons of UC patients [41]. The expression levels of these genes were correlated with bacterial genera that had been previously reported to be disease associated [42]. At a threshold of P≤0.05, exploratory analyses revealed potential correlations between transcript levels of specific genes with individual bacterial genera (e.g. Faecalibacterium, Bacteroidetes and Parabacteroides), that were modulated by disease phenotype. By honing in on these promising correlations identified by exploratory studies, we hope to be able to further confirm these observations in an expanded set of samples. Co-linearity between input variables may occur, despite our efforts to shrink the dimensions of the datasets. This may account for why *C. difficile* was not selected in this subset of the microbial dataset. Alternatively *C. difficile* may not have been selected because paired microarray and microbial data have been collected on a smaller number of subjects thus far. While the use of immunomodulators and anti-TNFα biologics were included as co-variates in the MANOVA [24], we cannot completely exclude the potential confounding effects of these drugs on the microbial composition and mucosal gene expression. Nevertheless our results demonstrate that integrating paired expression profiles and microbial data can lead to the discovery of biologically meaningful host-microbial interactions in inflammatory bowel diseases. We anticipate that as we expand the sample set, other associations will be detected.

Materials and Methods

Patients and Acquisition of Macroscopically Disease-unaffected Proximal Margin Ileal Tissue Samples

This study was approved by the Institutional Review Boards of Washington University-St. Louis and Stony Brook University. Ileal CD patients undergoing initial ileocolic resection, UC patients undergoing initial total colectomy and Control non-IBD patients undergoing either right hemicolectomy or total colectomy were prospectively enrolled in a consecutive fashion by the Washington University Digestive Diseases Research Core Center Tissue Procurement Facility to donate surgically resected tissue samples between April 2005 and February 2010. Patients who were unwilling or unable to give informed consent were excluded. Clinical information and patient samples were stripped of all identifying information and assigned a patient code and sample code. The de-identified patients were genotyped for the three major NOD2 and ATG16L1 genotypes and phenotyped as previously described [15]. All of the patients received antibiotics within one hour of incision. Ex-vivo biopsies were obtained of the disease unaffected proximal margin of the surgical resection specimens as previously described. RNA and DNA were extracted from the biopsy samples as previously described [15].

Human Ileal Mucosal Expression Profiles

The test RNA and a common reference ileal RNA were labeled and the resulting probes were hybridized to Agilent Whole Human Genome Arrays (Agilent No. G4410A) as previously described [15]. The pre-processing, filtering and normalization of the array data was conducted using the R package LIMMA [47], [48]. Probes with all Genepix flags less than −50 were treated as absent and removed from the dataset. There were technical duplicates on three samples and the log2 ratios for these three samples were averaged prior to analysis. Genes that were differentially expressed between ileal CD vs. Control, UC vs. Control, and ileal CD vs. UC were selected by conducting three two-class unpaired comparisons using SAM, with a cutoff of change >1.5 fold and false discovery rate (FDR) <0.05 [29]. The hierarchical clustering was carried out by using 1-r dissimilarity measurement and Ward linkage as previously described [32], [34]. The cluster number was decided based on inspection of the coefficient of determination (R2) plot [49], [50]. The biological significance of these clusters was assessed by using Ingenuity Pathway Analysis (IPA) software [51]. To select cluster-enriched IPA canonical pathways, we lowered the threshold of the *p*-value from 0.05 to 0.001, and included only pathways that included ≥4 genes in the cluster. The data discussed in this publication have been deposited in NCBI's Gene Expression Omnibus and are accessible through GEO Series accession number GSE24287 (http://www.ncbi.nlm.nih.gov/geo/query/acc.cgi?acc = GSE24287).

Assessment of Ileal-associated Microbial Composition

The V3–V5 region was targeted by using barcoded primers 357F (5′-CCTACGGGAGGCAGCAG-3′) and 907R (5′CCGTCAATTCMTTTRAGT) and were identical to the primers used by the Human Microbiome Project to characterize the microbiota in healthy human subjects. All sequences were screened for fidelity to a 16 S rRNA bacterial covariance model (CM) based on secondary structure using the Infernal software package [52] and were checked for chimerism with ChimeraSlayer [53] http://microbiomeutil.sourceforge.net/#A_CS). Potentially chimeric sequences and sequences lacking high fidelity to the CM were removed from subsequent analysis. Genera level taxonomic calls were produced by the *RDP Classifier* [53], which performs naïve Bayesian taxonomic classification versus a training set. This project used the code and training set provided by RDP (Version 2.1, http://sourceforge.net/projects/rdpclassifier/) April 6, 2010 respectively. The sequences were also classified into seven phyla/subphyla categories. The seven categories were 1) *Actinobacteria*, 2) *Bacteroidetes*, 3) *Firmicutes*.Clostridium Group IV, 4) *Firmicutes*. Clostridium Group XIVa, 5.) *Firmicutes*. Bacillus, 6.) *Proteobacteria*, and 7.) Other taxa. The subdivisions of the Firmicutes phyla were based on concordance between the RDP classifier and the Greengenes 16 S rRNA phylogenetic schema [54–56]. The Clostridium GroupIV and Clostridium Group XIVa taxa are subsets of the Lachnospiriciae taxon [22], [57]. The sequence screening, classification, final binning and enumeration operations described were performed within a python based analysis pipeline created for this project [24]. Assembled Sanger sequences were deposited in GenBank accession HQ739096-HQ821395. 454 V1–V3 and V3–V5 sequences were deposited in the Sequence Read Archive accession SRX021348-SRX021368, SRX037800-SRX037802. Clinical and genotyping data can be accessed through the dbGAP authorized access system. Request access to: phs000255. The study accession is SRP002479 "Effect of Crohn's disease risk alleles on enteric microbiota". In order to request access to any of the individual-level datasets within the controlled-access portions of the database, the Principal Investigator (PI) and the Signing Official (SO) at the investigator's institution will need to co-sign a request for data access, which will be reviewed by an NIH Data Access Committee at the appropriate NIH Institute or Center (https://dbgap.ncbi.nlm.nih.gov/aa/wga.cgi?page = login).

Statistical Analysis

In order to investigate the relationship between gene expression and bacteria composition, permutational MANOVA with stepwise variable selection was performed for a vector including six bacteria taxa, which served as the dependent variable [58]. Because the dependent variable is a vector of compositions, the centered log ratio transformation was used on the bacterial proportions [59]. The cluster medians [36], [37] were chosen to represent the cluster centroids and included as input variables along with clinical information (patients phenotype, age, race, smoking, BMI, gender, C._difficile, 5-ASA, steroids, immunomodulator, TNF) and genotypes (NOD2 and ATG16L1).

Supporting Information

Table S1   A. Gene-probes upregulated in CD compared to Control (n = 502). B. Gene-probes downregulated in CD compared to Control (n = 594). C. Gene-probes upregulated in UC compared to Control (n = 371).

Table S2   Gene-probes in the 43 clusters.

Table S3   Clusters obtained by after dimension reduction using SAM. The clusters are listed along with the

percentage of variation explained by the 1st PC of the cluster, which is related to the compactness of the cluster. The bolded clusters are the clusters in which >40% of the gene-probes were concentrated in two of the 265 clusters obtained without prior dimension reduction. The clusters were considered enriched for genes that were differentially expressed in CD vs. Control, UC vs. Control or CD vs. UC if ≥50% of the genes with a correlation of ≥0.75% to the 1st PC of the cluster demonstrated a significant fold change (see Supplementary Table 1). Clusters were considered enriched for genes in an IPA canonical pathway if P<0.01 and at least 4 genes were in the pathway. In addition we listed our interpretation of the biological significance of the pathway.

Acknowledgments

The authors thank the patients who have generously contributed their blood, tissue and medical information to the Washington University Digestive Diseases Research Core Center (DDRCC) Tissue Procurement Facility. We also thank the faculty in the Division of Colon Rectal Surgery and the Division of Gastroenterology at Washington University for their help and support in recruiting patients.

Author Contributions

Conceived and designed the experiments: SRH TD RDN DNF EL. Performed the experiments: QG GW ES. Analyzed the data: TZ RAD XJ FJR WZ CER DNF EL. Contributed reagents/materials/analysis tools: TZ XJ SRH TD RDN CER DNF EL. Wrote the paper: TZ RAD XJ FJR WZ QG SRH TD RDN GW ES CER DNF EL.

References

1. Ng SC, Woodrow S, Patel N, Subhani J, Harbord M (2011) Role of genetic and environmental factors in British twins with inflammatory bowel disease. Inflamm Bowel Dis doi: 10.1002/ibd.21747. [Epub ahead of print].
2. Khor B, Gardet A, Xavier RJ (2011) Genetics and pathogenesis of inflammatory bowel disease Nature 474: 307–317.
3. Abraham C, Cho J (2009) Mechanisms of disease: inflammatory bowel disease New Engl. J Medicine 361: 2066–2078.
4. Hancock L, Beckly J, Geremia A, Cooney R, Cummings F, et al. (2008) Clinical and molecular characteristics of isolated colonic Crohn's disease Inflamm Bowel Dis 14: 1667–1677.
5. Waterman M, Xu W, Stempak JM, et al. (2011) Distinct and overlapping genetic loci in Crohn's disease and ulcerative colitis: correlations with pathogenesis Inflamm Bowel Dis 17: 1936–1942.
6. Chen H, Lee A, Bowcock A, Zhu W, Li E, et al. (2011) Influence of Crohn's disease and smoking on disease location Dis Colon Rectum 54: 1020–1025.
7. Cuthbert A, Fisher S, Mirza MM, King K, Hampe J, et al. (2002) The contribution of NOD2 gene mutations to the risk and site of disease in inflammatory bowel disease. Gastroenterol 122: 867–874.
8. Lesage S, Zouali H, Cezard JP, Cézard JP, Colombel JF, et al. (2002) CARD15/NOD2 mutational analysis and genotype-phenotype correlation in 612 patients with inflammatory bowel disease. Am J Human Genet 70: 845–857.
9. Ogura Y, Lala S, Xin W, Smith E, Dowds TA, et al. (2003) Expression of NOD2 in Paneth cells: a possible link to Crohn's ileitis Gut 52: 1591–1597.
10. Bevins CL, Stange EF, Wehkamp J (2009) Decreased Paneth cell defensin expression in ileal Crohn's disease is independent of inflammation, but linked to the NOD2 1007fs genotype Gut 58: 882–883.
11. Simms LA, Doecke JD, Walsh MD, Huang N, Fowler EV, et al. (2008) Reduced alpha-defensin expression is associated with inflammation and not NOD2 mutation status in ileal Crohn's disease Gut 57: 903–910.
12. Prescott NJ, Fisher SA, Franke A, Hampe J, Onnie CM, et al. (2007) A nonsynonymous SNP in ATG16L1 predisposes to ileal Crohn's disease and is independent of CARD15 and IBD5 Gastroenterol. 132: 1665–1671.
13. Cadwell K, Liu JY, Brown SL, Miyoshi H, Loh J, et al. (2008) A key role for autophagy and the autophagy gene Atg16l1 in mouse and human intestinal Paneth cells. Nature. 456: 259–263.
14. Cadwell K, Patel KK, Maloney NS, Liu TC, Ng AC, et al. (2010) Virus-plus susceptibility gene interaction determines Crohn's disease gene Atg16L1 phenotypes in the intestine. Cell. 141: 1135–1145.
15. Hamm C, Reimers M, McCullough C, Gorbe EB, Lu J, et al. (2010) NOD2 status and human ileal gene expression. Inflamm Bowel Dis 16: 1649–1657.
16. Frank DN, St. Amand AL, Feldman RA, Boedeker EC, Harpaz N, et al. (2007) Molecular-phylogenetic characterization of microbial community imbalances in human inflammatory bowel diseases Proc Natl Acad Sci USA 104: 13780–13785.
17. Peterson DA, Frank DN, Pace N, Gordon JI (2008) Metagenomic approaches for defining the pathogenesis of inflammatory bowel diseases Cell Host Microbe 3: 417–427.
18. Sokol H, Lay C, Seksik P, Tannock GW (2008) Analysis of bacterial bowel communities of IBD patients: What has it revealed? Inflamm Bowel Dis 14: 858–867.
19. Sokol H, Pigneur B, Watterlot L, Lakhdari O, Bermúdez-Humarán LG, et al. (2008) Faecalibacterium prausnitzii is an anti inflammatory commensal bacterium identified by gut microbiota analysis of Crohn disease patients Proc Natl Acad Sci USA 105: 16731–16736.
20. Willing B, Halfvarson WB, Dicksved J, Rosenquist M, Järnerot G, et al. (2009) Twin studies reveal specific imbalances in the mucosal-associated microbiota of patients with ileal Crohn's disease Inflamm Bowel Dis 15: 653–660.
21. Qin J, Li R, Raes J, Arumugam M, Burgdorf KS, et al. (2009) A human gut microbial gene catalogue established by metagenomic sequencing Nature. 464: 59–65.
22. Frank DN, Robertson CE, Hamm CM, Kpadeh Z, Zhang T, et al. (2011) Disease phenotype and genotype are associated with shifts in intestinal-microbiota in inflammatory bowel diseases Inflamm Bowel Dis 17: 179–184.
23. Willing B, Dicksved J, Halfvarson J, Andersson AF, Lucio M, et al. (2010) A pyrosequencing study in twins shows that gastrointestinal microbial profiles vary with inflammatory bowel disease phenotypes Gastroenterol 139: 1844–1854.
24. Li E, Hamm CM, Gulati AS, Sartor RB, Chen H, et al. (2011) Inflammatory bowel diseases phenotype, C. difficile and NOD2 genotype are associated with shifts in human ileum associated microbial composition PLoS ONE, accepted for publication.
25. Frank DN, Zhu W, Sartor RB, Li E (2011) Investigating the biological and clinical significance of human dysbioses Trends Microbiol 19: 427–434.
26. Issa M, Vijaypal A, Graham MB, Beaulieu DB, Otterson MF, et al. (2007) Impact of Clostridium difficile on inflammatory bowel disease Clin Gastroenterol Hepatol 5: 345–351.
27. Rodemann JF, Dubberke ER, Reske KA, Seo da H, Stone CD (2007) The incidence of Clostridium difficile infection in inflammatory bowel disease. Clin Gastroenterol Hepatol. 5: 339–344.
28. Nelson RL, Glenny AM, Song F (2009) Antimicrobial prophylaxis for colorectal surgery Cochrane Database Syst Rev 1: CD001181.

29. Tusher VG, Tibshirani R, Chu G (2001) Significance analysis of microarrays applied to the ionizing radiation response Proc Natl Acad Sci USA 98: 5116–5121.

30. Lawrance IC, Fiocchi C, Chakravarti S (2001) Ulcerative colitis and Crohn's disease: distinctive gene expression profiles and novel susceptibility candidate genes Hum Mol Genet 10: 445–456.

31. Wu F, Dassopoulos T, Cope L, Maitra A, Brant SR, et al. (2007) Genome-wide gene expression differences in Crohn's disease and ulcerative colitis from endoscopic pinch biopsies: insights into distinctive pathogenesis Inflamm Bowel Dis 13: 807–821.

32. Ward RF, Werner SL Analysis of variance of the composition of a migmatite (1963) Science 140: 978–979.

33. Singh W (2008). Robustness of three hierarchical agglomerative clustering techniques for ecological data Thesis for the degree of Master of Science in Environment and Natural Resources, Department of Mathematics, University of Iceland.

34. Peterson J, Garges S, Giovanni M, et al. (2009) The NIH Human Microbiome Project Genome Res 19: 2317–2323.

35. Petrosino JF, Highlander S, Luna RA, et al. (2009) Metagenomic pyrosequencing and microbial identification Clin Chem 55: 856–866.

36. Ott RL, Longnecker M (2001) An introduction to statistical methods and data analysis Pacific Grove, CA Dyxbury.

37. Yeung SM, Zhou F-C, Ye F-C, Pan H-Y, Gao S-H (2005) Early and sustained expression of latent and host modulating genes in coordinated transcriptional program of KSHV productive primary infection of human primary endothelial cells Virology. 343: 47–64.

38. Vaughan IP, Omerod SJ (2005) Increasing the value of principal component analysis for simplifying ecological data: a case study for rivers and rive birds J Appl Ecol 42: 487–497.

39. Wehkamp J, Salzman NH, Porter E, Nuding S, Weichenthal M, et al. (2005) Reduced Paneth cell alpha-defensins in ileal Crohn's disease Proc Natl Acad Sci USA 102: 18129–18134.

40. Simms LA, Doecke JD, Walsh MD, Huang N, Fowler EV, et al. (2008) Reduced alpha-defensin expression is associated with inflammation and not NOD2 mutation status in ileal Crohn's disease Gut 57: 903–910.

41. Langmann T, Moehle C, Maurer R, Scharl M, Liebisch G, et al. (2004) Loss of detoxification in inflammatory bowel disease: dysregulation of pregnane X receptor target genes Gastroenterol 127: 26–40.

42. Lepage P, Häsler R, Spehlmann ME, Rehman A, Zvirbliene A, et al. (2011) Twin study indicates loss of interaction between microbiota and mucosa of patients with ulcerative colitis Gastroenterol 141: 227–236.

43. Salzman NH, Hung K, Haribhai D, et al. (2011) Enteric defensins are essential regulators of intestinal microbial ecology Nat Immunol 11: 76–83.

44. Hooper LV, Wong MH, Thelin A, Hansson L, Falk PG, et al. (2001) Molecular analysis of commensal host-microbial relationships in the intestine Science 291: 881–884.

45. Dieckgraefe B, Stenson W, Korzenik JR, Swanson PE, Harrington CA (2000) Analysis of mucosal gene expression in inflammatory bowel disease by parallel oligonucleotide arrays Physiol Genomics 4: 1–11.

46. Hartupee JC, Zhang H, Bonaldo MF, Soares MB, Dieckgraefe BK (2001) Isolation and characterization of a cDNA encoding a novel member of the human regenerating protein family: Reg IV. Biochim Biophys Acta. 1518: 287–293.

47. Smyth GK, Speed TP (2003) Normalization of cDNA microarray data. Methods. 31: 265–273.

48. Smyth GK (2005) Limma: linear models for microarray data. In Gentleman R, Carey V, Dudoit S, Irizarry R, Huber W eds. Bioinformatics and Computational Biology Solutions using R and Bioconductor. New York: Springer. 397–420.

49. Eisen MB, Spellman PT, Brown PO, Botstein D (1998) Cluster analysis and display of genome-wide expression patterns. Proc Natl. Acad Sci USA. 95: 14863–14868.

50. Sturn A, Quackenbush J, Trajanoski Z (2000) Genesis: cluster analysis of microarray data Bioinformatics 18: 207–208.

51. Sun J, Jia P, Fanous AH, van den Oord E, et al. (2010) Schizophrenia gene networks and pathways and their applications for novel candidate gene selection. PloS ONE. 5: e11351.

52. Nawrocki EP, Kolbe DL, Eddy SR (2009) Infernal 1.0: Inference of RNA alignments. Bioinformatics 25: 1335–1337.

53. Haas BJ, Gevers D, Earl A, Feldgarden M, Ward DV, et al. (2011) Chimeric 16 S rRNA sequence formation and detection in Sanger and 454-pyrosequenced PCR amplicons Genome Res 21: 494–504.

54. Wang Q, Garrity GM, Tiedje JM, Cole JR (2007) Naive Bayesian classifier for rapid assignment of rRNA sequences into the new bacterial taxonomy Appl Environ Microbiol 73: 5261–5267.

55. Cole JR, Wang Q, Cardenas E, Fish J, Chai B, et al. (2009) The Ribosomal Database Project: improved alignments and new tools for rRNA analysis Nucleic Acids Res 37: D141–145.

56. DeSantis TZ, Hugenholtz P, Larsen N, Rojas M, Brodie EL, et al. (2006) Greengenes, a chimera-checked 16 S rRNA gene database and workbench compatible with ARB Appl Environ Microbiol 72: 5069–5072.

57. Collins MD, Lawson PA, Willems A, Cordoba JJ, Fernandez-Garayzabal J, et al. (1994) The phylogeny of the genus Clostridium: proposal of five new genera and eleven new species combinations. Int J Syst Bacteriol 44: 812–826.

58. Anderson MJ (2001) A new method for non-parametric multivariate analysis of variance Austral Ecology 26: 32–46.

59. Aitchison J (1986) The Statistical Analysis of Compositional Data, Monographs on Statistics and Applied Probability. London: Chapman & Hall Ltd. 416p.

6

The Incidence of Inflammatory Bowel Disease in Northern China

Hong Yang[1,9], Yumei Li[2,9], Wei Wu[3], Qingwen Sun[2], Yunzhong Zhang[4], Wei Zhao[5], Hongbo Lv[2], Qing Xia[2], Pinjin Hu[6], Haihua Li[2], Jiaming Qian[1]*

1 Department of Gastroenterology, Peking Union Medical College Hospital, Beijing, China, 2 Department of Gastroenterology, Daqing Longnan Hospital, Daqing, China, 3 Department of Gastroenterology, Daqing Oilfield General Hospital, Daqing, China, 4 Department of Gastroenterology, Daqing People Hospital, Daqing, China, 5 Department of Gastroenterology, Daqing Fourth Hospital, Daqing, China, 6 Department of Gastroenterology, The First Affiliated Hospital of Sun Yat-sen University, Guangzhou, China

Abstract

Aims & Backgrounds: Although inflammatory bowel diseases (IBD) are emerging and increasing in China, epidemiologic data are rarely available. This study was to investigate the epidemiological and clinical characteristics of IBD in Northern China.

Methods: This is a prospective, population-based study of incidence of IBD in Daqing,Heilongjiang province of Northern China from March 1, 2012 to February 28, 2013. All incident patients with IBD were clinically identified by IBD specialist group from five main General Hospitals covering the healthcare service for 1,343,364 residents in the urban areas of Daqing. IBD cases included in this study were followed-up for three months for diagnosis confirmation.

Results: A total of 27 new IBD cases including 25 cases of ulcerative colitis (UC) and 2 cases of Crohn's disease (CD) were identified. The population at risk was 1,343,364 person years. Age-adjusted incidence for total IBD, CD and UC were 1.77, 0.13, and 1.64 per 100,000population, respectively. A male predominance was found in CD patients (male to female ratio was 2:0). In contrast, no obvious gender predominance was found in UC patients (male to female ratio was 1:1.1). CD patients were diagnosed at an average age of 39.5 years. The main disease phenotypes of UC were distal colitis with a 24% of proctitis and 56% of left-sided colitis. The mean diagnostic age of UC patients was 48.9 years.

Conclusions: This is the first report on the incidence of IBD in the Northern Chinese population. A lower incidence of IBD, similar male predominance for CD, similar disease phenotype of UC, and lower disease activity was observed in Daqing compared to that in Southern China.

Editor: Xiaoping Miao, MOE Key Laboratory of Environment and Health, School of Public Health, Tongji Medical College, Huazhong University of Science and Technology, China

Funding: This study was supported by Health Research & Special Projects Grant(No. 201002020). The funders had no role in study design,data collection and analysis,decision to publish,or preparation of the manuscript.

Competing Interests: The authors have declared that no competing interests exist.

* Email: qianjiaming1957@126.com

9 These authors contributed equally to this work.

Introduction

Inflammatory bowel diseases (IBDs), including ulcerative colitis (UC) and Crohn's disease (CD), frequently progress with long-term disability, morbidity and a variety of complications, which lead to low quality of life in patients [1]. Recent studies demonstrated that the incidence of IBD is increasing worldwide. The highest incidence rate of IBD was reported in North America and Europe. The annual incidence of CD in North America is 20.2 per 100,000 persons and the annual incidence of UC in Europe is 24.3 per 100,000 persons. However, considerable variations in IBD incidence have been reported around the world, which was proposed to be associated with different geographic regions, environmental factors and dietary factors [2–5]. Few epidemiologic studies have been conducted in developing countries, such as China, South Korea, India, Lebanon, Iran, Thailand, the French West Indies, and North Africa [6]. A population-based epidemiologic study of IBD in a country with a large demographic base, such as China with a population of 1.3 billion, is invaluable for understanding the burden of disease and formulating insurance policy for health care.

The incidence of IBD has been reported from two areas of Southern China recently [7–8]. However, there are a number of differences in climate, environment, lifestyle, diet and living conditions between Northern and Southern China. Based on a previous report from Europe, there are geographic variations in IBD risk [9]. Therefore, it is important to analyze the epidemiological characteristics of IBD in the Northern Chinese population and identify the clinical characteristics.

In this study, a prospective, population-based study was conducted to investigate the incidence and clinical characteristics of IBD in an area of Northern China and to give an overview of IBD between different geographic regions in China.

Materials and Methods

Study population

This study was approved by the Institutional Review Board of Peking Union Medical College Hospital. Written informed consent was obtained from all participants. Daqing, a prefectural-level city, is located in Heilongjiang province, Northern China with a total area of 22,161 square kilometers. This area is characterized by a relative low floating population. Therefore, it is easy to monitor and follow-up. Demographic data of the study population was extracted from the 2010 Population census published by the National Bureau of Statistics of China. Based on the data within the census, the total population of Daqing is 1,585,162 and 15.25% (241,798) of the population lived in rural areas, including the countryside and small towns. Thus, a population of 1,343,364 living in the urban areas was selected as the study population for this study. The sex and age proportional composition was calculated (female for 66 0,009, and male for 683,355).

1,343,364 residents in the urban areas of Daqing are served by five general hospitals and nine community hospitals. The specialists in the gastroenterology and qualified endoscopic equipments are essential in the five general hospitals, whereas they are not in community hospitals. The community hospitals usually refer symptomatic patients to a general hospital for the disease identification and confirmation. In the five general hospitals, specialists can be found in the gastroenterology units and endoscopic unit. All residents in Daqing city are covered by social health insurance. Each resident has a medical insurance number and detailed medical record.

Case selection procedure

The study protocol was mostly performed in adherence to published protocols in the studies of IBD in Guangzhou and Wuhan in Southern China [7–8] (Figure 1). Firstly, any patients with suspected or diagnosed IBD by any General Hospitals or community hospitals in Daqing were referred to Daqing Longnan Hospital for thorough Diagnosis. The demographic, clinical, endoscopic, and histologic data were collected by one of the gastroenterologists and checked by a group of gastroenterological specialists. Each participant completed the questionnaires including clinical characteristics, past history, family history, life style, and quality of life under the guidance of the IBD specialist group in Daqing Longnan Hospital.

Secondly, all the patients with suspected IBD were followed-up for 3 months. By the end of follow-up, two IBD experts determined the diagnosis for patients with suspected IBD. One pathologist reviewed pathologic results. Patients without definitive diagnosis of IBD were excluded.

Finally, to avoid missing cases, a retrospective search of local electronic medical records for endoscopic reports, medical charts, and histology reports at each hospital in Daqing was performed to find unreported incidence cases. A search using keywords such as "inflammatory bowel disease", "Crohn's disease", "ulcerative colitis", "chronic colitis" was conducted and matching patient records were identified and examined. Established registry, report and management systems in each hospital of Daqing provided support for periodic retrieval and tracking of IBD cases.

Case Definition and clinical evaluation

The diagnosis of IBD was determined according to the Lennard-Jones criteria [11]. The clinical diagnosis was confirmed on the basis of clinical symptoms, physical examination, colonoscopy, imaging (bariums studies, CT enterography), and histology. Enteric infections, intestinal tuberculosis, ischemia, non-steroidal anti-inflammatory drug induced ulceration, and radiation colitis were excluded.

Clinical classification was defined according to the Montreal Classification of IBD from [10]. Crohn's disease can be described using A, L and B classifications. A represents age at diagnosis, L represents the location of disease (A1:below 16 y; A2 between 17 and 40 y; A3 above 40 y L1: ileal;L2 colonic;L3 ileocolonic; L4 isolated upper disease). B represents disease behavior (B1:non-stricturing,non-penetrating;B2 stricturing; B3 penetrating;P perianal disease modifier). According to Montreal Classification of ulcerative colitis, the extent of UC was defined as proctitis (E1, lesions limited to the rectum), left-sided colitis (E2, lesions below the splenic flexure), and extensive/pancolitis (E3, lesions exceeded the splenic flexure).

The activity of IBD was classified according to Harvey-Bradshaw activity index for CD and SCCAI index for UC as mild, moderate and severe. The activity according to Harvey-Bradshaw was defined as remission (below 4 scores), moderate (5–8 scores), and severe (above 9 scores). The activity according to SCCAI index was defined as mild (3–5 scores), moderate (6–11 scores), and severe (above 12 scores).

Statistical analysis

The annual crude incidence rates were calculated for IBD, UC, and CD for 2012–2013, respectively, which were calculated by the number of incident patients diagnosed divided by the total population at risk. The Age-standardized incidence rates were adjusted by the national demographic structure from 6th nationwide census in 2010 (http://en.wikipedia.org/wiki/Daqing). Rates were reported with 95% confidence intervals (CI), assuming a Poisson distribution.

Results

1. Incidence and age-standardized incidence for new IBD cases

27 new IBD cases including 2 CD and 25UC were diagnosed (Table 1). The median age of diagnosis was 48.2±12.3years (range, 27–79 years) for all patients. Among patients, 14 were male and 13 were female, and the ratio of males to females was 1.1:1. Fifteen patients complete high school education or below and 12 patients completed a bachelor or higher degree. The median number of months from onset of symptoms to diagnosis of IBD was 11.0 months (interquartile range, 1–120 months).

The 2 patients with CD were diagnosed at38 and 41 years old. Both of them are male. The months from onset of symptoms to diagnosis was 2 and 120 months, respectively. Neither of them had appendectomy, a family history of IBD, or a history of tuberculosis. One patient had taken non-steroidal anti-inflmmatory drug (NSAIDs) before.

25 patients with UC were diagnosed at diagnostic age of 48.88±12.5 years. The average diagnostic age was 48.5±15.7 years for males, and 49.23±9.2 years for females. The ratio of males to females was 12:13. The median number of months from onset of symptoms to diagnosis of IBD was 7.04 (interquartile range, 1–48 months). None of the patients had appendectomy or a family history of UC. One patient had a history of tuberculosis. Two patients had taken NSAIDs before.

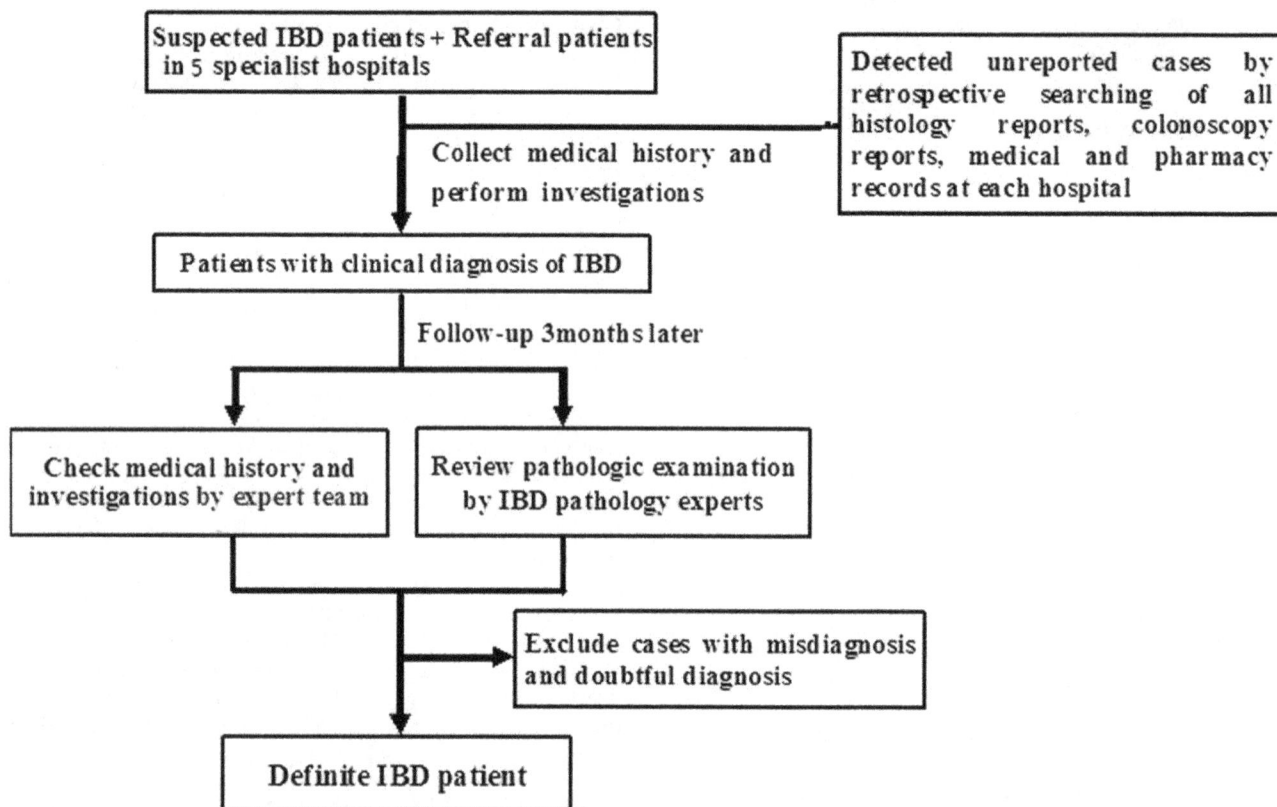

Figure 1. The flow chart of case capture. The flow chart described the procedure of case capture. Firstly, any patients with suspected or diagnosed IBD were checked medical history and investigations and then were follow-up for 3 months. Then expert team including IBD specialists and pathology experts determined the diagnosis. Finally, a retrospective search was performed to avoid missing cases.

Table 1. Demographic characteristics of new cases with IBD in North of China.

	IBD	UC	CD
Patients(n)	27	25	2
Gender,n(%)			
Females	13(48.1)	13(52.0)	0(0.0)
Males	14(51.9)	12(48.0)	2(100.0)
Median age at diagnosis,yr	48.2	48.9	39.5
Smoking history,n(%)			
Current	5(18.6)	4(16.0)	1(50.0)
Ex	6(22.2)	5(20.0)	1(50.0)
Never	16(59.2)	16(64.0)	0(0.0)
Education,n(%)			
Primary or below	1(3.7)	1(4.0)	0(0.0)
Secondary and apprentice	14(51.9)	13(52.0)	1(50.0)
Tetiary(university or college)	12(44.4)	11(44.0)	1(500.)
Appendectomy	0(0.0)	0(0.0)	0(0.0)
Family history	0(0.0)	0(0.0)	0(0.0)
NSAID	3(11.1	2(8.0)	1(50.0)
Tuberculosis history	1(3.7)	1(4.0)	0(0.0)

Table 2. Crude incidence rate (per 100,000) of IBD overall, CD, and UC in North of China.

	N	Crude incidence(per 100,000 persons)(95%CI)		
		Total	Male	Female
IBD	27	2.01(1.32–2.92)	2.12(1.16–3.56)	1.90(1.01–3.25)
UC	25	1.86(1.20–2.75)	1.82(0.94–3.18)	1.90(1.01–3.25)
CD	2	0.15(0.02–0.54)	0.30(0.04–1.09)	0.00(0.00–0.54)

The crude annual incidence of total IBD, CD, and UC was 2.01, 0.15, and 1.86 per 100,000 population, respectively. The crude annual incidence of IBD, CD, and UC for males was 2.12, 0.30, and 1.82 per 100,000 population, respectively. Crude annual incidence for females was 1.90, 0.00, and 1.90 per 100,000 population, respectively (Table 2). Age-adjusted incidence for total IBD, CD, and UC was 1.77, 0.13, and 1.64 per 100,000 population, respectively. The age-adjusted incidence for males was 1.96, 0.25, and 1.70 per 100,000 population, respectively. The age-adjusted incidence for females was 1.58, 0, and 1.58 per 100,000 population, respectively (Table 3). The median number of months from onset of symptoms to diagnosis of IBD was 11.04months (interquartile range, 1–120 months).

2. Clinical characteristics of new cases with IBD

The 2 CD patients experienced abdominal pain. Neither patient had diarrhea, blood or mucus in stool, but 1 patient had constipation. The median symptom duration before diagnosis was 61 months. All patients fall under L1 classification. Inflammation was found in both cases. One case was in remission and one case had moderate disease according to Harvey-Bradshaw activity index. One case had extra-intestinal manifestations of Arthralgia, but neither patient had other extra-intestinal manifestations like skin rashes, eye disease, ankylosing spondylitis, or primary sclerosing cholangitis (Table 4).

Among 25 UC patients, 13 cases (52%) experienced abdominal pain, 15 cases (60%) experienced diarrhea, and 3 cases (12%) experienced constipation. Bloody stool was observed in 14 cases (56%), and mucus in stool was observed in 15 cases (60%). Average symptom duration before diagnosis was 7.04±12.6 months. Among 25 cases (24%) with UC, 6 cases had proctitis, 14 cases (56%) had left-sided colitis, and 5 cases (20%) had extensive or pancolitis. 14 cases (56%) had mild disease and 11(44%) had moderate disease according to the Mayo clinical index. 4 patients had extra-intestinal manifestations including 2 cases had arthralgia, 1 case had skin rashes, and 1 case had eye disease. No patients had ankylosing spondylitis or primary sclerosing cholangitis (Table 4).

Discussion

In this study, we reported an annual incidence of IBD, CD, and UC for 1.77, 0.13, and 1.64 per 100,000 persons, respectively, in Northern China, which are obviously lower than that in western countries [2–5]. Moreover, the incidence of IBD, CD, and UC in Northern China is lower than that in Southern China [7–8]. For example, the incidence of IBD, CD, and UC in Guangzhou was 3.14, 1.09, and 2.05 per 100,000 persons, and 1.96, 0.51, and 1.45 per 100,000 persons in Wuhan. The reason of the lower IBD incidence in Daqing than in the other regions still need to be clarified, such as environmental factors, economic status and affordable medical service which will influence the case ascertainment. The variations on incidence of IBD from Northern China to Southern China may indicate a geographic difference. Guangzhou is located in Southern China on the Pearl River, having a humid subtropical climate, with a typical diet of seafood. Wuhan is located in Southern China at the intersection of the middle branches of the Yangtze and Han rivers, having humid subtropical climate with abundant rainfall. In contrast, Daqing is located in Northeastern China, known as the Oil Capital of China in the northern temperate zone, with a humid continental climate. Generally, winter is bitterly cold with occasional snowfalls, and spring and autumn are prevailed by monsoons. Therefore, there are many differences between Northern and Southern China including periods of sunshine, climate, diet, lifestyle, living conditions etc. However, this study provided no evidence to suggest which geographic features or environmental factors are responsible for the differences in incidence of IBD between Southern and Northern China. Although China has a large population of 1.3 billion, the incidence of IBD in China is obviously lower than that in western countries. IBD will place a heavy burden on medical costs, insurance, and quality of health care due to high relapse and remission rate of IBD patients.

Our study did not find the gender difference of UC occurrence, the ratio of male to female is 1.1:1, which is difference from the other studies [11–13]. Also, it is hard to estimate the gender difference of CD occurrence because only 2 cases were found in one year. In western countries, UC was found more frequently in

Table 3. Age-standardized incidence rate (per 100,000) of IBD overall, CD, and UC in North of China.

	N	age-standardized incidence(per 100,000 persons)(95%CI)		
		Total	Male	Femal
IBD	27	1.77(1.16–2.59)	1.96(1.06–3.30)	1.58(0.84–2.70)
UC	25	1.64(1.06–2.43)	1.70(0.87–2.99)	1.58(0.82–2.70)
CD	2	0.13(0.02–0.47)	0.25(0.03–0.91)	0.00(0.00–0.54)

Table 4. Clinical characteristics of new cases of IBD in North of China.

	UC(n = 25)	CD(n = 2)
Symptom(%)		
Abdominal pain	13(52.0)	2(100.0)
Diarrhea	15(60.0)	0(0.0)
Constipation	3(12.0)	1(50.0)
Bloody stool	14(56.0)	0(0.0)
Mucus	15(60.0)	0(0.0)
Median time from symptom onset to diagnosis(range)	7.0(1–48)	61.0(2–120)
Extra-intestinal manifestations (%)		
Arthralgia	2(8.0)	1(50.0)
Skin rashes	1(4.0)	0(0.0)
Eye disease	1(4.0)	0(0.0)
Ankylosing spondylitis (%)	0(0.0)	0(0.0)
Promarysclerosing cholangitis(%)	0(0.0)	0(0.0)
Severity of UC(%)		
Mild	14(56.0)	1(50.0)
Moderate	11(44.0)	1(50.0)
Severe	0(0.0)	0(0.0)

men (60%), whereas CD is 20%–30% more frequent in women [11–13]. Also, a similar male predominance of IBD was reported in the Southern Chinese population (male to female: 1.58 to 1 in UC and 2.4:1 in CD) [7]. Due to low numbers of new cases in this study, it is difficult to analyze the detailed reasons for different gender trends in IBD in China and the real gender predominance under different physiological age groups.

In this study, the analysis of clinical characteristics of new IBD cases in the Northern Chinese population showed that diarrhea and abdominal pain were the most common symptoms in UC, which was similar to that of the Southern Chinese population. The main disease phenotype in UC patients is left-side colitis (56%) followed by proctitis (24%), which was also similar to that in the Southern Chinese population (41.9% for left-side colitis, 35.5% for proctitis in Guangzhou; 41% for left-side colitis, 35% for proctitisin Wuhan). 5 patients (18.5%) showed extra-intestinal manifestations of IBD in the Northern Chinese population, which is less common compared to the study in Guangzhou in Southern China (38%). In addition, the severity of IBD in the Northern Chinese population was not as severe as that in the Southern Chinese population, such that no patient with severe IBD was observed in the Northern population, but 6.5% severe activity was observed in UC in the Southern Chinese population. We also observed significant differences in the median diagnostic age (48 years in UC, 39 years in CD in Northern Chinese population *vs.* 40.6 years in UC, and 25.5 years in CD in Southern Chinese population and the duration from symptom onset to diagnosis (61 months in CD and 7 months in UC in Northern Chinese population *vs.* 25.6 months in CD and 17.3 months in Southern

Chinese population) was different between Northern and Southern Chinese populations.

The major strengths of this study are the prospective population-based design, large sample size, and the completeness of IBD ascertainment and definition. However, this study still has some potential weaknesses. Although there is a well-established health care insurance system in Daqing, some patients do not take care of their health to see the doctor even though they have gastrointestinal symptoms, while some patients are more willing to acquire diagnosis and treatment from other cities with more skilled medical specialists. These problems may lead to possible selection bias and an underestimation in the proposed incidences. Understanding the most common clinical characteristics in different geographic areas may provide insights into possible etiologies of IBD. All of these observations highlight the need to compare environmental, dietary, and genotypic data in the future in different regions worldwide.

Acknowledgments

The study group is extremely grateful for substantial support from the contributed hospitals and the specialists. And the study group is appreciated to professor Hu for providing the Figure 1.

Author Contributions

Conceived and designed the experiments: JQ PH HHL. Performed the experiments: HY YL WW QS YZ WZ HL QX. Analyzed the data: HY. Contributed reagents/materials/analysis tools: HY YL JQ. Wrote the paper: HY JQ.

References

1. Molodecky NA, Soon IS, Rabi DM, Ghali WA, Ferris M, et al. (2012) Increasing incidence and prevalence of the inflammatory bowel disease with time, Based on systematic review. Gastroenterology 142:46–54.

2. Harvey RF, Bradshaw JM (1980) A simple index of Crohn's disease activity. Lancet 1:514.

3. Molodecky NA, Kaplan GG (2010) Environmental risk factors for inflammatory bowel disease. Gastroenterology hepatoloty 6:339–346.

4. Green C, Elliott L, Beaudoin C, Bernstein CN (2006) A population-based ecologic study of inflammatory bowel disease: searching for etiologic clues. Am J Epidemiol 164:615–23.

5. Lakatos PL (2006) Recent trends in the epidemiology of inflammatory bowel diseases: up or down? World J Gastroenterol 12:6102–8.

6. Ng SC, BernsteinCN VatnMH, Lakatos PL, Loftus EV Jr, et al. (2013) Geographical variability and environmental risk factors in inflammatory bowel disease. Gut62:630–649.

7. Zeng Z, Zhu Z, Yang Y, Ruan W, Peng X, et al. (2013) Incidence and clinical characteristics of inflammatory bowel disease in a developed region of Guangdong Province, China: a prospective population-based study. J GastroenterolHepatol 28:1148–53.

8. Zhao J, Ng SC, Lei Y, Yi F, Li J, et al. (2013) First prospective, population-based inflammatory bowel disease incidence study in mainland of China: the emergence of "western" disease. Inflamm Bowel Dis, 19:1839–45.

9. Loftus EV Jr (2004) Clinical epidemiology of inflammatory bowel disease:incidence, prevalence, and environmental influences. Gastroenterology 126:1504–1517.

10. Silverberg MS, Satsangi J, Ahmad T, Arnott ID, Bernstein CN, et al. (2005) Toward an integrated clinical, molecular and serological classification of inflammatory bowel disease:Report of a working party of the 2005 Montreal World Congress of Gastroenterology. Can J Gastroenterol 19(suppl A):5–36.

11. Prideaux L, Kamm MA, DeCruz PP, Chan FK, Ng SC (2012) Inflammatory bowel disease in Asia: a systematic review. J Gastroenterol Hepatol 27:1266–1280.

12. Kappelman MD, Rifas-Shiman SL, Kleinman K, Ollendorf D, Bousvaros A (2007) The prevalence and geographic distribution of Crohn's disease and ulcerative colitis in the United States. ClinGastroenterolHepatol 5:1424–1429.

13. Bernstein CN, Wajda A, Svenson LW, Mackenzie A, Koehoorn M (2006) The epidemiology of inflammatory bowel disease in Canada: a population-based study. Am J Gastroenterol 101:1559–1568.

7

Thrombospondin-1 Type 1 Repeats in a Model of Inflammatory Bowel Disease: Transcript Profile and Therapeutic Effects

Zenaida P. Lopez-Dee[1¤], Sridar V. Chittur[2], Bhumi Patel[1], Rebecca Stanton[1], Michelle Wakeley[1], Brittany Lippert[1], Anastasya Menaker[1], Bethany Eiche[1], Robert Terry[1], Linda S. Gutierrez[1]*

1 Department of Biology, Wilkes University, Wilkes-Barre, Pennsylvania, United States of America, 2 Center for Functional Genomics, University at Albany, State University of New York, Rensselaer, New York, United States of America

Abstract

Thrombospondin-1 (TSP-1) is a matricellular protein with regulatory functions in inflammation and cancer. The type 1 repeats (TSR) domains of TSP-1 have been shown to interact with a wide range of proteins that result in the anti-angiogenic and anti-tumor properties of TSP-1. To ascertain possible functions and evaluate potential therapeutic effects of TSRs in inflammatory bowel disease, we conducted clinical, histological and microarray analyses on a mouse model of induced colitis. We used dextran sulfate sodium (DSS) to induce colitis in wild-type (WT) mice for 7 days. Simultaneously, mice were injected with either saline or one form of TSP-1 derived recombinant proteins, containing either (1) the three type 1 repeats of the TSP-1 (3TSR), (2) the second type 1 repeat (TSR2), or (3) TSR2 with the RFK sequence (TSR2+RFK). Total RNA isolated from the mice colons were processed and hybridized to mouse arrays. Array data were validated by real-time qPCR and immunohistochemistry. Histological and disease indices reveal that the mice treated with the TSRs show different patterns of leukocytic infiltration and that 3TSR treatment was the most effective in decreasing inflammation in DSS-induced colitis. Transcriptional profiling revealed differentially expressed (DE) genes, with the 3TSR-treated mice showing the least deviation from the WT-water controls. In conclusion, this study shows that 3TSR treatment is effective in attenuating the inflammatory response to DSS injury. In addition, the transcriptomics work unveils novel genetic data that suggest beneficial application of the TSR domains in inflammatory bowel disease.

Editor: Anthony W. I. Lo, The Chinese University of Hong Kong, Hong Kong

Funding: This work was supported by grants from the National Institutes of Health (DK067901-12 02), the Howard Hughes Medical Institute (grant # 52006328) and a Wilkes Mentoring grant. The funders had no role in study design, data collection and analysis, decision to publish, or preparation of the manuscript.

Competing Interests: The authors have declared that no competing interests exist.

* E-mail: linda.gutierrez@wilkes.edu

¤ Current address: Department of Basic Sciences, The Commonwealth Medical College, Scranton, Pennsylvania, United States of America

Introduction

Thrombospondins (TSPs) are glycoproteins that are secreted into the extracellular matrix. They have important functions in development, inflammation, angiogenesis and cancer. The five members of this family (TSP-1 through 5) are all multimodular extracellular proteins. TSP-1 comprises a 450 kDA protein composed of three 150 kDA disulfide-linked polypeptide chains [1,2]. TSP-1 and TSP-2 organize into trimeric structures. Each subunit of the trimer consists of multiple domains: an N-terminal globular domain, a procollagen domain, three types of repeated sequence motifs (type 1, type 2, and type 3 repeats) and a C-terminal globular domain. TSP-1 and TSP-2 both have the thrombospondin type 1 repeat, also called thrombospondin structural repeats (TSRs). TSP-3, TSP-4 and TSP-5, on the other hand, lack the TSRs and procollagen domain; they also differ from TSP-1 and TSP-2 in their pentameric structure. The thrombospondins have been characterized in a variety of organisms, including Drosophila, other arthropods and vertebrates [3].

The TSRs are about 60 amino acids in length and are evolutionarily conserved (e.g., [2], [3–5]). TSRs have roles in cell attachment and have been implicated in binding a variety of transmembrane and extracellular proteins. They have been shown also to have functions in the regulation of cell proliferation, migration and apoptosis in a variety of physiological and pathological events, such as wound healing, inflammation and inhibition of angiogenesis [6]. For example, by interacting with CD36 [7,8] and integrins [9], TSRs inhibit endothelial cell migration.

The various functions of the TSRs have been attributed to several recognition motifs. Characterization of these motifs has led to the use of recombinant proteins that contain these motifs; these recombinant proteins are deemed useful in cancer therapy [10,11]. The TSP-1 3TSR (that is, all three TSRs of the type 1 repeat domain) can activate transforming growth factor beta 1 (TGFβ1) and inhibit endothelial cell migration, angiogenesis, and tumor growth [10,12]. In an efficacy study of 3TSR on human pancreatic cancer cells, 3TSR reduced tumor volume by 69% and induced extensive necrosis after 3 weeks of treatment. 3TSR treatment also reduced tumor microvessel density and increased apoptosis in the endothelia of tumors [12].

The TGFβ1 activating sequence RFK is located between the first and second TSR. When a squamous cell carcinoma cell line transfected with TSR2+RFK was injected into nude mice, TSR2+RFK inhibited *in vivo* tumor angiogenesis and growth in the mice. The tumors were shown to have increased levels of active TGFβ1. Treatment with TSR2 without RFK produced tumors that were slightly larger than the 3TSR and TSR2+RFK tumors [13]. However, mimetic peptides derived from TSR2, such as ABT-510 [14], decreased microvessel density and increased apoptosis in gliomas. ABT-510 was also effective in diminishing inflammation and angiogenesis in a murine model of inflammatory bowel disease (IBD) [15].

In this study, we evaluated the therapeutic effects of the subdomains of the TSP-1 TSRs using the DSS model of colitis and used a microarray approach to analyze the transcript profile of the mice treated with DSS and the TSRs. Our goals were to gain insight into the genes and pathways that are regulated upon TSR treatment and to determine the specific TSR treatment that would have the best potential for drug therapy. We were also interested in identifying novel genes not yet associated with and characterized in IBD, as well as putative intestinal stem cell genes. The results herein establish the efficacy of the 3TSR-containing recombinant protein in alleviating the inflammatory response to DSS injury as shown by improved clinical signs and lower perturbation of the transcriptome.

Materials and Methods

Mice

Wild-type (WT) mice (strain C57BL/6; n = 48) were purchased from Charles River Laboratories International (Wilmington, MA). Mice were bred at room temperature at the Wilkes University vivarium. All animal procedures were performed with the approval of the Wilkes University Institutional Animal Care and Use Committee and the U.S. National Institutes of Health (NIH) guidelines (Wilkes IACUC protocol # 189).

Dextran sulfate sodium (DSS) and TSR Treatments

DSS (MW: 36,000~50,000) (MP Biomedical, LLC, Aurora, OH) was dissolved in the drinking water (distilled) of the mice at a dilution of 2.5% (wt/vol) and administered to 6–7 week old mice for 7 days to induce acute colitis. Simultaneously, mice were subcutaneously injected daily with the following recombinant proteins: 3TSR (n = 10), TSR2 (n = 9) TSR2+RFK (n = 15). TSR doses were administered according to published results [10]. As a control for the TSR treatment, mice (n = 14) were injected with saline. Following 7 days of DSS administration, mice were sacrificed by CO_2 asphyxiation.

Recombinant proteins were obtained from Dr. Jack Lawler (Harvard Medical School, Boston, MA). The 3TSR contains amino acids 361–530 of TSP-1; TSR2, amino acids 416–473; TSR2+RFK, amino acids 411–473 [10].

Clinical parameters and Disease Activity Indices

The clinical severity of the colitis was determined daily by disease activity indices according to a published protocol [15]. Stool consistency was evaluated as follows: formed feces = 1, soft consistency = 2 and liquid feces = 3. Presence of fecal occult blood was tested using the stool guaiac test; scoring was done as follows: 1 for negative by guaiac paper, 2 for positive only with guaiac paper, 3 for bloody feces.

Histology and inflammation grading in colonic tissues

Intestines were removed, opened longitudinally, and rinsed with ice-cold PBS. For morphologic studies, tissues were fixed in Histochoice MB fixative (Electron Microscopic Sciences, Hatfield,

PA) overnight, processed and cut in serial 5-µm sections. Sections were stained with hematoxylin and eosin (H&E) for histopathological analysis. Inflammation was graded as follows: 0, no inflammation; 1, modest numbers of infiltrating leukocytes in the lamina propria; 2, infiltration of leukocytes leading to separation of crypts and mild mucosal hyperplasia; 3, massive infiltration of inflammatory cells accompanied by disrupted mucosal architecture and complete loss of goblet cells. Slides were double-coded before pictures were taken and frames blindly analyzed in a monitor.

RNA isolation

Colon segments (~1 cm long) were collected from treated and untreated mice and snap-frozen in liquid nitrogen. Total RNA was extracted from these tissues using the RNAqueous®-4PCR kit (Applied Biosystems), following the manufacturer's instructions. RNA was DNase I-treated and quantified using the Nanodrop ND1000 spectrometer (Thermo Scientific, Wilmington, DE). RNA integrity was checked on a non-denaturing agarose gel. The microarray experiments are described in the following sections following the MIAME guidelines.

Microarray Processing

Total RNA from colons of at least three mice from each treatment group were submitted to the Center for Functional Genomics, University at Albany, Rensselaer, New York, for microarray processing. Treatment groups included the mice treated with DSS and the TSR-containing recombinant proteins 3TSR, TSR2 and TSR2+RFK and mice treated with DSS+ saline injections as controls. Untreated WT were used as additional control. RNA integrity of the samples used for microarray hybridization was verified using Agilent's 2100 Bioanalyzer (Santa Clara, CA). The Affymetrix (Santa Clara, CA) Mouse Gene 1.0 ST Array was used for the transcript profiling. 20 ng total RNA per sample was processed using WT Ovation Pico RNA Amplification System (NuGEN Technologies, Inc., San Carlos, CA). Sense target cDNAs were generated using the standard NuGEN WT protocol and hybridized to the arrays. Arrays were washed, stained on a FS 450 station and scanned on a GeneChip 3000 7G scanner using GeneChip® Command Console® Software (AGCC).

Statistical Analysis

Statistical analysis of the CEL files was done using GeneSpring GX 11.5.1 (Agilent Technologies). Signals were quantile-normalized using PLIER16 algorithm and baseline-transformed to the median of all samples. The log2 normalized signal values were filtered to remove entities that show signal in the bottom 20th percentile across all samples. This list was further filtered to only include entities where at least 1 out of 6 conditions have CV<20.0% (that is, to remove probes that are highly variable across replicates in a condition). The list was then subjected to ANOVA (p<0.05) that compares all conditions to the WT-water or WT-DSS saline condition. A Benjamini-Hochberg False Discovery Rate correction (p<0.05) was also included in the analysis. A 1.5-fold filter was applied to identify genes that are differentially expressed between any two specific conditions. Microarray data have been deposited in the Gene Expression Omnibus (GEO) database under accession number GSE32697.

Real-Time Quantitative PCR Validation of Array Data

Real-time quantitative PCR (RT-qPCR) was performed on colonic total RNA isolated from another set of three mice. To obtain cDNAs, RNAs (2 ug) were reverse-transcribed using the High Capacity RNA-to-cDNA Kit (Applied Biosystems). This was followed by amplification of the undiluted cDNAs with the Fast SYBR Green master mix (Applied Biosystems) and real-time quantification in the StepOne Plus Real-time PCR system. Amplification was performed with 40 cycles of 95°C for 3 sec, and 60°C for 30 sec, using 150 nM of each primer.

The use of *Gapdh* as endogenous control gene in the RT-qPCR validation was problematic with samples that were treated with the recombinant proteins. Preliminary qPCR runs showed fluctuating levels of *Gapdh* among the TSR-treated samples. *Ubc*, *Gapdh*, *Rps23* and *Tpt1* have been evaluated for suitability as internal control in colon cancer studies [16]. Using the GeneMANIA [17] prediction server (www.genemania.org), we found that *Gapdh* interacts with *Igfbp5* (Figure S2). Our array data shows that *Igfbp5* is up-regulated in WT-DSS mice. The *Gapdh-Igfbp5* interaction suggests co-expression and could explain the high variability of *Gapdh* expression in our samples. On the other hand, query of *Tpt1* in GeneMANIA showed that it is unrelated to any of our genes of interest.

For the RT-qPCR validation, we selected (1) representative genes from the major pathways that are activated as a response to inflammation, (2) genes that code for acute phase proteins, and (3) genes that have not been extensively characterized, especially in IBD. The genes validated are: calcyphosine-like (*Capsl*), carbonyl reductase 3 (*Cbr3*), CXC chemokine ligand 5 (*Cxcl5*), epiregulin (*Ereg*), haptoglobin (*Hp*), inhibin A (*InhbA*), pentraxin related gene (*Ptx3*), insulin-like growth factor binding protein 5 (*Igfbp5*), matrix metallopeptidase 10 (*Mmp10*, also known as stromelysin-2), *Mmp13*, WAP four-disulfide core domain 12 (*Wfdc12*), serglycin (*Srgn*), Serine (or cysteine) peptidase inhibitor, clade A, member 3N (*Serpina3N*), formyl peptide receptor (*Fpr3*) and leucine-rich repeat-containing G-protein coupled receptor (*Lgr5*). Expression levels of the 15 genes were normalized to the internal control, *Tpt1* (tumor protein, translationally-controlled 1). The $2^{\wedge}$-ddCt method was used to quantify the expression levels of the genes. Details on the reference and target genes are given in the Table S1.

Immunohistochemistry (IHC)

IHC sections were incubated overnight with the following antibodies: cluster of differentiation 31 (CD31) and Ly-6G/Ly-6C (RB6-8C5) (BD Pharmingen, San Diego, CA), mouse panendothelial cell antigen (MECA-32) (BioLegend, San Diego, CA), Interleukin-6 (IL-6), cluster of differentiation 68 (Mac/CD68) and metalloproteinase 3 (MMP3) (Santa Cruz Biotechnologies Inc. Santa Cruz, CA), LGR5 and Calgranulin MRP8/S100A9 (Epitomics, Burlingame, CA). Sections were further incubated with biotinylated anti-rabbit, anti-goat or anti-rat IgG IMPRESS (Vector Laboratories, Burlingame, CA) respectively for 30 minutes. Finally, color was developed using a 3,3′-diaminobenzidine substrate kit (BD Pharmingen).

Evaluation of microvascular density (MVD)

MVD was determined in colon sections of the treated mice. Sections stained with CD31/MECA antibodies were screened for colitic lesions. Serial pictures were taken at high power (×400) using a digital camera (Olympus Corporation, Tokyo, Japan), covering both mucosa and submucosa. Images were blindly evaluated; MVD was assessed by counting the vessels in lesions in which endothelial cells were positive for MECA/CD31.

Evaluation of leukocytic infiltration

Slides stained with antibodies CD68 for macrophages and Ly-6G/Ly-6C for granulocytes were scanned at low magnification

and examined for areas with the highest number of leukocytic infiltration. The number of positive cells stained with Mac/CD68 or Ly-6G/Ly-6C was assessed at 400× magnification per field.

Results

Only 3TSR ameliorated clinical signs of colitis in the DSS-induced colitis

The presence of fecal blood was evaluated and rated in mice with DSS-induced colitis and treated with the TSRs (Figure 1A). While no significant differences were observed during the first 5 days of treatment, by days 6 and 7, 3TSR mice showed lesser fecal bleeding when compared with mice treated with saline, TSR2 and TSR2+RFK (day 6, 3TSR and saline p = 0.020; day 7, 3TSR and saline p = 0.045). Fecal consistency was also evaluated daily (Figure 1B). Again, by day 7, 3TSR mice displayed more solid feces compared to the liquid feces of saline-treated mice (p<0.0001) and TSR2+RFK (p<0.0001). TSR2 and TSR2+RFK mice showed more severe diarrhea than the controls (p<0.0001). Inflammation and epithelial injury were significantly decreased in colons of the 3TSR mice when compared with the saline-treated mice (p = 0.001) (Figure 1C). Differences between 3TSR and the other two recombinant proteins were statistically significant (3TSR and TSR2+RFK: p = 0.034; 3TSR and TSR2: p = 0.025) (Figure 1D).

Angiogenesis was not inhibited by the TSRs

By using CD31/Meca stained slides, endothelial cells lining blood vessels were analyzed in colonic sections (Figure S1) from the treated mice. Vessel counts were not statistically different across the treatments (p = 0.074; 3TSR, n = 29, vessels = 21.48±2.1 and TSR2+RFK, n = 35, vessels = 21.4±1.5). However, colonic sections from TSR2 mice showed a trend for lower counts (n = 20, vessels = 19.45±2.7) when compared to saline-treated colons (n = 16, vessels = 26.62±4.0) (Figure S1).

Colonic tissues from TSR-treated mice showed differential patterns of leukocytic infiltration

Sections stained with the antibody Ly-6G/Ly-6C were evaluated to identify granulocytes and monocytes (Figure 2A). Colonic sections from 3TSR- and TSR2-treated mice showed counts considerably lower than saline-treated colons, (with p = 0.030 and 0.047, respectively) (Figure 2B). Interestingly, counts obtained from the TSR2+RFK-treated colons were similar to the ones detected in saline-treated colons. The differences between TSR2 and TSR2+RFK were statistically significant (p = 0.021).

Macrophage infiltration was analyzed using Mac/CD68 antibody staining (Figure 2C). Though no differences were detected when each group was compared with the saline control, TSR2+RFK mice showed a significantly lower influx of macrophages compared with the controls and the TSR2 and 3TSR groups (p = 0.0006) (Figure 2D).

TSR treatment reduced the number of differentially expressed genes in the DSS induced colitis

Coincident treatment with 3TSR, TSR2+RFK and TSR2 show diminishing numbers of DE genes, with 3TSR showing the least number of DE genes (Figure 3A) when compared to either controls, WT-water or WT-DSS saline. The general trend of number of DE genes (when compared to WT-water) is as follows: WT-DSS-TSR2>WT-DSS-TSR2+RFK>WT-DSS-3TSR>WT-DSS-saline (Figure 3A). A heatmap of the top DE genes, eight up-regulated and four down-regulated, is shown in Figure 3B and the gene list is

A.

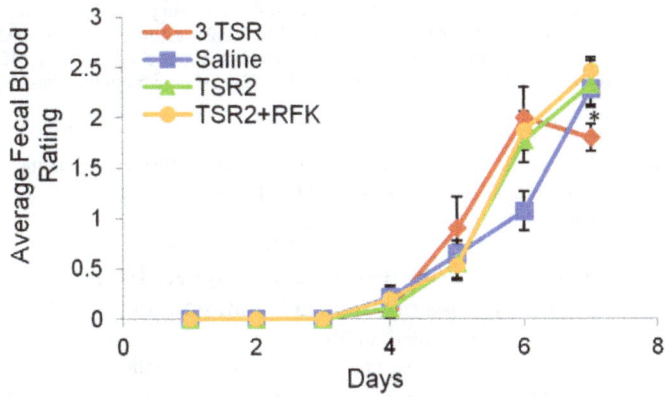

B.

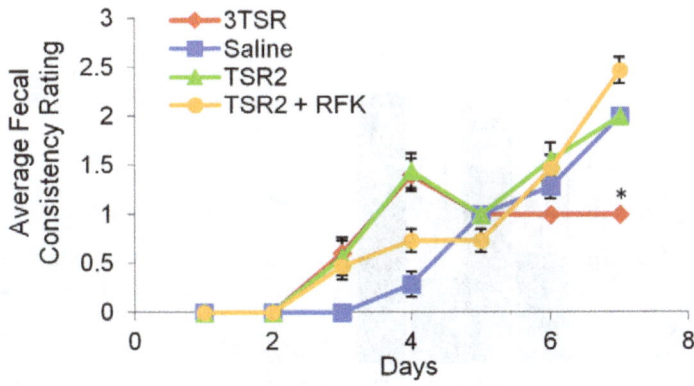

C.

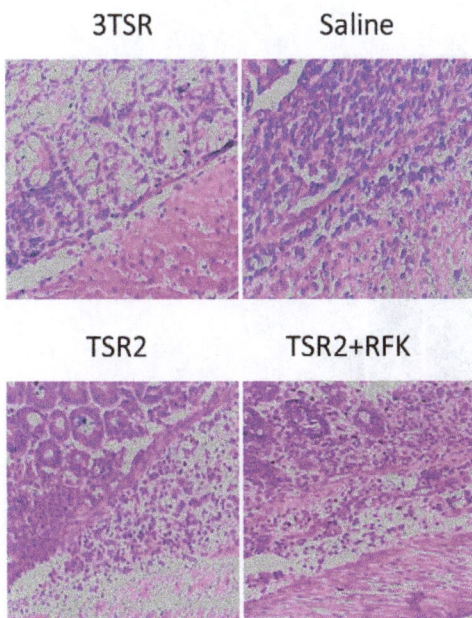

D.

Inflammation grade

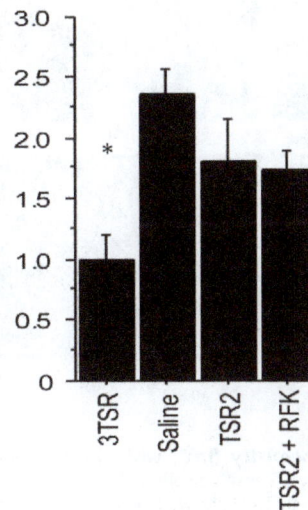

Figure 1. Fecal blood and consistency rating in mice treated with DSS and TSRs over one week. While no significant differences were observed during the first days of treatment, by days 6 and 7, mice treated with the 3TSR (n = 10) showed lesser fecal bleeding when compared with mice treated with the saline (n = 14), TSR2 (n = 9) and TSR2+RFK (n = 15), (day 6: p = 0.02; day 7: p = 0.045, asterisk) (A). Fecal consistency was also evaluated daily (B). By day 7, 3TSR mice displayed more solid feces compared to the liquid feces of saline-treated mice (p<0.0001, asterisk) and TSR2+RFK (p<0.0001). Inflammation grading (C, D) was assessed and H&E stained sections. Decreased inflammation was observed in sections of colons from 3TSR-treated mice (n = 9) compared to colons from mice treated with TSR2+RFK (n = 12), TSR2 (n = 10) and saline (n = 7). 400× original magnification.

presented in Table 1. Focusing on the 3TSR, only 43 genes were up-regulated and two genes were down-regulated in the 3TSR vs WT-DSS saline comparison. Figure 3C presents a heatmap of the top 14 DE genes in this pair. The numbers of up- and down-regulated genes in the 3TSR treatment group diminished when compared to either TSR2 or TSR+RFK (Figures 3D and 3E). Table 2 presents the top 12 genes that are up-regulated in the 3TSR-treated group and the two down-regulated genes, using the WT-DSS-saline as reference. Although some genes involved in the inflammatory response were up-regulated in 3TSR, their level of up-regulation was much lower

than in the other TSR treatment groups. The complete list of differentially expressed genes (FC>1.5; p<0.1) is provided in the Table S2.

DSS and the TSR treatments up-regulated key genes involved in inflammation, cell adhesion and apoptosis

Genes up-regulated in the DSS and TSR-treatment groups belong to the following pathways: (1) matrix metalloproteinases, (2) inflammatory response, (3) peptide GPCRs, (4) eicosanoid/prostaglandin synthesis regulation, (5) TGF-beta signaling, (6)

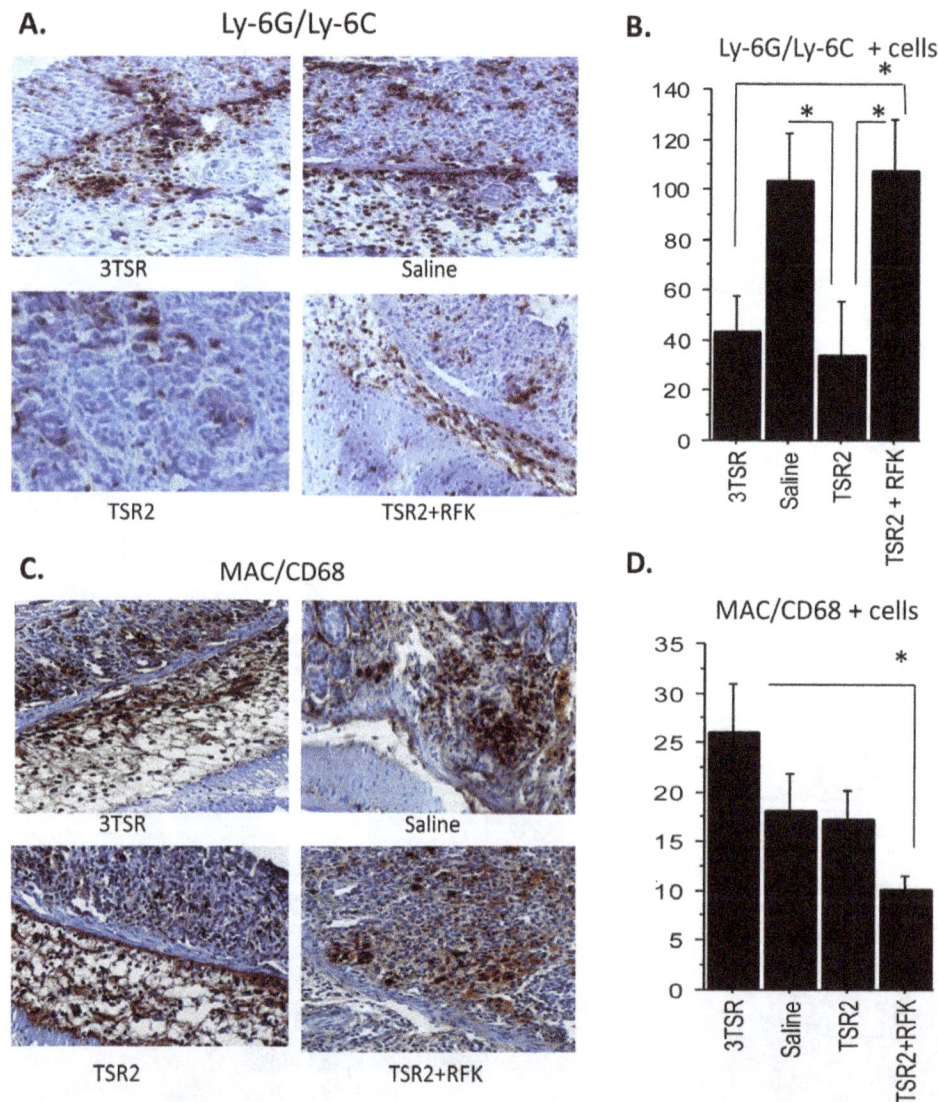

Figure 2. Immunohistochemistry (IHC) with the Ly-6G/Ly-6C antibody for detection of granulocytes and monocytes in colitic sections. Counts of Ly-6G/Ly-6C positive cells in TSR2 and 3TSR were considerably lower than in saline (n = 5 in each group) and TSR2+RFK-treated (n = 9) colons (A). However, only TSR2 showed lower counts that were statistically significant, p = 0.047 (B). IHC against Mac/CD68 (C) showed fewer CD68 positive cells (macrophages) in TSR2+RFK (n = 24) compared to TSR2 (n = 14) and saline (n = 18). These differences were statistically significant, p = 0.0006, when compared with 3TSR-treated (n = 18) colons (D). 400× magnification.

A.

	Total DE Genes
vs [WT-water]	
[WT-DSS-TSR2]	199
[WT-DSS-TSR2+RFK]	141
[WT-DSS-3TSR]	106
[WT-DSS saline]	65
vs [WT-DSS saline]	
[WT-DSS-TSR2]	163
[WT-DSS-TSR2+RFK]	96
[WT-DSS-3TSR]	45

B.

C.

D.

E.

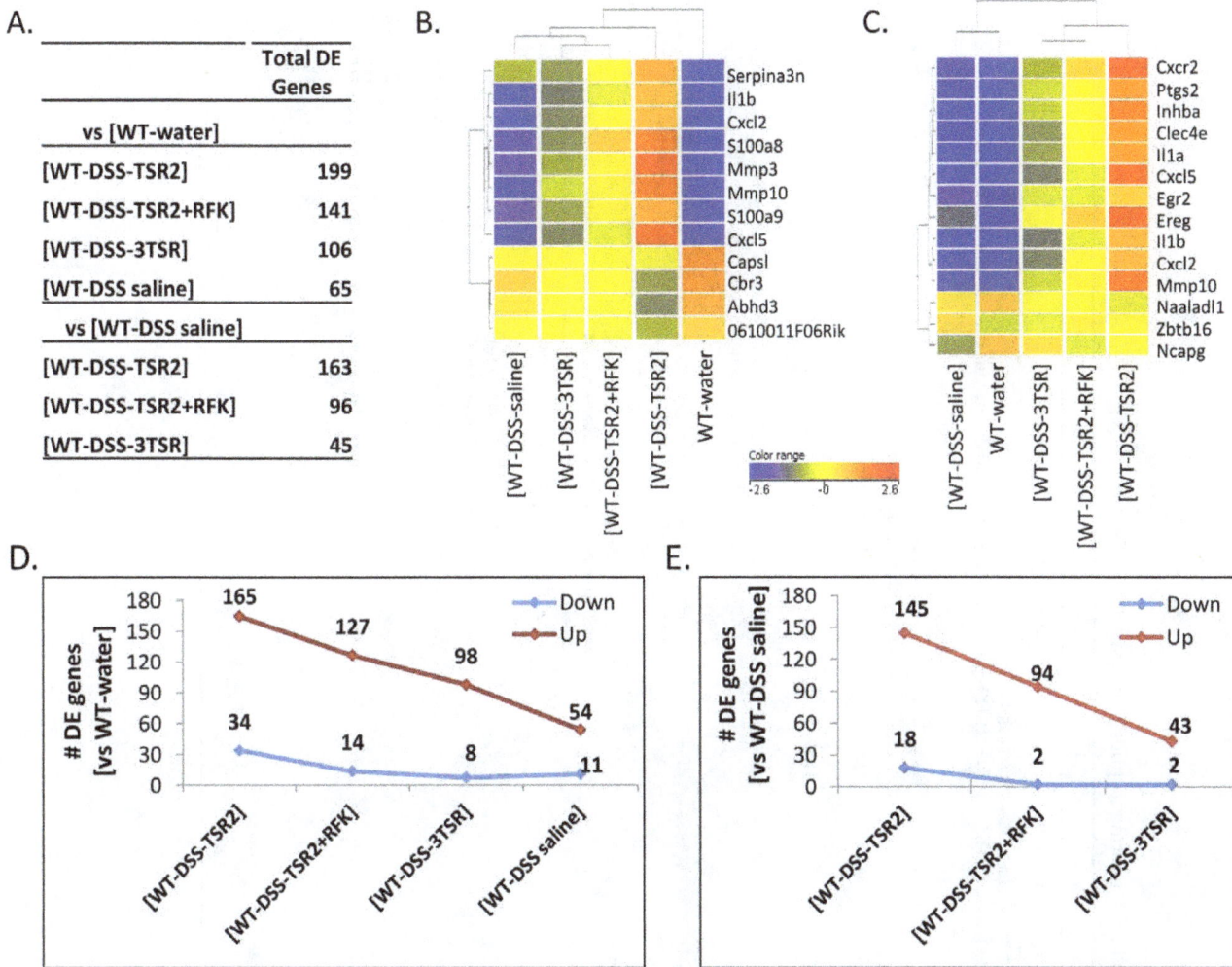

Figure 3. Differentially expressed genes in paired sets of comparison between the treatment and the control groups. Comparison of treatment groups with WT-water (A, upper panel of table) and WT-DSS saline controls (A, lower panel). Total DE genes refer to all genes that are up- or down-regulated by >1.5-fold at 95% confidence level. The 3TSR-treatment group clearly shows the least transcriptional perturbation among the TSR treatment groups. (B) A heatmap of the top 12 DE genes in the comparison that uses WT-water as the control. *Capsl*, *Cbr3*, *Abhd3* and *0610011F06Rik* are down-regulated in the TSR treatment groups. (C) A heatmap of the top DE genes in the 3TSR-treated group. The number of up- and down-regulated genes in the TSR treatment groups (when compared to the WT-water control) are presented in (D); (E) shows the breakdown of the DE genes in comparison to the WT-DSS saline.

smooth muscle contraction, (7) integrin-mediated cell adhesion and (8) apoptosis (Table 3). S100 calcium binding protein A9 (*S100a9*; also known as calgranulin B) had the highest transcript level in all treatment groups, with the WT-DSS group showing the highest FC (81), whereas the WT-DSS-3TSR has FC = 18 (Table S2). An inflammatory response was indicated by the high transcript levels of *Il-6* [WT-DSS-TSR2 (FC = 18)>WT-DSS-TSR2+RFK (FC = 7)>WT-DSS-3TSR (FC = 4)]. Chemokines, specifically *Cxcl2*, *Cxcl5*, *Cxcl13*, *Cxcl16*, *Ccl3* and *Ccl7*, were also up-regulated (FC = 2 to 60) in the treated samples. *Cxcl2*, in particular, had the greatest increase in the WT-DSS-TSR2 (FC = 55) compared to the other TSR-treated mice. Genes involved in inflammation and angiogenesis including *Adamts9*, *Tnf* alpha and the TNF receptor *Tnfrsf1b*, were enriched the most in the WT-DSS and WT-DSS-TSR2 groups.

Genes coding for proteins that are well known to interact with TSP-1 during inflammation were differentially expressed in DSS and TSR-treated mice, except in the 3TSR group. *Cd47* was only

slightly up-regulated in WT-DSS-TSR2 (1.8). It was not DE in TSR2+RFK and 3TSR. *Tgfβ1* was also slightly up-regulated in TSR2 (FC = 2.5) and TSR2+RFK (FC = 1.8), but not in 3TSR. None of the treatment samples showed differential expression of *Cd36*.

Real-time qPCR validation

Actual qPCR data revealed no fluctuation in expression of the internal control gene, *Tpt1*, which was consistent with the microarray data. We validated 15 DE genes to verify the array data. Figure 4 summarizes the validation for representative genes coding for acute phase proteins, growth factors and novel proteins. Validation for the metalloproteinases and genes coding for cytokines and a protein important for intestinal homeostasis are shown in Figure S3. Although *Srgn* and *Wfdc12* have p-values greater than 0.05, (*Srgn* p = 0.056, *Wfdc12* p = 0.065), the real-time qPCR validation shows that they are indeed differentially expressed.

Table 1. Top 12 differentially expressed genes (8 up- and 4 down-regulated) in the treatment groups compared to WT-water.

| Gene Name | Gene symbol | Refseq | Corrected p-value | Fold change (vs [WT-water]) | | | | Gene Ontology |
				[WT-DSS saline]	[WT-DSS 3TSR]	[WT-DSS-TSR2]	[WT-DSS-TSR2+RFK]	Biological process//Molecular function//Cellular component
Up-regulated genes								
S100 calcium binding protein A9 (calgranulin B)	S100a9	NM_009114	0.026	10.34	18.94	74.93	43.08	leukocyte chemotaxis/actin cytoskeleton reorganization/regulation of integrin biosynthetic process//calcium binding
S100 calcium binding protein A8 (calgranulin A)	S100a8	NM_013650	0.031	4.57	9.39	54.98	31.60	chemotaxis//calcium ion binding
Chemokine (C-X-C motif) ligand 2	Cxcl2	NM_009140	0.029	4.96	14.01	55.19	31.89	chemotaxis/inflammatory response/immune response/signal transduction//cytokine/chemokine activity//extracellular region/space
Matrix metallopeptidase 3	Mmp3	NM_010809	0.048	4.95	10.10	69.20	21.49	proteolysis/collagen catabolic process//catalytic/metalloendopeptidase/stromelysin 1 activity/calcium/Zn ion binding/hydrolase activity//proteinaceous extracellular matrix
Matrix metallopeptidase 10	Mmp10	NM_019471	0.036	4.54	17.11	74.14	29.54	proteolysis/metabolic/collagen catabolic process//catalytic/metalloendopeptidase activity/calcium/Zn binding/hydrolase/stromelysin 2 activity//proteinaceous extracellular matrix
Interleukin 1 beta	Il1b	NM_008361	0.030	3.07	9.59	39.65	15.96	fever/inflammatory/immune response/cell proliferation/neutrophil chemotaxis/positive regulation of I-kappaB kinase/NF-kappaB cascade/positive regulation of chemokine (IL-6) biosynthetic process/positive regulation of JNK cascade/leukocyte migration//IL-1 receptor binding/cytokine, growth factor activity//extracellular region/space
Chemokine (C-X-C motif) ligand 5	Cxcl5	NM_009141	0.030	1.30	3.33	24.56	5.37	chemotaxis/inflammatory/immune response/signal transduction//cytokine/chemokine activity//extracellular region/space
Serine (or cysteine) peptidase inhibitor, clade A, member 3N	Serpina3n	NM_009252	0.030	4.92	4.22	17.01	8.73	acute-phase response//serine-type endopeptidase inhibitor activity//extracellular region/space
Down-regulated genes								
Carbonyl reductase 3	Cbr3	NM_173047	0.044	−1.54	−2.22	−4.64	−2.31	metabolic process//carbonyl reductase (NADPH) activity/oxidoreductase activity//cytosol
Abhydrolase domain containing 3	Abhd3	NM_134130	0.046	−1.62	−2.13	−4.42	−2.43	no biological data available//carboxylesterase activity/hydrolase activity//integral to membrane
RIKEN cDNA 0610011F06 gene	0610011F06Rik	NM_026686	0.047	−1.55	−1.44	−2.63	−1.81	−−//methyltransferase activity/transferase activity
Calcyphosine-like	Capsl	NM_029341	0.028	−2.41	−2.26	−3.20	−2.93	−−//calcium ion binding//cytoplasm

Table 2. Top 14 differentially-expressed genes in the 3TSR group.

Gene name	Gene symbol Refseq	Corrected p-value	Fold change (vs [WT-DSS saline])				Pathway or [Gene Ontology]*
			[WT-DSS-3TSR]	[WT-DSS-TSR2+RFK]	[WT-DSS-TSR2]	[WT-water]	
Up-regulated							
Interleukin 1 alpha	Il1a NM_010554	0.036	3.84	6.97	15.18	−1.41	Inflammatory_Response_Pathway
Matrix metallopeptidase 10	Mmp10 NM_019471	0.036	3.77	6.51	16.33	−4.54	Matrix_Metalloproteinases
Inhibin beta-A	Inhba NM_008380	0.038	3.45	5.57	13.86	−1.40	TGF_Beta_Signaling_Pathway
Prostaglandin-endoperoxide synthase 2	Ptgs2 NM_011198	0.034	3.16	4.90	10.37	−1.59	Eicosanoid_Synthesis///Prostaglandin_synthesis_regulation
Interleukin 1 beta	Il1b NM_008361	0.030	3.13	5.21	12.94	−3.07	Inflammatory_Response_Pathway///Smooth_muscle_contraction
Chemokine (C-X-C motif) ligand 2	Cxcl2 NM_009140	0.029	2.82	6.43	11.12	−4.96	{inflammatory response/immune response/leukocyte/neutrophil chemotaxis///extracellular}
Epiregulin	Ereg NM_007950	0.039	2.68	3.84	8.80	−1.98	{angiogenesis///positive regulation of cytokine production//epidermal growth factor receptor signaling pathway}
Chemokine (C-X-C motif) ligand 5	Cxcl5 NM_009141	0.030	2.56	4.14	18.92	−1.30	{cytokine production///chemotaxis///inflammatory response//immune response}
Non-SMC condensin I complex, subunit G	Ncapg NM_019438	0.045	2.56	1.40	1.75	3.21	[no biological data available]
Chemokine (C-X-C motif) receptor 2	Cxcr2 NM_009909	0.040	2.55	6.18	16.62	−1.94	{apoptosis///chemotaxis///signal transduction//G-protein coupled receptor protein signaling pathway}
Early growth response 2	Egr2 NM_010118	0.038	2.45	2.49	5.05	−1.34	{regulation of ossification//response to insulin stimulus///positive regulation of transcription from RNA polymerase II promoter}
C-type lectin domain family 4, member e	Clec4e NM_019948	0.044	2.42	5.24	10.30	−1.51	{integral to membrane//sugar binding}
Down-regulated							
N-acetylated alpha-linked acidic dipeptidase-like 1	Naaladl1 NM_001009546	0.045	−1.55	−1.59	−1.84	1.26	{proteolysis///metallopeptidase activity//integral to membrane}
Zinc finger and BTB domain containing 16	Zbtb16 NM_001033324	0.038	−1.95	−1.22	−1.55	−2.13	{hemopoiesis///transcriptional repressor complex//protein C-terminus binding}

*The gene ontology is given, enclosed in brackets, where pathway has not been annotated in the microarray datasheet.

Table 3. Major pathways activated and genes enriched in the DSS- and TSR-treated mice.

Pathways	Genes up-regulated (fold change>2.0, p<0.05)
Matrix metalloproteinases	Matrix metallopeptidases 2, 3, 8, 10, 12, 13, 14
Inflammatory response	Interleukin 1 alpha (IL1a), IL1â, IL-6, Interleukin 4 receptor, alpha (Il4ra), Il1r2
Peptide GPCRs	Formyl peptide receptor 3 (Fpr3|2)
Eicosanoid/prostaglandin synthesis regulation	Prostaglandin-endoperoxide synthase 2 (Ptgs2)
TGF-beta signaling	Inhibin beta-A (Inhba)
Smooth muscle contraction	Insulin-like growth factor binding protein 5 (Igfbp5)
Blood clotting cascade/Wnt signaling	Plasminogen activator, urokinase (Plau)
Integrin-mediated cell adhesion	Integrins alpha M (Itgam), beta 2 (Itgb2), Itga4
Apoptosis	B-cell leukemia/lymphoma 2 related protein A1a (Bcl2a1a), Bcl2a1b, Bcl2a1c, Bcl2a1d; Tumor necrosis factor (Tnf), TNF receptor superfamily, member 1a (Tnfrsf1a), Tnfrsf1b
Ovarian Infertility Genes	Early growth response 2 (Egr2), CCAAT/enhancer binding protein (C/EBP), beta (Cebpb)

IHC validation of genes recognized in stem cell biology, cancer and inflammation

Array data show that *Lgr5*, an intestinal stem cell biomarker [18,19], was down-regulated in the TSR2-treated WT mice. *Lgr5* was not differentially expressed in the 3TSR and TSR2+RFK mice. However, results obtained in the RT-qPCR validation show that *Lgr5* was significantly down-regulated in the TSR2+RFK (Figure 4B).

MMP3, IL-6 and Calgranulin (MRP8) are relevant in angiogenesis and inflammation. Validation by IHC of these genes (Figure 5) showed the MMP3 protein localized in the cytoplasm of epithelial cells and endothelial cells. Strong positive staining for MMP3 was detected mainly in monocytes, polymorphonuclears, plasma and fibroblasts. Stromal staining was detected in the submucosa. Endothelial cells and the leukocytic infiltrate in inflamed areas were positive for IL-6. MRP8 staining was observed almost exclusively in polymorphonuclears.

Discussion

Our results indicate that 3TSR suppressed the inflammatory response induced by DSS injury and these data are supported by the array results. For pharmacological consideration, it is logical to assume that the lesser the perturbation of the transcriptome, the better the clinical outcome. Our results also confirm the finding that TSR2 is less effective than either 3TSR or TSR2+RFK [10]. 3TSR has been shown to induce endothelial cell apoptosis and inhibit tumor growth [11]. This function may be correlated to the modulation of VEGFR2 function by TSP-1 and 3TSR [20].

One of the unexpected findings when clinical parameters were evaluated was the severity of the bleeding and diarrhea in mice treated with TSR2 and TSR2+RFK. These results do not agree with previous studies using the ABT-510, a TSR2 mimetic peptide [15]. In the ABT-510 studies, osmotic mini-pumps were used for the continuous delivery of the peptide in contrast to the daily injections used in this study. Moreover, increased eNOS activity has been attributed to increased mucosal blood flow in induced colitis [21] and TSP-1 is known to regulate nitric oxide (NO) signaling [22]. Noteworthy is the lesser influx of granulocytes in the TSR2 mice compared to the TSR2+RFK and the 3TSR. This suggests that the TSR2 domain inhibits the influx of granulocytes independently of the RFK domain. TSR2 has been demonstrated to inhibit the secretion of NO during the acute phase of

inflammation, and therefore decreasing the trafficking of neutrophils [23]. On the other hand, RFK presumably inhibits inflammation by activating TGFß1. However, recent studies suggest that when there is a high secretion of IL-1 and IL-6, TGFß1 will favor the production of Th17 cells. Th17 cells secrete pro-inflammatory cytokines and metalloproteinases that exacerbate the inflammatory response [23].

Our array data showed that metalloproteases and chemokines such as MMP10, MMP13, the CCs and CXCs are involved in the pathogenesis of DSS colitis. Expression of *Cxcl2* and *Cxcl5* (Figure S3B), the proteins of which are known to target neutrophils and have suspected roles in IBD, was significantly increased in the DSS and TSR-treated mice during the acute phase of colitis. The increase in *Cxcl2* expression is the same observation reported for the leptin receptor-deficient mice that were treated with DSS [24]. An irregularity in chemokine signaling could jeopardize epithelial integrity, which could lead to the breakdown of defense against invading pathogens. Moreover, *Cxcl5* has a great potential in eliciting a pro-angiogenic phenotype [25].

The concentration of acute phase proteins is known to increase or decrease during inflammation. *Hp* and *Ptx3*, both of which are enriched in the DSS and TSR-treated mice, code for acute phase proteins. In a study of Hungarian patients with Crohn's disease (CD), *Hp* polymorphism was determined to be associated with CD and inflammatory disease behavior [26]. Hp has been suggested to have a protective role in inflammatory colitis [27]. *Ptx3* has been annotated to "positive regulation of nitric oxide biosynthetic process" and to "zymosan binding".

This study showed strong evidence for the alteration of gene expression in DSS-induced colitis that supports vulnerability to cancer. As an example, calgranulins, S100A8/A9 (calgranulins A and B, respectively), have been detected in various human cancers; hence they have been suggested to play a key role in inflammation-associated cancer [28]. They support epithelial barrier function and mediate responses to infection and inflammation [29] by amplifying pro-inflammatory responses [30]. In gastrointestinal epithelial cells, their expression is induced during inflammation and increased protein expression of S100A9 has been detected in colitis-related carcinogenesis in mice [31]. Key genes associated with colon tumor progression are reportedly activated by S100A8/A9 [32].

The 'novel' genes that we validated appear to have a role, one way or another, in inflammatory response and the promotion of inflammation-related cancer development. The function of these

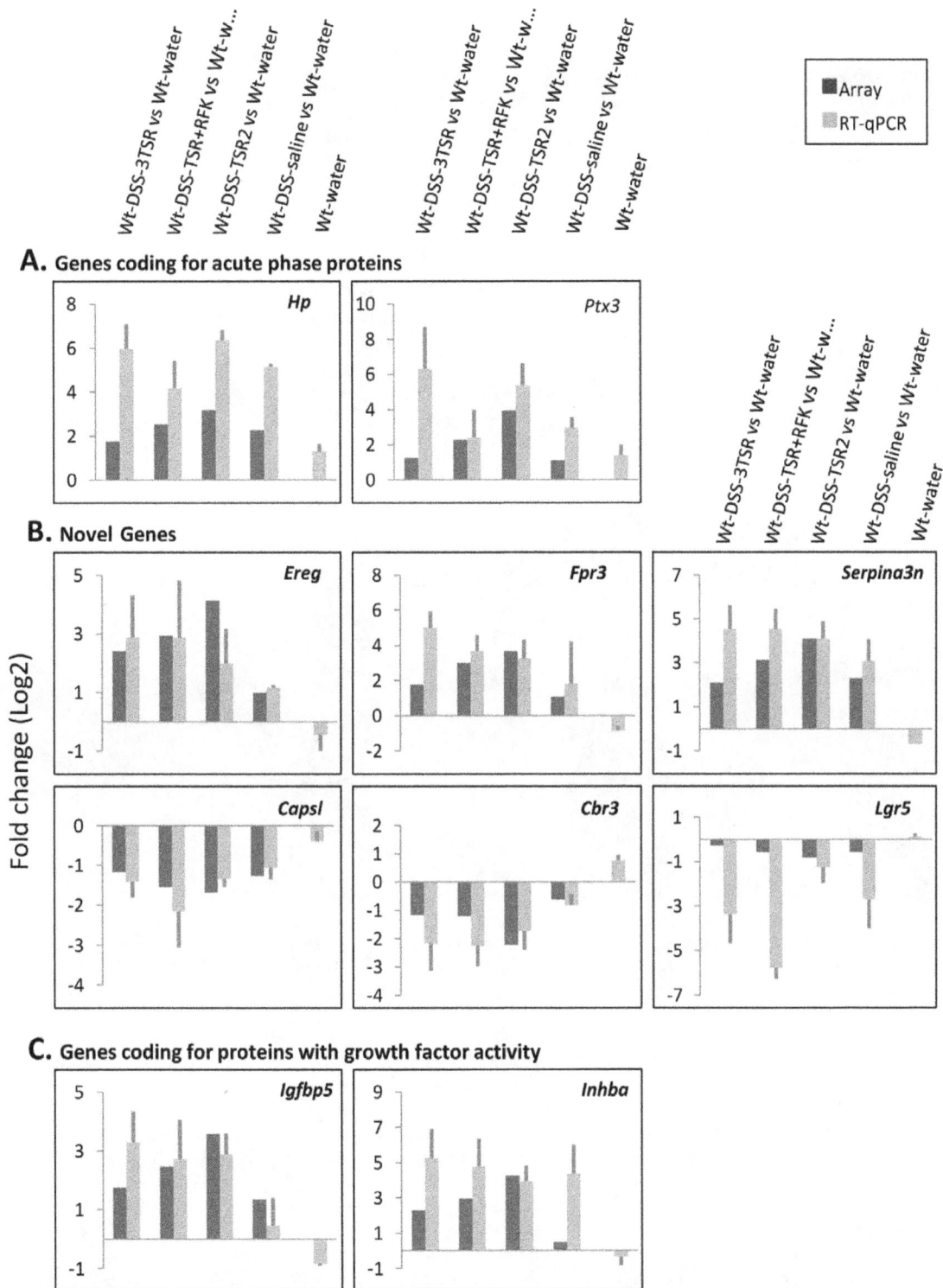

Figure 4. SyBR Green-based RT-qPCR validation of array data. Signal intensities were normalized to the endogenous control, *Tpt1*. Fold changes are the averages of three biological replicates different from those used in the microarrays. Linear FC values were log2-transformed. *Hp* and *Ptx3* code for acute phase proteins (A). We classified *Capsl*, *Cbr3*, *Ereg*, *Fpr3*, *Serpina3n* and *Lgr5* as novel genes (B) because they have not been characterized in IBD. Growth factors are clearly up-regulated (C).

genes as they relate to diseases and how these genes interact with other genes have not been extensively studied. The description ascribed to them in the gene ontology database, however, indicates some involvement in the development of physiological disorders.

Genome-wide association studies have identified *Capsl* to have association with type 1 diabetes [33] and the autoimmune thyroid disease Graves' disease [34]. *Cbr3*, an enzyme that reduces carbonyl groups in xenobiotics and endogenous compounds such

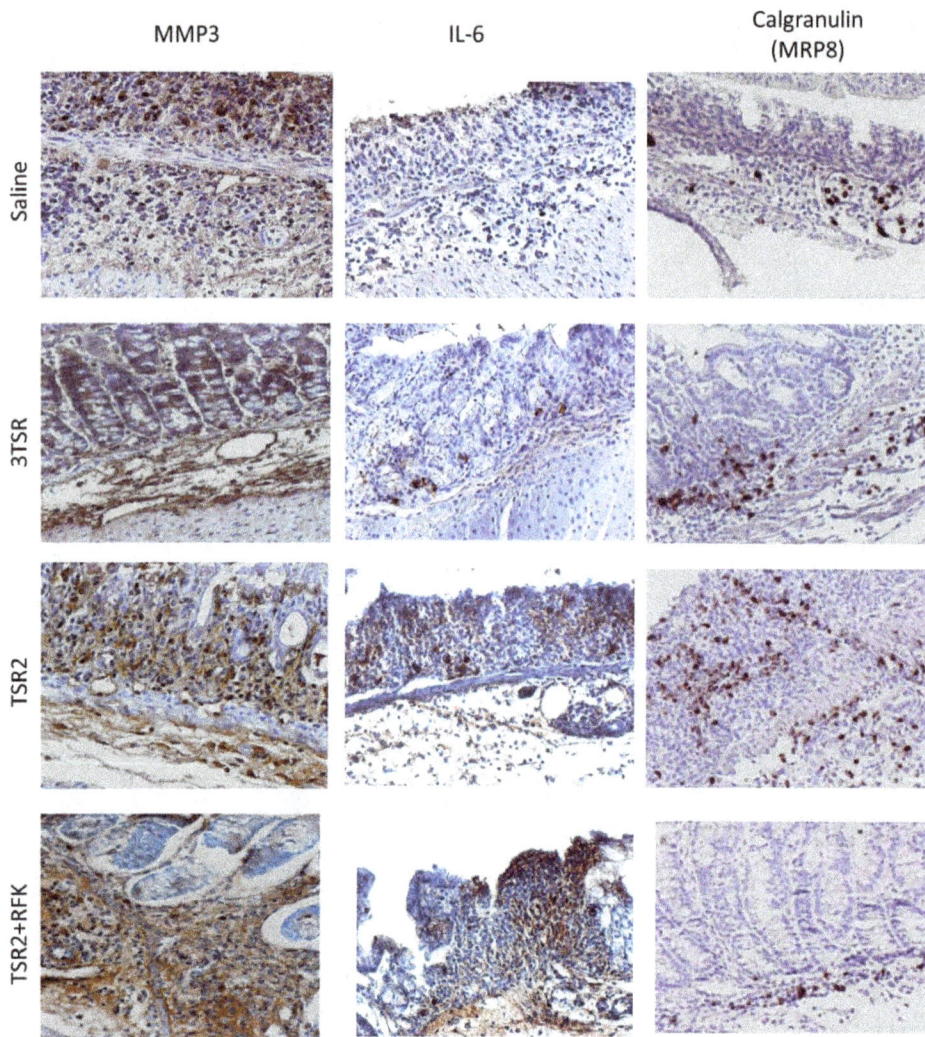

Figure 5. IHC of MMP3, IL-6 and MRP8. Protein expression of MMP3 was localized in colonocytes, leukocytes and endothelial cells. Staining was particularly intense in the submucosal stroma of colitic areas. IL-6 was detected in the leukocytic infiltrate and endothelial cells. Calgranulin or MRP8 also showed selective staining in the leukocytic infiltrate.

as steroids and eicosanoids, has been suggested to have a minor role in xenobiotic metabolism in humans [35]. *Ereg* is a growth factor that resides in the extracellular space and is a marker for ovarian cancer development [36]. *Fpr3* is a member of a G-protein coupled receptor family that controls immune responses such as leukocyte chemotaxis and activation [37]. *Serpina3n* has been found to inhibit human Granzyme B activity in sertoli cells as a mechanism to suppress the immune response [38].

SRGN is a proteoglycan that has important roles in inflammatory reactions [39]. In human endothelial cells, it co-localizes and interacts with tissue-type plasminogen activator (PLAT) [40]. In macrophages, where it is the major secreted proteoglycan, it regulates the secretion of TNF [41]. The up-regulation of *Srgn* (Figure S3B) in the DSS- and TSR-treated mice suggests that it is a component of the immune response in these mice.

The significance of *Wfdc12* up-regulation in the DSS- and TSR-treated mice (Figure S3C), lies in the fact that an altered microbiota composition in the intestinal tract characterizes the pathogenesis of IBD [42,43]. WFDC12 is an antibacterial protein that inhibits the growth of both *E. coli* and *S. aureus* at a IC90 of 10 μM [44]. With its anti-infective activity, it could serve as

mucosal defense against pathogenic bacterial strains, in conjunction with chemokine signaling.

Evidence for involvement of Insulin-like growth factor (IGF) signaling in cancer progression has been increasing [45]. IGF signaling plays a critical role in promoting cell survival and proliferation of embryonic and adult stem cells [46]. IGFBP5 is associated with "stemness" and its expression has been linked to LGR5, which has been shown to be expressed in cycling columnar epithelial cells at the intestinal crypt base [18,19]. LGR5-deficient mice showed decreased *Igfbp5* expression [47]. Erosive lesions in the intestinal epithelium due to DSS could account for the lower transcript levels of *Lgr5* in the DSS-treated mice. LGR5 deficiency was reported to deregulate the Wnt pathway and contribute to cancer [47].

In conclusion, this study showed that the 3TSR have anti-inflammatory properties that seem to be independent of any angiogenic inhibition or ability to activate TGFß1. These data highlight the anti-inflammatory functions of the 3TSR of TSP-1 in the mouse intestine and its potential use as novel therapeutic tool in IBD. The transcript profiles of the treatment groups showed a pool of genes involved in critical pathways of inflammation. The identification of these genes has implications in improving our understanding of the pathophysiology of IBD. Further characterization of their protein products and their interactions could provide leads in the development of other drug therapy for IBD.

Supporting Information

Figure S1 Assessment of microvessel counts. Using combined MECA/CD31 antibodies (A), fewer blood vessels were observed in sections from TSR2 mice (n = 20) compared to sections from mice treated with TSR2+RFK (n = 35), 3TSR (n = 29) or saline (n = 16), (B). 400× magnification.

Figure S2 A functional association network of selected mouse genes. GeneMANIA, a web interface for predicting gene function and determining usability of genes for functional assays (www.genemania.org) was used to determine suitability of endogenous control genes for validating array data by RT-qPCR. The following genes (grey circles) were inputted in GeneMANIA: *Ubc*; *Tpt1*; *Rps23*; *Gapdh*; *Capsl*; *Igfbp5*; *Fpr3*; *Srgn*; *Kcne3*; *Mmp10*; *Mmp13*; *Wfdc12*. The network generated shows interaction between *Gapdh* and *Igfbp5*; therefore, *Gapdh* expression is likely to be co-expressed with *Igfbp5* and show varying expression levels similar to that of *Igfbp5*. *Tpt1*, on the other hand, has no predicted interaction with any of the input genes.

Figure S3 Additional RT-qPCR validation of array data.

Table S1 Genes used for the RT-qPCR validation and their primers. *Tpt1* was used as the control gene after it was found to show no fluctuation compared to four other genes that were tested.

Table S2 ANOVA list of genes that were differentially expressed in the colons of DSS and TSR-treated mice.

Acknowledgments

We thank Dr. Jack Lawler (Beth Israel Deaconess Medical Center, Boston, MA) for providing the TSR recombinant proteins. We also thank Dr. Wilbur Hayes (Emeritus, Wilkes University) for his relevant comments on the manuscript.

Author Contributions

Conceived and designed the experiments: LG ZLD SVC. Performed the experiments: LG ZLD BP RS MW BL AM BE RT SVC. Analyzed the data: LG ZLD BP RS MW BL AM BE RT SVC. Contributed reagents/materials/analysis tools: LG SVC. Wrote the paper: ZLD LG SVC.

References

1. Lawler J (1986) The structural and functional properties of thrombospondin. Blood 67: 1197–1209.
2. Lawler J, Hynes RO (1986) The structure of human thrombospondin, an adhesive glycoprotein with multiple calcium-binding sites and homologies with several different proteins. J Cell Biol 103: 1635–1648.
3. Carlson CB, Lawler J, Mosher DF (2008) Structures of thrombospondins. Cell Mol Life Sci 65: 672–686.
4. Adams JC, Tucker RP (2000) The thrombospondin type 1 repeat (TSR) superfamily: diverse proteins with related roles in neuronal development. Dev Dyn 218: 280–299.
5. Tucker RP (2004) The thrombospondin type 1 repeat superfamily. Int J Biochem Cell Biol 36: 969–974.
6. Chen H, Herndon ME, Lawler J (2000) The cell biology of thrombospondin-1. Matrix Biol 19: 597–614.
7. Simantov R, Silverstein RL (2003) CD36: a critical anti-angiogenic receptor. Front Biosci 8: s874–882.
8. Simantov R, Febbraio M, Silverstein RL (2005) The antiangiogenic effect of thrombospondin-2 is mediated by CD36 and modulated by histidine-rich glycoprotein. Matrix Biol 24: 27–34.
9. Short SM, Derrien A, Narsimhan RP, Lawler J, Ingber DE, et al. (2005) Inhibition of endothelial cell migration by thrombospondin-1 type-1 repeats is mediated by beta1 integrins. J Cell Biol 168: 643–653.
10. Miao WM, Seng WL, Duquette M, Lawler P, Laus C, et al. (2001) Thrombospondin-1 type 1 repeat recombinant proteins inhibit tumor growth through Transforming growth factor-B-dependent and -independent mechanisms. Cancer Res 61: 7830–7839.
11. Ren B, Song K, Parangi S, Jin T, Ye M, et al. (2009) A double hit to kill tumor and endothelial cells by TRAIL and antiangiogenic 3TSR. Cancer Res 69: 3856–3865.
12. Zhang X, Galardi E, Duquette M, Delic M, Lawler J, et al. (2005) Antiangiogenic treatment with the three thrombospondin-1 type 1 repeats recombinant protein in an orthotopic human pancreatic cancer model. Clin Cancer Res 11: 2337–2344.
13. Yee KO, Streit M, Hawighorst T, Detmar M, Lawler J (2004) Expression of the type-1 repeats of thrombospondin-1 inhibits tumor growth through activation of transforming growth factor-beta. Am J Pathol 165: 541–552.
14. Haviv F, Bradley MF, Kalvin DM, Schneider AJ, Davidson DJ, et al. (2005) Thrombospondin-1 mimetic peptide inhibitors of angiogenesis and tumor growth: design, synthesis, and optimization of pharmacokinetics and biological activities. J Med Chem 48: 2838–2846.
15. Punekar S, Zak S, Kalter VG, Dobransky L, Punekar I, et al. (2008) Thrombospondin 1 and its mimetic peptide ABT-510 decrease angiogenesis and inflammation in a murine model of inflammatory bowel disease. Pathobiology 75: 9–21.
16. Andersen CL, Jensen JL, Orntoft TF (2004) Normalization of real-time quantitative reverse transcription-PCR data: a model-based variance estimation approach to identify genes suited for normalization, applied to bladder and colon cancer data sets. Cancer Res 64: 5245–5250.

17. Warde-Farley D, Donaldson SL, Comes O, Zuberi K, Badrawi R, et al. (2010) The GeneMANIA prediction server: biological network integration for gene prioritization and predicting gene function. Nucleic Acids Res 38: W214–220.
18. Barker N, van Es JH, Kuipers J, Kujala P, van den Born M, et al. (2007) Identification of stem cells in small intestine and colon by marker gene Lgr5. Nature 449: 1003–1007.
19. Sato T, van Es JH, Snippert HJ, Stange DE, Vries RG, et al. (2011) Paneth cells constitute the niche for Lgr5 stem cells in intestinal crypts. Nature 469: 415–418.
20. Zhang X, Kazerounian S, Duquette M, Perruzzi C, Nagy JA, et al. (2009) Thrombospondin-1 modulates vascular endothelial growth factor activity at the receptor level. FASEB J 23: 3368–3376.
21. Petersson J, Schreiber O, Steege A, Patzak A, Hellsten A, et al. (2007) eNOS involved in colitis-induced mucosal blood flow increase. Am J Physiol Gastrointest Liver Physiol 293: G1281–1287.
22. Isenberg JS, Martin-Manso G, Maxhimer JB, Roberts DD (2009) Regulation of nitric oxide signalling by thrombospondin 1: implications for anti-angiogenic therapies. Nat Rev Cancer 9: 182–194.
23. Feagins LA (2010) Role of transforming growth factor-beta in inflammatory bowel disease and colitis-associated colon cancer. Inflamm Bowel Dis 16: 1963–1968.
24. Gove ME, Rhodes DH, Pini M, van Baal JW, Sennello JA, et al. (2009) Role of leptin receptor-induced STAT3 signaling in modulation of intestinal and hepatic inflammation in mice. J Leukoc Biol 85: 491–496.
25. Moldobaeva A, Baek A, Eldridge L, Wagner EM (2010) Differential activity of pro-angiogenic CXC chemokines. Microvasc Res 80: 18–22.
26. Papp M, Lakatos PL, Hungarian IBDSG, Palatka K, Foldi I, et al. (2007) Haptoglobin polymorphisms are associated with Crohn's disease, disease behavior, and extraintestinal manifestations in Hungarian patients. Dig Dis Sci 52: 1279–1284.
27. Marquez L, Shen C, Cleynen I, De Hertogh G, Van Steen K, et al. (2011) Effects of haptoglobin polymorphisms and deficiency on susceptibility to inflammatory bowel disease and on severity of murine colitis. Gut.
28. Gebhardt C, Nemeth J, Angel P, Hess J (2006) S100A8 and S100A9 in inflammation and cancer. Biochem Pharmacol 72: 1622–1631.
29. Hsu K, Champaiboon C, Guenther BD, Sorenson BS, Khammanivong A, et al. (2009) ANTI-INFECTIVE PROTECTIVE PROPERTIES OF S100 CALGRANULINS. Antiinflamm Antiallergy Agents Med Chem 8: 290–305.
30. Sunahori K, Yamamura M, Yamana J, Takasugi K, Kawashima M, et al. (2006) The S100A8/A9 heterodimer amplifies proinflammatory cytokine production by macrophages via activation of nuclear factor kappa B and p38 mitogen-activated protein kinase in rheumatoid arthritis. Arthritis Res Ther 8: R69.
31. Yasui Y, Tanaka T (2009) Protein expression analysis of inflammation-related colon carcinogenesis. J Carcinog 8: 10.
32. Ichikawa M, Williams R, Wang L, Vogl T, Srikrishna G (2011) S100A8/A9 activate key genes and pathways in colon tumor progression. Mol Cancer Res 9: 133–148.

33. Santiago JL, Alizadeh BZ, Martinez A, Espino L, de la Calle H, et al. (2008) Study of the association between the CAPSL-IL7R locus and type 1 diabetes. Diabetologia 51: 1653–1658.

34. Todd JA, Walker NM, Cooper JD, Smyth DJ, Downes K, et al. (2007) Robust associations of four new chromosome regions from genome-wide analyses of type 1 diabetes. Nat Genet 39: 857–864.

35. Pilka ES, Niesen FH, Lee WH, El-Hawari Y, Dunford JE, et al. (2009) Structural basis for substrate specificity in human monomeric carbonyl reductases. PLoS One 4: e7113.

36. Amsterdam A, Shezen E, Raanan C, Slilat Y, Ben-Arie A, et al. (2011) Epiregulin as a marker for the initial steps of ovarian cancer development. Int J Oncol 39: 1165–1172.

37. Migeotte I, Communi D, Parmentier M (2006) Formyl peptide receptors: a promiscuous subfamily of G protein-coupled receptors controlling immune responses. Cytokine Growth Factor Rev 17: 501–519.

38. Sipione S, Simmen KC, Lord SJ, Motyka B, Ewen C, et al. (2006) Identification of a novel human granzyme B inhibitor secreted by cultured sertoli cells. J Immunol 177: 5051–5058.

39. Kolset SO, Tveit H (2008) Serglycin–structure and biology. Cell Mol Life Sci 65: 1073–1085.

40. Schick BP, Gradowski JF, San Antonio JD (2001) Synthesis, secretion, and subcellular localization of serglycin proteoglycan in human endothelial cells. Blood 97: 449–458.

41. Zernichow L, Abrink M, Hallgren J, Grujic M, Pejler G, et al. (2006) Serglycin is the major secreted proteoglycan in macrophages and has a role in the regulation of macrophage tumor necrosis factor-alpha secretion in response to lipopolysaccharide. J Biol Chem 281: 26792–26801.

42. Ott SJ, Musfeldt M, Wenderoth DF, Hampe J, Brant O, et al. (2004) Reduction in diversity of the colonic mucosa associated bacterial microflora in patients with active inflammatory bowel disease. Gut 53: 685–693.

43. Swidsinski A, Loening-Baucke V, Herber A (2009) Mucosal flora in Crohn's disease and ulcerative colitis - an overview. J Physiol Pharmacol 60 Suppl 6: 61–71.

44. Hagiwara K, Kikuchi T, Endo Y, Huqun, Usui K, et al. (2003) Mouse SWAM1 and SWAM2 are antibacterial proteins composed of a single whey acidic protein motif. J Immunol 170: 1973–1979.

45. Samani AA, Yakar S, LeRoith D, Brodt P (2007) The Role of the IGF System in Cancer Growth and Metastasis: Overview and Recent Insights. Endocrine Reviews 28: 20–47.

46. Li Y, Geng YJ (2010) A potential role for insulin-like growth factor signaling in induction of pluripotent stem cell formation. Growth Horm IGF Res 20: 391–398.

47. Garcia MI, Ghiani M, Lefort A, Libert F, Strollo S, et al. (2009) LGR5 deficiency deregulates Wnt signaling and leads to precocious Paneth cell differentiation in the fetal intestine. Dev Biol 331: 58–67.

8

Inflammatory Bowel Diseases Phenotype, *C. difficile* and NOD2 Genotype are Associated with Shifts in Human Ileum Associated Microbial Composition

Ellen Li[1,2,10]*, Christina M. Hamm[1], Ajay S. Gulati[6], R. Balfour Sartor[7], Hongyan Chen[3], Xiao Wu[3], Tianyi Zhang[1,3], F. James Rohlf[4], Wei Zhu[3], Chi Gu[12], Charles E. Robertson[5], Norman R. Pace[5], Edgar C. Boedeker[8], Noam Harpaz[9], Jeffrey Yuan[10], George M. Weinstock[11], Erica Sodergren[11], Daniel N. Frank[13]*

1 Department of Medicine, Stony Brook University, Stony Brook, New York, United States of America, 2 Department of Microbiology and Molecular Genetics, Stony Brook University, Stony Brook, New York, United States of America, 3 Department of Applied Mathematics and Statistics, Stony Brook University, Stony Brook, New York, United States of America, 4 Department of Ecology and Evolution, Stony Brook University, Stony Brook, New York, United States of America, 5 Department of Molecular, Cellular and Developmental Biology, University of Colorado, Boulder, Colorado, United States of America, 6 Department of Pediatrics, University of North Carolina, Chapel Hill, North Carolina, United States of America, 7 Departments of Medicine, Microbiology and Immunology, University of North Carolina, Chapel Hill, North Carolina, United States of America, 8 Department of Medicine, University of New Mexico, Albuquerque, New Mexico, United States of America, 9 Department of Pathology, Mount Sinai School of Medicine, New York, New York, United States of America, 10 Department of Medicine, Washington University, St. Louis, Missouri, United States of America, 11 Genome Institute, Washington University, St. Louis, Missouri, United States of America, 12 Division of Biostatistics, Washington University, St. Louis, Missouri, United States of America, 13 Department of Medicine, University of Colorado Anschutz Medical Campus, Aurora, Colorado, United States of America

Abstract

We tested the hypothesis that Crohn's disease (CD)-related genetic polymorphisms involved in host innate immunity are associated with shifts in human ileum–associated microbial composition in a cross-sectional analysis of human ileal samples. Sanger sequencing of the bacterial 16S ribosomal RNA (rRNA) gene and 454 sequencing of 16S rRNA gene hypervariable regions (V1–V3 and V3–V5), were conducted on macroscopically *disease-unaffected* ileal biopsies collected from 52 ileal CD, 58 ulcerative colitis and 60 control patients without inflammatory bowel diseases (IBD) undergoing initial surgical resection. These subjects also were genotyped for the three major NOD2 risk alleles (Leu1007fs, R708W, G908R) and the ATG16L1 risk allele (T300A). The samples were linked to clinical metadata, including body mass index, smoking status and *Clostridia difficile* infection. The sequences were classified into seven phyla/subphyla categories using the Naïve Bayesian Classifier of the Ribosome Database Project. Centered log ratio transformation of six predominant categories was included as the dependent variable in the permutation based MANCOVA for the overall composition with stepwise variable selection. Polymerase chain reaction (PCR) assays were conducted to measure the relative frequencies of the *Clostridium coccoides – Eubacterium rectales* group and the *Faecalibacterium prausnitzii* spp. Empiric logit transformations of the relative frequencies of these two microbial groups were included in permutation-based ANCOVA. Regardless of sequencing method, IBD phenotype, *Clostridia difficile* and NOD2 genotype were selected as associated (FDR ≤ 0.05) with shifts in overall microbial composition. IBD phenotype and NOD2 genotype were also selected as associated with shifts in the relative frequency of the *C. coccoides – E. rectales* group. IBD phenotype, smoking and IBD medications were selected as associated with shifts in the relative frequency of *F. prausnitzii* spp. These results indicate that the effects of genetic and environmental factors on IBD are mediated at least in part by the enteric microbiota.

Editor: Stefan Bereswill, Charité-University Medicine Berlin, Germany

Funding: This work was supported partially by National Institutes of Health (NIH) UH2DK083994, the Crohn's and Colitis Foundation of America, the Simons Foundation, and the Leona M. and Harry B. Helmsley charitable trust through the Sinai-Helmsley Alliance for Research Excellence Network and NIH R21HG005964. We acknowledge use of the Washington University Digestive Diseases Research Core Center Tissue Procurement Facility (P30 DK52574). No additional external funding was received for this study. The funders had no role in study design, data collection and analysis, decision to publish, or preparation of the manuscript.

Competing Interests: The authors have declared that no competing interests exist.

* E-mail: ellen.li@stonybrook.edu (EL); Daniel.frank@ucdenver.edu (DNF)

Introduction

Abnormal host-microbial interactions and genetic susceptibility are implicated in the pathogenesis of inflammatory bowel diseases (IBD) [1–4]. Culture-independent microbiological technologies coupled with high-throughput DNA sequencing have revolutionized the scale, speed, and economics of microbial ecological studies. When applied to IBD, these technologies have uncovered alterations in human intestine-associated microbial compositions ("dysbiosis") in IBD patients compared with controls [5–12]. To further investigate mechanisms and the biological and clinical significance of dysbiosis in IBD, we have begun integrating metagenomic and phenotype data with genotype and additional clinical metadata.

We focused on the three prevalent risk alleles of the nucleotide oligomerization domain 2 (NOD2; Leu1007fs, R702W, and G908R) and the ATG16L1 T300A genotype out of the ~100 IBD related genotypes identified thus far, because these loci have been linked to host innate immunity, particularly Paneth cell function, and ileal Crohn's disease (CD) phenotype [13–27]. We recently conducted an exploratory study that integrated NOD2 and ATG16L1 genotype data with a previously published 16S rRNA sequence dataset [5,11]. This analysis revealed potential associations between alterations in intestine-associated microbial composition and respectively disease phenotype, NOD2 and ATG16L1 genotype. One limitation was that the samples from IBD patients were collected from two separate anatomic sites (ileum and colon), and from both grossly disease-affected and disease unaffected regions. The CD patients were heterogeneous with respect to disease location and included patients with both ileal and colonic disease. There is evidence that patients with isolated colonic CD have distinct genetic characteristics from patients with ileal CD [28]. Genetic associations for Crohn's colitis patients overlap extensively with UC patients and differ from ileal CD patients [29]. For example, the relative frequency of patients with at least one of the three major NOD2 risk alleles is only 16% in Crohn's colitis patients, approaching the frequency observed in non-IBD control subjects [30]. Subphenotyping CD patients with respect to disease location would therefore facilitate biological interpretation of integrating metagenomic data with genotype data [31–33]. Another limitation of the previous study was that relatively limited clinical metadata was available for assessing the effects of potentially confounding variables, such as obesity [34].

In the current study, 16S rRNA sequence analysis was conducted on the proximal margins of resected ileum collected from a larger independent set of subjects with and without inflammatory disease to test the hypothesis that these genes affect ileum-associated microbiota in grossly *disease-unaffected* regions of the ileum, In contrast to the previous study, the subjects in the current study were restricted to three disease phenotypes that were unlikely to overlap with respect to disease location: 1.) Ileal CD patients undergoing ileocolic resection; 2.) colitis patients (without ileal disease) undergoing total colectomy or proctocolectomy; and 3.) control non-IBD patients undergoing either initial right hemicolectomy or total colectomy. Patients with ileocolic anastomoses from previous surgeries were excluded, because increased reflux of colonic luminal contents could potentially impact ileal mucosal microbial profiles. The samples were also linked to far more extensive clinical metadata than those used in the previous exploratory analysis [5,11].

Because the previous dataset we analyzed was generated by amplifying the entire 16S rRNA gene followed by Sanger sequencing, this methodology was also applied in the current study. However, to increase depth of coverage and corroborate results derived from Sanger sequencing datasets, we also performed 454 sequencing of two regions of the 16S rRNA gene (V1–V3 and V3–V5) using primers adopted by the ongoing Human Microbiome Project [35–38]. These three parallel datasets provide a unique opportunity for comparing the results of these three sequencing methods in a disease setting.

Materials and Methods

Patients and Acquisition of Macroscopically Disease-Unaffected Proximal Margin Ileal Tissue Samples

This study was approved by the Institutional Review Boards of Washington University-St. Louis and Stony Brook University. The

diagnosis of CD or UC was made ultimately on the basis of pathological criteria (surgical resection specimen) [31–33]. Ileal CD patients undergoing ileocolic resection, colitis patients undergoing total colectomy and control non-IBD patients undergoing either right hemicolectomy or total colectomy were prospectively enrolled in a consecutive fashion by the Washington University Digestive Diseases Research Core Center Tissue Procurement Facility to donate surgically resected tissue samples and clinical information between April 2005 and February 2010. The clinical information and patient samples were stripped of all identifying information and assigned a patient code and sample code.

The ileal CD patients were predominantly those falling within the Montreal classification of ileal disease with or without cecal disease (L1) [30]. Based on post-operative pathological diagnosis of the resected colon, 47 patients were diagnosed with UC, 9 patients were diagnosed with Crohn's colitis and 2 patients were diagnosed with indeterminate colitis. Fifty-eight percent of the control non-IBD patients underwent resection for benign colonic diseases (colonic inertia, diverticulosis, adenomas, etc.) and the remaining 42% underwent resection for primary colonic adenocarcinomas. Patients who were unwilling or unable to give informed consent were excluded. Patients who had undergone previous resection of ileum as evidence by the presence of an ileocolonic anastomosis were excluded from this study. The number of subjects (n = 170) included in this cross-sectional study was designed to exceed the number of subjects studied previously (n = 125) [5,11].

A minimum of 4 biopsies were taken from the macroscopically disease unaffected proximal ileal margin of fresh pathological specimens using Radial Jaw4 large-capacity biopsy forceps (Boston Scientific, Natick, MA), immediately placed in RNA stabilization solution (RNAlater, Applied Biosystems/Ambion, Austin, TX) and archived at −80°C [39]. The designation of *disease-unaffected* was based on the macroscopic appearance of the mucosa and the surgical pathology report of the adjacent biopsies ("no histopathologic abnormality"). The samples were de-identified and linked to a detailed clinical database by a patient study code.

Information on potential confounding variables was obtained by reviewing the medical records, including the pathological report of the resected intestine by a gastroenterologist (EL). Preoperative mechanical bowel preparations were not routinely ordered, particularly for the IBD patients. Also, adherence to bowel preparations was quite varied among participating subjects. For this reason, preoperative bowel preparation was not included in the analysis. A smoker was defined as smoking ≥7 cigarettes a week for at least a year [40–42]. The body mass index (BMI) was recorded for all individuals [34]. Concomitant *Clostridium difficile* infection was recorded as the presence of a positive fecal *C. difficile* toxin [43,44]. Most of these patients were treated with metronidazole or oral vancomycin [45]. All of the patients received intravenous antibiotic prophylaxis covering both aerobic and anerobic bacteria (e.g. ciprofloxacin and metronidazole, cefoxitin, cefotetan) within one hour of incision [46].

Genotyping of NOD2 and ATG16L1 Single Nucleotide Polymorphisms (SNPs)

Each patient was genotyped for the three major NOD2 SNPs, Leu1007fsInsC (rs2066847, SNP13), R702W (rs206884, SNP8) and G908R (rs2066845, SNP12) and for the autophagy like ATG16L1T300A SNP (rs2241880) by direct sequencing, and/or by a TaqMan MGB (Applied Biosystems, Foster City, CA) genotyping platform using genomic DNA prepared from peripheral blood and/or tissue by the Sequenom Technology Core within the Washington University Division of Human Genetics.(http://hg.wustl.edu/info/Sequenom_description.html) as previously described [39]. Because some combinations of individual NOD2 risk alleles, ATG16L1 risk alleles, and disease phenotype were not sampled in this study, the three NOD2 risk alleles were combined to form two composite categories: 1) $NOD2^{NR}$, subjects harboring none of the three risk alleles (i.e., $NOD2^{NR/NR}$); or 2) $NOD2^{R}$, subjects harboring at least one of the three risk alleles (i.e., $NOD2^{R/R} + NOD2^{R/NR}$). The three ATG16L1 genotype categories were: 1.) $ATG16L1^{NR/NR}$, no ATG16L1 risk allele; 2.) $ATG16L1^{R/NR}$, a single ATG16L1 risk allele; 3.) $ATG16L1^{R/R}$, two ATG16L1 risk alleles.

Library Construction and 16S rRNA Sequence Analysis

Parallel sequence datasets were generated for each of the samples at the Genome Institute at Washington University as previously described by 1.) broad-range PCR amplification of bacterial rRNA genes and Sanger sequencing and 2.) 454 sequencing of two separate segments of the 16S rRNA gene that encode either the V1 and V3 (V1–V3) or V3, V4, and V5 (V3–V5) hypervariable regions (see Methods S1) [35–37]. Of note, the 454 sequencing primers used in this current study were identical to the primers employed for characterizing the microbial communities in healthy individuals at different body sites, including the gastrointestinal tract by the Human Microbiome Project (http://hmpdacc.org/). The analysis software used to process the sequencing data consisted of established function specific tools that are described in greater detail in Methods S1. All sequences were screened for fidelity to a 16S rRNA bacterial covariance model (CM) based on secondary structure using the Infernal software package and were checked for chimerism with ChimeraSlayer [37,47]. Potentially chimeric sequences and sequences lacking high fidelity to the CM were removed from subsequent analysis. Patient DNA samples with less than 100 total screened sequences were excluded from the analysis.

The sequences were classified into seven phyla/subphyla categories using the Naïve Bayesian Classifier of the Ribosome Database Project as described in Methods S1 [5,11]: The seven categories were 1) *Actinobacteria*, 2) *Bacteroidetes*, 3) *Firmicutes*. Clostridium Group IV, 4) *Firmicutes*. Clostridium Group XIVa, 5.) *Firmicutes*. Bacillus, 6.) *Proteobacteria*, and 7.) Other taxa. The subdivisions of the Firmicutes phyla were based on concordance between the RDP classifier and the Greengenes 16S rRNA phylogenetic schema [5,11,48–51]. Six of these seven bacterial categories (Actinobacteria, Bacteroidetes, Firmicutes/Clostridium GroupIV, Firmicutes/Clostridium GroupXIVa, Firmicutes/Bacillus, and Proteobacteria) were selected as representing the overall microbial composition.

Assembled Sanger sequences were deposited in GenBank accession HQ739096-HQ821395. 454 V1–V3 and V3–V5 sequences were deposited in the Sequence Read Archive accession SRX021348-SRX021368, SRX037800-SRX037802. Clinical and genotyping data can be accessed through the dbGAP authorized access system. Request access to: phs000255. The study accession is SRP002479 "Effect of Crohn's disease risk alleles on enteric microbiota". In order to request access to any of the individual-level datasets within the controlled-access portions of the database, the Principal Investigator (PI) and the Signing Official (SO) at the investigator's institution will need to co-sign a request for data access, which will be reviewed by an NIH Data Access Committee at the appropriate NIH Institute or Center https://dbgap.ncbi.nlm.nih.gov/aa/wga.cgi?page=login.

Quantitative PCR (qPCR)

QPCR assays were performed for the *Clostridium coccoides – Eubacterium rectales Faecalibacterium prausnitzii* and total bacteria using established primers (see Methods S1) [52,53]. The assays were carried out in triplicate. Plasmid quantification standards were prepared from representative clones of the target organisms.

Statistical Analysis

Genotype and clinical categorical variables (e.g. disease phenotype, smoking, etc.) were compared between disease phenotypes using chi-square test for contingency tables. Clinical continuous variables, such as age and body mass index (BMI) were compared between disease phenotypes using the Kruskal-Wallis test. The relative frequencies of six of seven (excluding Other Taxa) categories selected to represent the overall microbial composition, were adjusted by adding 0.5 to all raw sequence counts in order to avoid 0% frequencies, and then subjected to centered log ratio transformation for the analysis of compositional data (see Methods S1) [54]. The effect of the independent variables and all first order interactions on these six bacterial categories (represented as a single vector), was analyzed in parallel for each sequencing platform by permutation based multivariate analysis of covariance (MANCOVA) with stepwise variable selection using the adonis function in R software (Version 2.12.1) package vegan (Version 1.17-2), Euclidean distances and a threshold significance level of 0.05 [55,56]. To address the multiple comparison issue, we applied the Benjamini-Hochberg method to adjust P-values to the false discovery rate (FDR) [57]. The effect of these independent variables and their first order interactions on individual bacteria categories was further analyzed by permutation based analysis of covariance (ANCOVA) with stepwise variable selection and a threshold significance of 0.05 [32,55,56]. Repeated measures ANCOVA was then used to assess the union of the variables and first order interactions selected by the parallel ANCOVAs conducted on the three sequencing platforms separately, in an effort to utilize all three data sets simultaneously [58,59]. The empirical logit transformations of the relative frequencies of the *C. coccoides – E. rectales* and the *F. prausnitzii* groups (measured by targeted qPCR) was used in the permutation-based ANCOVA. The Benjamini-Hochberg method was used to adjust P-values to the false discovery rate (FDR) [57]. The R codes are provided in Methods S1.

Results

Distribution of NOD2 and ATG16L1 Genotypes and Clinical Characteristics of Ileal CD, Colitis, and Non-IBD Control Subjects

As shown in Table 1, with the exception of race and gender, there were differences (FDR ≤0.05) in the distribution of the 11 remaining variables between the three disease phenotypes. For example, subjects who harbored at least one NOD2 risk allele, $NOD2^{R}$, were more prevalent among ileal CD patients [16,17,39]. Only two (4%) ileal CD patients were $ATG16L1^{NR/NR}$ Ileal CD patients were younger than the control patients at the time of surgery [23]. Actively smoking subjects were less prevalent in colitis patients [39–41]. The median BMI and age were lower in ileal CD subjects. *C. difficile* was more prevalent among subjects with colitis [43,45]. None of the control subjects were treated with5-ASA, immunomodulators, and/or anti-TNFα biologics. All of the patients received intravenous antibiotic prophylaxis that

Table 1. Distribution of NOD2 composite and ATG16L1 genotype and clinical characteristics of ileal CD, colitis and control non-IBD patients.

Variables	Ileal CD (n = 52)	Colitis (n = 58)	Control (n = 60)	P-value	FDR
NOD2^R (R/R + R/NR)	38%	15%	12%	**0.003**	**0.004**
ATG16L1T300A (NR/NR)	4%	28%	23%	**0.006**	**0.007**
Gender (male)	48%	57%	38%	0.130	0.14
Race (Caucasian)	92%	90%	83%	0.316	0.32
Median age (range) y	33 (18–72)	42 (17–68)	60 (32–64)	**<0.001**	**<0.001**
Current smoker	33%	3%	25%	**0.003**	**0.004**
Positive fecal *C. difficile* toxin	6%	28%	0%	**<0.001**	**<0.001**
Median BMI (range) kg/m^2	24 (16–41)	25 (16–45)	28 (18–47)	**0.006**	**0.007**
5-ASA	52%	59%	0%	**<0.001**	**<0.001**
Steroids	54%	72%	0%	**<0.001**	**<0.001**
Immunomodulators	44%	72%	0%	**<0.001**	**<0.001**
Anti-TNFα biologics				**<0.001**	**<0.001**
Current (≤8 weeks of surgery)	29%	29%	0%		
Past (>8 weeks of surgery)	6%	7%	0%		
Never	65%	64%	0%		

The variables shown above are included in the subsequent MANCOVA and ANCOVA analyses. Chi-square test for contingency table was used for categorical data and Kruskal-Wallis test was used for age and BMI. To address multiple comparison issues, the Benjamini-Hochberg method was applied to adjust P-values to the false discovery rate (FDR).

covered both aerobic and anaerobic bacteria within one hour prior to incision [46].

Comparison of the Relative Frequencies of Phyla/Subphyla Bacterial Categories between Ileal CD, Colitis and Control *Disease-Unaffected* Ileal Samples

Using the Sanger method, a total of 81,644 near full length 16S rRNA sequences with acceptable quality were obtained with an average of 500 reads/sample. A total of 1,191,278 454 V1–V3 sequences (mean 7260 reads/sample) and a total of 917,900 454 V3–V5 sequences (mean 5400 reads/sample) were obtained from *disease-unaffected* samples. Greater than 90% of the sequences were binned into six of seven phyla/subphyla categories as shown in Figure 1. The Clostridium Group IV and Group XIVa taxa correspond to two prominent subsets of the "*Lachnospiraceae*" taxonomic group previously discussed by Frank et al. [5,11]. As shown in Figure 1, and Table S1, the distribution of relative frequencies of the phyla/subphyla bacterial categories between the three disease phenotypes (ileal CD, colitis, control non-IBD) were very similar between the three datasets.

Disease Phenotype, *C. difficile* and NOD2 Genotype are Associated with Shifts in Overall Disease-Unaffected Ileum-Associated Microbial Composition (MANCOVA)

The three sequence datasets were analyzed in parallel using a vector that combined the relative iesof the six most prevalent of the seven phyla/subphyla categories (see Figure 1) as the dependent variable. Exploratory permutation based MANCOVA with stepwise variable selection including all first order interactions, was conducted with each of the datasets. The parallel analyses with each dataset selected disease phenotype among 13 variables, as associated (FDR ≤0.05) with overall changes in the composition of mucosal bacterial communities (see Table 2). In addition, *C. difficile* and NOD2 genotype were selected (FDR

≤0.05) as associated with shifts in microbial composition. These two variables had smaller effects (R^2) compared to the effect size of disease phenotype. Repeating the analysis with the 150 Caucasian subjects yielded similar results (see Table S2). Repeating the analysis after excluding subjects diagnosed with Crohn's colitis and indeterminate colitis also yielded similar results (see Table S3).

Disease Phenotype Is Associated with Shifts in the Relative Frequencies of Actinobacteria, Bacteroidetes, Firmicutes. Clostridium GroupIV and Firmicutes. Bacillus Categories

In order to explore whether these variables were associated with particular microbial groups, permutation based ANCOVA with stepwise variable selection was carried out in parallel for each of the three datasets for each of the six phyla/subphyla categories (see Table S4). The union of the significant independent variables and first order interactions identified by these parallel analyses was then reanalyzed by permutation based repeated measures ANCOVA, in which the data from each sequence dataset was treated as a repeated measure (see Table 3). Analyzing the three datasets in parallel and as repeated measures (See Table 3 and Table S4), disease phenotype was selected as associated (FDR ≤0.05) with shifts in the relative frequencies of four of the six phyla/subphyla categories (Actinobacteria, Bacteroidetes, Firmicutes. Clostridium GroupIV and Firmicutes.Bacillus). Repeated measures ANCOVA also provided a means of comparing the results of the three sequencing methods. The three sequencing methods demonstrated good agreement (FDR>0.05) for the Actinobacteria and Bacteroidetes categories. Differences between the three sequencing methods may have the biggest effect ($R^2 = 0.040$) on assessing the relative frequency of Proteobacteria.

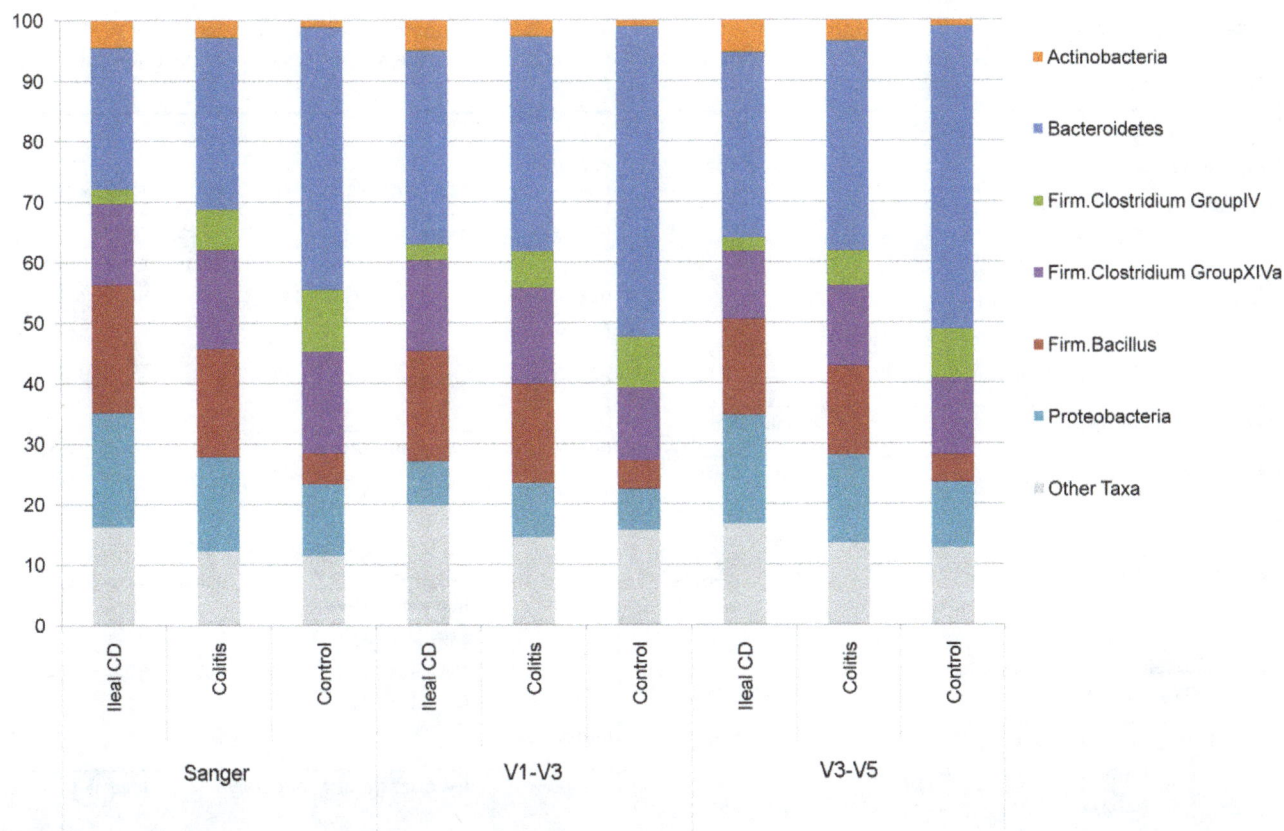

Figure 1. Phyla/subphyla comparison of three disease phenotypes (ileal CD, colitis, using the Sanger, 454 V1–V3 and 454 V3–V5 data sets. The average relative frequency of each taxa is shown for ileal CD, colitis and control subjects for each of the three sequencing data sets, (see also Table S1 for means ± standard deviations).

Quantification of Clostridium Coccoides – Eubacterium Rectales and Fecalibacterium Prausnitzii by qPCR

QPCR analyses were conducted on total bacteria, the *C. coccoides-E. rectales* group and *F. prausnitzii* using previously established primers (see Figure 2).[52-53] The relative frequency of the *C. coccoides-E. rectales* group, which overlaps the "*Lachnospiraceae*" taxonomic group (Clostridium GroupIV and XIVa are prominent subsets) was previously shown to be reduced in a subset of IBD subjects.[5] *F. prausnitzii* is a major species within the Clostridium Group IV category. Low relative frequency of *F. prausnitzii* has been reported to be reduced in patients with ileal CD and has been associated with an increased risk of ileocolonoscopic recurrence of ileal CD [8,9,12].

As shown in Figure 2, the relative frequency of the *C. coccoides-E. rectales* group was significantly higher in NOD2[R] ileal CD subjects than in NOD2[NR] ileal CD subjects. In contrast, the relative frequency of the *C. coccoides-E. rectales* group was lower in ileal CD subjects compared to control non-IBD subjects, consistent with previous analysis of an independent set of tissues [5]. As shown in Table 4, IBD phenotype, NOD2 genotype and IBD medications were selected by ANCOVA with stepwise variable selection as associated (FDR ≤0.05) with shifts in the relative frequency of *C. coccoides-E. rectales* group. First order interactions between IBD phenotype and race, and between NOD2 genotype and steroids, were also selected. Unfortunately 13 DNA samples were exhausted before the qPCR assays for *F. prausnitzii* were conducted, reducing the total samples analyzed from 170 to 157. IBD phenotype, smoking and steroids were selected by ANCOVA with stepwise

variable selection as associated (FDR ≤0.05) with shifts in the relative frequency of *F. prausnitzii* (see Table 4). First order interactions between NOD2 and smoking, and between age and gender were also selected.

Comparison of Non-IBD Control Samples from Subjects with and without Primary Colon Adenocarcinoma

Because a major proportion (42%) of the non-IBD control subjects underwent surgery for resection of right sided primary colon adenocarcinoma, we performed exploratory analyses comparing the relative frequencies of the seven phyla/subphyla clades as well as other clinical variables. As shown in Table S5, the only variable that was different (FDR ≤0.05) between the two groups of patients was the age of surgery, which is consistent with the observation that the incidence of colon cancer increases with patient age [60].

Discussion

In this study we report the results of multiple regression analysis of the largest 16S rRNA sequence datasets reported thus far on ileal tissues collected from IBD subjects. This analysis demonstrates that IBD phenotype has a predominant effect on microbial composition associated with the macroscopically normal appearing proximal margin of resected ileum. The changes in intestinal microbiota that were observed in ileal CD may have occurred early in the pathogenic process before overt disease was manifest. Alternatively, chronic enteric dysbiosis that arises as a conse-

Table 2. Permutation based MANCOVA with stepwise variable selection results for Sanger, 454 V1–V3 and 454 V3–V5 sequencing.

Sequencing	Sanger (n = 164)	R^2	P value	FDR
Main effects	Disease phenotype	0.151	0.001	0.008
	C. difficile	0.019	0.019	0.04
	NOD2	0.018	0.011	0.03
Interactions	Disease phenotype * 5-ASA	0.022	0.012	0.03
	Steroids * Immunomodulators	0.022	0.006	0.03
	Disease phenotype * Age	0.033	0.008	0.03
Sequencing	**454 V1–V3** (n = 164)	R^2	**P value**	**FDR**
Main effects	Disease phenotype	0.126	0.001	0.008
	C. difficile	0.019	0.016	0.03
	NOD2	0.017	0.029	0.05
Interactions	Disease phenotype * 5-ASA	0.022	0.011	0.03
	Steroids * Immunomodulators	0.022	0.006	0.03
	Disease phenotype * Age	0.032	0.009	0.03
Sequencing	**454 V3–V5** (n = 169)	R^2	**P value**	**FDR**
Main effects	Disease phenotype	0.119	0.001	0.008
	C. difficile	0.020	0.014	0.03
	NOD2	0.029	0.004	0.02
Interactions	Disease phenotype * 5-ASA	0.020	0.015	0.03
	Steroids * Immunomodulators	0.030	0.001	0.008
	NOD2 * ATG16L1	0.024	0.028	0.05
	5-ASA * ATG16L1	0.024	0.040	0.06

The dependent variable was the vector generated by the centered log ratio of the relative frequencies of six phyla/subphyla categories (see text). The significant main effects and first order interactions selected by analysis of each of the three data sets as well as the R^2, P values are listed here. To address multiple comparison issues, the Benjamini-Hochberg method was applied to adjust P-values to the false discovery rate (FDR). The number of samples (total = 170 samples) that yielded results suitable for analysis is listed for each method.

Table 3. Permutation-based repeated measures ANCOVA results for each of the six phyla/subphyla bacterial categories (Clade).

Category/Clade	**ACTINOBACTERIA**	R^2	P value	FDR
Main effects	**Disease phenotype**	**0.126**	**0.001**	**0.01**
	Steroids	0.021	0.029	0.08
Interactions	Age of Surgery * ATG16L1	0.041	0.014	0.07
Measurements		0.001	0.328	0.47
Category/Clade	**BACTEROIDETES**	R^2	**P value**	**FDR**
Main effects	**Disease phenotype**	**0.117**	**0.001**	**0.01**
	Smoking	0.018	0.034	0.09
	5-ASA	0.021	0.025	0.08
	Steroids	0.023	0.013	0.07
Interactions	**Steroids * Immunomodulators**	**0.040**	**0.006**	**0.04**
	Disease phenotype * 5-ASA	0.019	0.023	0.08
	5-ASA * Age	0.016	0.050	0.12
	5-ASA * C. difficile	0.019	0.023	0.08
Measurements		0.002	0.047	0.12
Category/Clade	**FIRM.CLOSTRIDIUM GROUPIV**	R^2	**P value**	**FDR**
Main effects	**Disease phenotype**	**0.161**	**0.001**	**0.01**
	Gender	**0.038**	**0.003**	**0.02**
	Smoking	0.025	0.015	0.07
	NOD2	0.021	0.027	0.08
Interactions	**Disease phenotype * Age**	**0.040**	**0.003**	**0.02**
	BMI * 5-ASA	0.025	0.010	0.06
Measurements		0.008	0.001	0.01
Category/Clade	**FIRM.CLOSTRIDIUM GROUPXIVa**	R^2	**P value**	**FDR**
Main effects	Gender	0.023	0.019	0.08
Interactions	**Disease phenotype * Age**	**0.049**	**0.004**	**0.03**
	Steroids * BMI	0.030	0.011	0.06
Measurements		0.006	0.006	0.04
Category/Clade	**FIRM.BACILLUS**	R^2	**P value**	**FDR**
Main effects	**Disease phenotype**	**0.175**	**0.001**	**0.01**
	NOD2	0.016	0.046	0.12
Interactions	**Disease phenotype * Steroids**	**0.040**	**0.002**	**0.02**
	Disease phenotype * Age	0.027	0.032	0.09
	5-ASA * ATG16L1	0.025	0.025	0.08
	Steroids * Immunomodulators	0.019	0.027	0.08
Measurements		0.008	0.001	0.01
Category/Clade	**PROTEOBACTERIA**	R^2	**P value**	**FDR**
Main effects	NOD2	0.027	0.016	0.07
Interactions	**Steroids * NOD2**	**0.040**	**0.002**	**0.02**

quence of pathologic inflammation at one location within the GI tract may be propagated to unaffected sites. The observed alterations in ileal microbiota could have an impact on regional inflammation or metabolic properties (e.g., butyrate metabolism), however the functional implications of these shifts remain to be determined.

NOD2 genotype was also selected albeit with more modest effect for all three 16S rRNA sequence datasets and for targeted qPCR assays of the *C. coccoides- E. rectales* group. The bacterial 16S rRNA sequences assayed by the *C. coccoides – E. rectales* qPCR assay likely overlap with some but not all the 16S rRNA sequences included in Group XIVa and IV. The observation that ileal CD phenotype and NOD2 risk alleles, which presumably contribute to this phenotype, had opposite effects on this microbial group, suggests that the effect of the NOD2 risk allele on the relative frequency of the *C. coccoides-E. rectales* group is not simply mediated through an association with ileal CD phenotype. Thus the results of targeted QPCR assays and 16S rRNA sequence analysis both demonstrate a significant effect of NOD2 genotype on ileum associated microbial composition. Our results in disease –unaffected ileal tissues

Table 3. Cont.

Category/ Clade	ACTINOBACTERIA	R^2	P value	FDR
	5-ASA * Race	**0.032**	**0.007**	**0.04**
	Steroids * Immunomodulators	0.021	0.030	0.08
	NOD2 * ATG16L1	0.056	0.019	0.08
Measurements		**0.040**	**0.001**	**0.01**

Sequencing results for all three platforms were available for 157 samples (44 ileal CD, 53 colitis and 60 control non-IBD). The variables and first order interactions with P≤0.05 are listed above. To address multiple comparison issues, the Benjamini-Hochberg method was applied to adjust P-values to the false discovery rate (FDR). The variables and first order interactions with FDR ≤0.05 are bolded.

support our previous analysis of an independent set of intestinal tissues that were more heterogeneous with respect to anatomic location and inflammation. Our findings are consistent with the report that the relative frequency of *Firmicutes* spp., as determined by targeted qPCR, is higher in NOD2 knockout mice than in wild type mice [20,21]. However, it is important to note that the patient-based studies are not directly comparable to the mouse studies because 1) the NOD2 knockout mouse may differ phenotypically from the NOD2Leu1007fs knock-in mouse [61], and 2) only 4% of the ileal CD patients compared to 28% of colitis and 23% of control non-IBD patients, were homozygous for the ATG16L1 T300A nonrisk allele (ATG16L1$^{NR/NR}$). These findings are also consistent with the recent report that the relative frequency of Firmicutes measured by targeted qPCR is higher in three CD patients that were homozygous for the Leu1007fs (SNP13) compared to 11 CD patients that were homozygous for the wild type allele [21]. Since only two of the ileal CD patients were homozygous for the Leu1007fs allele in our dataset, a parallel comparison could not be made (see Table S6).

C. difficile infections, particularly recurrent *C. difficile* infections have been associated with altered fecal microbial composition [62,63]. Patients with inflammatory bowel diseases are more likely to develop *C. difficile* infections, which are also associated with clinical exacerbation of their disease [43,44]. It is possible that the shifts in microbial composition associated with IBD contribute to these patients' susceptibility to *C. difficile* and other infections that may exacerbate inflammation. Alternatively antibiotic treatment of subjects with *C. difficile* could contribute to the observed shifts in microbial composition [64,65].

Sanger sequencing of the entire 16S rRNA gene permits accurate phylogenetic identification of bacteria, whereas 454 pyrosequencing generates much greater depth of coverage, but with lesser phylogenetic resolution. While the results of all three sequencing methodologies demonstrated associations of disease phenotype, *C. difficile* infection and NOD2 genotype to the overall microbial composition in parallel analyses, they differed with respect to the main effects and first order interactions associated with individual phyla/subphyla categories. Methodological differences may reflect biases introduced during the initial PCR amplification step, as noted by Olsen and coworkers for the 27F forward primer [66]. In addition, there are likely differences in the phylogenetic resolution/assignment of the complete 16S sequence as opposed to different hypervariable regions (V1–V3 and V3–V5) of the gene sequence. Although the results from each sequencing method may converge with increasing the sample size, differences

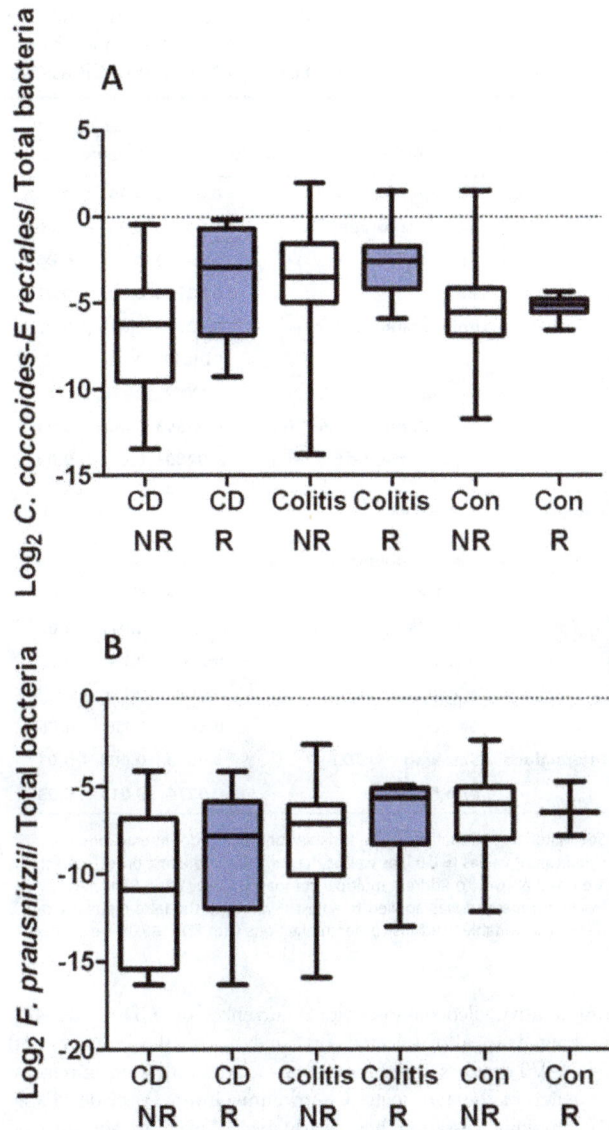

Figure 2. Targeted qPCR results for the *C. coccoides-E. rectales* group and for *F. prausnitzii* spp. Boxplots of (panel A) the $\log_2$ *C. coccoides-E. rectales* group/total bacteria and (panel B) the $\log_2$ *F. prausnitzii*/total bacteria as a function of disease phenotype and NOD2 genotype assayed using qPCR are shown. The middle line represents the median, and the lower edge and the upper edge of the box represent the 25% and 75% quartiles. The bottom and top lines represent the minimum and maximum values, respectively. For the *C. coccoides-rectales* group, all 170 samples were assayed. For *F. prausnitzii*, 157 of 170 samples were assayed.

in the microbial composition data generated by different sequencing methods will make it challenging to compare results from studies using different primers for the initial PCR amplification.

The *F. prausnitzii* 16 S rRNA sequences assayed by targeted qPCR form a major subset of all the sequences grouped within the Firmicutes.Clostridium Group IV clade. The selection of smoking as a potentially significant covariate is intriguing, since smoking has been associated with ileal CD phenotype and with early postoperative recurrence in ileal CD patients, and is consistent with the observations of Sokol and coworkers that low ileal mucosal concentrations of *F. prausnitzii* is associated with early

Table 4. ANCOVA with stepwise variable selection results for relative frequencies of the *C. coccoides-E. rectales* microbial group and *F. prausnitzii* spp. based on targeted qPCR assays.

Category	*C. coccoides-E. rectales* n = 170	R^2	P value	FDR
Main effects	**Disease phenotype**	**0.06368**	**0.001**	**0.006**
	NOD2 genotype	**0.08250**	**0.001**	**0.006**
	Anti-TNFα	**0.08216**	**0.001**	**0.006**
	ASA	**0.02904**	**0.009**	**0.02**
	Immunomodulator	**0.02548**	**0.019**	**0.03**
	Race	0.01050	0.125	0.16
	Steroids	0.00002	0.954	0.95
Interactions	**Disease phenotype * Race**	**0.05563**	**0.003**	**0.01**
	NOD2 * steroids	**0.02605**	**0.056**	**0.03**

Category	*F. prausnitzii* n = 157	R^2	P value	FDR
Main effects	**Disease phenotype**	**0.0662**	**0.002**	**0.008**
	Smoking	**0.0284**	**0.018**	**0.03**
	Steroids	**0.0270**	**0.017**	**0.03**
	NOD2	0.0033	0.394	0.48
	Age	0.0020	0.500	0.51
	Gender	0.0025	0.456	0.52
Interactions	**Smoking * NOD2**	**0.0528**	**0.004**	**0.01**
	Age * Gender	**0.0274**	**0.019**	**0.03**

See Materials and Methods. The variables and first order interactions with significant P values ($\leq$0.05) as well as the variables in the first order interactions are listed above. To address multiple comparison issues, the Benjamini-Hochberg method was applied to adjust P-values to the false discovery rate (FDR). The variables and first order interactions with FDR $\leq$0.05 are bolded.

postoperative ileocolonoscopic recurrence of CD [8,34–42]. Smoking was also selected by analysis of the Sanger and 454V1–V3 datasets as significantly associated with shifts in relative frequency of the Firmicutes.Clostridium Group IV clade (Table S4). Smoking cessation has clearly been linked to altering the subgingival microbial profile [67], but has not been previously linked to altering the ileum associated microbial profile.

Although pathologic review of the resected tissues provided rigorous phenotyping of the samples, the use of surgically resected tissues may bias the results by sampling of IBD patients with relatively severe disease who have been treated for various lengths of time with antibiotics and different IBD medications. Although the focus of this study was ileal CD, it is likely that other human diseases will exhibit similar links between genetically determined defects in mucosal immunity and alterations of resident microbiota. As we further expand these datasets by analyzing more samples, we anticipate that further associations between microbial composition, IBD subphenotypes, IBD polymorphisms and environmental factors will emerge.

Supporting Information

Table S1 A. Relative frequencies of the six phyla/subphyla categories selected to represent overall microbial composition based on the Sanger dataset. The mean value ± standard deviation is shown for each of the three disease phenotypes, ileal CD, colitis and control non-IBD. **B. Relative frequencies of the six phyla/subphyla categories select-** ed to represent the overall microbial composition based on the 454 V1–V3 dataset. The mean value ± standard deviation is shown for each of the three disease phenotypes, ileal CD, colitis and control non-IBD. **C. Relative frequencies of the six phyla/subphyla categories selected to represent the overall microbial composition based on the 454 V3–V5 dataset.** The mean value ± standard deviation is shown for each of the three disease phenotypes, ileal CD, colitis and control non-IBD.

Table S2 Permutation-based MANCOVA with stepwise variable selection results for Caucasian patients. Because NOD2 risk alleles are rarely observed in subjects of Asian and African descent, the analysis was repeated for the 150 Caucasian subjects in the study (48 ileal CD, 52 colitis, 50 non-IBD control subjects). The dependent variable was the vector generated by the centered log ratio of the relative frequencies of six phyla/subphyla categories (see text). The significant main effects and first order interactions selected by analysis of each of the three data sets as well as the R^2, P values are listed below. To address multiple comparison issues, the Benjamini-Hochberg method was applied to adjust P-values to the false discovery rate (FDR). The number of samples (total = 150 samples) that yielded results suitable for analysis is listed for each method.

Table S3 Permutation-based MANCOVA with stepwise variable selection results for Sanger, 454 V1–V3 and 454 V3–V5 sequencing. Samples with Crohn's colitis and indeterminate colitis were excluded in this analysis. The dependent variable was the vector generated by the centered log ratio of the relative frequencies of six phyla/subphyla categories (see text). The significant main effects and first order interactions selected by analysis of each of the three data sets as well as the R^2, P values are listed below. To address multiple comparison issues, the Benjamini-Hochberg method was applied to adjust P-values to the false discovery rate (FDR). The number of samples (around 150 samples) that yielded results suitable for analysis is listed for each method.

Table S4 Permutation based ANCOVA with stepwise variable selection results for each of the six individual phyla/subphyla categories. Permutation based ANCOVA with step wise variable selection was carried out for the individual phyla/subphyla categories. in parallel for each of the datasets. A total of 164 samples were analyzed for the Sanger and the 454 V1–V3 datasets respectively. A total of 169 samples were analyzed for the 454 V3–V5 dataset. Listed below are the main effects, first order interactions with P-values $\leq$0.05, as well as the main effects of first order interactions with P values $\leq$0.05. To address multiple comparison issues, the Benjamini-Hochberg method was applied to adjust P-values to the false discovery rate (FDR). The main effects and first order interactions with FDR $\leq$0.05 are bolded.

Table S5 Comparison between nonIBD control subjects with primary colon adenocarcinoma with non-IBD subjects without primary colon adenocarcinoma. Continuous variables (e.g. age, BMI, relative frequency of bacterial groups) were compared using the Wilcoxon rank sum test and categorical variables (e.g. genotype, smoking, race) were compared using the chi-square test. Note that none of the non-IBD control subjects had a positive C. difficile toxin or were taking any IBD medications. To address multiple comparison issues, the Benjamini-Hochberg method was applied to adjust P-values to the false discovery rate (FDR). Variables with FDR ≤ 0.05 are bolded.

Table S6 Distribution of the three common NOD2 genotypes in ileal CD, colitis and non-IBD control subjects.

The three major NOD2 risk alleles that account for 80% of the NOD2 variants, are Leu1007fs (SNP13, rs2066847), R702W (SNP8, rs2066844), and G908W (SNP12, rs2066845).

Methods S1

Acknowledgments

The authors thank the patients who have contributed their medical information, blood and tissue samples to the Digestive Diseases Research Core Center (DDRCC) Clinical Database, the faculty of the Section of Colon and Rectal Surgery and the Division of Gastroenterology at Washington University. We thank Yanjiao Zhou in the Genome Center at Washington University for facilitating the 16S rRNA sequencing of the samples. We thank Drs. William Shannon and Phillip Tarr at Washington University and Drs. Kenny Ye and Tao Wang at Albert Einstein College of Medicine for many helpful discussions.

Author Contributions

Conceived and designed the experiments: EL RBS ECB NH GW ES DNF. Performed the experiments: EL CMH AG JY ES. Analyzed the data: EL CMH AG HC XW TZ FJR WZ CG CER JY DNF. Contributed reagents/materials/analysis tools: EL CMH HC XW TZ FJR WZ CER DNF. Wrote the paper: EL CMH AG RBS HC XW TZ FJR WZ CG CER NRP ECB NH JY GMW ES DNF.

References

1. Frank DN, Zhu W, Sartor RB, Li E (2011) Investigating the biological and clinical significance of human dysbioses. Trends Microbiol. 19: 427–434.
2. Sartor RB (2008) Microbial influences in inflammatory bowel diseases. Gastroenterology. 134: 577–594.
3. Eckburg PB, Relman DA (2007) The role of microbes in Crohn's disease. Clin Infect. Dis. 454: 256–262.
4. Abraham C, Cho J (2009) Mechanisms of disease: inflammatory bowel disease. New Engl. J Medicine. 361: 2066–2078.
5. Frank DN, St. Amand AL, Feldman RA, Boedeker EC, Harpaz N, et al. (2007) Molecular-phylogenetic characterization of microbial community imbalances in human inflammatory bowel diseases. Proc Natl Acad Sci USA. 104: 13780–13785.
6. Peterson DA, Frank DN, Pace N, Gordon JI (2008) Metagenomic approaches for defining the pathogenesis of inflammatory bowel diseases. Cell Host Microbe. 3: 417–427.
7. Sokol H, Lay C, Seksik P, Tannock GW (2008) Analysis of bacterial bowel communities of IBD patients: What has it revealed? Inflamm Bowel Dis 14: 858–867.
8. Sokol H, Pigneur B, Watterlot L, Lakhdari O, Bermúdez-Humarán LG, et al. (2008) Faecalibacterium prausnitzii is an anti inflammatory commensal bacterium identified by gut microbiota analysis of Crohn disease patients. Proc Natl Acad Sci U S A. 105: 16731–16736.
9. Willing B, Halfvarson WB, Dicksved J, Rosenquist M, Järnerot G, et al. (2009) Twin studies reveal specific imbalances in the mucosal-associated microbiota of patients with ileal Crohn's disease. Inflamm Bowel Dis. 15: 653–660.
10. Qin J, Li R, Raes J, Arumugam M, Burgdorf KS, et al. (2009) A human gut microbial gene catalogue established by metagenomic sequencing. Nature 464: 59–65.
11. Frank DN, Robertson CE, Hamm CM, Kpadeh Z, Zhang T, et al. (2011) Disease phenotype and genotype are associated with shifts in intestinal-microbiota in inflammatory bowel diseases. Inflamm Bowel Dis. 17: 179–84.
12. Willing B, Dicksved J, Halfvarson J, Andersson AF, Lucio M, et al. (2010) A pyrosequencing study in twins shows that gastrointestinal microbial profiles vary with inflammatory bowel disease phenotypes. Gastroenterology 139: 1844–1854.
13. Anderson CA, Boucher G, Lees CW, Franke A, D'Amato M, et al. (2011) Meta-analysis identifies 29 additional ulcerative colitis risk loci, increasing the number of confirmed associations to 47. Nat Genet. 43: 246–252.
14. Hugot JP, Chamaillard M, Zouali H, Lesage S, Cézard JP, et al. (2001) Association of NOD2 leucine-rich repeat variants with susceptibility to Crohn's disease. 411: 599–603.
15. Ogura Y, Bonen DK, Inohara N, Nicolae DL, Chen FF, et al. (2001) A frameshift mutation in NOD2 associated with susceptibility to Crohn's disease. Nature 411: 603–6.
16. Cuthbert A, Fisher S, Croucher PJ, King K, Hampe J, et al. (2002) The contribution of NOD2 gene mutations to the risk and site of disease in inflammatory bowel disease. Gastroenterology 122: 867–74.
17. Lesage S, Zouali H, Cézard JP, the EPWG-IBD group, Colombel JF, et al. (2002) CARD15/NOD2 mutational analysis and genotype-phenotype correlation in 612 patients with inflammatory bowel disease. Am J Human Genet 70: 845–57.
18. Ogura Y, Lala S, Xin W, Smith E, Dowds TA, et al. (2003) Expression of NOD2 in Paneth cells: a possible link to Crohn's ileitis. Gut. 52: 1591–7.
19. Salzman NH, Underwood MA, Bevins CL (2007) Paneth cells, defensins, and the commensal microbiota: a hypothesis on intimate interplay at the intestinal mucosa. Seminars in Immunology. 19: 70–83.
20. Petnicki-Ocwieja T, Hrncir T, Liu YJ, Biswas A, Hudcovic T, et al. (2009) Nod2 is required for the regulation of commensal microbiota in the intestine. PNAS 106: 15813–15818.
21. Rehman A, Sina C, Gavrilova O, Häsler R, Ott S, et al. (2011) Nod2 is essential for temporal development of intestinal microbial communities. Gut. 60: 1354–1362.
22. Rioux JD, Xavier RJ, Taylor KD, Silverberg MS, Goyette P, et al. (2007) Genome-wide association study identifies new susceptibility loci for Crohn disease and implicates autophagy in disease pathogenesis. Nat Genet. 39: 596–604.
23. Prescott NJ, Fisher SA, Franke A, Hampe J, Onnie CM, et al. (2007) A nonsynonymous SNP in ATG16L1 predisposes to ileal Crohn's disease and is independent of CARD15 and IBD5. Gastroenterology. 132: 1665–1671.
24. Cadwell K, Liu JY, Brown SL, Miyoshi H, Loh J, et al. (2008) A key role for autophagy and the autophagy gene Atg16l1 in mouse and human intestinal Paneth cells. Nature. 456: 259–263.
25. Cadwell K, Patel KK, Maloney NS, Liu TC, NG ACY, et al. (2010) Virus-plus-susceptibility gene interaction determines Crohn's disease gene Atg16L1 phenotypes in the intestine. Cell. 141: 1135–1145.
26. Bevins CL, Stange EF, Wehkamp J (2009) Decreased Paneth cell defensin expression in ileal Crohn's disease is independent of inflammation, but linked to the NOD2 1007fs genotype. Gut. 58: 882–883.
27. Simms LA, Doecke JD, Walsh MD, Huang N, Fowler EV, et al. (2008) Reduced alpha-defensin expression is associated with inflammation and not NOD2 mutation status in ileal Crohn's disease. Gut. 57: 903–910.
28. Hancock L, Beckly J, Geremia A, Cooney R, Cummings F, et al. (2008) Clinical and molecular characteristics of isolated colonic Crohn's disease. Inflamm Bowel Dis. 14: 1667–1677.
29. Waterman M, Xu W, Stempak JM, Milgrom R, Bernstein CN, et al. (2011) Distinct and overlapping genetic loci in Crohn's disease and ulcerative colitis: correlations with pathogenesis. Inflamm Bowel Dis. 17: 1936–1942.
30. Chen H, Lee A, Bowcock A, Zhu W, Li E, et al. (2011) Influence of Crohn's disease and smoking on disease location. Dis Colon Rectum 54: 1020–1025.
31. Satsangi J, Silverberg MS, Vermeire S, Colombel JF (2006) The Montreal classification of inflammatory bowel disease: controversies, consensus, and implications. Gut. 55: 749–753.
32. Stange EF, Travis SP, Vermeire S, Colombel JF (2006) European evidence based consensus on the diagnosis and management of Crohn's disease: definitions and diagnosis. Gut 55 (suppl 1): i1–i15.
33. Geboes K, Van Eyken (2009) Inflammatory bowel disease unclassified and indeterminate colitis: the role of the pathologist. J. Clin Pathol. 62: 201–205.
34. Ley RE, Turnbaugh PJ, Klein S, Gordon JI (2006) Microbial ecology: human gut microbes associated with obesity. Nature. 444: 1022–1023.
35. Peterson J, Garges S, Giovanni M, McInnes P, Wang L, et al. (2009) The NIH Human Microbiome Project. Genome Res. 19: 2317–2323.
36. Petrosino JF, Highlander S, Luna RA, Gibbs RA, Versalovic J (2009) Metagenomic pyrosequencing and microbial identification. Clin Chem. 55: 856–866.
37. Salzman NH, Hung K, Haribhai D, Chu H, Karlsson-Sjöberg J, et al. (2010) Enteric defensins are essential regulators of intestinal microbial ecology. Nat Immunol. 11: 76–83.
38. Haas BJ, Gevers D, Earl A, Feldgarden M, Ward DV, et al. (2011) Chimeric 16S rRNA sequence formation and detection in Sanger and 454-pyrosequenced PCR amplicons. Genome Res 21: 494–504.
39. Hamm C, Reimers M, McCullough C, Gorbe EB, Lu J, et al. (2010) NOD2 status and human ileal gene expression. Inflamm Bowel Dis. 16: 1649–1657.
40. Aldhous MC, Drummond HE, Anderson N, Smith LA, Arnott ID, et al. (2007) Does cigarette smoking influence the phenotype of Crohn's disease? Analysis using the Montreal classification. Am J Gastroenterol. 102: 577–588.
41. Mahid SS, Minor KS, Soto RE, Hornung CA, Galandiuk S (2006) Smoking and inflammatory bowel disease: a meta-analysis. Mayo Clin Proc. 81: 1462–1471.

42. Unkart JT, Anderson L, Li E, Miller C, Yan Y, et al. (2008) Risk factors for surgical recurrence after ileocolic resection of Crohn's disease. Dis Colon Rectum. 51: 1211–1216.

43. Issa M, Vijaypal A, Graham MB, Beaulieu DB, Otterson MF, et al. (2007) Impact of Clostridium difficile on inflammatory bowel disease. Clin Gastroenterol Hepatol 5: 345–351.

44. Rodemann JF, Dubberke ER, Reske KA, Seo DH, Stone CD (2007) The incidence of Clostridium difficile infection in inflammatory bowel disease. Clin Gastroenterol Hepatol 5: 339–44.

45. Cohen SH, Gerding DN, Johnson S, Kelly CP, Loo VG, et al. (2010) Clinical practice guidelines for Clostridium difficile infection in adults: 2010 update by the society for healthcare epidemiology of America (SHEA) and the infectious diseases society of America (IDSA). Infect Control Hosp Epidemiol. 31: 431–555.

46. Nelson RL, Glenny AM, Song F (2009) Antimicrobial prophylaxis for colorectal surgery. Cochrane Database Syst Rev. (1): CD001181.

47. Nawrocki EP, Kolbe DL, Eddy SR (2009) Infernal 1.0: Inference of RNA alignments. Bioinformatics. 25: 1335–7.

48. Wang Q, Garrity GM, Tiedje JM, Cole JR (2007) Naive Bayesian classifier for rapid assignment of rRNA sequences into the new bacterial taxonomy. Appl Environ Microbiol 73: 5261–7.

49. Cole JR, Wang Q, Cardenas E, Fish J, Chai B, et al. (2009) The Ribosomal Database Project: improved alignments and new tools for rRNA analysis. Nucleic Acids Res. 37: D141–145.

50. DeSantis TZ, Hugenholtz P, Larsen N, Rojas M, Brodie EL, et al. (2006) Greengenes, a chimera-checked 16S rRNA gene database and workbench compatible with ARB. Appl Environ Microbiol 72: 5069–5072.

51. Collins MD, Lawson PA, Willems A, Cordoba JJ, Fernanadez-Garayzabal J, etal. (1994) The phylogeny of the genus Clostridium: proposal of five new genera and eleven new species combinations. Int J Syst Bacteriol. 44: 812–826.

52. Rinttilä T, Kassinen A, Malinen E, Krogius L, Palva A (2004) Development of an extensive set of 16S rDNA-targeted primer for quantification of pathogenic and indigenous bacteria in faecal samples by real-time PCR. J. Appl. Microbiol. 97: 1166–1177.

53. Maeda H, Fujimoto C, Haruki Y, Maeda T, Kokequchi S, et al. (2003) Quantitative real-time PCR using TaqMan and SYBR Green for Actinobacillus actinomycetemcomitans, Porphyromonas gingivalis, Prevotella intermedia, tetQ gene and total bacteria. (2003) FEMS Immunol Med Microbiol. 39: 81–86.

54. Aitchison J (1986) The statistical analysis of compositional data, Monographs on Statistics and Applied Probability. London (UK): Chapman and Hall Ltd.

55. Anderson MJ (2001) A new method for non-parametric multivariate analysis of variance. Austral Ecology. 26: 32–46.

56. McArdle BH, Anderson MJ (2001) Fitting multivariate models to community data: a comment on distance-based redundancy analysis. Ecology 82: 290–297.

57. Benjamini Y, Hochberg Y (1995) Controlling the false discovery rate: a practical and powerful approach to multiple testing. J R Statist Soc B 57: 289–300.

58. Anderson MJ, Legendre P (1999) An empirical comparison of permutation methods for tests of partial regression coefficients in a linear model. J Stat Comput Simul 62: 271–303.

59. Manly BFJ (1997) Randomization, bootstrap, and Monte Carlo methods in biology, 2nd ed. London (UK): Chapman and Hall Ltd.

60. Rim SH, Seeff L, Ahmed F, King JB, Coughlin SS (2009) Colorectal cancer incidence in the United States, 1999–2004 : an updated analysis of data from the National Program of Cancer Registries and the Surveillance, Epidemiology, and End Results Program. Cancer. 115: 1967–1976.

61. Maeda S, Hsu LC, Liu H, Bankston H, Iimura LA, et al. (2005) Nod2 mutation in Crohn's disease potentiates NF-kappaB activity and IL-1beta processing. Science. 307: 734–738.

62. Hopkins MJ, MacFarlane GT (2002) Changes in predominant bacterial populations in human faeces with age and with Clostridium difficile infection. J Med Microbiol. 51: 448–454.

63. Chang JY, Antonopoulos DA, Kalra A, Tonelli A, Khalife WT, et al. (2008) Decreased diversity of the fecal microbiome in recurrent Clostridium difficile-associated diarrhea. J Infect Dis. 197: 435–438.

64. Croswell A, Amir E, Teggatz P, Barman M, Salzman NH (2009) Prolonged impact of antibiotics on intestinal microbial ecology and susceptibility to enteric Salmonella infection. Infect Immun. 77: 2741–2753.

65. Dethlefsen L, Huse S, Sogin ML, Relman DA (2008) The pervasive effects of an antibiotic on the human gut microbiota, as revealed by deep 16S rRNA sequencing. PLoS Biol. 6: e280.

66. Frank JA, Reich CI, Sharma S, Weisbaum JS, Wilson BA, et al. (2008) Critical evaluation of two primers commonly used for amplification of bacterial 16S rRNA genes. Appl. Environ. Microbiol. 74: 2461–70.

67. Delima SL, McBride RK, Preshaw PM, Heasman PA, Kumar PS (2010) Response of subgingival bacteria to smoking cessation. J Clin Microbiol. 48: 2344–2349.

9

Investigation of the Enteric Pathogenic Potential of Oral *Campylobacter concisus* Strains Isolated from Patients with Inflammatory Bowel Disease

Yazan Ismail[1][⑨], Vikneswari Mahendran[1][⑨], Sophie Octavia[1], Andrew S. Day[2,3,4], Stephen M. Riordan[5,7], Michael C. Grimm[6], Ruiting Lan[1], Daniel Lemberg[2], Thi Anh Tuyet Tran[1], Li Zhang[1]*

1 The School of Biotechnology and Biomolecular Sciences, University of New South Wales, Sydney, Australia, 2 Department of Gastroenterology, Sydney Children's Hospital, Sydney, Australia, 3 School of Women's and Children's Health, University of New South Wales, Sydney, Australia, 4 Department of Paediatrics, University of Otago, Christchurch, New Zealand, 5 Gastrointestinal and Liver Unit, The Prince of Wales Hospital, Sydney, Australia, 6 St. George Clinical School, University of New South Wales, Sydney, Australia, 7 Faculty of Medicine, University of New South Wales, Sydney, Australia

Abstract

Background: *Campylobacter concisus*, a bacterium colonizing the human oral cavity, has been shown to be associated with inflammatory bowel disease (IBD). This study investigated if patients with IBD are colonized with specific oral *C. concisus* strains that have potential to cause enteric diseases.

Methodology: Seventy oral and enteric *C. concisus* isolates obtained from eight patients with IBD and six controls were examined for housekeeping genes by multilocus sequence typing (MLST), Caco2 cell invasion by gentamicin-protection-assay, protein analysis by mass spectrometry and SDS-PAGE, and morphology by scanning electron microscopy. The whole genome sequenced *C. concisus* strain 13826 which was isolated from an individual with bloody diarrhea was included in MLST analysis.

Principal Findings: MLST analysis showed that 87.5% of individuals whose *C. concisus* belonged to Cluster I had inflammatory enteric diseases (six IBD and one with bloody diarrhea), which was significantly higher than that in the remaining individuals (28.6%) ($P<0.05$). Enteric invasive *C. concisus* (EICC) oral strain was detected in 50% of patients with IBD and none of the controls. All EICC strains were in Cluster 1. The *C. concisus* strain colonizing intestinal tissues of patient No. 1 was closely related to the oral *C. concisus* strain from patient No. 6 and had gene recombination with the patient's own oral *C. concisus*. The oral and intestinal *C. concisus* strains of patient No. 3 were the same strain. Some individuals were colonized with multiple oral *C. concisus* strains that have undergone natural recombination.

Conclusions: This study provides the first evidence that patients with IBD are colonized with specific oral *C. concisus* strains, with some being EICC strains. *C. concisus* colonizing intestinal tissues of patients with IBD at least in some instances results from an endogenous colonization of the patient's oral *C. concisus* and that *C. concisus* strains undergo natural recombination.

Editor: Stefan Bereswill, Charité-University Medicine Berlin, Germany

Funding: This work was supported by the Broad Medical Research Program of the Broad Foundation (Grant no: IBD0273-R) and a research grant awarded to Dr Li Zhang from the Faculty of Science, University of New South Wales (FRG2011). Yazan Ismail is supported by a PhD scholarship from Al-Balaq' Applied University, Jordan. The funders had no role in study design, data collection and analysis, decision to publish, or preparation of the manuscript.

Competing Interests: The authors have declared that no competing interests exist.

* E-mail: L.Zhang@unsw.edu.au

⑨ These authors contributed equally to this work.

Introduction

Campylobacter oncisus is a Gram-negative bacterium with a curved shape and a polar flagellum, which was first isolated from human gingival plaques in 1981 [1]. *C. concisus* is a fastidious bacterium, requiring hydrogen enriched microaerobic conditions for growth [2,3].

Recently, *C. concisus* has been shown to be associated with inflammatory bowel disease (IBD). IBD is a chronic inflammatory disorder of the gastrointestinal tract; the two major forms of IBD are Crohn's disease (CD) and ulcerative colitis (UC) [4,5]. The

aetiology of IBD is unknown. Studies have shown that multiple factors including genetic factors, environmental factors and intestinal microflora are involved in the development of IBD [4,5]. Despite strong evidence showing that the intestinal microbiota plays a key role in the pathogenesis of IBD, the exact causative or triggering agent still remains unknown [6,7,8].

A significantly higher prevalence of *C. concisus* in intestinal biopsies and fecal samples of patients with IBD as compared with controls were reported by a number of research groups [9,10,11,12]. Using *in vitro* cell culture models, *C. concisus* was shown to increase intestinal epithelial permeability and induce intestinal epithelial production of IL-8 and apoptosis [13,14,15]. Some *C. concisus* strains cultured from intestinal biopsies of patients with IBD and diarrheal stool samples were shown to be invasive to Caco2 cells [14]. The presence of bacterial virulence factors such as phospholipase A2 and a cytolethal distending toxin (CDT)-like toxin in some *C. concisus* strains has been reported [16,17].

C. concisus is a commensal bacterium of the human oral cavity. Zhang *et al* isolated *C. concisus* from 75% of saliva samples obtained from healthy individuals aged 3 to 60 years old and detected *C. concisus* by PCR in 95% of these samples [18]. The prevalence of *C. concisus* in the oral cavity of patients with IBD and healthy controls was not statistically different [18]. Furthermore, this study noted some bacterial protein banding similarities between a *C. concisus* strain colonizing the oral cavity and the *C. concisus* strain colonizing the intestinal tissues of a patient with IBD and proposed that specific oral *C. concisus* strains are involved in human IBD [18].

Currently, whether patients with IBD are colonized with specific oral *C. concisus* strains is not known. It is also not clear whether oral *C. concisus* strains have enteric pathogenic potential and whether *C. concisus* colonizing intestinal tissues of a given patient with IBD results from an endogenous colonization of the patient's own oral *C. concisus*. To investigate these issues, we compared the housekeeping genes and protein profiles of oral *C. concisus* isolated from patients with IBD and controls, as well as *C. concisus* isolated from intestinal biopsies of patients with IBD. In addition, we examined the invasiveness of oral *C. concisus* isolates to Caco2 cells and identified a number of bacterial proteins that may be important to *C. concisus* invasion of Caco2 cells.

Results

Analysis of Housekeeping Genes of Oral and Enteric *C. Concisus* Isolated from Patients with IBD and Controls by Multilocus Sequence Typing

Six housekeeping genes amplified from 70 *C. concisus* isolates, which were obtained from eight patients with IBD and six controls (details of these *C. concisus* isolates were described in Materials and Methods section), were analysed by multilocus sequence typing (MLST). The six housekeeping genes amplified were *aspA* (aspartase A), *glnA* (glutamine synthetase), *tkt* (transkelotase), *asd* (aspartate semialdehyde dehydrogenase), *atpA* (ATP synthase alpha subunit) and *pgi* (glucose-6-isomerase). MLST analysis was based on the sequences of six housekeeping genes with a total of 2,561 bp from each isolate analysed. The sequence types (ST) and allelic profiles of *C. concisus* isolates analysed are shown in Table 1. The polymorphic nucleotides were submitted as supplementary data (Figure S1). The criteria to define strains and variants were described in the Materials and Methods section.

MLST Analysis of Oral *C. Concisus* Isolated from Patients with IBD and Controls

Among the 21 oral *C. concisus* isolates (P1CDO1-P1CDO21) obtained from patient No. 1, five sequence types (ST1- ST5) of *C. concisus* were identified (Table 1). ST1 included 16 isolates (P1CDO1, P1CDO5-O12, P1CDO14-O17 and P1CDO19-O21). ST2 included two isolates (P1CDO3 and P1CDO18). ST3, ST4 and ST5 each contained a single isolate (P1CDO4, P1CDO13 and P1CDO2) respectively. ST1 and ST2 differed in all six housekeeping genes (showing different allelic numbers at all six housekeeping genes), representing two different strains (Table 1). ST3 (P1CDO4) had four housekeeping genes (*asd, atpA, glnA,* and *pgi*) identical to ST1, *aspA* gene identical to ST2 and *tkt* gene

identical to ST5, suggesting that this isolate resulted from genomic recombination between ST1, ST2 and ST5 (Table 1). ST4 (P1CDO13) had five housekeeping genes identical to ST1 and its *asd* gene was different from the patient's oral *C. concisus* isolates, suggesting that ST4 is a recombinant of ST1 and an unsampled *C. concisus* isolate (Table 1). ST5 had housekeeping genes identical to ST1 except for one nucleotide mutation in *tkt* gene, suggesting that ST5 is a mutational variant of ST1 (Table 1 and Figure S1). Thus, two oral strains (ST1 and ST2), two recombinant variants (ST3 and ST4) and one mutational variant (ST5) were identified from patient 1.

Five STs (ST7-ST11) were identified in oral *C. concisus* isolates obtained from patient No. 2 (Table 1). ST7 contained two isolates (P2CDO1 and P2CDO4). ST8 contained two isolates (P2CDO3 and P2CDO7). ST7 and ST8 differed at all six housekeeping genes, representing two different strains (Table 1). ST9 contained one isolate (P2CDO5), which had five housekeeping genes identical to ST7 and *tkt* gene identical to ST8, suggesting that ST9 is a recombinant of ST7 and ST8 (Table 1). ST10 contained one isolate (P2CDO2), which had five housekeeping genes identical to ST8 and *aspA* gene identical to ST7, suggesting that ST10 is also a recombinant of ST7 and ST8 (Table 1). ST11 (P2CDO6) had five housekeeping genes identical to ST8, and *tkt* gene identical to ST7, suggesting that ST11 is another recombinant of ST7 and ST8 (Table 1). Thus, two oral strains (ST7 and ST8) and three recombinant variants (ST9, ST10 and ST11) were identified from patient 2 (Table 1).

The sequences of all six housekeeping genes of the 10 oral isolates (P3UCO1-O10) of patient No. 3 were identical, suggesting that this patient was colonized with a single oral *C. concisus* strain (ST12) (Table 1).

One oral *C. concisus* isolate was available from each of the remaining four patients (patients No. 5 to No. 8). The four *C. concisus* isolates from these four patients differed at all six housekeeping genes, each representing a different strain.

The nine isolates (H1O1-O9) obtained from the healthy individual No. 1 had identical housekeeping genes, suggesting that this individual was colonized with a single oral *C. concisus* strain (ST15) (Table 1). One oral *C. concisus* isolate was available from each of the remaining five healthy controls (H2-H6). Four of these healthy controls were colonized with a different *C. concisus* strain (differing at six housekeeping genes), except for H2O1 which had *atpA* and *tkt* genes identical to *C. concisus* ST12 (Table 1).

MLST Analysis of Enteric *C. Concisus* Isolated from Patients with IBD

The intestinal biopsy *C. concisus* isolate (P1CDB1(UNSWCD)) of patient No. 1 (designated as ST6) had five unique housekeeping genes (Table 1). However, its *asd* gene was identical to the patient's own oral ST1, ST3 and ST5, suggesting that ST6 has acquired its *asd* gene from the patient's own oral *C. concisus* isolates (Table 1).

The 10 intestinal biopsy *C. concisus* isolates (P3UCB1-B10) obtained from patient No. 3 had six housekeeping genes identical to that of the patient's own oral *C. concisus* isolates, indicating that the oral and intestinal biopsy *C. concisus* isolates are the same strain (ST12) (Table 1). Two luminal-washout isolates (P3UCLW1 and P3UCLW2) were obtained from patient No. 3. P3UCLW2 (ST13) had five housekeeping genes identical to the patient's own oral and intestinal biopsy isolates (ST12) and differed only by one base in *pgi*, suggesting that ST13 is a mutational variant of ST12 (Table 1). P3UCLW1 (ST14) had six housekeeping genes that were different from the patient's own oral and intestinal biopsy *C. concisus* isolates, representing a different *C. concisus* strain (Table 1).

Table 1. Sequence types (ST) and allelic profiles of *C. concisus* isolated from patients with IBD and controls.

Isolate ID	Total No. of isolate	ST	asd	aspA	atpA	glnA	pgi	tkt
P1CDO1, P1CDO5-O12, P1CDO14-O17, P1CDO19-O21	16	1	8	7	4	6	1	1
P1CDO3, P1CDO18	2	2	2	5	3	7	7	5
P1CDO4	1	3*	8	5	4	6	1	2
P1CDO13	1	4*	1	7	4	6	1	1
P1CDO2	1	5*	8	7	4	6	1	2
P1CDB1(UNSWCD)	1	6@	8	4	2	8	4	3
P2CDO1,P2CDO4	2	7	7	8	5	5	8	7
P2CDO3,P2CDO7	2	8	6	6	6	4	9	8
P2CDO5	1	9*	7	8	5	5	8	8
P2CDO2	1	10*	6	8	6	4	9	8
P2CDO6	1	11*	6	6	6	4	9	7
P3UCO1-P3UCO10, P3UCB1-P3UCB10	20	12	5	1	1	1	3	4
P3UCLW2	1	13	5	1	1	1	2	4
P3UCLW1	1	14	4	2	8	3	6	4
H1O1-H1O9	9	15	3	3	7	2	5	6
H5O1	1	16	10	18	16	9	12	10
P5CDO1	1	17	11	14	14	14	10	17
H2O1	1	18	12	16	1	3	15	4
P6CDO1	1	19	13	9	15	13	19	9
H6O1	1	20	14	12	9	16	14	16
P8UCO1	1	21	15	17	13	12	18	15
P7UCO1	1	22	16	15	11	10	11	11
H3O1	1	23	17	13	12	11	17	13
P4CDO1	1	24	18	10	16	17	13	12
H4O1	1	25	9	11	10	15	16	14
C. concisus strain 13826		26	19	19	17	18	20	18

*Recombinant or mutational variants of the patient's own oral *C. concisus* **strains.**
@This strain, which was isolated from a patient with CD, had asd gene identical to the patient's own oral *C. concisus* isolates.

The Genetic Relationship of Oral and Enteric *C. Concisus* Isolated from Patients with IBD and Controls

To further illustrate the genetic relationship between oral and enteric *C. concisus* strains isolated from patients with IBD and controls, a phylogenetic tree was constructed based on the sequences of the six housekeeping genes analysed (Figure 1). The housekeeping genes of the whole genome sequenced *C. concisus* strain 13826 were also included.

C. concisus isolates obtained from the majority of the patients with IBD (6/8) formed one cluster (Cluster 1). The *C. concisus* strain (P1CDB1(UNSWCD)) isolated from intestinal biopsies of patient No. 1 with CD, *C. concisus* strain 13826 (a strain isolated from fecal sample of a patient with bloody diarrhea) and the oral *C. concisus* isolate obtained from healthy individual No. 3 were also grouped into Cluster 1. All enteric invasive *Campylobacter concisus* (EICC) strains (see results in Table 2) were grouped into Cluster 1 (Figure 1). Seven of the eight individuals (7/8, 87.5%) whose isolates belonged to Cluster 1 had inflammatory enteric diseases (six patients with IBD and one had bloody diarrhea), which was significantly higher than the remaining individuals (2/7, 28.6%) (P<0.05). Among the *C. concisus* isolates that did not belong to Cluster 1, six isolates were genetically closely related, forming a second cluster (Cluster 2). The oral *C. concisus* isolate obtained from

a healthy control (H6O1) was genetically distinct from the other *C. concisus* isolates (Figure 1).

The intestinal biopsy isolate of patient 1 (P1CDB1(UNSWCD)) was genetically most closely related to the oral *C. concisus* isolate of a patient with CD (P6CDO1) (Figure 1). The intestinal biopsy isolates of patient No. 3 (P3UCB1-B10) were identical to the patient's own oral isolates (P3UCO1-10). One luminal-washout isolate (P3UCLW2) of patient No. 3 was very closely related to the patient's own oral and intestinal biopsy isolates. The second luminal-washout *C. concisus* isolate (P3UCLW1) of this patient was different from the patient oral and intestinal *C. concisus* isolates, but was more closely related to the oral isolates of healthy control No. 1 (Figure 1).

Comparison of Protein Profiles of Different *C. Concisus* Isolates

All 70 *C. concisus* isolates analyzed by MLST were also subjected to whole cell protein profile analysis. The protein profile types of all 70 *C. concisus* isolates were shown in Figure 1 and the representative protein profiles of *C. concisus* isolates from each individual are shown in Figure 2. The 21 oral *C. concisus* isolates (P1CDO1-O21) of patient 1 showed two different protein profiles (P1-1 and P1-2). Thus, the different strains showed different

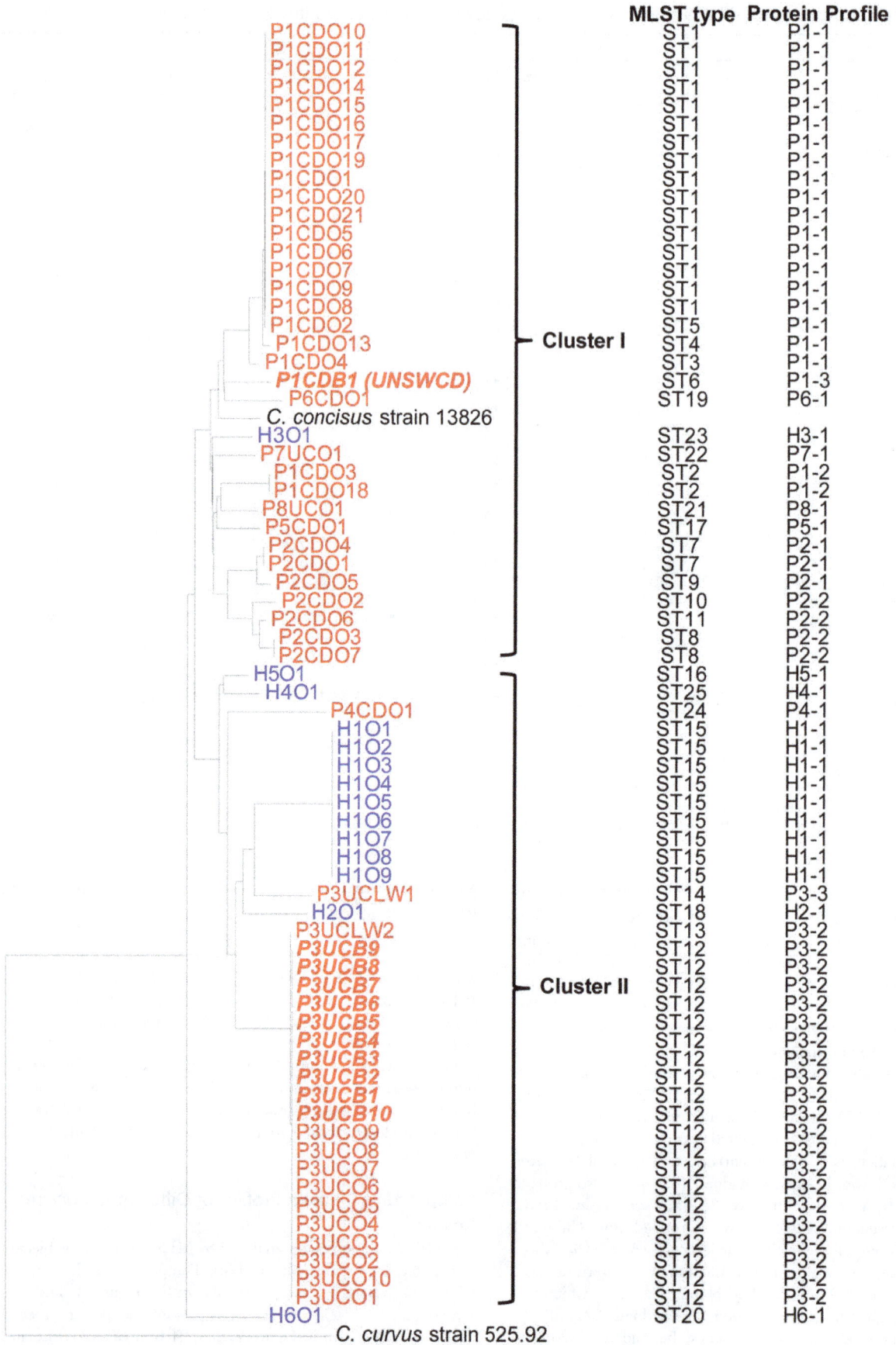

	MLST type	Protein Profile
P1CDO10	ST1	P1-1
P1CDO11	ST1	P1-1
P1CDO12	ST1	P1-1
P1CDO14	ST1	P1-1
P1CDO15	ST1	P1-1
P1CDO16	ST1	P1-1
P1CDO17	ST1	P1-1
P1CDO19	ST1	P1-1
P1CDO1	ST1	P1-1
P1CDO20	ST1	P1-1
P1CDO21	ST1	P1-1
P1CDO5	ST1	P1-1
P1CDO6	ST1	P1-1
P1CDO7	ST1	P1-1
P1CDO9	ST1	P1-1
P1CDO8	ST1	P1-1
P1CDO2	ST1	P1-1
P1CDO13	ST5	P1-1
P1CDO4	ST4	P1-1
P1CDB1 (UNSWCD)	ST3	P1-1
P6CDO1	ST6	P1-3
C. concisus strain 13826	ST19	P6-1
H3O1	ST23	H3-1
P7UCO1	ST22	P7-1
P1CDO3	ST2	P1-2
P1CDO18	ST2	P1-2
P8UCO1	ST21	P8-1
P5CDO1	ST17	P5-1
P2CDO4	ST7	P2-1
P2CDO1	ST7	P2-1
P2CDO5	ST9	P2-1
P2CDO2	ST10	P2-2
P2CDO6	ST11	P2-2
P2CDO3	ST8	P2-2
P2CDO7	ST8	P2-2
H5O1	ST16	H5-1
H4O1	ST25	H4-1
P4CDO1	ST24	P4-1
H1O1	ST15	H1-1
H1O2	ST15	H1-1
H1O3	ST15	H1-1
H1O4	ST15	H1-1
H1O5	ST15	H1-1
H1O6	ST15	H1-1
H1O7	ST15	H1-1
H1O8	ST15	H1-1
H1O9	ST15	H1-1
P3UCLW1	ST14	P3-3
H2O1	ST18	H2-1
P3UCLW2	ST13	P3-2
P3UCB9	ST12	P3-2
P3UCB8	ST12	P3-2
P3UCB7	ST12	P3-2
P3UCB6	ST12	P3-2
P3UCB5	ST12	P3-2
P3UCB4	ST12	P3-2
P3UCB3	ST12	P3-2
P3UCB2	ST12	P3-2
P3UCB1	ST12	P3-2
P3UCB10	ST12	P3-2
P3UCO9	ST12	P3-2
P3UCO8	ST12	P3-2
P3UCO7	ST12	P3-2
P3UCO6	ST12	P3-2
P3UCO5	ST12	P3-2
P3UCO4	ST12	P3-2
P3UCO3	ST12	P3-2
P3UCO2	ST12	P3-2
P3UCO10	ST12	P3-2
P3UCO1	ST12	P3-2
H6O1	ST20	H6-1
C. curvus strain 525.92		

Cluster I

Cluster II

0.02

Figure 1. Neighbour-Joining tree based on the sequences of six housekeeping genes (*asd, aspA, atpA, glnA, pgi* and *tkt*) **illustrating the phylogenetic relationships of oral and enteric** *Campylobacter concisus* **isolates analysed in this study.** Isolates from patients with IBD are coloured red. Isolates from a healthy control are coloured blue. Clusters are indicated in roman numerals. *Campylobacter curvus* is used as an outgroup. Alongside the tree on the right are the MLST sequence types (ST) and protein profiles. *Campylobacter concisus* strain 13826 is the whole genome sequenced strain (Accession No.: CP000792.1).

protein profiles, the variants did not generate new protein profiles (see MLST data). The intestinal biopsy isolate (P1CDB1(UNSWCD)) of patient No. 1 showed a protein profile (P1-3) that was different from the patient's oral strains. The seven oral *C. concisus* isolates (P2CDO1-O7) from patient No. 2 revealed two protein profiles (P2-1 and P2-2). Again, individual strains showed different protein profiles, the recombinant variants did not generate new protein profiles. The oral *C. concisus* isolates of patient No. 3 (P3UCO1-O10) showed an identical protein profile (P3-1), consistent with the finding that all oral *C. concisus* isolates of this patient had identical sequences of housekeeping genes and representing a single strain. The intestinal biopsy *C. concisus* isolates (P3UCB1-B10) and one luminal-washout isolate of patient 3 (P3UCLW2) showed the same protein profile (P3-2), which was identical to the protein pattern of the patient's oral *C. concisus* isolates except for the disappearance of a 210 kD band (band A in Figure 2). The second luminal-washout *C. concisus* isolate (P3UCLW1) showed a different protein profile (P3-3) (Figures 1 and 2).

Sequencing of the 210 kD band of P3UCO5 (oral isolate) identified 47 *C. concisus* proteins, the majority of which were ribosomal proteins and various proteins involved in metabolism. Interestingly, one protein was a bacterial virulence protein S-layer-RTX.

All oral *C. concisus* isolates of the healthy control No. 1 showed an identical *C. concisus* protein profile (H1-1) (Figure 2), consistent with the finding that all oral *C. concisus* isolates from this individual had identical housekeeping genes.

The *C. concisus* isolates obtained from the remaining patients and controls showed individual protein patterns (Figure 2).

Disease associated protein profiles were not identified.

Detection of Enteric Invasive *C. Concisus* (EICC) Oral Strains in Patients with IBD

The invasiveness of all 70 *C. concisus* isolates to Caco2 cells was examined and expressed as invasive index. EICC strains, which have an invasive index ≥1, are shown in Table 2. EICC oral strains were detected in 50% (4/8) patients with IBD and none of the controls (0/6) (Table 2). However, the prevalence of EICC oral strains in patients with IBD was not statistically

different from that in controls ($P>0.05$). The remaining *C. concisus* isolates had an invasive index <1. The positive control invasive *C. concisus* strain (P1CDB1(UNSWCD)) showed an invasion index of 1.3.

Identification of Bacterial Proteins that may be Associated with *C. Concisus* Enteric Epithelial Invasion

Given that patient 1 was colonized with both EICC and non-EICC oral *C. concisus* isolates, we sequenced the most abundantly expressed protein band (band B shown in Figure 2) of an EICC isolate (P1CDO3) and its corresponding band (band C shown in Figure 2) of a non-EICC oral isolate (P1CDO2), attempting to identify some bacterial proteins that may be associated with *C. concisus* invasion to intestinal epithelial cells.

Twenty-three and 21 *C. concisus* proteins were identified from the protein band of the EICC isolate and the non-EICC isolate respectively. Seventeen proteins were common proteins identified from both the EICC isolate and the non-EICC isolate, and these proteins are involved in protein transport, metabolism and protein synthesis. General glycosylation pathway protein and Type II secretion system protein E, which were previously shown to be associated with bacterial virulence, were identified only from the protein band of EICC isolate. The distinctive proteins identified from the EICC isolate and the non-EICC isolate are listed in Table 3.

Bacterial Morphology of EICC and Non-EICC *C. Concisus* Isolates

To observe whether EICC isolates and non-EICC isolates are morphologically different, an EICC oral isolate (P1CDO3), a non-EICC oral isolate (P1CDO2) and an EICC enteric isolate (P1CDB1(UNSWCD)) were examined using electron microscopy. Both EICC and non-EICC isolates showed a similar morphology. Flagellum was present in all isolates (Figure 3).

Discussion

This study examined whether patients with IBD are colonized with specific oral *C. concisus* strains and whether oral *C. concisus* strains have enteric pathogenic potential. Furthermore, this study

Table 2. Enteric invasive *C. concisus* (EICC) oral isolates detected in patients with IBD.

Individual ID and Clinical condition	Sample source	EICC isolates identified	Invasion Index* mean±SE
Patient No. 1, CD	Saliva	P1CDO3 P1CDO18	2.0±0.9 1.5±0.2
Patient No. 1, CD	Intestinal biopsy	P1CDB1 (UNSWCD)#	1.3±0.2
Patient No. 2, CD	Saliva	P2CDO1 P2CDO2 P2CDO3 P2CDO4 P2CDO5 P2CDO6 P2CDO7	9.5±0.9 6.5±1.4 11.1±3.0 6.4±1.0 5±0.9 12.3±3.2 11.2±2.8
Patient No. 5, CD	Saliva	P5CDO1	4.0±1.1
Patient No. 8, UC	Saliva	P8UCO1	3.0±0.9

*The invasion index was the average of triplicate experiments
#Positive control strain used in this study.

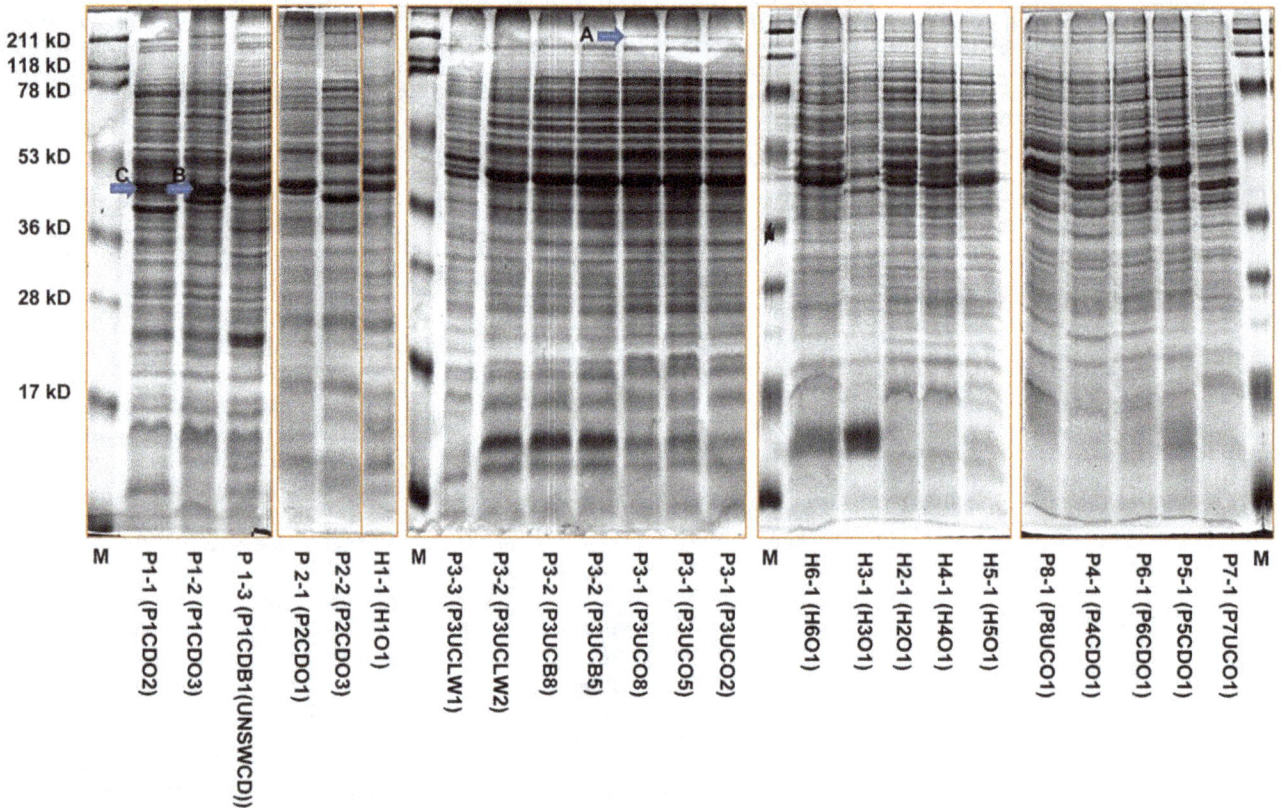

Figure 2. Representative whole cell protein profiles of oral and enteric *C. concisus* isolates obtained from patients with IBD and healthy controls. Arrows indicate protein bands that have been sequenced for protein identification. M: molecular weight Marker. Each lane was labelled as Protein profile (Isolate ID).

investigated whether *C. concisus* colonizing intestinal tissues of a given patient with IBD results from the endogenous colonization of the patient's own oral *C. concisus* strain.

MLST analysis revealed an association between Cluster I *C. concisus* strains and enteric inflammatory diseases including IBD (see results section). The oral *C. concisus* strains isolated from patients with IBD were predominantly grouped into Cluster I (Figure 1). EICC oral *C. concisus* strains were detected in 50% of patients with IBD and none of the controls (Table 2). All EICC oral *C. concisus* strains were in Cluster I. *C. concisus* colonizing intestinal tissues of patients with IBD, at least in some instances, originated from the colonization of the patients own oral *C. concisus* strain (Figure 1 and Table 1). Taken together, these results suggest that patients with IBD are colonized with a specific group of oral *C. concisus* strains that have enteric pathogenic potential if colonizing the intestinal tract.

Patient No. 1 was colonized with both EICC strain and non-EICC oral strains, which were morphologically indistinguishable (Figure 3). We attempted to identify proteins that may be associated with *C. concisus* intestinal epithelial invasion by sequencing the most abundantly expressed protein band of an EICC isolate and its corresponding protein band of a non-EICC isolate (Table 3 and Figure 2). Use of EICC and non-EICC *C. concisus* strains isolated from the oral cavity of the same individual would minimize the influence of environmental factors on bacterial protein expressions. We found that two of the proteins that were identified from the EICC isolate, including general glycosylation pathway protein and type II secretion system protein E, are particularly interesting in relation to bacterial virulence.

General glycosylation system has been reported to be important for *C. jejuni* to attach to and invade human epithelial cells [19]. The

Table 3. Distinctive proteins identified from the most abundantly expressed protein band[#] of an oral EICC isolate and the corresponding band of a non-EICC oral *C. concisus* isolate obtained from patient 1.

EICC isolate (P1CDO3)	Non-EICC isolate (P1CDO2)
General glycosylation pathway protein* Pyridoxal phosphate-dependent enzyme Outer membrane protein Peptide chain release factor 2 Hypothetical protein CCC13826_1624 Type II secretion system protein E*	3-isopropylmalate dehydratase large subunit Glutamate dehydrogenase Signal recognition particle protein Threonine dehydratase

[#]Protein bands were shown in Figure 3.
*Proteins related to bacterial virulence.

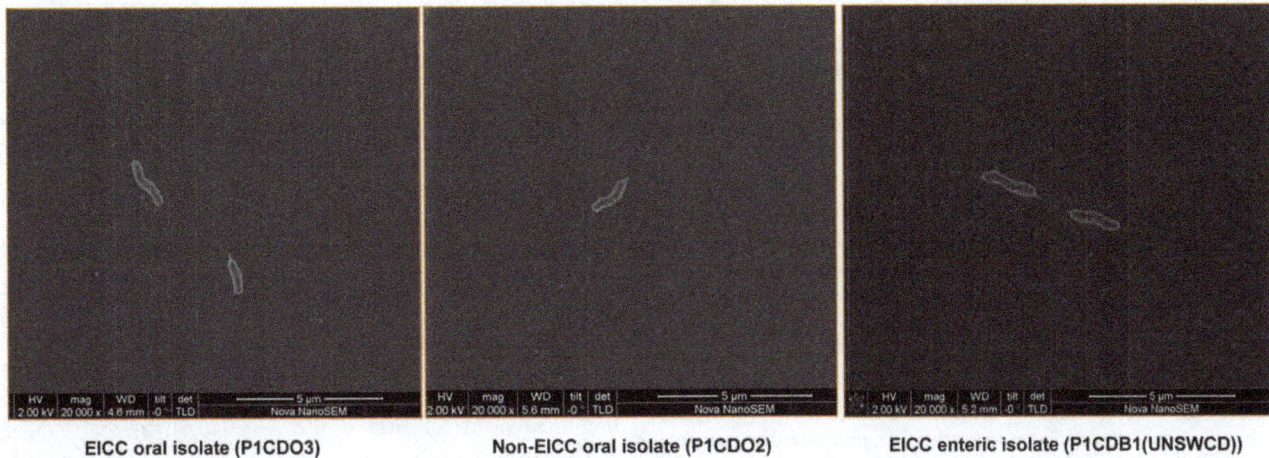

EICC oral isolate (P1CDO3)	Non-EICC oral isolate (P1CDO2)	EICC enteric isolate (P1CDB1(UNSWCD))

Figure 3. Electron Microscopic image of an oral EICC isolate, an oral non-EICC isolate and an enteric EICC isolate. All isolates were cultured from Patient No. 1.

Type II secretion system (T2SS), consisting of at least 12 core components including T2SS protein E, is one of the five protein secretion systems that Gram-negative bacteria use to export proteins from within the bacterial cell to the extracellular environment or into host cells [20,21]. T2SS has been shown to be important in bacterial pathogenesis [22]. A study by Iwobi *et al* showed that a novel type II secretion gene cluster is present only in high-pathogenicity *Yersinia enterocolitica* strains [23]. In our study, the fact that General glycosylation system protein and T2SS protein E were identified only from the protein band of the EICC isolate, not from the corresponding protein band of the non-EICC isolate indicates a difference of these proteins in EICC and non-EICC isolates. Future studies examining genes coding for these proteins in EICC and non-EICC isolates will further illustrate whether General glycosylation system and T2SS play a role in *C. concisus* invasion to intestinal epithelial cells.

A recent study by Kaakoush *et al* detected exotoxin 9 gene which is located in the plasmid in four enteric *C. concisus* strains that were invasive to Caco2 cells including the UNSWCD strain [24]. The presence of plasmid and the exotoxin 9 gene in oral *C. concisus* strains isolated from patients with IBD and controls should be examined in future studies. There are other evidence supporting that specific oral *C. concisus* strains may be enteric pathogenic. For example, Nielsen *et al* showed that both oral and fecal *C. concisus* strains induced epithelial barrier dysfunction [13].

The oral cavity is the primary colonization site of *C. concisus* in humans. Using a filtration method, we previously isolated *C. concisus* from 75% of saliva samples collected from healthy individuals and 85% of saliva collected from patients with IBD [18]. In comparison to the human oral cavity, the human intestine represents a less favourable environment for *C. concisus* growth. Using the same filtration method, Engberg *et al* isolated *C. concisus* from 2.8% of fecal samples collected from healthy individuals [25]. *C. concisus* requires H_2-enriched microaerobic condition for growth [3]. H_2 in the human intestine is generated by bacterial fermentation of unabsorbed carbohydrates; the amount of H_2 available in an individual's intestine is influenced by the ingested food and the composition of the local intestinal microbial community [26,27]. Thus, whether oral *C. concisus* strains are able to establish intestinal colonization and multiply to a sufficient number to cause enteric disorders will be determined by both the properties of *C. concisus* strains and the local intestinal environ-

ment, the latter may fluctuate due to the change of ingested food and the composition of an individual's intestinal microbial community.

Humans were previously considered as the only host of *C. concisus*, however, recently *C. concisus* was detected in fecal and saliva samples of domestic dogs and cats [28,29]. Whether domestic pets are an additional source of human intestinal *C. concisus* infection needs to be investigated. A study by Lynch *et al* isolated *C. concisus* from chicken and beef meat [30]. While chicken and beef meat may serve as a source of human infection, it is unable to conclude whether chicken and cattle are a natural host of *C. concisus*.

Oral and intestinal biopsy *C. concisus* isolates of patient 3 revealed identical protein profiles, except for the disappearance of a 210 kD protein band in the intestinal biopsy *C. concisus* isolates (Figure 2). Interestingly, S-layer-RTX protein was identified from this 210 kD protein band of the oral isolate. S-layer is a cell surface protein found in a range of bacterial species. RTX proteins are a family of proteins secreted by a variety of Gram-negative bacteria, which exhibit various biological functions including formation of the S-layer protein in some bacterial species [31]. S-layer contributes to bacterial pathogenesis by adhering to host cells and immune evasion [32]. *Campylobacter fetus* and *Campylobacter rectus* possess S-layer [33]. High frequency antigenic variation of S-layer in *C. fetus*, resulting from DNA inversion, has been reported [33,34]. Future studies are required to examine whether the disappearance of S-layer-RTX protein in intestinal biopsy *C. concisus* isolates in this patient is due to antigenic variation. S-layer RTX protein was previously detected in the P1CDB1(UNSWCD) strain [35]. Kalischuk *et al* reported that the gene coding for S-layer RTX was detected in two *C. concisus* strains isolated from fecal samples of healthy individuals, but not in *C. concisus* strains isolated from fecal samples of patients with diarrhea [15].

This study showed that the genome of *C. concisus* species is highly diverse. All individuals included in this study were colonized with different *C. concisus* strains, demonstrated by the findings that these *C. concisus* isolates differed at all six housekeeping genes (except for H2O1 strain, which had *atpA* and *tkt* genes identical to that of ST12) and showed unique protein profiles. This is consistent with the finding by Aabenhus *et al* [36]. Aabenhus *et al* examined 62

C. concisus strains using amplified fragment length polymorphism (AFLP) and found that all *C. concisus* strains gave unique AFLP profiles [36]. Our finding that *C. concisus* strains undergo natural recombination (Table 1) offer an explanation for the high genetic diversity of *C. concisus* species, as observed by other research groups [36,37,38,39].

From the luminal-washout of patient No. 3, two *C. concisus* isolates were isolated. While one isolate (P3UCLW2) was the variant of the *C. concisus* strain colonizing the intestinal tissues of this patient, the other isolate (P3UCLW1) was a different strain which was closely related to the oral *C. concisus* strain of healthy control No. 1 (Figure 1 and Table 1). This suggests that *C. concisus* detected in fecal samples may contain both *C. concisus* strains colonizing the intestinal tissues and *C. concisus* strains transiently colonizing the fecal materials.

In summary, this study provides the first evidence that patients with IBD are colonized with a group of specific oral *C. concisus* strains that may have enteric pathogenic potential. In addition, this study showed that *C. concisus* colonizing intestinal tissues of patients with IBD, at least in some instances, results from an endogenous colonization of the patient's own oral *C. concisus* and that *C. concisus* strains undergo natural recombination.

Materials and Methods

Ethics Statement

Saliva samples were obtained at the Prince of Wales Hospital, the St George Hospital and Sydney Children's Hospital, Sydney, Australia. Ethics approvals for this study were granted by the Ethics Committees of the University of New South Wales and the South East Sydney Area Healthy Service (Ethics Nos: HREC 09237/SESIAHS 09/078, HREC08335/SESIAHS(CHN)07/48 and HREC 06233/SESAHS (ES) 06/164). Written informed consent was obtained from all subjects in this study.

C. Concisus Isolates and Cultivation

A total of 70 *C. concisus* isolates obtained from eight patients with IBD and six controls were included in this study. Enteric *C. concisus* refers to isolates cultured from intestinal biopsies or luminal-washout fluid. Oral *C. concisus* refers to isolates cultured from saliva. Luminal-washout fluid was the fluid collected from luminal fluid draining tube prior to the start of the colonoscopy, which contains fecal bacteria and the mucosa associated bacteria flushed out from the intestinal mucus due to the severe diarrhoea induced during the preparation for colonoscopy. The enteric *C. concisus* isolate of patient 1 (P1CDB1) was isolated by Zhang *et al* [9], which was named as UNSWCD in a following study by Man *et al* [14]. To maintain the consistency with the previous publications and the naming system in this study, we used P1CDB1 (UNSWCD) to label this strain in this study. The enteric *C. concisus* isolates of patient 3 were isolated by Mahendran *et al* [11]. The oral *C. concisus* isolates were either isolated in our previous studies or in this study [18]. The identities of these *C. concisus* isolates were confirmed by microscopic examination of bacterial morphology and *C. concisus* specific PCR [12]. Details of the *C. concisus* isolates used in this study are listed in Table 4.

C. concisus isolates were cultured on Horse blood agar (HBA), prepared using Blood Agar Base No. 2 supplemented with 6% (v/v) defibrinated horse blood and 10 μg/ml vancomycin (Oxoid Australia Pty Limited, South Australia). Culture plates were incubated at 37°C for 48 hours under microaerobic conditions generated using a *Campylobacter* gas generating kit (Oxoid).

The clinical information of patients included in this study is shown in Table 5.

Bacterial DNA Extraction

C. concisus DNA was extracted using the Puregene DNA Extraction kit (Gentra, Minneapolis, USA) following the manufacturer's instructions.

Comparison of the Sequences of Housekeeping Genes of Oral and Enteric *C. Concisus* Isolates by Multilocus Sequence Typing

Choice of housekeeping genes and primer design. Six housekeeping genes (*aspA*, *glnA*, *tkt*, *asd*, *atpA* and *pgi*) were selected for MLST analysis. These housekeeping genes have previously been used for MLST analysis of *C. jejuni* [40,41,42].

The polymerase chain reaction (PCR) primers used to amplify each of the above genes were designed using the software Primer 3 plus, based on the genome sequence of *C. concisus* strain 13826 (Accession No. CP000792.1). The sequences of the PCR primers used are shown in Table 6.

Amplification and sequencing of MLST genes. To amplify the MLST genes, hot start PCR reactions were performed in a 25 μl reaction mixture containing $1\times$ PCR buffer, 200 nM of deoxynucleotide triphosphate, 2.5 mM $MgCl_2$, 5.5 U of Taq polymerase (Fisher Biotech, Subiaco, Australia), 10 pmol of each primer and 10 ng of bacterial DNA extracted from each *C. concisus* isolates. The thermal cycling conditions consist of denaturing at 96°C for 2 minutes, followed by 40 cycles of 94°C for 10 seconds, annealing for 10 seconds and 72°C for 45 seconds. The annealing temperatures were 55°C for *aspA* and *atpA*, 51°C for *tkt* and *asd*. The annealing temperatures for *gln* and *pgi* were 55°C–57°C, depending on individual isolates. Both strands of all PCR products were sequenced using BigDye™ terminator chemistry (Applied Biosystems, Foster City, CA) and separated on an ABI Capillary DNA Sequencer ABI3730 (Applied Biosystems).

MLST analysis. Sequences of housekeeping genes of *C. concisus* isolates were aligned and compared using software programs of MEGA 4 [43] and an in-house script MULTICOMP [44]. PHYLIP was used to generate neighbour-joining trees [45]. *Campylobacter curvus* (Accession No. CP000767.1) was used as an outgroup.

For each housekeeping gene, the different sequences present in different isolates were assigned distinct allele numbers. The allele numbers at each of the housekeeping genes defined the allelic profiles. Each isolate with a distinct allelic profile was referred as an individual sequence type (ST). Isolates with identical sequences at all six housekeeping genes were defined as the same strain. Isolates with different sequences at all six housekeeping genes were defined as different strains. In the case that a given individual was colonized with multiple *C. concisus* strains (more than one *C. concisus* strain), if evidence suggesting that some *C. concisus* isolates were generated due to gene recombination or mutations of the *C. concisus* strains colonizing the same individual, the generated *C. concisus* isolates were defined as recombinant or mutational variants.

GenBank Sequence Submission

Sequences of housekeeping genes amplified by PCR were submitted to GenBank. The accession numbers of the sequences of the PCR products of housekeeping genes submitted to GenBank were JQ683402-JQ683505.

Table 4. *C. concisus* isolates used in this study.

Isolate ID	Number of isolates[#]	Sample source*	Individual ID and diagnosis
P1CDO1-P1CDO21	21	Saliva	Patient No. 1, CD
P1CDB1(UNSWCD)	1	Intestinal biopsies	Patient No. 1, CD
P2CDO1-P2CDO7	7	Saliva	Patient No. 2, CD
P3UCO1-P3UCO10	10	Saliva	Patient No. 3, UC
P3UCB1-P3UCB10	10	Intestinal biopsies	Patient No. 3, UC
P3UCLW1-P3UCLW2	2	Luminal-washout fluid	Patient No. 3, UC
P4CDO1	1	Saliva	Patient No. 4, CD
P5UCO1	1	Saliva	Patient No. 5, UC
P6CDO1	1	Saliva	Patient No. 6, CD
P7UCO1	1	Saliva	Patient No. 7, UC
P8UCO1	1	Saliva	Patient No. 8, UC
H1O1-H1O9	9	Saliva	Healthy individual No. 1
H2O1	1	Saliva	Healthy individual No. 2
H3O1	1	Saliva	Healthy individual No. 3
H4O1	1	Saliva	Healthy individual No. 4
H5O1	1	Saliva	Healthy individual No. 5
H6O1	1	Saliva	Healthy individual No. 6

[#]A total of 70 *C. concisus* isolates were examined in this study.
C. concisus isolated from intestinal biopsies and luminal-washout fluid was referred as enteric *C. concisus* and *C. concisus* isolated from saliva was referred as oral *C. concisus*.

Comparison of Whole Cell Protein Profiles of Oral and Enteric *C. Concisus* Isolates

Whole cell proteins of *C. concisus* isolates were prepared. Briefly, *C. concisus* was harvested from HBA plates following cultivation for two days. After washing three times with PBS, the pellet was frozen-thawed three times using liquid nitrogen, then suspended in 600 μl of PBS. The bacterial mixtures were sonicated on ice for 3 minutes with 0.5 seconds intervals (40% amplitudes). The protein concentrations were determined using the BCA™ protein assay kit (Pierce, Rockford, USA). 15 μg whole cell proteins of each isolate were loaded on to 12% sodium dodecyl sulphate polyacrylamide gel electrophoresis (SDS-PAGE) to examine the whole cell protein profiles as described previously [46].

Investigation of Enteric Invasiveness of *C. Concisus* Isolates

Invasive abilities of *C. concisus* isolates to Caco2 cells were examined using previously described gentamicin protection assay with modifications [14,47,48].

Briefly, Minimum Essential Medium (MEM) supplemented with 10% heat inactivated fetal bovine serum (HI-FBS), 1 mM Sodium

Table 5. Clinical information of patients included in this study.

Patient ID-Sex- Age at diagnosis*	Diagnosis and disease activity at the time of sample collection	Montreal classification [50,51,52]
Patient No. 1-F-2y	CD, new case, active	L2, L4
Patient No. 2-M-19y	CD, relapse, active	L3, L4
Patient No. 3-M-23y	UC, new case, active	Extensive E3/S1
Patient No. 4-M-16y	CD, remission	L3,L4
Patient No. 5-M-13y	CD, remission	L2,L4
Patient No. 6-M-13y	CD, remission	L3, L4
Patient No. 7-M-65y	UC, new case, active	Left sided E2/S2
Patient No. 8-M-16y	UC, remission	Left sided E2/S1

C. concisus strains were previously isolated from biopsies of patients No. 1 and No. 3 [9,11]. The intestinal biopsies collected from patients No. 1 and No. 3 were from caecum and descending colon respectively, sampled from areas next to inflamed mucosa. *C. concisus* was detected in intestinal biopsies collected from patients No. 2 and No. 7 by PCR [11]. No intestinal biopsies were available from patients in remission.
Patients No. 2, No. 5, No. 6 and No. 8 were being treated with anti-inflammatory drugs (infliximab, aminosalicylates, methotrexate or azathioprine) at the time of saliva collection. Patient No. 4 had ileocolonic resection and antibiotics treatment (metronidazone and ciprofloxacin) two years ago. None of the patients were receiving antibiotics treatment at the time of sample collection for this study.

Table 6. PCR primers used for amplification of MLST genes in this study.

Gene	Forward sequence (5′–3′)	Reverse sequence (5′–3)
aspA	ACCATGCTCGGATTTAGC	CCATCCAAACGATCACAC
glnA	ATGAAGCCAGAAGCGACATC	GCGTTCTCTGATCTCATCTAGG
Tkt	CACCGATACCTTGCTCAG	GGACACGACTACAACCAG
Asd	TAGAGTTATGGAGGAGGTTG	AGATAGTAGGCATCGGATAC
atpA	GCGGTATCACAGAAGGAAG	GCGGAGAATATGGAGGTTG
Pgi	GCAAGCAGCGAGGTCATC	TAGTGGCGTAGTGGTAGGC

PCR primers were designed based on the whole genome sequenced *C. concisus* strain 13826 (Accession No: CP000792.1).

pyruvate, 0.1 mM non-essential amino acids, 100 Unit/ml Penicillin, 100 µg/ml streptomycin and 225 mg/l Sodium Bicarbonate (Invitrogen Australia Pty Limited, Mulgrave, Australia) was used for routine maintenance of Caco2 cells. For gentamicin protection assay, Caco-2 cells (5×10^5 cells/well) were seeded onto 24-well cell culture plates pre-treated with rat tail collagen type 1 (0.05 mg/ml) (BD Australia, North Ryde, Australia) and incubated at 37°C with 5% CO_2 for 4 days to form a monolayer. The monolayer was washed 4 times using Phosphate Buffer Saline (PBS) and incubated with *C. concisus* isolates at a multiplicity of infection (MOI) of 100 for 2 hours in MEM media containing no antibiotics. Six wells of Caco2 cells were infected with each *C. concisus* isolate. Following the 2 hour incubation, the wells were washed 4 times with PBS. The Caco2 monolayer of three wells was lysed with 1% Triton X-100 for 5 minutes. Serial dilutions of cell lysates were inoculated onto HBA plates and incubated as described above. Colony-forming units (CFU) of *C. concisus* were recorded, which were regarded as the numbers of *C. concisus* that have adhered to Caco2 cells. The remaining three wells of Caco2 cells infected with *C. concisus* were incubated with 1 ml of MEM containing 200 µg/ml of gentamicin to kill the extracellular bacteria. Following washing of the Caco2 monolayer for 5 times using PBS, the cells were lysed with 1% Triton X-100. Serial dilutions of cell lysates were inoculated onto HBA plates and incubated for two days. CFU of *C. concisus* were recorded, which were regarded as the numbers of *C. concisus* that have been internalised into Caco2. Gentamicin assay was repeated three times.

Invasive index, which is the number of internalized *C. concisus*/number of adherent *C. concisus* × 100, was calculated using the formula described by Larson *et al* [49]. A *C. concisus* strain that has an invasive index ≥1 was defined as an enteric-invasive *C. concisus* (EICC) strain. This definition was based on previous studies showing that the established human enteric pathogen *Campylobacter jejuni* with an invasive index ≥1 causes symptoms in infected pigs similar to human symptoms [49]. The UNSWCD strain, which

was previously shown to invasive to Caco2 cells [14], was used as the positive control.

Mass Spectrometry Analysis

A number of *C. concisus* protein bands separated on SDS-PAGE were subjected to mass spectrometry analysis to identify proteins that may be important for *C. concisus* invasion to Caco2 cells and for *C. concisus* intestinal colonization. Briefly, protein bands of interest were excised from Commassie Blue stained polyacrylamide gel and were digested with trypsin. Digested peptides were separated by nano-liquid chromatography (LC) using an Ultimate 3000 HPLC and autosampler system (Dionex, Amsterdam, The Netherlands) and then subjected to analysis using a LTQ-FT Ultra mass spectrometer (Thermo Electron, Bremen, Germany). All MS/MS spectra were searched against NCBI database using MASCOT (version 2.3). Mass spectrometric analysis was carried out at the Bioanalytical Mass Spectrometry Facility, University of New South Wales, Australia.

Scanning Electron Microscopy

Scanning electron microscopy was used to examine the morphology of two different oral *C. concisus* isolates, one shown to have an invasive index >1 (defined as EICC in this study) and another shown to have an invasive index <1 (defined as non-EICC in this study). *C. concisus* suspension prepared using MEM containing 10% HI-FBS was placed on glass cover slips. The glass cover slips were incubated at 37°C with 5% CO_2 for 2 hours, the bacteria were fixed with 2% glutaraldehyde and 2.5% paraformadehyde in 0.1 mol/L phosphate buffer (pH 7.4). Following dehydration in ethanol and critical point drying, *C. concisus* was mounted on carbon tabs, gold-coated then observed using Nova™ NanoSEM 230 high resolution scanning electron microscope (FEI, Oregon, USA). Scanning electron microscopic examination was performed at the Electron Microscope Unit at the University of New South Wales, Australia.

Statistic Analysis

Fisher's exact test (two tailed) was used in this study. Statistical analysis was performed using GraphPad Prism 5 software (San Diego, CA).

Acknowledgments

We would like to thank Ms Jenny Norman for her help in performing scanning electron microscopic examination of *C. concisus*.

Author Contributions

Conceived and designed the experiments: LZ YI VM. Performed the experiments: YI VM TATT. Analyzed the data: YI VM LZ. Wrote the paper: LZ VM YI SO AD RL SR MG DL. MLST analysis: SO RL. Obtained clinical samples and clinical information: AD SR MG DL.

References

1. Tanner ACR, Badger S, Lai CH, Listgarten MA, Visconti RA, et al. (1981) *Wolinella* gen-nov, *Wolinella-succinogenes* (vibrio-succinogenes-wolinet-al) Comb-nov, and description of *Bacteruides-gracilis* sp-nov, *Wolinella-recta* sp-nov, *Campylobacter-concisus* sp-nov and *Eikenella-corrodens* from humans with periodontal-disease. Int J Syst Bacteriol 31: 432–445.

2. Vandamme P, Dewhirst FE, Paster BJ, On SLW (2005) Genus I. *Campylobacter*. In: Garrity GM, Brenner DJ, Krieg NR, Staley JT, eds. Bergey's Manual of Systematic Bacteriology. 2 ed. New York: Springer. pp 1147–1160.

3. Lastovica AJ (2006) Emerging *Campylobacter* spp.: the Tip of the Iceberg. Clin Microbiol Newsl 28: 7.

4. Fiocchi C (1998) Inflammatory bowel disease: etiology and pathogenesis. Gastroenterology 115: 182–205.

5. Sartor RB (2006) Mechanisms of disease: pathogenesis of Crohn's disease and ulcerative colitis. Nature Clinical Practice Gastroenterology & Hepatology 3: 390–407.

6. Sartor RB (2008) Microbial influences in inflammatory bowel diseases. Gastroenterology 134: 577–594.

7. D'Haens GR, Geboes K, Peeters M, Baert F, Penninckx F, et al. (1998) Early lesions of recurrent Crohn's disease caused by infusion of intestinal contents in excluded ileum. Gastroenterology 114: 262–267.

8. Rutgeerts P, Goboes K, Peeters M, Hiele M, Penninckx F, et al. (1991) Effect of faecal stream diversion on recurrence of Crohn's disease in the neoterminal ileum. Lancet 338: 771–774.

9. Zhang L, Man SM, Day AS, Leach ST, Lemberg DA, et al. (2009) Detection and isolation of Campylobacter species other than *C. jejuni* from children with Crohn's disease. J Clin Microbiol 47: 453–455.

10. Mukhopadhya I, Thomson JM, Hansen R, Berry SH, El-Omar EM, et al. (2011) Detection of *Campylobacter concisus* and Other *Campylobacter* Species in Colonic Biopsies from Adults with Ulcerative Colitis. Plos One 6(6): e21490.

11. Mahendran V, Riordan S, Grimm M, Tran T, Major J, et al. (2011) Prevalence of *Campylobacter* species in adult Crohn's disease and the preferential colonization sites of *Campylobacter* species in the human intestine. Plos One 6(9): e25417.

12. Man SM, Zhang L, Day AS, Leach ST, Lemberg DA, et al. (2010) *Campylobacterconcisus* and Other *Campylobacter* Species in Children with Newly Diagnosed Crohn's Disease. Inflamm Bowel Dis 16: 1008–1016.

13. Nielsen HL, Nielsen H, Ejlertsen T, Engberg J, Gunzel D, N, et al. (2011) Oral and fecal *Campylobacter concisus* strains perturb barrier function by apoptosis induction in HT-29/b6 intestinal epithelial cells. Plos One 6(8): e23858.

14. Man SM, Kaakoush NO, Leach ST, Nahidi L, Lu HK, et al. (2010) Host Attachment, Invasion, and Stimulation of Proinflammatory Cytokines by *Campylobacter concisus* and Other Non-*Campylobacter jejuni* *Campylobacter* Species J Infect Dis 202: 1855–1865.

15. Kalischuk LD, Inglis GD (2011) Comparative genotypic and pathogenic examination of *Campylobacter concisus* isolates from diarrheic and non-diarrheic humans. Bmc Microbiol 11: 53–66.

16. Istivan TS, Coloe PJ, Fry BN, Ward P, Smith SC (2004) Characterization of a haemolytic phospholipase A(2) activity in clinical isolates of *Campylobacter concisus*. J Med Microbiol 53: 483–493.

17. Engberg J, Bang DD, Aabenhus R, Aarestrup FM, Fussing V, et al. (2005) *Campylobacter concisus*: an evaluation of certain phenotypic and genotypic characteristics. Clin Microbiol Infect 11: 288–295.

18. Zhang L, Budiman V, Day AS, Mitchell H, Lemberg DA, et al. (2010) Isolation and Detection of *Campylobacter concisus* from Saliva of Healthy Individuals and Patients with Inflammatory Bowel Disease. J Clin Microbiol 48: 2965–2967.

19. Karlyshev AV, Everest P, Linton D, Cawthraw S, Newell DG, et al. (2004) The *Campylobacter jejuni* general glycosylation system is important for attachment to human epithelial cells and in the colonization of chicks. Microbiol-Sgm 150: 1957–1964.

20. Cianciotto NP (2005) Type II secretion: a protein secretion system for all seasons. Trends Microbiol 13: 581–588.

21. Russel M (1998) Macromolecular assembly and secretion across the bacterial cell envelope: Type II protein secretion systems. J Mol Biol 279: 485–499.

22. Sandkvist M (2001) Type II secretion and pathogenesis. Infect Immun 69: 3523–3535.

23. Iwobi A, Heesemann J, Garcia E, Igwe E, Noelting C, et al (2003) Novel virulence-associated type II secretion system unique to high-pathogenicity *Yersinia enterocolitica*. Infect Immun 71: 1872–1879.

24. Kaakoush NO, Deshpande NP, Wilkins MR, Tan CG, Burgos-Portugal JA, et al. (2011) The pathogenic potential of *Campylobacter concisus* strains associated with chronic intestinal diseases. PLoS ONE 6(12): e29045.

25. Engberg J, On SLW, Harrington CS, Gerner-Smidt P (2000) Prevalence of *Campylobacter, Arcobacter, Helicobacter,* and *Sutterella* spp. in human fecal samples as estimated by a reevaluation of isolation methods for campylobacters. J Clin Microbiol 38: 286–291.

26. Levitt MD (1969) Production and excretion of hydrogen gas in man. New Engl J Med 281: 122–127.

27. Cummings JH (1983) Fermentation in the human large-intestine-evidence and implications for healthy. Lancet 1: 1206–1209.

28. Chaban B, Ngeleka M, Hill JE (2010) Detection and quantification of 14 *Campylobacter* species in pet dogs reveals an increase in species richness in feces of diarrheic animals. BMC Microbiol 10: 73–79.

29. Petersen RF, Harrington CS, Kortegaard HE, On SLW (2007) A PCR-DGGE method for detection and identification of *Campylobacter, Helicobacter, Arcobacter* and related Epsilobacteria and its application to saliva samples from humans and domestic pets. J Appl Microbiol 103: 2601–2615.

30. Lynch OA, Cagney C, McDowell DA, Duffy G (2011) Occurrence of fastidious *Campylobacter* spp. in fresh meat and poultry using an adapted cultural protocol. Int J Food Microbiol 150: 171–177.

31. Linhartova I, Bumba L, Masin J, Basler M, Osicka R, et al. (2010) RTX proteins: a highly diverse family secreted by a common mechanism. Fems Microbiol Rev 34: 1076–1112.

32. Thompson S (2002) *Campylobacter* surface-layers (S-layers) and immune evasion. Ann Periodontol 7: 43–45.

33. Blaser MJ, Wang E, Tummuru MKR, Washburn R, Fujimoto S, et al. (1994) High-frequency s-layer protein variation in *Campylobacter-fetus* revealed by sapa mutagenesis. Mol Microbiol 14: 453–462.

34. Garcia MM, Lutzewallace CL, Denes AS, Eaglesome MD, Holst E, et al. (1995) Prtein shift and antigenic variation in the S-layer of *Campylobacter-fetus* subsp *venerealis* during bovine infection accompanied by genomic rearrangement of sapa homologs. J Bacteriol 177: 1976–1980.

35. Kaakoush NO, Man SM, Lamb S, Raftery MJ, Wilkins MR, et al. (2010) The secretome of *Campylobacter concisus*. FEBS Journal 277: 1606–1617.

36. Aabenhus R, On S LW, Siemer BL, Permin H, Andersen, LP (2005) Delineation of *Campylobacter concisus* genomospecies by amplified fragment length polymorphism analysis and correlation of results with clinical data. J Clin Microbiol 43: 5–91–5096.

37. Vandamme P, Falsen E, Pot B, Hoste B, Kersters K, et al. (1989) Identification of ef group-22 campylobacters from gastroenteritis cases as *Campylobacter-concisus*. J Clin Microbiol 27: 1775–1781.

38. Matsheka MI, Lastovica AJ, Elisha BG (2001) Molecular identification of *Campylobacter concisus*. J Clin Microbiol 39: 3684–3689.

39. Bastyns K, Chapelle S, Vandamme P, Goossens H, Dewachter R (1995) Specific detection of *Campylobacter-concisus* by PCR amplification of 23 s rDNA areas. Mol Cell Probe 9: 247–250.

40. Dingle KE, Colles FM, Wareing DRA, Ure R, Fox AJ, et al. (2001) Multilocus sequence typing system for *Campylobacter jejuni*. J Clin Microbiol 39: 14–23.

41. Miller WG, On SLW, Wang GL, Fontanoz S, Lastovica AJ, et al. (2005) Extended multilocus sequence typing system for *Campylobacter coli, C lari, C-upsaliensis,* and *C-helveticus*. J Clin Microbiol 43: 2315–2329.

42. Suerbaum S, Lohrengel M, Sonnevend A, Ruberg F, Kist M (2001) Allelic diversity and recombination in *Campylobacter jejuni*. J Bacteriol 183: 2553–2559.

43. Tamura K, Dudley J, Nei M, Kumar S (2007) MEGA4: Molecular evolutionary genetics analysis (MEGA) software version 4.0. Mol Biol Evol 24: 1596–1599.

44. Reeves PR, Farnell L, Lan RT (1994) MULTICOMP - A program for preparing sequence data for phylogenetic analysis. Bioinformatics 10: 281–284.

45. Felsenstein J (1989) PHYLIP-phylogeny inference package. Cladistics 5: 164–166.

46. Laemmli U (1970) Cleavage of Structural Proteins during the Assembly of the Head of Bacteriophage T4. Nature 227: 680–685.

47. Hale TL, Bonventre PF (1979) Shigella infection of henle intestinal epithelial-cells - role of the bacterium. Infect Immun 24: 879–886.

48. Misawa N, Blaser MJ (2000) Detection and characterization of autoagglutination activity by *Campylobacter jejuni*. Infect Immun 68: 6168–6175.

49. Larson CL, Christensen JE, Pacheco SA, Minnich SA, Konkel ME (2008) *Campylobacter jejuni* secretes proteins via the flagellar type III secretion system that contribute to host cell invasion and gastroenteritis. In: Nachamkin I, Szymanski CM, Blaser MJ, eds. *Campylobacter*. 3rd. ed. Washington DC.: ASM press.

50. Silverberg MS, Satsangi J, Ahmad T, Arnott IDR, Bernstein CN, et al. (2005) Toward an integrated clinical, molecular and serological classification of inflammatory bowel disease: Report of a Working Party of the 2005 Montreal World Congress of Gastroenterology. Can J Gastroenterol 19: 5A–36A.

51. Satsangi J, Silverberg MS, Vermeire S, Colombel JF (2006) The Montreal classification of inflammatory bowel disease: controversies, consensus, and implications. Gut 55: 749–753.

52. Levine A, Griffiths A, Markowitz J, Wilson DC, Turner D, et al. (2011) Pediatric Modification of the Montreal Classification for Inflammatory Bowel Disease: The Paris Classification. Inflamm Bowel Dis 17: 1314–1321.

10

NKX2-3 Transcriptional Regulation of Endothelin-1 and VEGF Signaling in Human Intestinal Microvascular Endothelial Cells

Wei Yu[1], John P. Hegarty[1], Arthur Berg[2], Xi Chen[4], Gail West[5], Ashley A. Kelly[1], Yunhua Wang[1], Lisa S. Poritz[1,3], Walter A. Koltun[1]*, Zhenwu Lin[1]*

1 Department of Surgery, Pennsylvania State University, Hershey, Pennsylvania, United States of America, 2 Center for Statistical Genetics, Department of Public Health Sciences, Pennsylvania State University, Hershey, Pennsylvania, United States of America, 3 Department of Cellular & Molecular Physiology, Pennsylvania State University, Hershey, Pennsylvania, United States of America, 4 Department of Biostatistics, Vanderbilt University, Nashville, Tennessee, United States of America, 5 Department of Pathobiology, Lerner Research Institute, the Cleveland Clinic Foundation, Cleveland, Ohio, United States of America

Abstract

Background: NKX2-3 is associated with inflammatory bowel disease (IBD). NKX2-3 is expressed in microvascular endothelial cells and the muscularis mucosa of the gastrointestinal tract. Human intestinal microvascular endothelial cells (HIMECs) are actively involved in the pathogenesis of IBD and IBD-associated microvascular dysfunction. To understand the cellular function of NKX2-3 and its potential role underlying IBD pathogenesis, we investigated the genes regulated by NKX2-3 in HIMEC using cDNA microarray.

Methodology/Principal Findings: NKX2-3 expression was suppressed by shRNA in two HIMEC lines and gene expression was profiled by cDNA microarray. Pathway Analysis was used to identify gene networks according to biological functions and associated pathways. Validation of microarray and genes expression in intestinal tissues was assessed by RT-PCR. NKX2-3 regulated genes are involved in immune and inflammatory response, cell proliferation and growth, metabolic process, and angiogenesis. Several inflammation and angiogenesis related signaling pathways that play important roles in IBD were regulated by NKX2-3, including endothelin-1 and VEGF-PI3K/AKT-eNOS. Expression levels of NKX2-3, VEGFA, PI3K, AKT, and eNOS are increased in intestinal tissues from IBD patients and expression levels of EDN1 are decreased in intestinal tissues from IBD patients. These results demonstrated the important roles of NKX2-3, VEGF, PI3K, AKT, eNOS, and EDN1 in IBD pathogenesis. Correlation analysis showed a positive correlation between mRNA expression of NKX2-3 and VEGFA and a negative correlation between mRNA expression of NKX2-3 and EDN1 in intestinal tissues from IBD patients.

Conclusion/Relevance: NKX2-3 may play an important role in IBD pathogenesis by regulating endothelin-1 and VEGF signaling in HIMECs.

Editor: Christian Schönbach, Kyushu Institute of Technology, Japan

Funding: This work was supported by a grant from the Philadelphia Health Care Trust (WAK), the Carlino fund for IBD research at the Milton S. Hershey Medical Center (WAK), Penn State College of Medicine, and the Milton S. Hershey Penn State College of Medicine Surgery Research Feasibility Grant (WY). Budget: 942-82HY, Fund: 1940. The funders had no role in study design, data collection and analysis, decision to publish, or preparation of the manuscript.

Competing Interests: The authors have declared that no competing interests exist.

* E-mail: wkoltun@hmc.psu.edu (WAK); zlin@hmc.psu.edu (ZL)

Introduction

Crohn's disease (CD) and ulcerative colitis (UC), the two main subtypes of inflammatory bowel disease (IBD), are chronic, relapsing inflammatory disorders of the gastrointestinal tract. Genetics play an important role in the development of IBD [1]. *NKX2-3* (NK2 transcription factor related, locus 3) has been shown to be associated with both CD and UC by recent genome-wide association studies [2,3].

NKX2-3 is a member of the Nkx family of homeodomain transcription factors that play critical roles in regulating tissue-specific gene expression essential for determining tissue differentiation, as well as the temporal and spatial patterns of development [4,5]. During development, *NKX2-3* is primarily expressed in the midgut and hindgut mesoderm and spleen, as well as in

pharyngeal endoderm [6,7,8]. Analysis of *NKX2-3*-deficient mice has revealed a critical role for this homeobox transcription factor in spleen development and organization [9], and in establishing the correct environment for normal B cell development and T cell dependent immune response [10]. *NKX2-3* is also essential for normal small intestine development and function [11]. *NKX2-3* is also expressed in microvascular endothelial cells within the lamina propria and submucosa of the intestine, where it is required for expression of the lymphocyte adhesion molecule MAdCAM-1 in the mouse [9].

Microvascular endothelial cells have a critical "gatekeeper" role in the inflammatory process through their ability to recruit circulating immune cells to foci of inflammation. Endothelial activation in response to cytokines and bacterial products results in cell adhesion molecule expression and chemokine production, which mediate increased binding and transmigration of leukocytes across the vascular wall. Intestinal microvascular endothelial cells are recognized as a cell population actively involved in the pathogenesis of inflammatory bowel diseases (IBD) and IBD-associated microvascular dysfunction [12].

Transcription factors can regulate the expression of downstream genes. Recently, we found that the expression of *NKX2-3* is up-regulated in intestinal tissues and B cells from CD patients [13] and subsequently identified many inflammation and immune-response genes regulated by *NKX2-3* in B cell lines from a CD patient. These included several genes which also have important functions in endothelial cells, such as endothelin-1 (*EDN1*), *ASS1*, and *KLF2* [14]. Since endothelial cells play a key role in mucosal immune homeostasis and *NKX2-3* is expressed in intestinal endothelial cells, we further performed cDNA microarray to identify genes regulated by *NKX2-3* in two human intestinal microvascular endothelial cell lines (HIMEC).

Results

Suppression of *NKX2-3* expression in 2 HIMEC lines

pSUPER.retro.puro.shRNA-*NKX2-3* and empty vector were transfected into 21B and 432 HIMEC. RT-PCR results showed that mRNA expression levels of *NKX2-3* in the two shRNA-*NKX2-3* cells were significantly reduced compared with the empty vector cells (control cells) 48 hours after transfection (Fig. 1).

Identification of genes regulated by *NKX2-3*

To analyze the effects of *NKX2-3* knockdown on gene expression and identify genes with altered expression levels, cDNA microarray analysis was conducted with *NKX2-3* knockdown and control cells from two HIMEC. Stringent criteria (fold change ≥1.5, up or down, $p<0.0005$) were used to filter the differentially expressed genes. The expression levels of 1746 genes were affected by *NKX2-3* knockdown (935 down-regulated and 811 up-regulated) in the HIMEC 21B cell line as compared to control, and 1603 genes were affected by *NKX2-3* knockdown (741 down-regulated and 862 up-regulated) in the HIMEC 432 cell line as compared to control. A total of 1000 shared genes were found to be affected by *NKX2-3* knockdown in both HIMEC, including 996 (99.6%) genes in the same direction (432 genes down-regulated and 564 genes up-regulated by *NKX2-3* knockdown in both HIMEC), and only 4 genes in the opposite direction. Taken together, the transcriptional profile of genes affected by *NKX2-3* knockdown was highly consistent for both HIMEC. Table 1 shows the top 100 down-regulated and top 100 up-regulated genes by *NKX2-3* knockdown with average fold changes in the two cell lines.

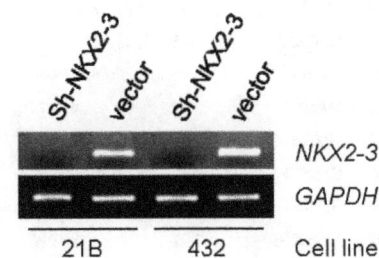

Figure 1. *NKX2-3* mRNA expression is suppressed by shRNA in 21B and 432 HIMEC. pSUPER.retro.puro.shRNA-*NKX2-3* and empty vector were transfected into two HIMEC. 48 hours after transfection, RNA was isolated and analyzed by RT-PCR in two knockdown HIMEC compared with controls. GAPDH expression served as a control.

In order to characterize the top genes affected by *NKX2-3* knockdown, they were assigned to ontological functional groups based on IPA and references in the literature. These 200 genes grouped primarily within the following functional categories, which are listed as such in Table 1: immune and inflammatory response; cell growth and proliferation; metabolic process; cell adhesion; transcription regulation; transport and structure; and angiogenesis. Since the *NKX2-3* transcription factor is associated with IBD and is up-regulated in CD patients [13], it is reasonable to assume that *NKX2-3* could play a role in IBD pathogenesis by regulating inflammation-related genes. In fact, among the 200 genes regulated by *NKX2-3*, 70 genes were immune and inflammatory response genes, including *IL8* (array ratio 0.4) and *KLF2* (array ratio 3.92). Angiogenesis plays an important role in endothelial cell participation in inflammation [15], *ANGPT2* is down-regulated (array ratio 0.18) and *FGF2* is up-regulated (array ratio 4.0) by *NKX2-3* knockdown.

Identification of pathways regulated by *NKX2-3*

To assess the global effects of *NKX2-3* on gene expression, IPA was used to systematically visualize the relationships among genes regulated by *NKX2-3* knockdown. The 25 pathways most affected by *NKX2-3* are shown in Fig. 2A. G-Protein Coupled Receptor Signaling ($p = 1.71 \times 10^{-14}$), Axonal Guidance Signaling ($p = 5.80 \times 10^{-11}$), and ERK/MAPK Signaling ($p = 5.42 \times 10^{-9}$) were the top three canonical pathways affected by *NKX2-3* knockdown.

We previously found that knockdown of *NKX2-3* in human B cells [14] significantly affected the expression of genes, including *EDN1* and *NOS*, known to have important roles in endothelial cell function. We sought to investigate whether *NKX2-3* knockdown would affect important genes and signaling pathways in HIMEC.

EDN1 was found to be up-regulated by *NKX2-3* knockdown in both HIMEC (array ratio 1.2/1.3, $p<0.05$). *NKX2-3* knockdown significantly affected genes within the endothelin-1 pathway ($p = 1.02 \times 10^{-4}$), which was among the top 25 pathways affected by *NKX2-3* (Fig. 2A). Fig. 2B illustrates the genes in the endothelin-1 pathway affected by *NKX2-3* knockdown. *NKX2-3* knockdown activated MAPK through EDN1-PLCβ-PLC pathway, thus regulated inflammation response and cell proliferation.

Nitric oxide (NO) which is generated by NO synthase (NOS) may play an important role in the pathogenesis of IBD [15]. Production of NO (in macrophages) is among the top 10 pathways affected by *NKX2-3* (Fig. 2A). *eNOS* is down-regulated by *NKX2-3* knockdown in both HIMEC (array ratio −1.3/−2.7, $p<0.0001$). IPA analysis showed that the regulation of eNOS can be through VEGF-PI3K/AKT pathway and that this pathway is significantly affected by *NKX2-3* knockdown ($p = 5.45 \times 10^{-3}$) (Fig. 2C). Fold changes of key genes in this pathway regulated by *NKX2-3* knockdown in HIMEC are: *VEGF* (−1.3/−1.3), *PI3K* (−1.5/−1.7), and *AKT* (−1.35/−1.35).

Validation of cDNA microarray by RT-PCR

RT-PCR on 10 genes (involved in or affected by EDN1 and VEGF pathways) was carried out as an independent verification method of the microarray results. Among the 10 genes, seven (*MAdCAM1*, *AKT*, *VCAM1*, *VEGF*, *PLCB1*, *PI3K*, and *eNOS*) were down-regulated by *NKX2-3* knockdown in both HIMEC, and three (*EDN1*, *ADM*, and *CASP1*) were up-regulated by *NKX2-3* knockdown in 2 HIMEC detected by cDNA microarray. All RT-PCR results were consistent with the microarray data. The fold changes in microarray between the 2 *NKX2-3* knockdown cell lines and 2 control HIMEC lines were: *MAdCAM1* (−1.2;−1.2), *AKT*

Table 1. Top 200 genes regulated by NKX2-3 knockdown in HIMEC.

Gene	Fold	p-value	Gene	Fold	p-value	Gene	Fold	p-value	Gene	Fold	p-value
Cell growth and proliferation			*Transport and structure*			*Inflammation and immune response*			*Inflammation and immune response*		
PIM3	0.3	2.31E-06	SYT11	0.35	3.66E-07	TNFRSF10D	0.31	3.54E-07	SAMD9	7.31	2.01E-10
TFPI2	0.32	3.94E-06	KRT81	0.4	3.31E-07	TNFSF18	0.32	6.43E-05	STAT1	7.72	1.98E-09
NR2F1	0.37	4.64E-07	RPS23	0.4	2.97E-07	CERK	0.33	1.39E-06	TAP2	7.83	7.33E-10
EIF4B	0.38	2.68E-07	EXOC6	0.47	2.09E-06	FAM172A	0.37	1.94E-07	PSMB8	8.22	1.84E-10
GHR	0.39	3.69E-07	RPL23	0.47	1.33E-06	YPEL2	0.39	0.000952	UBE2L6	8.33	9.08E-10
HMMR	0.39	3.79E-06	RPS29	0.48	2.41E-06	PAPSS2	0.39	8.84E-06	PTGS2	8.63	2.77E-11
REEP1	0.4	2.86E-07	ADAP1	3.29	2.36E-08	IL8	0.4	7.63E-06	GBP1	9.24	2.23E-08
ZMAT3	0.41	3.60E-07	SLC25A28	3.71	1.99E-07	UACA	0.4	3.05E-05	PARP9	9.46	6.09E-10
MMP7	0.42	3.43E-06	RTP4	6.47	0.000111	GIMAP7	0.41	9.24E-07	SP110	9.83	1.31E-10
GDF15	0.42	1.22E-05	GJD3	7.95	0.000154	HES2	0.41	2.05E-07	TAP1	10.62	7.18E-11
MFNG	0.42	2.32E-05				SLC40A1	0.41	2.59E-07	USP18	11.2	9.63E-11
AGAP3	0.43	6.31E-07				TNFAIP8L1	0.43	3.66E-07	DDX58	11.39	3.09E-08
TMEM158	0.44	1.25E-05	*Cell adhesion*			F2RL1	0.43	0.000121	HLA-B	11.89	8.66E-12
UNC5A	0.44	7.44E-05				CD36	0.43	5.14E-07	PRIC285	12.35	1.67E-10
SHMT2	0.44	1.55E-06	POSTN	0.22	6.28E-09	PLD1	0.44	2.12E-07	PSMB9	14.18	1.73E-10
FAM198B	0.45	3.44E-06	MMRN1	0.35	3.33E-06	CBS	0.46	3.70E-06			
HNRNPA0	0.46	6.11E-05	CXADR	0.36	7.75E-07	CEP55	0.47	3.69E-06			
PAWR	0.46	4.71E-05	SRPX	0.37	7.57E-06	GNG12	0.48	5.21E-05	*Others*		
DCLK1	0.47	7.04E-07	FLRT2	0.46	8.02E-06	TNFSF4	0.48	1.00E-05	ANKRD55	0.18	1.07E-07
TTC3	0.47	5.53E-07	AIF1L	3.41	8.77E-08	ARHGDIB	0.49	2.55E-05	C2CD4B	0.22	2.48E-08
TFF3	0.47	1.73E-05				CLEC1A	0.49	1.96E-05	KIAA0114	0.27	2.03E-08
PTPRE	0.47	4.31E-06				CXCL16	3.19	1.04E-05	NT5DC2	0.28	8.23E-09
UBE4B	0.47	2.02E-06	*Transcription regulation*			GCH1	3.32	5.31E-05	EIF4BP7	0.29	3.73E-07
CDKN3	0.48	0.000101				UNC93B1	3.46	1.36E-06	FLJ41200	0.29	2.64E-08
CCNB2	0.49	2.92E-05	SDPR	0.44	1.95E-06	CD68	3.51	3.49E-07	C13orf33	0.34	7.43E-06
ANLN	0.49	3.85E-05	HOXD1	0.45	0.000147	TRIM21	3.62	9.21E-06	EIF4BP3	0.38	1.42E-07
LGMN	3.23	4.42E-07	ZNFX1	3.52	2.22E-06	APOBEC3G	3.67	5.26E-06	FBN2	0.39	5.49E-06
SEMA3A	3.25	2.19E-06	BATF2	4.11	1.75E-06	TRIM5	3.82	4.78E-05	C7orf41	0.4	5.68E-07
PNPT1	3.44	2.45E-05				KLF2	3.92	7.66E-06	SNHG9	0.41	0.000156
MAP2	3.57	4.49E-09				PLSCR1	4.05	2.58E-08	WRB	0.42	1.18E-06
PMAIP1	3.65	3.66E-08	*Metabolic process*			MYD88	4.28	1.98E-06	BCYRN1	0.42	0.000157
EIF2AK2	3.73	9.30E-09				CD38	4.28	6.55E-08	ZNF704	0.44	5.90E-07
HEY1	3.85	2.33E-07	ACO1	0.2	8.00E-07	CX3CL1	4.33	0.000209	ANKRD37	0.46	5.41E-06
CSRNP1	3.87	1.55E-06	HSD17B2	0.23	2.48E-06	STAT2	4.34	1.08E-05	HNRPA1L-2	0.46	8.27E-06
C8orf4	3.95	5.53E-06	PHGDH	0.29	1.86E-08	PLEKHA4	4.37	1.83E-05	TCTEX1D2	0.47	0.000153
XAF1	4.17	2.88E-06	PSAT1	0.3	1.24E-07	IFNB1	4.37	3.68E-06	CENPW	0.48	7.38E-05
SERPINE2	4.33	2.29E-08	ASNS	0.31	1.09E-07	FCN3	4.38	0.000198	NETO2	0.48	1.93E-05
HEY2	4.6	4.55E-08	GALNTL2	0.33	7.00E-06	F2RL3	4.44	2.45E-07	C8orf45	0.48	8.75E-05
PARP10	5.54	5.42E-08	PKIA	0.34	7.05E-05	ZC3HAV1	4.6	5.95E-07	MAMDC2	3.19	6.34E-07
CRYAB	6.8	8.25E-06	MYO5A	0.38	5.34E-05	HCG4	4.61	2.85E-09	FBXO6	3.26	7.21E-08
KLF4	6.86	6.09E-10	TXNDC12	0.4	1.43E-07	HLA-C	4.63	1.63E-09	C1orf74	3.48	0.000186
LY6E	7.47	1.94E-10	SNCAIP	0.41	0.000257	GBP2	4.71	4.44E-08	USP41	3.52	3.72E-06
TMEM100	15.53	3.36E-07	CHST7	0.44	7.79E-07	SMAD7	4.78	1.31E-06	C19orf66	3.92	2.77E-08
			MCTP1	0.46	0.000231	NT5C3	4.8	1.92E-07	HIST2H2AC	4.18	5.43E-08
			FAR2	0.48	0.000238	HLA-H	5.39	4.83E-10	GCA	5.14	5.15E-06
Angiogenesis			PRSS12	0.48	1.43E-06	TRIM22	5.49	9.22E-08	HIST2H2AA3	5.17	2.92E-09
			BCHE	0.49	3.81E-06	DHX58	5.58	1.57E-06			

NKX2-3 Transcriptional Regulation of Endothelin-1 and VEGF Signaling in Human Intestinal Microvascular...

89

Table 1. Cont.

Gene	Fold	p-value	Gene	Fold	p-value	Gene	Fold	p-value	Gene	Fold	p-value
ANGPT2	0.18	1.42E-05	ADAMTSL2	3.2	1.26E-06	IL18BP	5.66	3.92E-09	HIST2H2AA4	5.28	2.11E-09
SRPX2	0.33	0.000284	TIPARP	3.28	1.18E-07	HLA-F	5.79	2.68E-10	RNF213	6.6	1.03E-06
TRPC6	0.33	1.08E-07	PLA1A	4.75	3.24E-08	CASP1	5.82	5.35E-10	DDX60L	6.75	1.14E-06
BTG1	0.43	3.66E-05	GMPR	4.8	5.63E-08	PARP12	6.28	1.97E-09	LYPD1	6.75	3.01E-05
BMP4	0.48	2.53E-05	LAP3	6.07	9.20E-09	IDO1	6.93	1.77E-08	DDX60	7.87	2.71E-09
ANGPTL4	3.37	1.01E-08	UBA7	6.64	9.54E-08	HCP5	6.99	3.95E-10	FAM46A	8.63	4.81E-06
TYMP	3.38	1.13E-08	CMPK2	10.3	5.63E-08	PARP14	7.01	1.24E-08	MT1M	8.77	6.76E-11
FGF2	4	5.16E-05	ALPL	12.12	0.000474	IL7R	7.06	3.94E-05	SAMD9L	9.07	1.22E-08

($-1.35;-1.35$), *VCAM1* ($-1.3;-1.14$), *VEGFA* ($-1.3;-1.3$), *PLCB1* ($-1.6;-1.5$), *PI3K* ($-1.5;-1.7$), *eNOS* ($-1.3;-2.7$), *EDN1* ($1.2;1.3$), *ADM* ($1.9;2.1$), and *CASP1* ($4.6;5$). The PCR ratios between the 2 *NKX2-3* knockdown cell lines and 2 control

HIMEC lines were: *MAdCAM1* ($-3;-4$), *AKT* ($-3;-3.5$), *VCAM1* ($-3;-3$), *VEGFA* ($-4;-3$), *PLCB1* ($-3.5;-3.5$), *PI3K* ($-3;-2.8$), *eNOS* ($-3;-4.5$), *EDN1* ($2.5;3$), *ADM* ($3.5;3$), and *CASP1* ($4.5;4.8$) (Fig. 3).

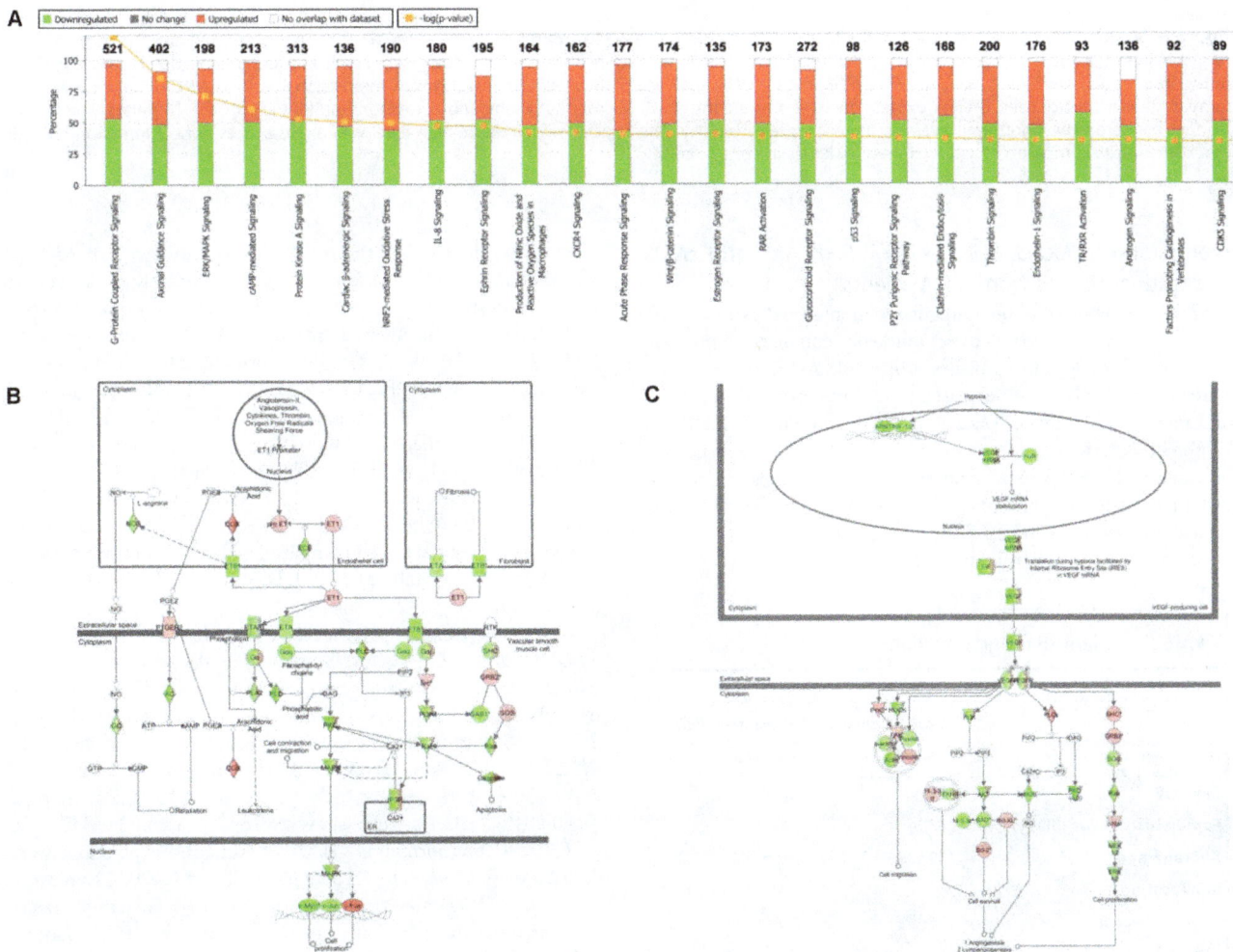

Figure 2. An interaction network generated using IPA analysis shows genes regulated by *NKX2-3* in HIMEC. (A) The top 25 signaling pathways affected by *NKX2-3* knockdown. (B) The EDN1 pathway is regulated by *NKX2-3* in 2 HIMEC. IPA analysis shows genes up-regulated (red) and down-regulated (green) by *NKX2-3* knockdown. (C) The VEGF-PI3K/AKT-eNOS pathway is regulated by *NKX2-3* in 2 HIMEC. IPA analysis shows genes up-regulated (red) and down-regulated (green) by *NKX2-3* knockdown in the VEGF-PI3K/AKT-eNOS pathway.

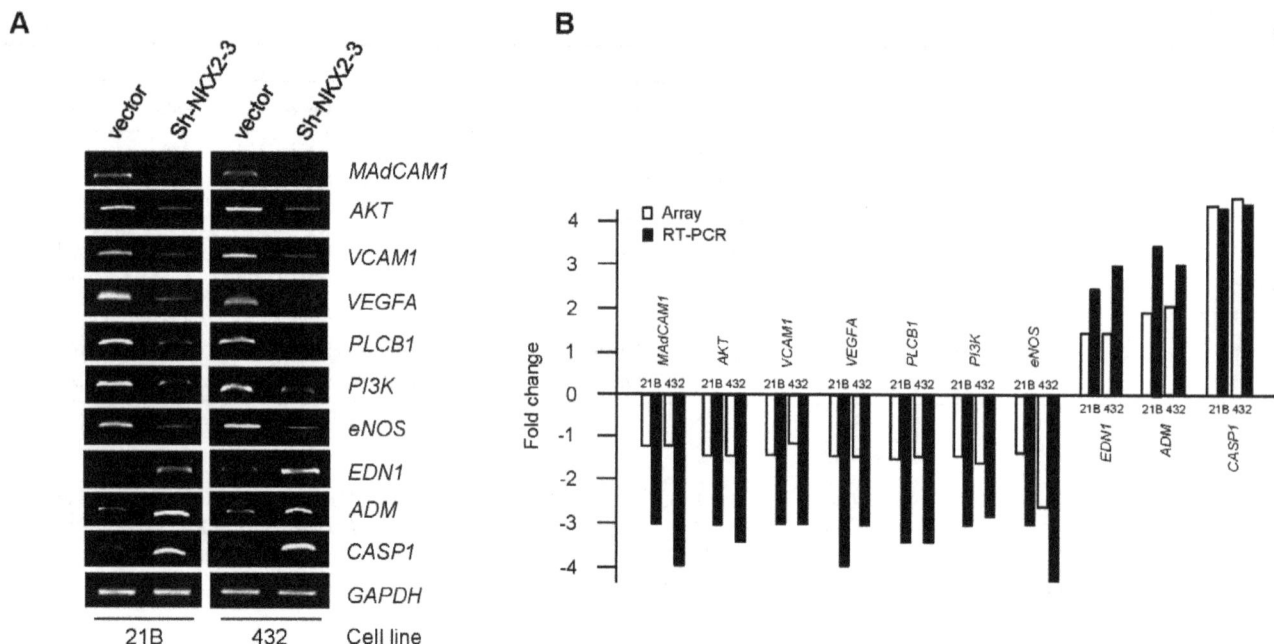

Figure 3. Validation of microarray results by RT-PCR in two *NKX2-3* knockdown HIMEC. (A) RT-PCR analysis of mRNA expression levels of 10 genes in knockdown and control cells. *EDN1, ADM,* and *CASP1* showed increased mRNA expression levels in *NKX2-3* knockdown cells compared with control cells; *MAdCAM1, AKT, VCAM1, VEGF, PLCB1, PI3K,* and *eNOS* showed decreased mRNA expression levels in *NKX2-3* knockdown cells compared with control cells. *GAPDH* expression served as a control. (B) Microarray results and corresponding RT-PCR for the 10 genes. The RT-PCR product bands on the photograph were scanned by densitometry. The relative mRNA expression level was expressed as gene expression levels in knockdown cells compared to gene expression levels in control cells.

Expression of *NKX2-3, EDN1, VEGFA, PI3K, AKT,* and *eNOS* in intestinal tissues from IBD patients

NKX2-3 is reported to be up-regulated in intestinal tissues in CD patients [13] and VEGF showed markedly enhanced expression levels in both CD and UC tissues [16], while *EDN1* showed both increased levels [17] and decreased levels in intestinal tissues from IBD patients [18]. Since *NKX2-3* can affect the endothelin-1 and VEGF-PI3K/AKT-eNOS pathways (Fig. 2B and C) in HIMEC, we examined mRNA expression levels of the 6 genes in diseased and adjacent normal intestinal tissues from IBD patients to study clinical implication of *NKX2-3* and its regulated genes. 31 CD and 32 UC patients are for this study (Table 2).

Table 2. Patient demographic data.

	Crohn's disease (n = 31)	Ulcerative colitis (n = 32)
Sex M/F	14/17	16/16
Family history for IBD (yes/no)	8/23	5/27
Average age	39.9±15.1	48.4±16.3
IBD location		
terminal ileum	16	1
small bowel	5	1
colon	8	26
cecum	2	3
rectum	0	1

As shown in Fig. 4A, the mRNA expression levels of *NKX2-3, VEGFA, PI3K, AKT,* and *eNOS* are significantly increased in diseased intestinal tissues compared with adjacent normal tissues in CD patients. The overall mean *NKX2-3* expressions were: 3.88±2.42 (CD) vs. 2.11±1.4 (normal) ($p = 0.0065$); *VEGFA* expressions were: 4.8±15.57(CD) vs. −0.55±7.43 (normal) ($p = 0.0036$); *PI3K* expressions were: 15.78±35.76 (CD) vs. 1.91±7.61 (normal) ($p = 0.0078$); *AKT* expressions were: 10.32±30.75 (CD) vs. −5.05±24.58 (normal) ($p = 0.0164$); and *eNOS* expressions were: 11.13±48.31(CD) vs. −20.22±55.52 (normal) ($p = 0.0088$). Expression levels of *EDN1* are decreased in diseased intestinal tissues compared with adjacent normal tissues in CD patients: −16.82±83.13 (CD) vs. −10.77±26.94 (normal) ($p = 0.7196$).

As shown in Fig. 4B, the mRNA expression levels of *NKX2-3, VEGFA, PI3K, AKT,* and *eNOS* are increased in diseased intestinal tissues compared with adjacent normal tissues in UC patients. The overall mean *NKX2-3* expressions were: 4.26±3.39 (UC) vs. 2.78±1.68 (normal) ($p = 0.0387$); *VEGFA* expressions were: 1.7±1.53 (UC) vs. 0.65±3.13 (normal) ($p = 0.3572$); *PI3K* expressions were: 6.46±7.63 (UC) vs. 3.73±5.22 (normal) ($p = 0.2942$); *AKT* expressions were: −3±5.63 (UC) vs. −26.79±45.65 (normal) ($p = 0.5701$); and *eNOS* expressions were: 0.62±2.04 (UC) vs. −1.67±5.19 (normal) ($p = 0.4203$). Expression levels of *EDN1* are decreased in diseased intestinal tissues compared with adjacent normal tissues in UC patients: −1.85±8.7 (UC) vs. 0.97±4.29 (normal) ($p = 0.0653$).

Taken together, expression levels of *NKX2-3, VEGFA, PI3K, AKT,* and *eNOS* are increased in intestinal tissues from IBD patients. On the other hand, expression levels of *EDN1* are decreased in intestinal tissues from IBD patients. These results demonstrated the important roles of these genes in IBD pathogenesis.

A

B

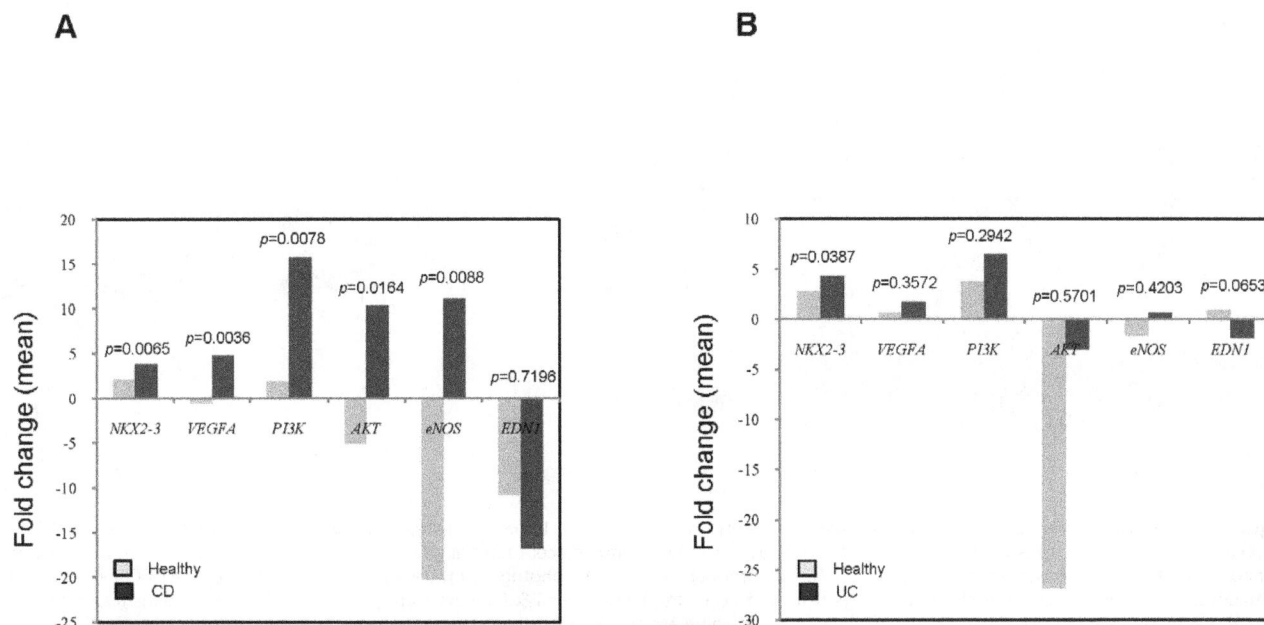

Figure 4. mRNA expression levels of 6 genes in intestinal tissues from CD and UC patients. (A) Comparison of mRNA expression levels of 6 genes in diseased vs. adjacent normal intestinal tissues from CD patients: *NKX2-3* (n = 30), *VEGFA* (n = 30), *PI3K* (n = 31), *AKT* (n = 28), *eNOS* (n = 24), and *EDN1* (n = 30). RT-PCR was carried out on surgically excised diseased and adjacent normal intestinal tissues from CD patients. The RT-PCR product bands on the photograph were scanned by densitometry. RT-PCR results were normalized by *GAPDH* as fold change for each patient. Data are presented as the means. (B) Comparison of mRNA expression levels of 6 genes in diseased vs. adjacent normal intestinal tissues from UC patients: *NKX2-3* (n = 30), *VEGFA* (n = 32), *PI3K* (n = 32), *AKT* (n = 21), *eNOS* (n = 23), and *EDN1* (n = 27). RT-PCR was carried out on surgically excised diseased and adjacent normal intestinal tissues from UC patients. Data are presented as the means.

Positive correlation of gene expression of *NKX2-3* with *VEGFA* in intestinal tissues from IBD patients

There are seven members of the vascular endothelial growth factors (VEGFs) family, ie, VEGF-A, -B, -C, -D, -E, -F, and placental growth factor. *VEGFA* is crucially involved in several chronic inflammatory disorders in which it not only promotes pathologic angiogenesis but directly fosters inflammation [19,20]. VEGFA has been reported to over-express in humans with IBD [21,22,23]. *VEGFA* was down-regulated by *NKX2-3* knockdown in 2 HIMEC (Fig. 2C and 3). Since both *NKX2-3* and *VEGFA* are up-regulated in intestinal tissues from IBD patients (Fig. 4), next we examined whether *NKX2-3* expression was correlated with *VEGFA* expression in IBD patients. We examined mRNA expression levels of *NKX2-3* and *VEGFA* in diseased and adjacent normal intestinal tissues from 30 CD and 30 UC patients. Fold change results of normalized *NKX2-3* or *VEGFA* were summarized as a ratio of medians (CD or UC: adjacent normal tissue) in every patient. Correlation analysis showed a positive correlation between expression of *NKX2-3* and *VEGFA* ($r = 0.681$, $p < 0.0001$) for CD (Fig. 5A) and for UC ($r = 0.509$, $p < 0.0001$) (Fig. 5B).

Negative correlation of gene expression of *NKX2-3* with *EDN1* in intestinal tissues from IBD patients

Endothelin-1 (*EDN1*) is a vasoactive peptide implicated in a number of pathological conditions, including human IBD [17]. *EDN1* was up-regulated by *NKX2-3* knockdown in 2 HIMEC by cDNA microarray analysis (Fig. 2B) and this observation was confirmed by RT-PCR (Fig. 3). Since *NKX2-3* is up-regulated and *EDN1* is down-regulated in intestinal tissues from IBD patients (Fig. 4), we examined whether *NKX2-3* expression was correlated with *EDN1* expression in IBD patients. We examined mRNA expression levels of *NKX2-3* and *EDN1* in diseased intestinal tissues

from 30 CD and 25 UC patients. Correlation analysis showed a negative correlation between expression of *NKX2-3* and *EDN1* for CD ($r = -0.353$, $p < 0.01$) (Fig. 6A) and for UC ($r = -0.442$, $p < 0.005$) (Fig. 6B).

Discussion

Pathogenesis of IBD is not only restricted to those mediated by classic immune cells, such as T and B cells [24], but also involves nonimmune cells, including endothelial cells [15]. Endothelial cells play a key role in mucosal immune homeostasis by regulating the leukocytes migrating from the intravascular to the interstitial space, thus highlighting the endothelium as one of the pillars in inflammation pathogenesis [25]. The vascular response is a key component of inflammation. Microvascular endothelial cells could form capillary-like structures and display different functional sets of adhesion molecules, distinct chemokine secretory patterns, and activation of unique sets of genes in response to stress and inflammatory stimuli [26].

In this study, we performed genome-wide gene expression microarray analysis using two HIMEC with *NKX2-3* knockdown, and identified 1746 genes in 21B cells and 1603 genes in 432 cells regulated by *NKX2-3* knockdown. The regulation of these genes is highly consistent between the two HIMEC. Most of the *NKX2-3* regulated genes are involved in immune and inflammatory response, cell proliferation and growth, metabolic process, and angiogenesis. Various aspects of immunity contribute to the development of an overall inflammatory immune response. Chemokines control leukocyte trafficking during homeostasis as well as inflammation. The migration of leukocytes into sites of inflammation is crucial in the pathogenesis of IBD. The CXC chemokine IL8/CXCL8 is down-regulated by *NKX2-3* knock-down in HIMEC. IL8 is expressed in leucocytes and endothelial

A

B

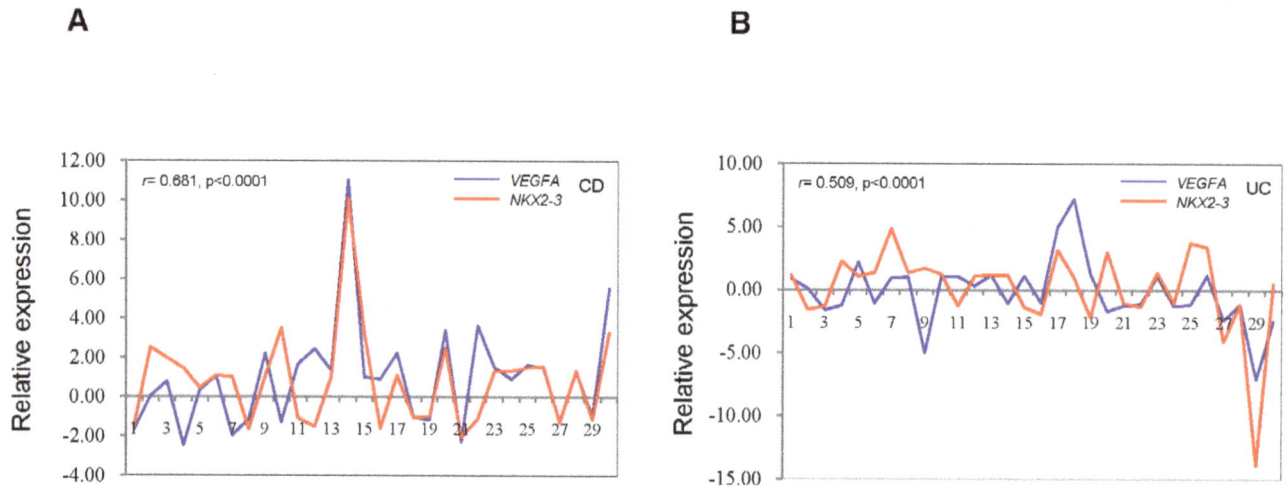

Figure 5. The correlation between the expression levels of *NKX2-3* **and** *VEGFA* **in intestinal tissues from IBD patients.** (A) The correlation between the expression levels of *NKX2-3* and *VEGFA* in diseased and adjacent normal intestinal tissues from 30 CD patients. RT-PCR was carried out on surgically excised intestinal tissues. The RT-PCR product bands on the photograph were scanned by densitometry. RT-PCR results were normalized by *GAPDH* for each sample. Fold change results of normalized *NKX2-3* or *VEGFA* were summarized as a ratio of medians (CD: adjacent normal tissue) in every patient. Correlation coefficient (*r*) and *p* value are shown. (B) The correlation between the expression levels of *NKX2-3* and *VEGFA* in diseased and adjacent normal intestinal tissues from 30 UC patients.

cells and plays an important role in inflammation and angiogenesis [27]. The expression level of IL8 is up-regulated in tissues after ischaemic injury [28]. One of the most novel aspects that directly implicates endothelial cell participation in inflammation is the process of angiogenesis. It is now well established that angiogenesis and microvascular remodeling are intrinsic components of the tissue remodeling in chronic inflammatory diseases [15]. ANGPT2 (angiopoietin 2) is down-regulated by *NKX2-3* knockdown in HIMEC. ANGPT2 is responsible for the initiation of angiogenesis through recruitment and proliferation of endothelial cells [29]. Elevated serum ANGPT2 levels in IBD patients have been reported [30].

We used pathway analysis to systematically visualize the relationships of genes regulated by *NKX2-3* knockdown. The top 25 pathways affected by *NKX2-3* knockdown included those involved in inflammation and immune response, including the EDN1 and NO pathways. Generation of nitric oxide (NO) by NO synthase (NOS) is a central feature of chronic inflammatory diseases in the gastrointestinal tract [15]. *eNOS* is down-regulated by *NKX2-3* knockdown in HIMEC. We identified that *NKX2-3* regulated *eNOS* through the VEGF-PI3k/AKT pathway in HIMEC. *VEGF, PI3K, and AKT* are all down-regulated by *NKX2-3* knockdown in HIMEC. A few reports have described overexpression of VEGFA in human intestinal tissues with IBD [21,22,23], but the functional significance of such up-regulation is not yet understood. In murine colonic-derived endothelial cells, VEGFA triggers an inflammatory phenotype by up-regulating CAMs and inducing adhesion of neutrophils and T cells, thus

A

B

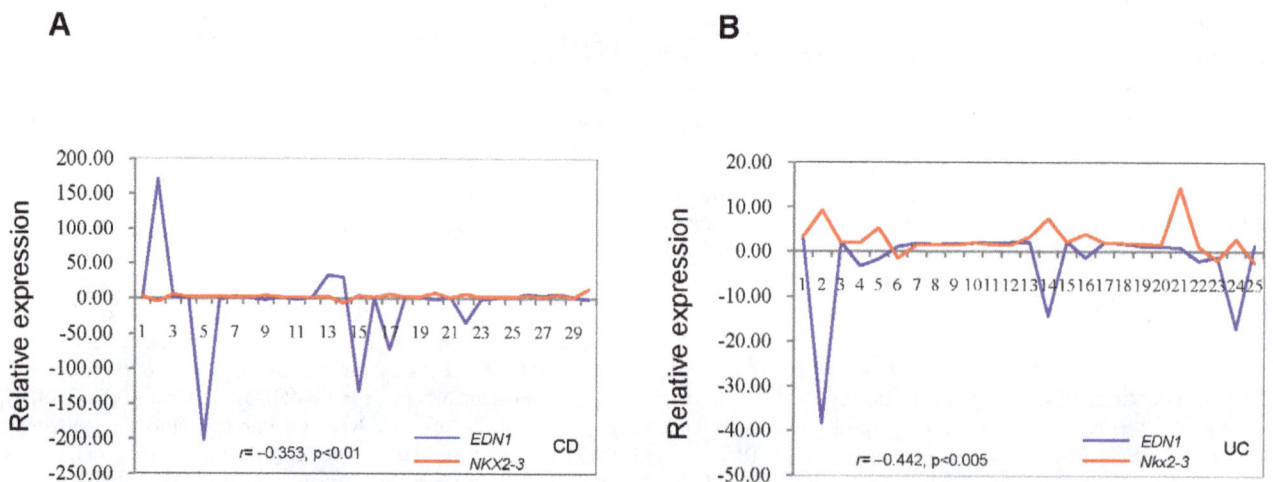

Figure 6. The correlation between the expression levels of *NKX2-3* **and** *EDN1* **in intestinal tissues from IBD patients.** (A) The correlation between the expression levels of *NKX2-3* and *EDN1* in diseased intestinal tissues from 30 CD patients. RT-PCR was carried out on surgically excised intestinal tissues. The RT-PCR product bands on the photograph were scanned by densitometry. RT-PCR results were normalized by *GAPDH* in every patient. Correlation coefficient (*r*) and *p* value are shown. (B) The correlation between the expression levels of *NKX2-3* and *EDN1* in diseased intestinal tissues from 25 UC patients.

supporting an inflammatory role for this cytokine in the intestine [31]. One recent study showed that in vitro, VEGF-A induces both angiogenic activity and an inflammatory phenotype in human intestinal microvascular endothelial cells (HIMEC), whereas overexpression in vivo increases disease severity and blockade decreases disease severity in colitic mice [23]. Given that the activation of this VEGF–eNOS angiogenesis pathway results in maintenance production of NO, it is most likely to be implicated in the regulation of NO-controlled gene expression, as well as the NO-mediated angiogenic responses to VEGF. VEGF is known to be a potent activator of endothelial cells and a critical factor for the induction of angiogenesis during IBD development [23]. The importance of the VEGF–eNOS pathway for regulating angiogenesis and vascular remodeling makes these genes important for IBD pathogenesis. Our results showed that mRNA expression levels of *NKX2-3, VEGFA, PI3K, AKT, and eNOS* were increased in intestinal tissues from IBD patients. And the positive correlation between the expression levels of *NKX2-3* and *VEGFA* in intestinal tissues from IBD patients (Fig. 5) suggests a regulatory role of *NKX2-3* in *VEGFA* gene expression. The mechanism of regulation of *VEGF* by *NKX2-3* is not clear. *NKX2-3* could regulate expression of *IL8, ANGPT2, KLF2, and KLF4* in HIMEC. IL8 Stimulates VEGF expression in endothelial cells [32] and ANGPT2 stimulates the synthesis of VEGF [33]. The KLF2 and KLF4 transcription factors have been shown to coordinate transcriptional programs important for the establishment of an anti-inflammatory, vasodilatory, and anti-thrombotic vascular endothelial phenotypes, thus acting as critical regulators of endothelial homeostasis [34]. KLF2 and KLF4 regulate expression of VEGF and eNOS in vascular endothelial cells [34]. It is reasonable to speculate that *NKX2-3* regulates *VEGF* expression through *IL8, ANGPT2, KLF2, and KLF4* or direct regulation of *VEGF*. Although the role of *NKX2-3* in IBD is still unclear, its regulatory role in VEGF-eNOS strongly suggests that *NKX2-3* could be involved in IBD pathogenesis by regulating the VEGF-PI3K/AKT-eNOS pathway.

Endothelin-1 (*EDN1*) is one of several vasoconstrictors that may play a role in the progression of IBD. Endothelin-1 is expressed by endothelial cells as a precursor peptide (proET-1) that is first cleaved to bigET-1 and then to the mature 21-amino acid peptide. *EDN1* acts through two receptors, ET-A and ET-B. EDN1 binding to ET-B receptors in endothelial cells initiates a signaling cascade that leads to nitric oxide (NO) and endothelial-derived relaxing factor production. The signaling of NO production through ET-B receptors via the G-protein βγ subunit dimer has been linked to AKT phosphorylation of eNOS. The G-protein Galpha12 has been linked to increased levels of eNOS [35]. EDN1 increases leukocyte adhesion to intestinal microvasculature [36], resulting in oxidant stress and mucosal dysfunction [37]. Increased levels of EDN1 in intestinal tissues from IBD patients have been reported [17]. However, other reports have indicated that EDN1 levels were decreased in IBD [18,38]. We showed that expression of EDN1 was down-regulated in intestinal tissues from IBD patients. Correlation study confirmed the negative correlation between the expression levels of *NKX2-3* and *EDN1* in intestinal tissues from IBD patients (Fig. 6), suggesting a regulatory role of *NKX2-3* in *EDN1* gene expression. *NKX2-3* could negatively regulate *EDN1* expression and is thus involved in IBD pathogenesis.

In summary, this work identified many inflammation-related genes and microvascular endothelial cell function related genes that are regulated by *NKX2-3* in HIMEC. Our present results demonstrate that a decrease in *NKX2-3* gene expression level can profoundly affect the signaling pathways relevant to the pathogenesis and progression of IBD such as the EDN1 and VEGF signaling and PI3K/AKT-eNOS pathways. Further functional

studies of the genes and pathways affected by *NKX2-3* using HIMEC are underway to confirm and expand upon the current work.

Materials and Methods

Cell lines

Two HIMEC (432 and 21B) were isolated from normal ileal intestinal tissue from patients undergoing surgery at the Cleveland Clinic Lerner Research Institute as approved by the Institutional Review Board of University Hospitals of Cleveland. Cell lines were cultured in MCDB131 medium (Invitrogen, USA) supplemented with 20% fetal bovine serum (FBS), heparin, endothelial cell growth factor and antibiotics. HIMEC were incubated at 37°C in an atmosphere of 5% CO_2.

Transfection

A small hairpin RNA (shRNA) vector targeting human *NKX2-3* was generated using the pSUPER vector system as described previously [14,39]. The 19-nucleotide sequence within *NKX2-3* targeted by the shRNA oligonucleotide pair was 5'-AGGAA-CATGAAGAGGAGCC-3'. Forward and reverse primers were synthesized containing this sequence in sense and antisense orientations with an intervening linker. Forward and reverse primers were annealed and ligated into the pSUPER.retro.puro vector according to the manufacturer's instructions (OligoEngine, WA, USA).

pSUPER.retro.puro.shRNA-*NKX2-3* and empty vector were transfected into two HIMEC lines with TransPass™ HUVEC transfection reagent (New England BioLabs, USA) according to the manufacturer's instructions. Forty-eight hours posttransfection, to confirm the suppression of *NKX2-3* expression, mRNA from was isolated from the transfected HIMEC lines for further examination.

Microarray and data analysis

Illumina Human HT12 v 3 Expression BeadChips (Illumina, CA) were used in this study. This BeadChip targets >25,000 genes with >48,000 probes derived from the RefSeq (Build 36.2, rel22) and UniGene (Build 99) databases. 300 ng of total RNA collected from two independent cultures of control and sh*NKX2-3*-expressing HIMEC cells was reverse transcribed into cRNA and biotin-UTP labeled using the Illumina Total Prep RNA Amplification Kit (Ambion, Austin, TX). Microarray hybridization, data collection, and analysis were performed at the Genomics Core of the Cleveland Clinic Lerner Research Institute.

Raw data filtering and quantile normalization were performed using the Bioconductor package *lumi*, a Beadarray specific software package for Illumina microarray data. Due to the small sample size, the moderated t-statistic implemented in the Bioconductor *LIMMA* package was used to detect differentially expressed genes. This statistic has the same interpretation as the standard t-statistic; however, standard errors were calculated to shrink toward a common value by empirical Bayes model to borrow information across all genes [40]. The *p*-values from moderated t-tests were adjusted by Benjamini and Hochberg's method to control false discovery rate. All data is MIAME (Minimum Information About a Microarray Experiment) compliant and that the raw data has been deposited in a MIAME compliant database (GEO at NCBI, accession number GSE28656).

Ingenuity pathway analysis (IPA)

IPA was used to identify gene networks according to biological functions and/or diseases in the Ingenuity Pathways Knowledge

Table 3. Primers for RT-PCR.

Gene	Primer sequences	Sizes	Accession
EDN1	F: 5'- ctttgagggacctgaagctg-3'	392 bp	NM_001955
	R: 5'- ctgttgcctttgtgggaagt-3'		
ADM	F: 5'- acttcggagtttttgccattg-3'	230 bp	NM_001124
	R: 5'- ctcttcccacgactcagagc-3'		
PI3K	F: 5'- tgctttgggacaaccataca-3'	394 bp	NM_006218
	R: 5'- cggttgcctactggttcaat-3'		
AKT	F: 5'- ggtgatcctggtgaaggaga-3'	379 bp	NM_005163
	R: 5'- cttaatgtgcccgtccttgt-3'		
eNOS	F: 5'- tgctggcatacaggactaag-3'	385 bp	NM_000603
	R: 5'- taggtcttggggttgtcagg-3'		
PLCB1	F: 5'- cgtggctttccaagaagaag-3'	305 bp	NM_015192
	R: 5'- ggcaaaggttgttgaggaaa-3'		
CASP1	F: 5'- acctctgacagcacgttcct-3'	329 bp	NM_033292
	R: 5'- ggtgtggaagagcagaaagc-3'		
VCAM1	F: 5'- attgacttgcagcaccacag-3'	391 bp	NM_001078
	R: 5'- ttccaggggacttcctgtctg-3'		
VEGFA	F: 5'- tcctcacaccattgaaacca-3	379 bp	NM_001171623
	R: 5'- caccgatcagggagagagag-3'		
NKX2-3	F: 5'-ccacccctttctcagtcaaa-3'	210 bp	NM_145285
	R: 5'-ctgcggctagtgagttcaaa-3'		
GAPDH	F: 5'-tgatgacatcaagaaggtggtgaag-3'	236 bp	NM_002046
	R: 5'-tccttggaggccatgtgggccat-3'		

Base (Ingenuity Systems, Redwood City, CA). Known genes' expression levels served as input to the Ingenuity Pathways Analysis (IPA) Knowledge Base v4.0. Lists of top pathways associated with genes with changes in expression relative to controls were generated with corresponding Benjamini and Hochberg's p values. Expression data was overlaid upon canonical pathways associated with altered gene expression.

Patients and intestinal tissue samples

Intestinal tissues were obtained from IBD patients undergoing surgery at the Penn State Hershey Medical Center. All human tissues were approved by the Human Subjects Protection Offices of The Pennsylvania State University College of Medicine, and were undertaken with the understanding and written consent of each subject. Macroscopically normal areas of intestine and areas of intestine with obvious disease were classified by a pathologist. The intestinal tissues were immediately submerged in RNA*later* Solution (Ambion, CA, USA) and stored at 4°C overnight. Tissues were stored frozen at −70°C until total RNA extraction.

RNA isolation and reverse transcription PCR

Total RNA was extracted from HIMEC and intestinal tissues using the RNeasy mini kit (QIAGEN Sciences, MD, USA) according to the manufacturer's instructions. cDNA was synthesized from 1.0 μg of total RNA using a Superscript III 1st Strand Synthesis Kit (Invitrogen, CA, USA).

Primer sequences are listed in table 3. Primers were designed using Primer3 software. PCR amplifications were performed at 94°C for 30 seconds, 60°C for 45 seconds, and 72°C for 45 seconds for 35 cycles (all genes except GAPDH) or 26 cycles (GAPDH), followed by a final extension at 72°C for 5 min. PCR products were visualized on 2% agarose gels stained with ethidium bromide. RT-PCR product bands were scanned by densitometry and results were normalized by GAPDH for each cell line.

Statistical analysis

The paired data (RT-PCR results) were analyzed with a one sample permutation t-test with 500,000 permutations. The analysis was performed using R (version 2.12.0) and the onet.permutation function in the R library DAAG (version 1.03).

Acknowledgments

We thank Dr. Claudio Fiocchi (Department of Pathobiology, the Cleveland Clinic Foundation) for kindly providing two HIMEC lines. Gene expression profiling microarray experiments were performed at the Genomics Core of the Cleveland Clinic Lerner Research Institute (contact P.W. Faber, Ph.D., faberp@ccf.org). We thank Dr. Faber for his assistance with the cDNA microarray experiments.

Author Contributions

Conceived and designed the experiments: WK ZL. Performed the experiments: WY. Analyzed the data: AB XC. Wrote the paper: WY ZL. Cell Culture: JPH GW. Tissue Collection: AK LP WK. Collected and prepared tissue samples for RT-PCR: YW.

References

1. Cho JH (2008) The genetics and immunopathogenesis of inflammatory bowel disease. Nat Rev Immunol 8: 458–466.
2. Wellcome Trust Case Control Consortium (WTCCC) (2007) Genome-wide association study of 14,000 cases of seven common diseases and 3,000 shared controls. Nature 447: 661–678.
3. Franke A, Balschun T, Karlsen TH, Hedderich J, May S, et al. (2008) Replication of signals from recent studies of Crohn's disease identifies previously unknown disease loci for ulcerative colitis. Nat Genet 40: 713–715.
4. Krumlauf R (1994) Hox genes in vertebrate development. Cell 78: 191–201.
5. Lawrence PA, Morata G (1994) Homeobox genes: their function in Drosophila segmentation and pattern formation. Cell 78: 181–189.
6. Buchberger A, Pabst O, Brand T, Seidl K, Arnold HH (1996) Chick NKx-2.3 represents a novel family member of vertebrate homologues to the Drosophila homeobox gene tinman: differential expression of cNKx-2.3 and cNKx-2.5 during heart and gut development. Mech Dev 56: 151–163.
7. Fu Y, Yan W, Mohun TJ, Evans SM (1998) Vertebrate tinman homologues XNkx-2-3 and XNkx-2-5 are required for heart formation in a functionally redundant manner. Development 125: 4439–4449.
8. Pabst O, Schneider A, Brand T, Arnold HH (1997) The mouse Nkx-2-3 homeodomain gene is expressed in gut mesenchyme during pre- and postnatal mouse development. Dev Dyn 209: 29–35.
9. Wang CC, Biben C, Robb L, Nassir F, Barnett L, et al. (2000) Homeodomain factor Nkx2-3 controls regional expression of leukocyte homing coreceptor MAdCAM-1 in specialized endothelial cells of the viscera. Dev Biol 224: 152–167.
10. Tarlinton D, Light A, Metcalf D, Harvey RP, Robb L (2003) Architectural defects in the spleens of Nkx2-3-deficient mice are intrinsic and associated with defects in both B cell maturation and T cell-dependent immune responses. J Immunol 170: 4002–4010.
11. Pabst O, Zweigerdt R, Arnold HH (1999) Targeted disruption of the homeobox transcription factor Nkx2-3 in mice results in postnatal lethality and abnormal development of small intestine and spleen. Development 126: 2215–2225.
12. Hatoum OA, Binion DG (2005) The vasculature and inflammatory bowel disease: contribution to pathogenesis and clinical pathology. Inflamm Bowel Dis 11: 304–313.
13. Yu W, Lin Z, Kelly AA, Hegarty JP, Poritz LS, Wang Y, Li T, Schreiber S, Koltun WA (2009) Association of a Nkx2-3 polymorphism with Crohn's disease and expression of Nkx2-3 is up-regulated in B cell lines and intestinal tissues with Crohn's disease. Journal of Crohn's and Colitis 3: 189–195.
14. Yu W, Lin Z, Hegarty JP, John G, Chen X, et al. (2010) Genes regulated by Nkx2-3 in siRNA-mediated knockdown B cells: implication of endothelin-1 in inflammatory bowel disease. Mol Genet Metab 100: 88–95.

15. Deban L, Correale C, Vetrano S, Malesci A, Danese S (2008) Multiple pathogenic roles of microvasculature in inflammatory bowel disease: a Jack of all trades. Am J Pathol 172: 1457–1466.

16. Tsiolakidou G, Koutroubakis IE, Tzardi M, Kouroumalis EA (2008) Increased expression of VEGF and CD146 in patients with inflammatory bowel disease. Dig Liver Dis 40: 673–679.

17. Murch SH, Braegger CP, Sessa WC, MacDonald TT (1992) High endothelin-1 immunoreactivity in Crohn's disease and ulcerative colitis. Lancet 339: 381–385.

18. Rachmilewitz D, Eliakim R, Ackerman Z, Karmeli F (1992) Colonic endothelin-1 immunoreactivity in active ulcerative colitis. Lancet 339: 1062.

19. Takahashi H, Shibuya M (2005) The vascular endothelial growth factor (VEGF)/VEGF receptor system and its role under physiological and pathological conditions. Clin Sci (Lond) 109: 227–241.

20. Lee YC (2005) The involvement of VEGF in endothelial permeability: a target for anti-inflammatory therapy. Curr Opin Investig Drugs 6: 1124–1130.

21. Danese S (2007) Inflammation and the mucosal microcirculation in inflammatory bowel disease: the ebb and flow. Curr Opin Gastroenterol 23: 384–389.

22. Koutroubakis IE, Tsiolakidou G, Karmiris K, Kouroumalis EA (2006) Role of angiogenesis in inflammatory bowel disease. Inflamm Bowel Dis 12: 515–523.

23. Scaldaferri F, Vetrano S, Sans M, Arena V, Straface G, et al. (2009) VEGF-A links angiogenesis and inflammation in inflammatory bowel disease pathogenesis. Gastroenterology 136: 585–595 e585.

24. Fiocchi C (1997) Intestinal inflammation: a complex interplay of immune and nonimmune cell interactions. Am J Physiol 273: G769–775.

25. Danese S, Dejana E, Fiocchi C (2007) Immune regulation by microvascular endothelial cells: directing innate and adaptive immunity, coagulation, and inflammation. J Immunol 178: 6017–6022.

26. Binion DG, West GA, Ina K, Ziats NP, Emancipator SN, et al. (1997) Enhanced leukocyte binding by intestinal microvascular endothelial cells in inflammatory bowel disease. Gastroenterology 112: 1895–1907.

27. Koch AE, Polverini PJ, Kunkel SL, Harlow LA, DiPietro LA, et al. (1992) Interleukin-8 as a macrophage-derived mediator of angiogenesis. Science 258: 1798–1801.

28. Kocher AA, Schuster MD, Bonaros N, Lietz K, Xiang G, et al. (2006) Myocardial homing and neovascularization by human bone marrow angioblasts is regulated by IL-8/Gro CXC chemokines. J Mol Cell Cardiol 40: 455–464.

29. Ramsauer M, D'Amore PA (2002) Getting Tie(2)d up in angiogenesis. J Clin Invest 110: 1615–1617.

30. Oikonomou KA, Kapsoritakis AN, Kapsoritaki AI, Manolakis AC, Tiaka EK, et al. Angiogenin, angiopoietin-1, angiopoietin-2, and endostatin serum levels in inflammatory bowel disease. Inflamm Bowel Dis.

31. Goebel S, Huang M, Davis WC, Jennings M, Siahaan TJ, et al. (2006) VEGF-A stimulation of leukocyte adhesion to colonic microvascular endothelium: implications for inflammatory bowel disease. Am J Physiol Gastrointest Liver Physiol 290: G648–654.

32. Martin D, Galisteo R, Gutkind JS (2009) CXCL8/IL8 stimulates vascular endothelial growth factor (VEGF) expression and the autocrine activation of VEGFR2 in endothelial cells by activating NFkappaB through the CBM (Carma3/Bcl10/Malt1) complex. J Biol Chem 284: 6038–6042.

33. Kang YS, Park YG, Kim BK, Han SY, Jee YH, et al. (2006) Angiotensin II stimulates the synthesis of vascular endothelial growth factor through the p38 mitogen activated protein kinase pathway in cultured mouse podocytes. J Mol Endocrinol 36: 377–388.

34. Villarreal G, Jr., Zhang Y, Larman HB, Gracia-Sancho J, Koo A, et al. Defining the regulation of KLF4 expression and its downstream transcriptional targets in vascular endothelial cells. Biochem Biophys Res Commun 391: 984–989.

35. Andreeva AV, Vaiskunaite R, Kutuzov MA, Profirovic J, Skidgel RA, et al. (2006) Novel mechanisms of G protein-dependent regulation of endothelial nitric-oxide synthase. Mol Pharmacol 69: 975–982.

36. Boros M, Massberg S, Baranyi L, Okada H, Messmer K (1998) Endothelin 1 induces leukocyte adhesion in submucosal venules of the rat small intestine. Gastroenterology 114: 103–114.

37. Oktar BK, Coskun T, Bozkurt A, Yegen BC, Yuksel M, et al. (2000) Endothelin-1-induced PMN infiltration and mucosal dysfunction in the rat small intestine. Am J Physiol Gastrointest Liver Physiol 279: G483–491.

38. McCartney SA, Ballinger AB, Vojnovic I, Farthing MJ, Warner TD (2002) Endothelin in human inflammatory bowel disease: comparison to rat trinitrobenzenesulphonic acid-induced colitis. Life Sci 71: 1893–1904.

39. Yu W, Lin Z, Pastor DM, Hegarty JP, Chen X, et al. (2010) Genes Regulated by Nkx2-3 in Sporadic and Inflammatory Bowel Disease-Associated Colorectal Cancer Cell Lines. Dig Dis Sci 55: 3171–3180.

40. Smyth GK, Michaud J, Scott HS (2005) Use of within-array replicate spots for assessing differential expression in microarray experiments. Bioinformatics 21: 2067–2075.

11

Intestinal Cell Barrier Function *In Vitro* is Severely Compromised by Keratin 8 and 18 Mutations Identified in Patients with Inflammatory Bowel Disease

Tina Zupancic[1], Jure Stojan[2], Ellen Birgitte Lane[3], Radovan Komel[1,2], Apolonija Bedina-Zavec[1], Mirjana Liovic[1,2]*

1 National Institute of Chemistry, Ljubljana, Slovenia, 2 Medical Centre for Molecular Biology, Faculty of Medicine, University of Ljubljana, Ljubljana, Slovenia, 3 Institute of Medical Biology, Immunos, Singapore

Abstract

Keratin 8 and 18 (K8/K18) mutations have been implicated in the aetiology of certain pathogenic processes of the liver and pancreas. While some K8 mutations (K8 G62C, K8 K464N) are also presumed susceptibility factors for inflammatory bowel disease (IBD), the only K18 mutation (K18 S230T) discovered so far in an IBD patient is thought to be a polymorphism. The aim of our study was to demonstrate that these mutations might also directly affect intestinal cell barrier function. Cell monolayers of genetically engineered human colonocytes expressing these mutations were tested for permeability, growth rate and resistance to heat-stress. We also calculated the change in dissociation constant (K_d, measure of affinity) each of these mutations introduces into the keratin protein, and present the first model of a keratin dimer L12 region with *in silico* clues to how the K18 S230T mutation may affect keratin function. Physiologically, these mutations cause up to 30% increase in paracellular permeability *in vitro*. Heat-stress induces little keratin clumping but instead cell monolayers peel off the surface suggesting a problem with cell junctions. K18 S230T has pronounced pathological effects *in vitro* marked by high K_d, low growth rate and increased permeability. The latter may be due to the altered distribution of tight junction components claudin-4 and ZO-1. This is the first time intestinal cells have been suggested also functionally impaired by K8/K18 mutations. Although an *in vitro* colonocyte model system does not completely mimic the epithelial lining of the intestine, nevertheless the data suggest that K8/K18 mutations may be also able to produce a phenotype *in vivo*.

Editor: Markus M. Heimesaat, Charité, Campus Benjamin Franklin, Germany

Funding: This work was supported by the Slovenian Research Agency grants J3-2274 and J3-3617 to M. Liovic and P1-0104 to R. Komel. The funders had no role in study design, data collection and analysis, decision to publish, or preparation of the manuscript.

Competing Interests: The authors declare that no competing interests exist.

* E-mail: mirjana.liovic@mf.uni-lj.si

Introduction

In the last 20 years intermediate filaments (IF) have been recognized as an important component of the cytoskeleton filament system and to have a variety of functions, far beyond the initial simplistic view of a mechanical support to cells. IF proteins have been shown to contribute to the overall cell architecture, migration, cell cycle and proliferation [1–4], and to have a role in cell signalling that can even affect target gene expression [5–8]. IF proteins are also being used in diagnostics as markers of distinct physiological changes in tissues during tumorigenesis [9], [10]. In addition, 93 pathological conditions have been associated with some 700 mutations in 73 IF proteins. The amazing progress made on IF protein biology started in the early 90's, when the first keratin gene mutations were identified and linked to a group of skin blistering disorders [11], [12]. Keratins are the largest family of IF proteins and are specific to epithelial tissues. The vast majority of the discovered several hundred keratin gene mutations are linked to hereditary disorders of the skin and skin appendages (nail, hair, teeth). However a number of mutations have been also identified in the simple

epithelia keratins K8, K18 and K19 [13]. These are associated with pathologies of the liver, pancreatitis and inflammatory bowel disease (IBD). On the contrary to epidermal keratins, which when mutated mostly have a dominant-negative effect, the simple epithelia keratins appear to act as a susceptibility factor.

Crohn's disease and ulcerative colitis are the major types of IBD. Both are complex and chronic inflammatory conditions of the gastrointestinal tract, which are considered a combination of an altered immune response to luminal microbial flora, genetic factors (over 150 associated loci), and the effects of life style, diet and environment [14], [15]. The main symptoms are diarrhoea, abdominal pain, intolerance to certain types of food and fever. Both diseases are characterized by frequent ulcerations of the intestinal epithelium, which are considered important for the pathogenesis of IBD by causing altered barrier function and further exacerbating the immune response to toxins and pathogens normally present in the gut [16]. Therefore, intestinal fragility and altered barrier function are as important to the aetiology of IBD, as epidermal fragility and perturbed barrier function are to a large number of keratin-related skin disorders [17], [18].

Several years ago we published that severe K5/K14 gene mutations, which are associated with a severe skin blistering phenotype in patients with epidermolysis bullosa simplex, cause a down-regulation of cell junction proteins [19]. Since then several other reports indicated that keratin IFs are necessary for proper targeting and assembly of cell junction complexes at the cell membrane [20–22]. While this helps explain the fragility and diminished epidermal barrier function of a variety of genetic skin conditions, it also reminds us of some clinical features of IBD. We now know that a mutation in a cytoskeletal protein may affect its function on different levels, and not only affect protein structure *per se*. Although a mutation may not alter the structure of a protein to affect its primary function, it may still hinder the binding of associated proteins or interfere its interaction with other cytoskeletal components, as well as affect post-translational modification by obstructing site-specific changes like phosphorylation, glycosylation, acetylation and sumoylation. This may well be the case for mutations in simple epithelia keratins [23–25].

In this study we show that both K8 (G62C, K464N) and K18 (S230T) substitutions can severely affect the barrier function of a colonocyte monolayer *in vitro*. An important aspect of our findings is that these mutations were tested in the background of a pre-existent wild type K8/K18 filament network, as we compared mutant and wild type genetically engineered cell lines in the same genetic background of HT-29 colonocytes (isogenic cell lines). The data on K18 S230T are particularly interesting as it causes a high increase in K_d and a decrease in cell growth rate, despite a normal cell cycle profile. Exposure of K8/K18 mutants to heat-stress does not appear to induce much keratin aggregation and filament bundling as seen for mutant epidermal keratins, but instead causes the intestinal cell monolayers to detach from the surface as a sheet of cells. Tight junction proteins ZO-1 and claudin-4 are in the case of K18 S230T displaced, which has the potential to directly interfere with the epithelial barrier function. To further assess this data we developed a computer-generated model of the L12 linker region of the K8/K18 dimer. This was used for *in silico* testing of the impact the K18 S230T mutation has on the structure of this domain. Though the S230T substitution may not structurally alter the L12 domain in a major way, it may introduce a new hydrogen bond within the K18 chain, setting additional constraints to the flexibility of this region. We believe that K18 S230T is a mutation in its own right and similar to the mutations in K8 may rightfully predispose carriers to pathologies of the gastrointestinal tract by affecting the barrier function of the intestinal epithelium. Our data demonstrates for the first time that K8/K18 mutations may be able on their own to interfere with colonocyte function *in vitro*.

Material and Methods

Isogenic cell lines, design and cloning

HT-29 cells (HTB-38 from ATCC), a human colorectal adenocarcinoma cell line, were grown in culture at 37°C, 5% CO2, using DMEM (PAA, Austria) supplemented with 10% FBS (PAA, Austria), 1x antibiotic/antimycotic solution (Gibco, Life technologies, USA) and 1 x MEM non-essential amino acids (Gibco, Life technologies, USA), as culture medium. Cells were passaged at 70% confluence. K8 and K18 clones were generated as described previously [26]. In brief, site-directed mutagenesis was performed using the QuikChange kit (Stratagene, USA) to generate K8/K18 cDNA constructs with IBD patient mutations (K8 wild type (WT), K8 G62C, K8 K464N, K18 WT and K18 S230T). cDNA constructs were tagged at the N-terminus with a FLAG epitope and cloned into pcDNA3 vector (Invitrogen, Life technologies, USA). HT-29 cells were subsequently transfected

using FuGene (Roche), according to manufacturers instructions. Wild type and mutant construct expressing cells were initially selected using 1 mg/ml of G418 (Gibco, Life technologies, USA). This was followed by two additional rounds of selection of stably transfected single clones in the presence of G418 at 0.5 mg/ml. To confirm that newly generated cell lines express the K8/K18 mutations above, we sequenced KRT8 and KRT18 from genomic DNA isolated from these cells, and assessed K8/K18 protein expression by immunoblotting. The following antibodies were used: anti-FLAG mouse monoclonal antibody M2 and anti-K8 mouse monoclonal antibody M20 (both from Sigma-Aldrich, USA), and anti-K18 mouse monoclonal antibody LDK-18 (gift from E.B. Lane). Mouse monoclonal antibody LJ4 was used to detect phosphorylated K8 (gift from B. Omary). The resulting cell lines were designated as HT-29+K8 WT (K8 WT control), HT-29+K8 G62C, HT-29+K8 K464N, HT-29+K18 WT (K18 WT control) and HT-29+K18 S230T, but for easier reading will be from now on referred to according to the construct they express.

Permeability assay

In this assay 24-well cell culture inserts (ThinCert, Greiner BioOne, Germany) with a 0.4 μm pore size were used. Cells were grown on inserts for 2 weeks, at which point transepithelial membrane conductance (TEER) was measured to ensure that the colonocyte monolayer was confluent and tight junctions assembled. Lucifer yellow (LY, 444 Da), a small fluorescent molecule routinely used in permeability studies, was added at 0.1 mg/ml final concentration to the medium in the upper chamber of the ThinCert system. Cells were further incubated at 37°C for 2 hours, after which the medium in the bottom chamber was collected and its fluorescence measured on a spectrophotometer. The resulting data was used to calculate the permeability coefficient (Papp) of each cell line. All experiments were done in triplicate repeats and the standard deviation was calculated accordingly.

Growth rates

K8 and K18 cell lines were plated at 20,000 cells per well on 24-well plates. Cells were grown in HT-29 growth media supplemented with 0.5 mg/ml of G418. After 1 week in culture cells were detached from the plates using trypsin and counted with an automated cell counter (Scepter cell counter, Millipore, USA). Experiments were done in triplicate repeats and the standard deviation was calculated accordingly.

Heat-stress assay

Heat-stress assay was performed as previously described [27]. At regular time intervals (0 time point, 1 hour, 2 hours, 4 hours and 16 hours of recovery after stress) cells were fixed and stained using either the anti-K18 antibody LDK-18 or anti-K8 antibody M20 as primary, and fluorescently labelled goat anti-mouse (488 nm) as secondary antibody (Molecular Probes, Life technologies, USA). Images were acquired using a fully motorized Zeiss Axioplan 2 fluorescent microscope running of Axiovision software (Carl Zeiss, Germany).

Immunolabelling of tight junction proteins

K8 WT and K18 S230T cells were grown on 13 mm coverslips over 2 weeks, after which they were fixed and stained according to manufacturer's instructions using as primary antibodies the anti-claudin-4 mouse monoclonal 3E2C1 antibody, and the N-terminus anti-ZO-1 polyclonal rabbit antibody (both from Invitrogen, Life technologies, USA). As secondary fluorescently labelled (488 nm) antibodies we used goat anti-mouse and goat anti-rabbit antibodies (Molecular Probes, Life technologies, USA).

Total protein extracts

Cells were cultured as described above. After reaching 70–80% confluence cells were washed with PBS and lysed in extraction buffer containing: 50 mM Tris/HCl pH 7.5, 1 mM EDTA, 1 mM EGTA, 50 mM NaF, 5 mM sodium pyrophosphate, 10 mM β-phosphoglycerate and 1% Triton X-100, plus the following which were freshly added immediately prior to use: 1 mM Na-orthovanadate, 0.1% β-mercaptoethanol, 1 mM PMSF, 1 mM benzamidine, 10 µg/ml leupeptin and 10 µg/ml pepstatin A. Protein concentration was determined using the Bradford assay (Bio-Rad protein assay, Bio-Rad Gmbh, Germany) and 10 µg of total protein per sample was loaded per track on denaturing protein gels. Immunoblotting was carried out using monoclonal antibodies described above (against K8, K18, phospho-K8, ZO-1 and claudin-4).

Calculation of dissociation constants (K_d)

We re-analysed the previously published surface plasmon resonance data on K8 and K18 wild type and mutant recombinant proteins by Owens and colleagues [26] using ENZO: Enzyme Kinetics [28]. ENZO is a free web tool for building kinetic models of enzyme-catalysed reactions, evaluation of rival reaction schemes and routine tests in enzyme kinetics. ENZO allowed us to calculate the K_d of K8 and K18 mutants and compare them with wild type proteins (Table 1).

Computer modelling of K8/K18 L12 region dimer

Modelling was performed using the crystal structures of vimentin (PDB code 3TRT) and Maf-G transcription factor (PDB code 3A5T) as the templates for the coil and linker regions, respectively [29], [30]. According to the alignment the residues were mutated with the Whatif molecular modelling tool. After structure optimization, a 1 ns constant pressure and temperature (CPT) dynamic simulation (300 K, 1 bar, time step 1 fs) invoking the EWALD summation for calculating the electrostatic interactions was run for each structure (wild type and the mutant). For averaging purposes the simulation was repeated four times in the case of wild type K8/K18 fragment and five times for the K8 WT/K18 S230T mutant. In all dynamic simulations 10240 water molecules were included. All molecular simulations and analyses were performed with CHARMM, a versatile molecular simulation program.

Results

Increased paracellular permeability of K8 and K18 mutant cell lines

Clones of HT-29 colonocytes stably transfected with K8 and K18 wild type and mutant constructs (K8 WT, K8 G62C, K8 K464N, K18 WT and K18 S230T) were engineered and selected according to the methodology described in Materials and Methods. Clones with similar levels of K8 and K18 expression were selected for further experiments (Fig.1). As shown, no major differences in K8 and K18 protein levels could be observed between the clones selected. However, the level of keratin phosphorylation appears somewhat altered in two of the three mutants analysed (Fig.1), i.e. increased in the K8 G62C and K8 K464N clones in comparison to their K8 WT control cells, and decreased in K18 S230T in comparison to K18 WT control cells. Cells were grown on cell culture inserts commonly used for permeability studies. The "leakiness" of confluent cell monolayers was measured by following the diffusion rate of lucifer yellow (LY), a small fluorescent molecule. As small molecules are more likely to cross sheets of epithelial cells by simple diffusion than by a receptor or energy dependent mechanism, any detected LY in the basal compartment of this culture system is due to the paracellular transport mechanism. The tighter tight junctions lock colonocytes together into a monolayer the lower is the permeability of the epithelial sheet, and vice-versa. The results of the permeability assays are presented in Fig. 2. As shown, in vitro cell monolayers of the two K8 mutants (K8 G62C and K8 K464N, Fig. 2A) have a significantly higher permeability coefficient (Papp) from the K8 WT control cell line. Surprisingly, a similar result was also obtained for colonocytes expressing the K18 S230T mutation, which have a much higher permeability for LY than K18 WT control cells (Fig. 2B).

Distribution of tight junction proteins ZO-1 and claudin-4 is altered in K18 S230T cells

The increased permeability rate of the K8/K18 mutants prompted us to check the protein levels of certain components of tight junctions, namely ZO-1 and claudin-4 (Fig. 3). While protein levels of ZO-1 appear similar between these cell lines, the levels of claudin-4 differ substantially. As shown, the K8 G62C and K8 K464N mutants display an increase in claudin-4 in comparison to K8 WT, while in the K18 S230T mutant this appears decreased in comparison to the K18 WT control. We found the data on K18 S230T particularly interesting and so also examined the distribution of ZO-1 and claudin-4 in these cells by immunofluorescent labelling (Fig. 4). Figure 4A, B are the K18 WT and K18 S230T cells respectively, stained with an antibody

Table 1. K8/K18 mutations induce an increase in protein dissociation constants (K_d).

Cell line	K_d
K8 WT	8.5 nM
K8 K464N	13.4 nM
K8 G62C	26.2 nM
K18 WT	8.5 nM
K18 S230T	161 nM

The surface plasmon resonance data published by Owens and colleagues [26] was re-analysed using ENZO software (enzo.cmm.ki.si) to calculate the dissociation constants of the different recombinant proteins. The K_d of K18 S230T recombinant protein resulted to be the highest, suggesting a significantly lower affinity of K18 S230T for wild type K8 than in the case of K8 G62C and K8 K464N for wild type K18.

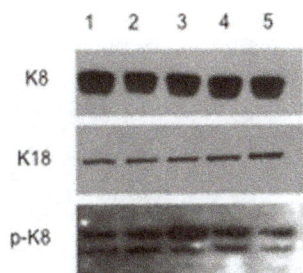

Figure 1. Western blot analysis of protein extracts from isogenic K8 and K18 cell lines. Tracks: (1) K8 WT cells; (2) K8 G62C cells; (3) K8 K464N cells; (4) K18 WT cells; (5) K18 S230T cells. Total protein extracts (10 μg) from selected clones were run on a 5% denaturing polyacrylamide gel, transferred to a PVDF membrane, and incubated with antibodies against K8 (M20), K18 (LDK-18) and phosphorylated keratin (LJ4) protein. As shown, K8 and K18 expression levels are very similar between the selected clones, while phosphorylated keratin levels are altered in the mutants, up-regulated in the K8 G62C (track 2) and K8 K464N (track 3) cells and down-regulated in the K18 S230T cells (track 5).

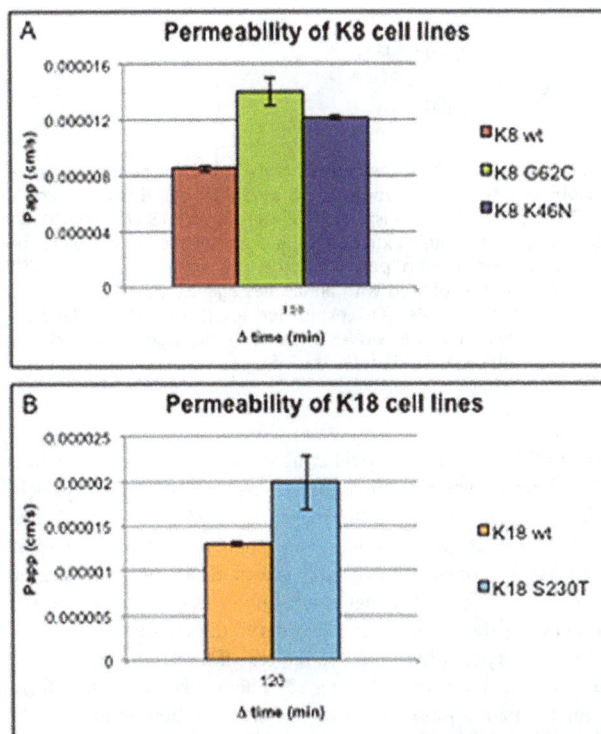

Figure 2. K8/K18 mutants have higher paracellular permeability. Isogenic K8/K18 cell lines were grown on cell culture inserts with a 0.4 μm pore size. Lucifer yellow was used to test the permeability of tight junctions after cells reached confluence and matured over a period of 2 weeks in culture. (A) Permeability coefficient (Papp) of K8 cell lines. Both mutants have a much higher permeability than the K8 control cell line. (B) Papp of K18 cell lines, where the K18 S230T mutant (similar to K8 mutants) displays a 30% higher permeability from the K18 control cell line.

against ZO-1, while in Figure 4C, D are the same cells stained with an antibody against claudin-4. In both cases the staining is more regular in K18 WT overexpressing cells, where it traces the cell membrane as expected for tight junctions (see arrows). In contrast, ZO-1 and claudin-4 seem to have a diffuse distribution in K18 S230T mutants, with visible speckles and aggregates (arrows). Hence, tight junctions of an epithelial sheet consisting of colonocytes expressing the K18 S230T mutation may have a compromised function, just as previously indicated by the permeability assay.

K18 S230T colonocytes have low growth rates

Next we decided to test whether these mutations interfere with cell growth. Although all cell lines appear to have normal cell cycle profiles (based on flow cytometry with propidium iodide staining, data not shown), their growth rates differ significantly. The results of these assays are summarized in Fig. 5. Both control cell lines (K8 WT and K18 WT) display similar growth rates, suggesting that the extra copy of the wild type gene on its own does not interfere with growth. The two K8 mutants (K8 G62C and K8 K464N) grow considerably faster, with a growth rate that is almost the double of the wild type. On the contrary, the K18 S230T cells differ greatly as they grow much slower than the K18 WT control cells.

Heat-stress causes K8/K18 mutants to detach from the surface as a sheet of cells

As the effect of the K18 S230T mutation appears to act more severely on cell function than previously concluded based on recombinant IF protein polymerization experiments [26], we decided to challenge these cells with heat-stress. The heat-stress assay proved useful in testing the IF network resilience for epidermal keratins. Cells were grown on coverslips for several days to allow them to attach firmly and form larger groups of cells. Cells were then subjected to heat stress and left to recover at normal growth temperature. At regular time intervals coverslips were fixed and immunofluorescently labelled to visualize the keratin cytoskeleton. The greatest differences between wild type and mutant cells were observed at 1 hour of recovery after heat-stress. Figure 6A, B are representative images of K18 WT and K18 S230T cells, while Figure 6C, D are representative images for K8

G62C and K8 K464N cells respectively. As shown, at this stage the free edges of islands of K8/K18 mutant cells (see arrows) appear much thicker in comparison to wild type cells. This is due to the detachment of border cells from the surface whilst remaining attached one another, causing the monolayers to curl up against the sheet of attached cells.

The K_d of K18 S230T is significantly higher than of K8 mutants

As the dissociation constant (K_d) is used in chemistry as measure of affinity between two molecules, we re-analysed surface plasmon resonance data previously published [26]. The web tool ENZO allowed us to calculate the K_d of K8 and K18 wild type and mutant proteins (Table 1). The higher the K_d, the lower the affinity between two molecules. Although all mutations appear to decrease the affinity of the mutant protein to their respective wild type partner, the data on K18 S230T is striking, having the highest K_d among these mutations.

Molecular modelling of the K8/K18 L12 dimer region

To test the effect of the K18 S230T mutation on the L12 region of the K8/K18 keratin heterodimer, we generated a 3D model of the L12 linker along with several adjacent residues of the 2A and 1B helices (from amino acid 181 to 315 of both K8 and K18, in total 134 residues of each chain). The linker domain was modelled according to the crystal structure of Maf-G transcription factor (PDB code 3A5T), while the helices according to vimentin (PDB

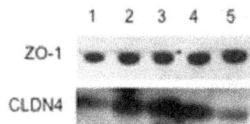

Figure 3. Western blot analysis of tight junction components in protein extracts from isogenic K8 and K18 cell lines. Tracks: (1) K8 WT cells; (2) K8 G62C cells; (3) K8 K464N cells; (4) K18 WT cells; (5) K18 S230T cells. Total protein extracts (10 μg) from selected clones were run on a 4–12% denaturing polyacrylamide gel, transferred to a PVDF membrane, and incubated with antibodies against ZO-1 (N-term) and claudin-4 (3E2C1). While ZO-1 expression levels are similar, claudin-4 levels are elevated in the two K8 mutants (tracks 2 and 3) and down-regulated in the K18 S230T cells (track 5).

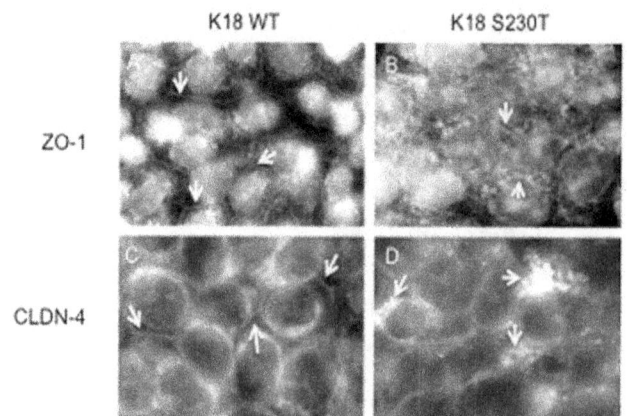

Figure 4. The distribution of ZO-1 and claudin-4 is altered in the K18 S230T mutant. Colonocytes stably expressing the K18 S230T mutation were immunofluorescently labelled for ZO-1 (upper panels, A and B) and claudin-4 (bottom panels, C and D), important components of tight junctions. In both cases the K18 control cells (panels A and C) show a more regular pattern of staining that traces the cell membrane. In contrast, the K18 S230T mutant (panels B and D) has a very diffuse pattern of staining for ZO-1 and claudin-4, and smaller protein aggregates are also visible (see arrows). Images were acquired with a 60x objective lens.

code 3TRT). Since the crystal structure of any keratin protein is still unknown, we identified three possible L12 linker models, which are based on the following concepts (Figure 7A): (1) The linker region is just a linear continuation of the coiled-coil, disrupting the coiled-coil in a similar fashion like the stutter region of coil 2B; (2) The linker region is a bubble between coils 2A and 1B, allowing the main chain to conserve the characteristic seven amino acid repeat (this would be the case if the entire protein had only one origin of protein folding; (3) The two keratin chains form an interchanging loop with a short four helix bundle in the L12 linker region (this is the case of a protein having several origins of protein folding). In the resulting structures the K18 S230T mutation is positioned at the beginning of the linker region. Models (1) and (2) were discarded. Model 1 seemed unlikely as the 23 amino acid long (the L12 region) disruption of the heptad repeat within the helical domains would introduce great instability into the K8/K18 heterodimer coiled-coil. On the other hand model 2 is not realistic as it predicts only one origin of protein folding, and keratin monomers are between 400 and 600 amino acids long. Therefore such a simplified model would also disregard any possible influence of the loop region to the coiled-coil structure of the K8/K18 heterodimer. However in model 3 the K18 S230T mutation lies at the beginning of the four-helix bundle region, which can only form if the keratin monomer has several origins of folding, and it also suggests having impact on the structure's dynamics. We performed molecular dynamics on model 3, which indicated the possibility that the K18 S230T mutation introduces an additional hydrogen bond into the structure (Fig. 7B). From the molecular dynamics data we calculated two key parameters: the average distance between the hydroxyl group of SER/THR230 and the backbone oxygen of ALA226 in K18 (Figure 8A), and the relative root-mean-square along the run, which is a measure of dimer stability (Fig. 8B). Both parameters suggested an additional hydrogen bond in the T230 mutant, stabilizing the structure and increasing the rigidity of the mutant L12 linker region.

Discussion

We have here shown that not only some K8 variations, but also the disputed K18 S230T change, are able to produce a phenotype in an *in vitro* intestinal epithelium model system. By introducing the K8 (G62C and K464N) and K18 (S230T) mutations into the background of the same wild type HT-29 colonocyte cell line, we created isogenic cell lines and eliminated potential variations arising from different genetic backgrounds. We observed increased paracellular permeability in all three mutants compared to their corresponding isogenic wild type control cells (HT-29 cells with an extra copy of the K8 or K18 wild type genes). Unlike mutant

epidermal keratins, where heat-stress generally induces keratin aggregation and filament bundling, the K8/K18 mutations we tested appear to affect cell adhesion and perturb tight junctions. The paracellular route of transport is primarily dependent on tight junctions. We already demonstrated that severe K5/K14 mutations (giving rise to a skin fragility disorder in humans) affect the expression and distribution of cell junction proteins, principally desmosomal components [19]. Like desmosomes, tight junctions are also multiprotein intercellular adhesion complexes with a defined stoichiometry, which is necessary to ensure their primary function: locking epithelial cells tightly together into a selective barrier that protects underlying tissues from pathogens and toxins. As we were particularly interested in the K18 S230T mutant, we tested by Western blotting and immunofluorescence if tight junction proteins were affected. We found that proteins ZO-1 and claudin-4 have a diffuse distribution in the K18 S230T mutant, and that claudin-4 is down-regulated in these cells, suggesting impaired function of tight junctions. Therefore, under in vitro conditions mutant keratins K8/K18 appear able to affect two major roles of intestinal epithelia: tissue permeability and tissue fragility. The mechanism how these mutations interfere with cell function is unclear, however it seems to be linked to cell junction complexes. The keratin IF network assembly, dynamics and maintenance are dependent on the interaction of the keratin network and precursors with both microtubules and actin filaments [6], [31]. As the three cytoskeletal filament systems interact between them and bind to cell junction proteins, changes in one filament system may be able to interfere with the function and/or distribution of distant proteins through their binding partners [32], [33]. An interesting aspect of this is that the K8 and K18 mutant cell lines analysed here do show some differences in keratin phosphorylation status, which is reflected by alterations in protein levels of claudin-4.

Evidence of a link between simple epithelial keratins and IBD has been previously shown on animal models. K8 null mice develop colitis, rectal prolapse and hyperplasia of the colon. Histological analysis suggests that the colonic inflammation seen in

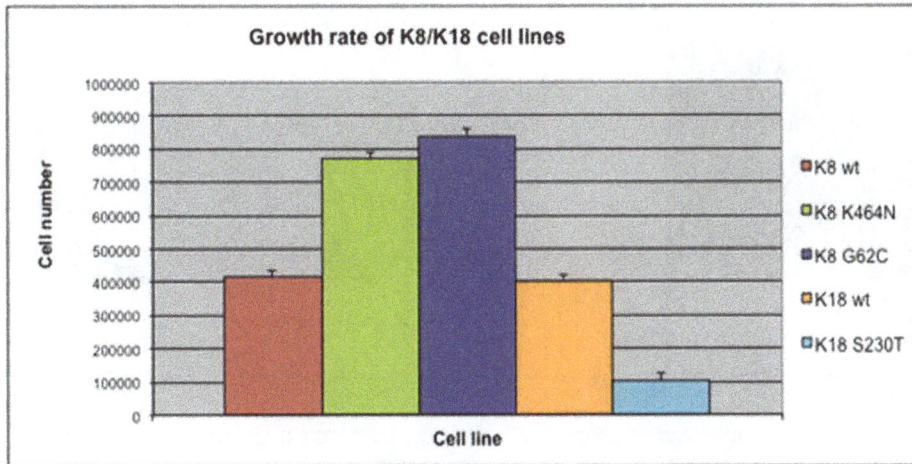

Figure 5. K8/K18 mutants have altered growth rates. Cells were grown on 24-well cell culture plates. After a week in culture cells were trypsinized and counted. As shown, the K8 mutants grow at a much higher rate than the K8 WT cell line, while the K18 S230T cells grow very slow, having only a quarter of the growth rate of K18 WT cells. All cell lines (mutant and wild type) have a normal cell cycle profile (not shown).

K8 null mice might be the result of an epithelial rather than immune system defect [34]. In addition, K8 null mouse colonocytes display a resistance to apoptotic stimuli, which is considered a protective function [35]. Both inflammation and resistance to apoptosis was treatable with antibiotics, suggesting the primary defect lies in the intestinal epithelium, while inflammation is the result of a subsequent immune response to luminal bacteria. It has also been shown that colons of K8 null

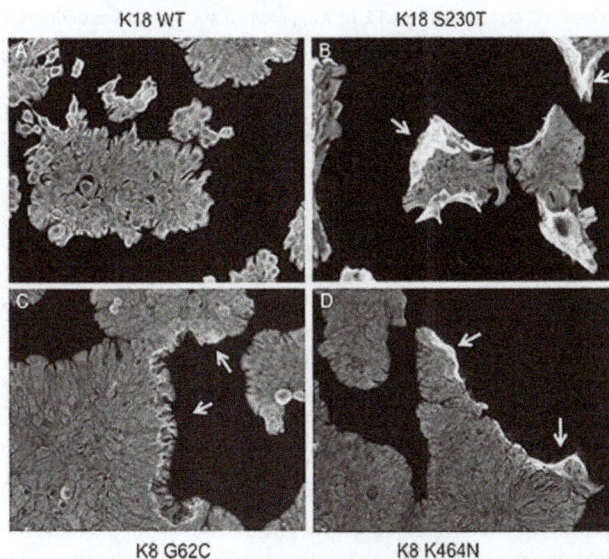

Figure 6. Effect of heat-stress on K8/K18 mutants. Cells were grown on coverslips until they formed smaller patches of cells, after which they were exposed to heat-stress for a brief period of time. At 0 time, 1 hour, 2 hours, 4 hours and 16 hours of recovery, cells were fixed and immmunofluorescently labelled for either K8 or K18 protein. Images shown are representative for the 1 hour time point of recovery, when the biggest differences were observed. In panel A are the K18 wild type control cells and these appear unaffected by heat stress. Panels B, C and D are the K18 S230T, K8 G62C and K8 K464N mutants respectively. Arrows mark border regions where cell sheets have detached from barrier surface and curled up against it. Images were acquired with a 20x objective lens.

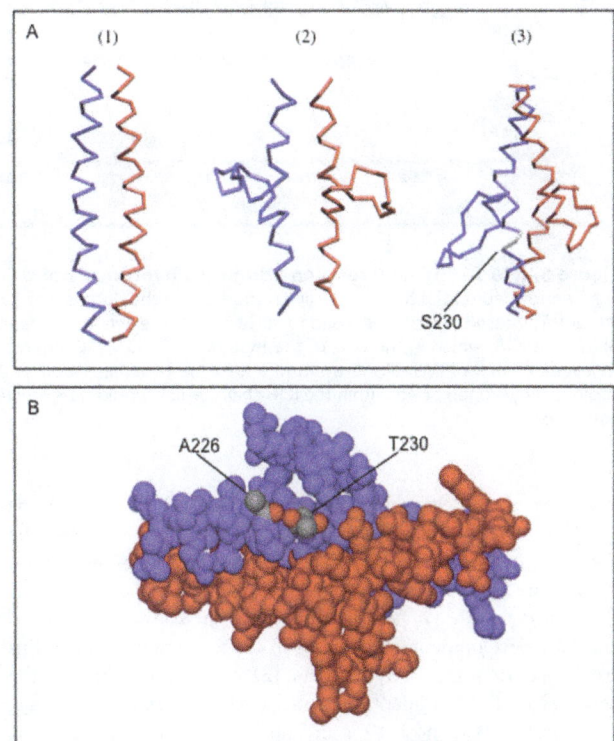

Figure 7. Molecular modelling of the K8/K18 L12 domain. We used 134 residues from the K8 and K18 polypeptides, which span the end part of helix 2A, the L12 linker and the beginning of helix 1B. The helical regions in our model were built based on the crystal structure of vimentin (PDB code 3TRT), while the linker domain on Maf-G protein (PDB code 3A5T). (A) The three possible models of the L12 region of K8/K18 protein folding. Models 1 and 2 were discarded, as they do not take into account many of the known keratin heterodimer structural features. Model 3 was further refined as the K8/K18 chains form in the L12 linker region an interchanging loop with a short four-helix bundle. The position of the S230 residue of K18 is labelled white. (B) In case of the S230T substitution the threonine residue cannot rotate freely as serine due to its size. Also, a new hydrogen bond may form between residues T230 and A226 of K18, thus stabilizing this part of the protein.

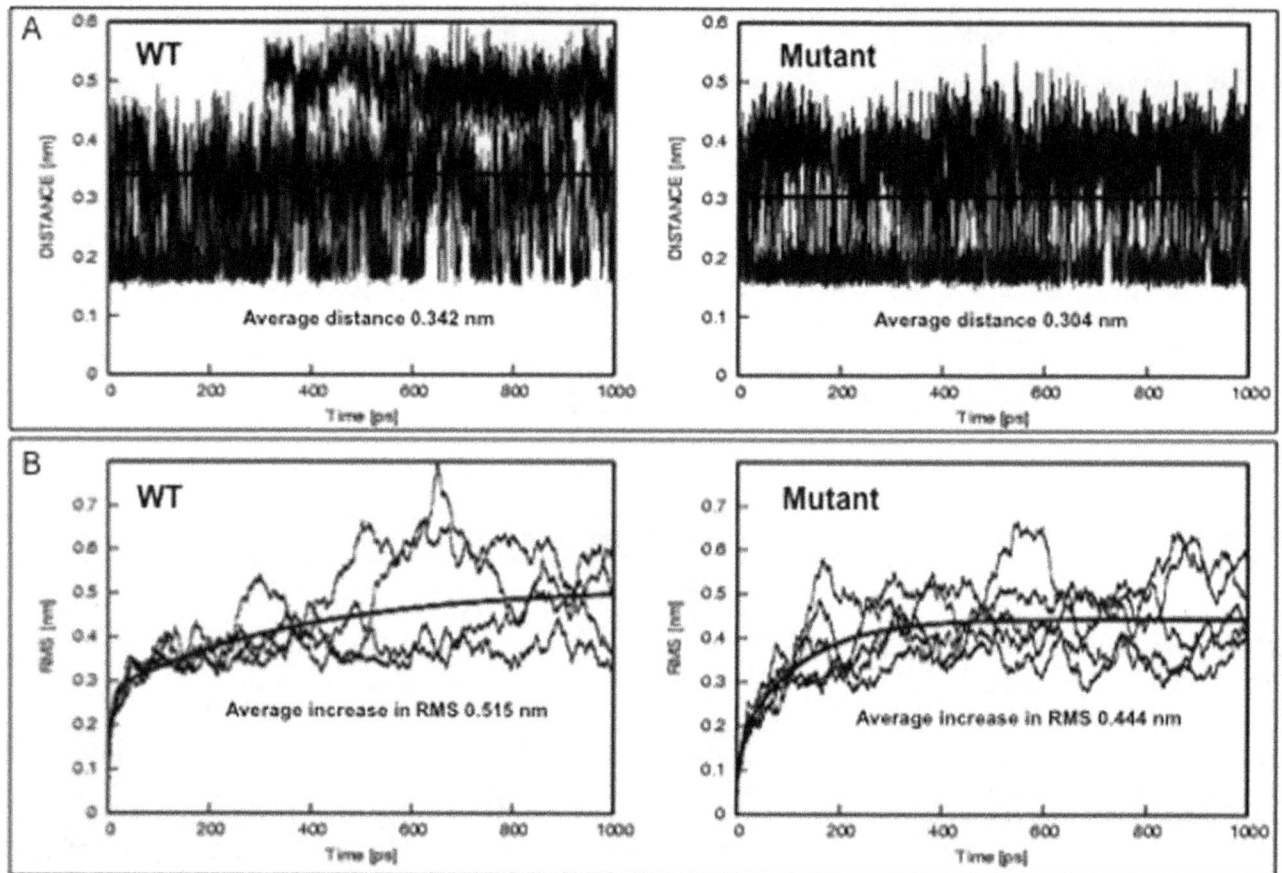

Figure 8. K18 S230T may form an additional hydrogen bond within the K18 chain in the L12 linker. Molecular dynamics experiments were performed on the K8/K18 L12 linker model with the duration of 1 ns. This was repeated 4 times for the wild type sequence and 5 times for the mutant. The resulting data was used to calculate: (A) the average distances between the hydroxyl group of SER/THR230 and the backbone oxygen of ALA226 in K18, which in the case of the mutant (THR230) falls within the range of a moderately strong hydrogen bond (2.5–3.2 Å); (B) the relative root mean square (RMS) along the run, a measure of dimer stability. Both parameters indicate that the K18 S230T mutation may be forming an additional hydrogen bond within the K18 chain, which would be expected to increase the rigidity of this part of protein to additional conformational pressures.

mice have altered electrolyte transport across the barrier caused by ion transporter mistargeting, which probably accounts for the diarrhoea in these animals [36], [37]. However studies focused on the genetic analysis of genomic DNA of groups of patients with IBD failed to show an explicit link between K8/K18 mutations and IBD development, at least not in the way epidermal keratins are linked to some skin disorders [27], [38], [39]. Firstly, the percentage of IBD patients carrying a K8/K18 mutation is low, somewhere between 2–10% of the total number of patients involved in the study. Secondly, in contrast to epidermal keratins, where mutations predominantly affect the helical domains of the protein and physically perturb the IF network, the K8/K18/K19 mutations found in IBD patients lie in the non-helical end domains, generally expected to produce a milder phenotype. It was therefore presumed that mutations in simple epithelial keratins act indirectly and in concert with some other susceptibility factors, making carriers susceptible to IBD development.

In 2004, Owens and colleagues [26] identified the first K8 mutations in IBD patients (G62C, I63V and K464N). These are situated in the end domains of K8 and accounted for only 5% of the patients included in the study. A K18 mutation (S230T) was also found within the L12 linker domain, which in epidermal keratins is associated with milder disease phenotypes. Experiments

(surface plasmon resonance, sedimentation assay, *in vitro* filament assembly, de novo filament polymerization) with purified recombinant wild type and mutant K8/K18 protein led to the conclusion that K8 mutations may interfere with keratin filament assembly. This was in particular true for the G62C mutation, which is now also associated with cryptogenic cirrhosis, pancreatitis, liver disease and primary biliary cirrhosis. On the other hand, although the K18 S230T variation was found in surface plasmon resonance experiments to interfere with the binding of monomeric K18 S230T to immobilized wild type K8, it was the only change to affect a non-conserved residue, not to affect *in vitro* filament assembly and was also found in four individuals from the control group. Consequently it was designated as a polymorphism. By using ENZO: Enzyme Kinetics software [28] we now calculated the dissociation constants (K_d) from the published surface plasmon resonance graphs [26]. The highest K_d and therefore the lowest affinity for the immobilized keratin partner was determined for the K18 S230T protein, followed by K8 G62C and K8 K464N. Nevertheless it has been shown that once bound these K8/K18 heterodimer complexes are relatively stable [26].

In this study we also developed the first computer-generated model of the keratin L12 linker region and analysed the potential effects of K18 S230T *in silico*. Our model suggests that T230 establishes a new hydrogen bond with residue A226 of the same K18 chain. In theory the resulting stabilization of the protein could slow down protein turnover and thus affect the rate of cell growth. Interestingly, our K18 S230T colonocytes do have a lower growth rate than control cells.

To conclude, this is the first time intestinal cells expressing K8 or K18 mutations have been proposed as directly functionally impaired by these. We have shown that although in the background of endogenous wild type keratin protein, certain K8 and K18 mutations may be able to affect the permeability of intestinal epithelium and its resilience to stress. Although our data is based on an *in vitro* colonocyte model system, which may not exactly reproduce the situation found in the epithelial lining of the intestine *in vivo*, this still suggests that K8 and K18 mutations may

be able to produce a phenotype on their own. The combined action of these with the immune response may certainly induce a variety of symptoms frequently found in patients with IBD.

Acknowledgments

We would like to thank Mateja Ozir, Spela Peternel and Jelka Lenarcic for their technical help.

Author Contributions

Conceived and designed the experiments: TZ ABZ JS EBL ML. Performed the experiments: TZ ABZ JS EBL ML. Analyzed the data: TZ ABZ JS EBL RK ML. Contributed reagents/materials/analysis tools: JS EBL. Wrote the paper: RK ML.

References

1. Lane EB, Goodman SL, Trejdosiewicz LK (1982) Disruption of the keratin filament network during epithelial cell division. EMBO J 1: 1365–1372.
2. Galarneau L, Loranger A, Gilbert S, Marceau N (2007) Keratins modulate hepatic cell adhesion, size and G1/S transition. Exp Cell Res 313: 179–194.
3. Magin TM, Vijayaraj P, Leube RE (2007) Structural and regulatory functions of keratins. Exp Cell Res 313: 2021–2032.
4. Chung BM, Rotty JD, Coulombe PA (2013) Networking galore: intermediate filaments and cell migration. Curr Opin Cell Biol 25: 600–612.
5. D'Alessandro M, Russell D, Morley SM, Davies AM, Lane EB (2002) Keratin mutations of epidermolysis bullosa simplex alter the kinetics of stress response to osmotic shock. J Cell Sci 115(Pt 22): 4341–4351.
6. Liovic M, Mogensen MM, Prescott AR, Lane EB (2003) Observation of keratin particles showing fast bidirectional movement colocalized with microtubules. J Cell Sci 116(Pt 8): 1417–1427.
7. Liovic M, Lee B, Tomic-Canic M, D'Alessandro M, Bolshakov VN, et al. (2013) Dual-specificity phosphatases in the hypo-osmotic stress response of keratin-defective epithelial cell lines. Exp Cell Res 314: 2066–2075.
8. Russell D, Ross H, Lane EB (2010) ERK involvement in resistance to apoptosis in keratinocytes with mutant keratin. J Invest Dermatol 130: 671–681.
9. Majumdar D, Tiernan JP, Lobo AJ, Evans CA, Corfe BM (2012) Keratins in colorectal epithelial function and disease. Int J Exp Pathol 93: 305–318.
10. Valentin MD, da Silva SD, Privat M, Privat M, Alaoui-Jamali M, et al. (2012) Molecular insights on basal-like breast cancer. Breast Cancer Res Treat 134: 21–30.
11. Coulombe PA, Hutton ME, Letai A, Hebert A, Paller AS, et al. (1991) Point mutations in human keratin 14 genes of epidermolysis bullosa simplex patients: genetic and functional analyses. Cell 66: 1301–1311.
12. Lane EB, Rugg EL, Navsaria H, Leigh IM, Heagerty AH, et al. (1992) A mutation in the conserved helix termination peptide of keratin 5 in hereditary skin blistering. Nature 356: 244–246.
13. Szeverenyi I, Cassidy AJ, Chung CW, Lee BT, Common JE, et al. (2008) The Human Intermediate Filament Database: comprehensive information on a gene family involved in many human diseases. Hum Mut 29: 351–360.
14. Kucharzik T, Maaser C, Lügering A, Lügering A, Kagnoff M, et al. (2006) Recent understanding of IBD pathogenesis: implications for future therapies. Inflamm Bowel Dis 12: 1068–1083.
15. Xavier RJ, Podolsky DK (2007) Unravelling the pathogenesis of inflammatory bowel disease. Nature 448: 427–434.
16. Sartor RB (2206) Mechanisms of disease: pathogenesis of Crohn's disease and ulcerative colitis. Nat Clin Pract Gastroenterol Hepatol 3: 390–407.
17. Roth W, Kumar V, Beer HD, Richter M, Wohlenberg C, et al (2012) Keratin 1 maintains skin integrity and participates in an inflammatory network in skin through interleukin-18. J Cell Sci 125: 5269–5279.
18. Lessard JC, Piña-Paz S, Rotty JD, Hickerson RP, Kaspar RL, et al. (2013) Keratin 16 regulates innate immunity in response to epidermal barrier breach. Proc Natl Acad Sci USA 110: 19537–19542.
19. Liovic M, D'Alessandro M, Tomic-Canic M, Bolshakov VN, Coats SE, et al. (2009) Severe keratin 5 and 14 mutations induce down-regulation of junction proteins in keratinocytes. Exp Cell Res 315: 2995–3003.
20. Wallace L, Roberts-Thompson L, Reichelt J (2012) Deletion of K1/K10 does not impair epidermal stratification but affects desmosomal structure and nuclear integrity. J Cell Sci 125(Pt 7): 1750–1758.

21. Bär J, Kumar V, Roth W, Schwarz N, Richter M, et al. (2013) Skin fragility and Inpaired Desmosomal Adhesion in mice Lacking all keratins. J Invest Dermatol doi: 10.1038/jid.2013.416
22. Kröger C, Loschke F, Schwarz N, Windoffer R, Leube RE, et al. (2013) Keratins control intercellular adhesion involving PKC-?-mediated desmoplakin phosphorylation. J Cell Biol 201: 681–692.
23. Ku NO, Toivola DM, Strnad P, Omary MB (2010) Cytoskeletal keratin glycosylation protects epithelial tissue from injury. Nat Cell Biol 12: 876–885.
24. Snider NT, Weerasinghe SV, Iñiguez-Lluhí JA, Herrmann H, Omary MB (2011) Keratin hypersumoylation alters filament dynamics and is a marker for human liver disease and keratin mutation. J Biol Chem 286: 2273–2284.
25. Busch T, Armacki M, Eiseler T, Joodi G, Temme C, et al. (2012) Keratin 8 phosphorylation regulates keratin reorganization and migration of epithelial tumor cells. J Cell Sci 125(Pt 9): 2148–2159.
26. Owens DW, Wilson NJ, Hill AJ, Rugg EL, Porter RM, et al. (2004) Human keratin 8 mutations that disturb filament assembly observed in inflammatory bowel disease patients. J Cell Sci 117(Pt 10): 1989–1999.
27. Morley SM, D'Alessandro M, Sexton C, Rugg EL, Navsaria H, et al. (2003) Generation and characterization of epidermolysis bullosa simplex cell lines: scratch assays show faster migration with disruptive keratin mutations. Br J Dermatol 149: 46–58.
28. Bevc S, Konc J, Stojan J, Hodoscek M, Penca M, et al. (2011) ENZO: a web tool for derivation and evaluation of kinetic models of enzyme catalyzed reactions. PLoS One 6:e22265
29. Kurokawa H, Motohashi H, Sueno S, Kimura M, Takagawa H, et al. (2009) Structural basis of alternative DNA recognition by Maf transcription factors. Mol Cell Biol 29: 6232–6244.
30. Chernyatina AA, Strelkov SV (2012) Stabilization of vimentin coil2 fragment via an engineered disulfide. J Struct Biol 177: 46–53.
31. Kölsch A, Windoffer R, Leube RE (2009) Actin-dependent dynamics of keratin filament precursors. Cell Motil Cytoskeleton 66: 976–985.
32. Maniotis AJ, Chen CS, Ingber DE (1997) Demonstration of mechanical connections between integrins, cytoskeletal filaments, and nucleoplasm that stabilize nuclear structure. Proc Natl Acad Sci USA 94: 849–854.
33. Jefferson JJ, Leung CL, Liem RK (2004) Plakins: goliaths that link cell junctions and the cytoskeleton. Nature Rev Mol Cell Biol 5: 542–553.
34. Baribault H, Penner J, Iozzo RV, Wilson-Heiner M (1994) Colorectal hyperplasia and inflammation in keratin 8-deficient FVB/N mice. Genes Dev 8: 2964–2973.
35. Habtezion A, Toivola DM, Asghar MN, Kronmal GS, Brooks JD, et al. (2011) Absence of keratin 8 confers a paradoxical microflora-dependent resistance to apoptosis in the colon. Proc Natl Acad Sci USA 108: 1445–1450.
36. Toivola DM, Krishnan S, Binder HJ, Singh SK, Omary MB (2004) Keratins modulate colonocyte electrolyte transport via protein mistargeting. J Cell Biol 164: 911–921.
37. Habtezion A, Toivola DM, Butcher EC, Omary MB (2005) Keratin-8-deficient mice develop chronic spontaneous Th2 colitis amenable to antibiotic treatment. J Cell Sci 118: 1971–1980.
38. Buning C, Halangk J, Dignass A, Ockenga J, Deindl P, et al. (2004) Keratin 8 Y54H and G62C mutations are not associated with inflammatory bowel disease. Dig Liver Dis 36: 388–391.
39. Tao GZ, Strnad P, Zhou Q, Kamal A, Zhang L, et al. (2007) Analysis of keratin polypeptides 8 and 19 variants in inflammatory bowel disease. Clin Gastroenterol Hepatol 5: 857–864.

12

Relevance of TNBS-Colitis in Rats: A Methodological Study with Endoscopic, Histologic and Transcriptomic Characterization and Correlation to IBD

Øystein Brenna[1,2]*, Marianne W. Furnes[2], Ignat Drozdov[3], Atle van Beelen Granlund[2], Arnar Flatberg[2], Arne K. Sandvik[1,2], Rosalie T. M. Zwiggelaar[2], Ronald Mårvik[2,4], Ivar S. Nordrum[2,5], Mark Kidd[6], Björn I. Gustafsson[1,2]

1 Department of Gastroenterology and Hepatology, St. Olavs Hospital, Trondheim University Hospital, Trondheim, Norway, 2 Department of Cancer Research and Molecular Medicine, Norwegian University of Science and Technology, Trondheim, Norway, 3 Bering Limited, Richmond, United Kingdom, 4 Department of Gastrointestinal Surgery, St. Olavs Hospital, Trondheim University Hospital, Trondheim, Norway, 5 Department of Pathology and Medical Genetics, St. Olavs Hospital, Trondheim University Hospital, Trondheim, Norway, 6 Department of Surgery, Section of Gastroenterology, Yale School of Medicine, New Haven, Connecticut, United States of America

Abstract

Background: Rectal instillation of trinitrobenzene sulphonic acid (TNBS) in ethanol is an established model for inflammatory bowel disease (IBD). We aimed to 1) set up a TNBS-colitis protocol resulting in an endoscopic and histologic picture resembling IBD, 2) study the correlation between endoscopic, histologic and gene expression alterations at different time points after colitis induction, and 3) compare rat and human IBD mucosal transcriptomic data to evaluate whether TNBS-colitis is an appropriate model of IBD.

Methodology/Principal Findings: Five female Sprague Daley rats received TNBS diluted in 50% ethanol (18 mg/0.6 ml) rectally. The rats underwent colonoscopy with biopsy at different time points. RNA was extracted from rat biopsies and microarray was performed. PCR and *in situ* hybridization (ISH) were done for validation of microarray results. Rat microarray profiles were compared to human IBD expression profiles (25 ulcerative colitis Endoscopic score demonstrated mild to moderate colitis after three and seven days, but declined after twelve days. Histologic changes corresponded with the endoscopic appearance. Over-represented Gene Ontology Biological Processes included: *Cell Adhesion, Immune Response, Lipid Metabolic Process,* and *Tissue Regeneration.* IL-1α, IL-1β, TLR2, TLR4, PRNP were all significantly up-regulated, while PPARγ was significantly down-regulated. Among genes with highest fold change (FC) were SPINK4, LBP, ADA, RETNLB and IL-1α. The highest concordance in differential expression between TNBS and IBD transcriptomes was three days after colitis induction. ISH and PCR results corresponded with the microarray data. The most concordantly expressed biologically relevant pathways included *TNF signaling, Cell junction organization,* and *Interleukin-1 processing.*

Conclusions/Significance: Endoscopy with biopsies in TNBS-colitis is useful to follow temporal changes of inflammation visually and histologically, and to acquire tissue for gene expression analyses. TNBS-colitis is an appropriate model to study specific biological processes in IBD.

Editor: Benoit Foligne, Institut Pasteur de Lille, France

Funding: Kontaktutvalget, St. Olavs Hospital, Trondheim University Hospital and DMF/NTNU (Project number 96990)(BIG); MK is supported by NIH DK080871; The microarray work was carried out with support from the National Technology Microarray Platform (Norwegian Microarray Consortium) funded the Functional Genomics Programme (FUGE) of the Norwegian Research Council. The funders had no role in study design, data collection and analysis, decision to publish, or preparation of the manuscript.

Competing Interests: The authors have the following interests. Ignat Drozdov is employed by Bering Limited and was paid was paid by NTNU as a consultant to do this work. Bering Limited was involved in data analysis. There are no patents, products in development or marketed products to declare.

* E-mail: Oystein.Brenna@stolav.no

Introduction

Inflammatory bowel disease (IBD) is the common denomination of ulcerative colitis (UC) and Crohn's disease (CD). The etiology is unknown and the pathogenesis is complex and incompletely understood. The interplay between genetic and immunological host factors and the gut microbiota are important factors in the development of disease [1,2].

The inflammatory response in IBD is characterized by mucosal barrier dysfunction, microbial invasion and activation of immune response [3,4]. In genetically predisposed individuals, microbial activation via toll-like receptors (TLRs) and induction of an inflammatory response accompanied by high levels of pro-inflammatory cytokines such as interleukins (ILs) (IL-1, IL-6, IL-13 and IL-17) and tumor necrosis factor alpha (TNF-α), seem to be critical [1,5–9]. However, the exact molecular basis of IBD remains poorly understood.

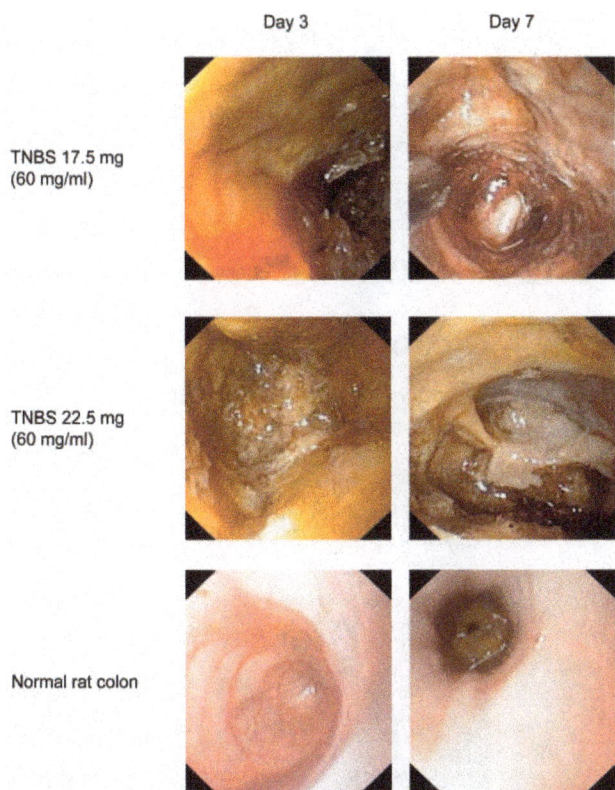

Figure 1. **Endoscopic images demonstrating the effect of different doses of TNBS in a fixed concentration of 60 mg/ml.** Severe colitis with a yellowish membrane and coprostasis was noted at day 3, and mucosal shedding, stenosis and necrosis was evident at day 7 in rats given TNBS 17.5 mg and 22.5 mg (0.29 ml and 0.38 ml, respectively). The bottom panel depicts examples of normal rat colon.

Experimentally induced colitis with trinitrobenzene sulphonic acid (TNBS) is used to generate models that are used to examine the pathogenesis of gut inflammation, and determine the mechanisms and efficacy of therapies [10]. TNBS is diluted in ethanol which disrupts the mucosal barrier. Usually, the TNBS-solution is rectally instilled. Inflammation is induced by TNBS-induced haptenization of colonic mucosal proteins [11]. The use of TNBS to generate colitis was originally described and histologically characterized by Morris *et al.* in rats. Granulomas were observed in over 50% of animals two to three weeks after induction of colitis [12]. TNBS-ethanol administration is characterized by Th1-driven inflammation [11], and has primarily been regarded as a model for CD [10,13]. The clinical features include weight loss and bloody diarrhea, while morphologically the model is characterized by mucosal, submucosal and transmural inflammation. Consequently, the model has been used to investigate the role and mechanistic action of drugs including 5-aminosalisylic acid, steroids and anti-tumor necrosis factor (TNF) in IBD [14–16]. The administration and doses of TNBS differ significantly between studies; the methodology is inconsistent and no standardized protocol exists [14,17–20].

Both TNBS-colitis and IBD include disturbances in basic physiological processes like immune activation, metabolism and mucosal repair [21]. Microbial regulation of TLRs and induction of an inflammatory response is accompanied by regulation of pro- and anti-inflammatory cytokines and the shaping of the intestinal immune response [22]. Down-regulation of the peroxisome proliferator-activated receptor (PPAR) gamma involved in the regulation of fatty acid metabolism and inflammation, has been demonstrated in IBD and is associated with maintenance of defensin expression [23–25]. The cellular Prion protein (PrP^c) is expressed in brain and various extra cerebral tissues including neuroendocrine cells and lymphoid tissue of the gut [26–28]. PrP^c can have an anti-inflammatory effect in the colon [29].

We report the development and characterization of TNBS-colitis in rats using colonoscopy and temporal gene expression profiling. The aim was to standardize TNBS administration to achieve a moderate inflammation. Achieving a moderate colitis allowed for the study of epithelial alterations upon mucosal damage, while temporal gene expression profiling identified longitudinal transcriptomic changes that were associated with these abnormalities. We further aimed to compare the genome-wide changes in TNBS-colitis to a human transcriptome to determine whether TNBS at this dose was an appropriate model for IBD.

Materials and Methods

Animals

The study was approved by the National Animal Research Authority (NARA). The general care and use of the animals were in accordance with the European Convention for the protection of Vertebrate Animals used for Experimental and other Scientific purposes. We used female Sprague Dawley rats weighing 200–250 g from Taconic (Taconic Farms, Inc., Hallingore, Denmark). They were housed in individually ventilated cages (IVC) with aspen bedding (Tapvei) in a specific pathogen free (SPF) environment with temperature 19–22°C and humidity 50–60% and 12 hr day and night cycle with 1 hr dusk and dawn. All rats had access to water and standard chow (RM1 maintenance, SDS, UK) *ad libitum*, apart from the 24 hr fasting periods before each colonoscopy to allow voiding of the left colon, when they had access only to glucose 2% fluid mixture and were kept in wired bottom cages. Rat colonoscopy was performed under general gas anesthesia using isoflurane. At termination, the rats were sacrificed by exsanguination during general isoflurane anesthesia.

Initial studies and main study

Initial studies to optimize TNBS dose and concentration. Sixteen rats weighing 264.9 g (standard deviation [SD] ±14.5) were divided into two groups. Group 1 received 17.5 and group 2 received 22.5 mg TNBS (1 M, 293.17 mg/ml, product number 92822, Fluka, Buchs, Switzerland) diluted in 50% ethanol to a concentration of 60 mg/ml. The total volume instilled was ~0.29 ml and ~0.38 ml respectively for group 1 and 2. In a subsequent study, eight rats received TNBS in eight different doses (7–31.5 mg) diluted in 50% ethanol, to a total volume of 0.7 ml with concentrations ranging from 10–45 mg/ml.

TNBS was rectally instilled via a female urinary catheter (DCT Ch 10, Servoprax GmbH, Wesel, Germany). After removal of residual rectal fecal pellets, the catheter was advanced approximately to the splenic flexure. After instillation, the rats were held with the head down for one minute to prevent TNBS from leaking out. The colitis was evaluated with colonoscopy (Olympus ureterorenoscope, URF Type V) with picture documentation at Day 3, Day 7 and at Day 12. Biopsies were obtained using an Olympus biopsy forceps (FB-56 D-1, Olympus, Norway).

Main study. Eight female Sprague Dawley rats, age eight weeks and weighing 196.9 g (SD±14.3) were used. Based on the initial studies, TNBS dissolved in 50% ethanol to a concentration of 30 mg/ml in a total volume of 0.6 ml was instilled. Animal

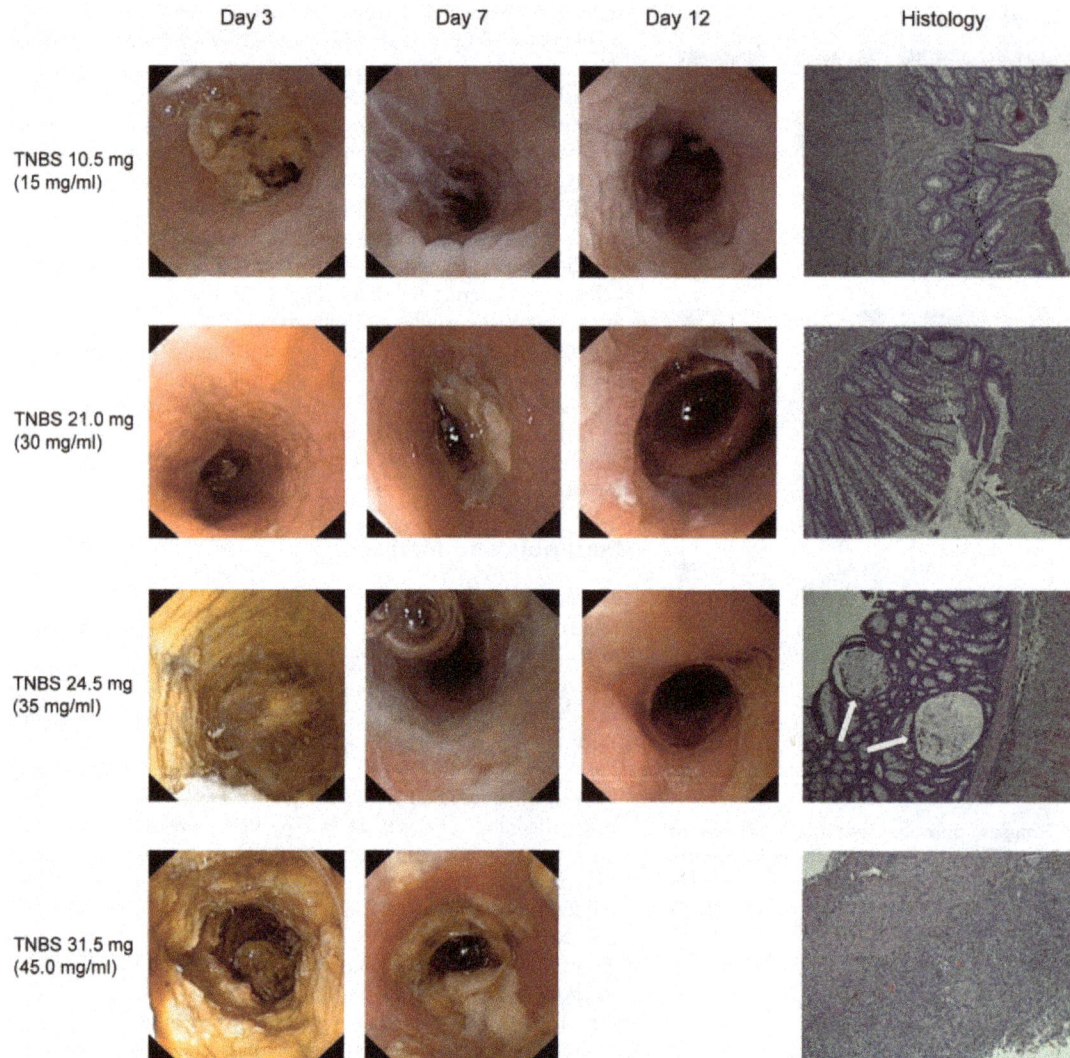

Figure 2. Endoscopic images demonstrating the effect of TNBS at different concentrations instilled rectally in a total volume of 0.7 ml. TNBS 10.5 mg (15 mg/ml) was associated with minimal mucosal inflammation and edema. TNBS 21.0 mg (30 mg/ml) resulted in an erythematous and edematous mucosa at day 3 and 7. At day 12 mucosal granulation and ulcerations were seen. TNBS 24.5 mg (35 mg/ml) and 31.5 mg (45 mg/ml) resulted in a more severe acute inflammation, and at day 7, larger areas of ulceration with fibrin cover were visible. At day 12, stenotic strictures developed in the rat receiving TNBS 24.5 mg. The rat receiving 31.5 mg was euthanized after the second endoscopy and consequently no endoscopic picture from day 12 can be shown. In the right column, histological pictures corresponding to mild, moderate and severe TNBS-colitis are included. TNBS 10.5 mg (15 mg/ml) resulted in only minimal inflammation with some architectural changes. TNBS 21.0 mg (30 mg/ml) resulted in ulceration that bordered the mucosa with inflammatory cell infiltration. In TNBS 24.5 mg (35 mg/ml), crypt distortion and abscesses (arrows) with mucosal and submucosal inflammatory infiltration were visible. Severe TNBS colitis is seen in the lower hitstologic picture with transmural inflammatory cell infiltration and total denudation of the mucosa. Objective x10 in all histological images.

weights and clinical status were monitored throughout the study. Colonoscopy with photo documentation and tissue sampling was performed two days before (T0), and three (T3), seven (T7) and twelve (T12) days after induction of colitis. A modified Murine Endoscopic Index of Colitis Severity [30] (MEICS, 0–12, *Thickening of the colon* was not considered) was used for endoscopic evaluation and grading of the colitis. Five animals that developed similar endoscopically moderate colitis in the left colon were chosen for further studies.

During each colonoscopy, three biopsies were collected and snap frozen in liquid nitrogen for later RNA extraction. Another two biopsies were fixed in 4% buffered formaldehyde and then embedded in paraffin. The study was terminated at T12. The colon was divided longitudinally and one part fixed in formalde-

hyde for histologic examination and the other frozen in liquid nitrogen.

Animal weight data were compared using Student's t-test with equal variances after confirming this with f-test. The significance level was set at $\alpha = 0.05$.

RNA extraction, microarray amplification, hybridization, scanning and quantification

Rat mucosal samples. From each animal, three biopsies were collected at every time point in the main study (TNBS 30 mg/ml, 0.6 ml). Samples were pooled and RNA was extracted using the RNeasy Mini RNA extraction Kit (cat.no. 74106, Qiagen, Hilden, Germany) according to the manufacturer's protocol. Quality of extracted RNA was controlled using

A

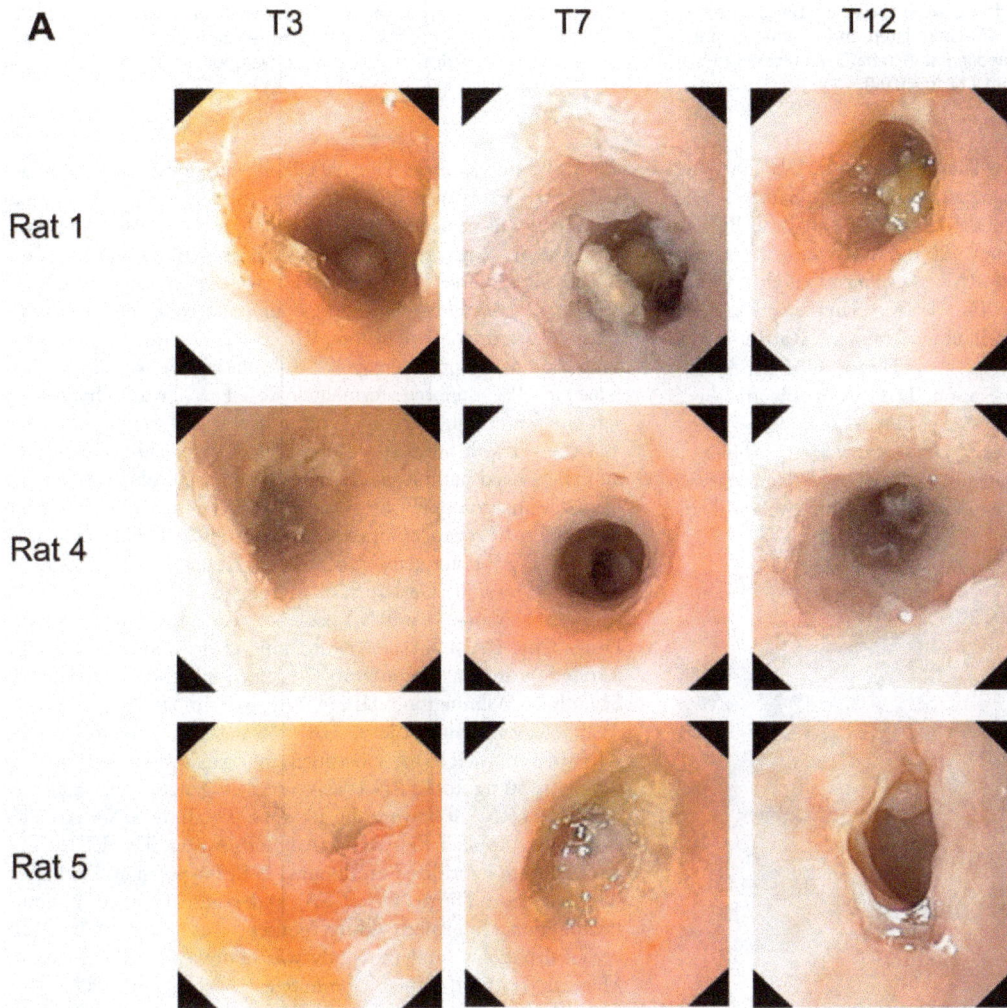

B

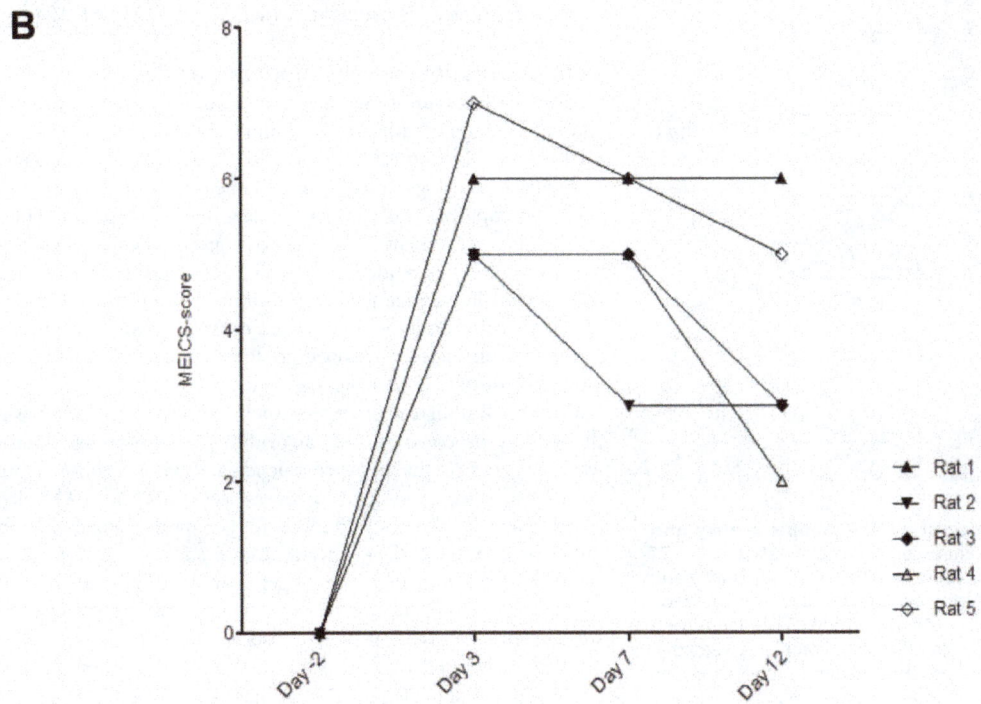

Figure 3. Representative endoscopic images of TNBS (30 mg/ml, 0.6 ml) associated changes at different time points and MEICS-score at T0, T3, T7 and T12. (A) Granulated and edematous mucosa at T3 and T7, and ulcerations at T12 were evident in Rat 1. At T7, small ulcerations/erosions were identified in Rat 4. In Rat 5, an ulceration is visible at T7 and at T12, a stricturing ulcer has developed. (B) The MEICS-score at T3 was significantly different from T12 ($p = 0.02$).

NanoDrop Spectrophotometer (Thermo Scientific, DE, USA) and Bioanalyzer (Agilent Technologies, CA, USA). Samples with RIN>7 were deemed suitable for downstream analysis. Biotinylated cRNA was prepared from 400 ng RNA for each sample using the Illumina TotalPrep RNA Amplification kit (Applied Biosystems/Ambion, Austin, TX, USA). Sample cRNA was subsequently hybridized on Illumina human RatRef-12 v1 expression BeadChips (Illumina, San Diego, CA, USA) and scanned on an Illumina BeadStation. Data from this analysis is publicly available at ArrayExpress, E-MTAB-1263.

Human mucosal samples. Gene expression profiles in mucosal samples from 25 patients with UC, 11 patients with CD, and 25 healthy controls were used for comparison with the

Figure 4. Histologic appearance of an endoscopic biopsy and whole colon specimen. (A) Endoscopic biopsy collected at T7 showing evidence of a crypt abscess (arrow), and mucosal gland distortion. Objective x40. (B) Histologic image of a whole colon specimen collected at termination of the study (T12) identifying distorted mucosal glands, and an ulceration with completed reepithelialization and underlying submucosal inflammation (arrow). Objective x4. The slides were stained with hematoxylin and eosin.

TNBS-transcriptomes. The data used was drawn from a larger IBD gene expression analysis study performed at Norwegian University of Science and Technology/St. Olavs Hospital, Trondheim, Norway. All IBD samples were obtained from maximally inflamed colonic mucosa, while normal controls were taken from the hepatic flexure. Four endoscopic pinch biopsies were collected from each area. Three biopsies were immediately snap frozen in liquid nitrogen, while the remaining sample was fixed in 4% buffered formaldehyde. The formaldehyde-fixed samples were embedded in paraffin and 4 µm sections were cut and stained with hematoxylin-eosin for histological evaluation by an experienced pathologist. In cases where the evaluation differed from the macroscopic observations, samples were removed from the analysis. Frozen biopsies were homogenized using an Ultra-Turrax T 25 homogenizer (Zanke & Kunkel IKA-Laboratorie Technik, Staufen, Germany). Total RNA was extracted using Ambion mirVana^{TM} miRNA Isolation Kit (Applied Biosystems, Foster City, CA, USA). RNA quantity, purity and integrity were assessed using a NanoDrop^{TM} Spectrophotometer (Thermo Scientific, Wilmington, DE, USA) and Bioanalyzer (Agilent Technologies, Santa Clara, CA, USA). Only samples with a RIN>7 were used in the subsequent microarray analysis. For each sample, 250 ng total RNA was used to generate biotinylated, amplified cRNA following the Illumina TotalPrer RNA Amplification Kit (Applied Biosystems/Ambion, Austin, TX, USA). The samples were hybridized on Illumina HT12 expression BeadChips (Illumina, San Diego, CA, USA) and scanned on an Illumina BeadStation. Informed written consent was obtained from all involved patients, and the study was approved by the Regional Medical Research Ethics Committee (approval no 5.2007.910). The study was registered in the Clinical Trials Protocol Registration System (identifier NCT00516776). Data from this analysis is publicly available at ArrayExpress, E-MTAB-184.

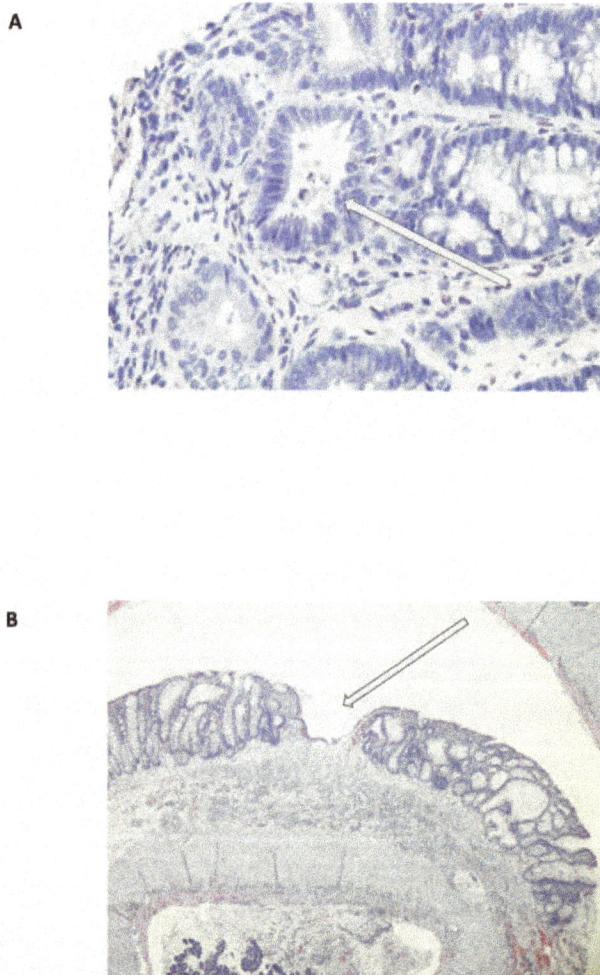

Data preparation and bioinformatic analysis

Gene expression analysis. Raw data was exported from the Illumina GenomeStudio software and normalized using the $lumi$ package for Bioconductor suite [31]. The data was quantile normalized and log2 transformed. Time course differential gene expression analysis was performed using the BETR package for R statistical environment [32]. Pairwise group comparisons were performed using a Student's t-test. The (FC) was used to express the changes in average gene expressions between studied groups. To standardize annotation across microarray platforms, Illumina probe identifiers were mapped to their corresponding Ensembl (accessed March 23, 2011) gene identifiers (IDs) [33].

Clusters of similar gene expression profiles were identified using the Affinity propagation (AP) algorithm [34], where dissimilarity was expressed as the negative Euclidian distance. Subsequently, gene clusters were enriched for over-represented Gene Ontology (GO) Biological Process (BP) terms [35] using the hypergeometric test. For a cluster with n genes and an $a priori$ defined functional category with K genes, the hypergeometric test was used to evaluate the significance of overlap k between the cluster and GO-BP category [36,37]. All N genes on a microarray were used as reference. To ensure specificity of annotation within a gene cluster, functional categories containing <5 or >1000 genes were removed.

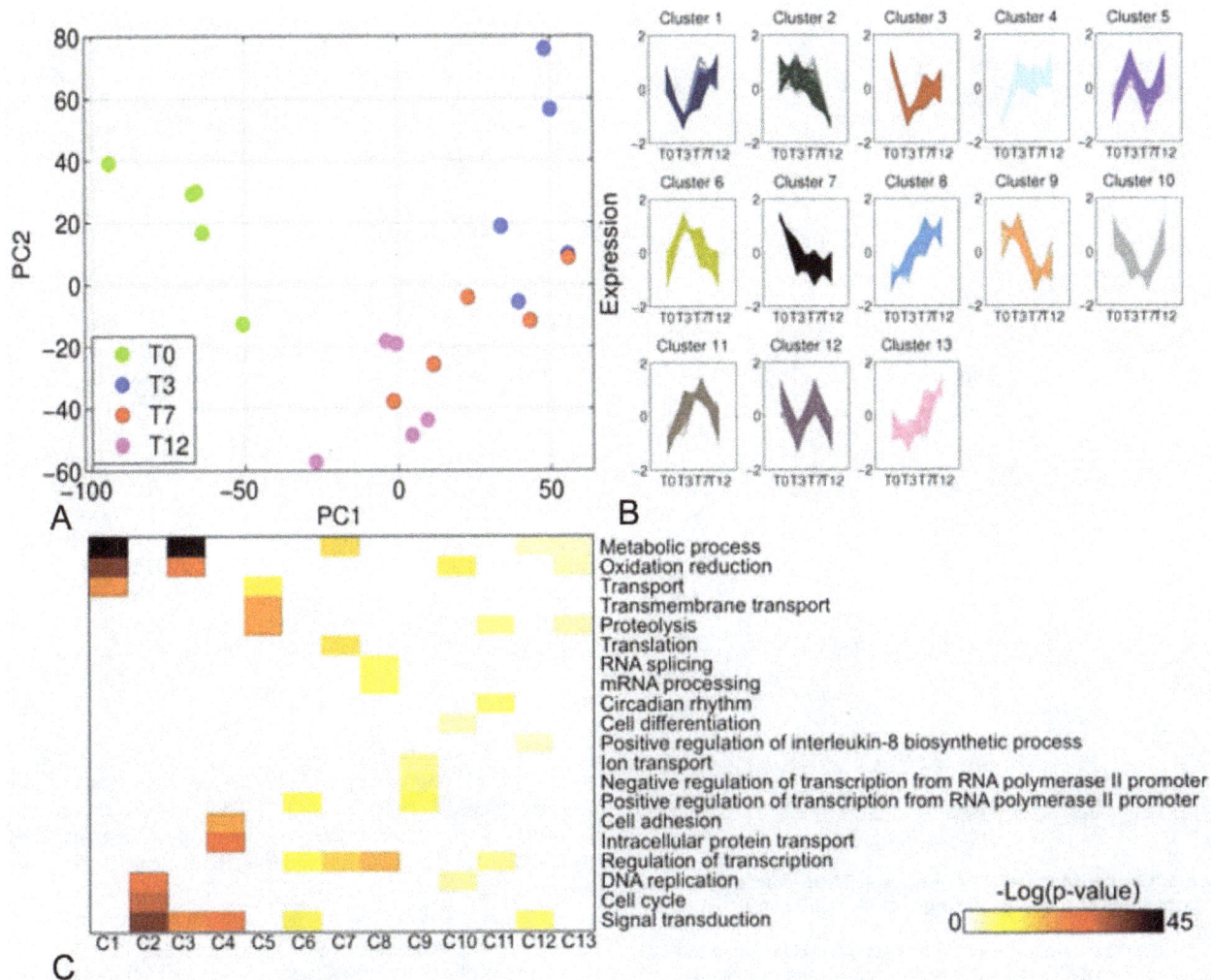

Figure 5. Differential expression analysis of the TNBS transcriptome. (A) Scatter plot of the Principal Component Analysis of 8316 genes in response to TNBS. (B) Expression profiles of genes assigned to the 13 clusters of similar expression (see Table S1). Only differentially expressed genes are included. (C) Heat map visualizing functional enrichment of the 13 clusters for over-represented Gene Ontology Biological Process terms. Darker shades represent a greater degree of enrichment.

Comparison of TNBS to IBD transcriptomes

Concordance between TNBS-colitis and IBD transcriptomes was assessed at the level of individual gene loci as well as at the level of KEGG [38] and Reactome pathways [39]. To standardize comparisons between rat and human data, rat gene Ensembl IDs were mapped to respective human orthologs. In total, 6142 genes were considered. TNBS-colitis FCs were calculated by comparing gene expression profiles at T3, T7, and T12 to T0. Similarly, IBD FCs were computed by comparing CD and UC samples to normal (N) tissue. At the level of single gene loci, concordance tests were carried out by correlating FCs of the TNBS-colitis and IBD transcriptomes. Gene expression profiles with Student's t-test $p < 0.05$ and absolute log2 FC ≥ 1.1 were considered differentially regulated.

To assess concordance at the level of biological pathways, gene expression FCs in TNBS-colitis and IBD transcriptomes were mapped to respective Reactome and KEGG pathways. To ensure that only well-characterized cascades were studied, pathways with fewer than 5 genes were excluded. Subsequently, a pathway-level FC was computed by averaging FCs of all genes that mapped to a

specific pathway. Finally, TNBS-colitis and IBD pathway level FCs were correlated.

For all comparisons, Spearman's rho was used to estimate correlations between TNBS-colitis and IBD FCs. Respective p-values were computed for testing the hypothesis of no correlation against the alternative that there is a nonzero correlation and $p < 0.05$ was called statistically significant. Analysis was performed using the Statistics toolbox for Matlab (2009a, The MathWorks, Natick, MA, USA).

Candidate genes

Interleukin 1 alpha (IL-1α) and interleukin 1 beta (IL-1β) were chosen as general markers of inflammation. TLR2 and TLR4 were considered markers of bacterial regulation of inflammatory responses. In addition, based on the degree of regulation and statistical significance, genes encoding the peroxisome proliferator-activated receptor gamma (PPARγ) and the endogenous prion protein (PRNP [PrP^c]) were further evaluated.

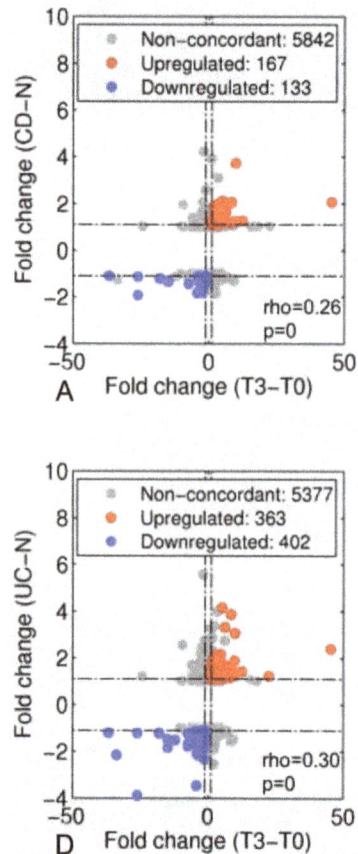

Figure 6. Concordance analysis between TNBS-colitis and IBD transcriptomes at the level of single gene loci. *T3 vs. T0, T7 vs. T0 and T12 vs. T0 compared to CD vs. normal* (top) *and UC vs. normal* (bottom). (A–F) Scatterplots of FCs in rat data (x-axis) compared to FCs in the human data (y-axis). Rho values correspond to Spearman correlation coefficients with p-values representing the level of significance of the correlation. Concordant up- and down-regulated genes are represented as red and blue circles respectively. Non-concordant genes are shown as grey circles. Numbers in the legend correspond to the total number of genes assigned to each category. B, C, E and F are only shown in the supplemental section (Figure S1).

Histological evaluation

Endoscopic biopsies and whole colon specimens were fixed in 4% buffered formaldehyde, placed in standard plastic briquettes for tissue specimens and processed via standard protocols (dehydration, clearing and paraffinization overnight). Sections from each block were cut in 4 µm thickness and stained with hematoxylin-eosin. The slides were examined by a surgical pathologist (ISN) and the degree and type of inflammation, ulceration and degree of regeneration/architectural distortion was assessed.

In situ hybridization

In situ hybridization (ISH) on endoscopic biopsies was performed using RNA-probes for the following genes: IL-1α (NM_017019), IL-1β (NM_031512), TLR2 (NM_198769), TLR4 (NM_019178), PPARγ (NM_001145367) and PRNP (NM_012631) with the RNAscope® 2.0 assay kit (Advanced Cell Diagnostics Inc., Hayward CA, USA.), according to the manufacturer's protocol. Briefly, endoscopic biopsies were fixed in 4% buffered formaldehyde for five days and embedded in paraffin.

Sections from each block were cut in 4 µm thickness and baked 1 hr at 60°C prior to use. After de-paraffinization and dehydration, the biopsies were air dried and treated with peroxidase blocker before gentle boiling in a pretreat solution for 15 min. Then, protease was applied for 30 min at 40°C. After pretreatment steps, the target probe was applied and hybridized for 2 hr at 40°C. Thereafter, the amplification steps including application of a horseradish peroxidase (HRP)-linked labeling probe were performed prior to DAB-visualization.

PCR

RNA from 18 biopsies (no residual RNA was available from rat 2 and 4 at T3 and T7, respectively), was converted to cDNA with High Capacity RNA-to-cDNA Kit (Applied Biosystems, Foster City, CA, USA) according to the manufacturer's manual. PCR was performed using TaqMan® Array Plates (Life Technologies™, Carlsbad, CA, USA) on a Step One Plus™ Real Time PCR System. Genes with the largest FC alteration in the microarray data, serine peptidase inhibitor of the Kazal type 4 (SPINK4), adenosine deaminase (ADA), and fatty acid binding protein (FABP) 1 were analyzed. Actin beta (ACTB) was used as housekeeping gene. For each time point relative differential expression was calculated using the ddCT method followed by two-tailed paired t-test, T0 served as control.

Results

Optimization of the TNBS protocol

In order to standardize the TNBS-protocol to achieve a moderate colitis, we initially instilled TNBS in two doses (17.5 and 22.5 mg) at a fixed concentration of 60 mg/ml. The inflammation was severe in seven out of 16 rats in both treatment groups. MEICS-score ranged from 8–11 (9.9 ± 0.9) at T7 (Figure 1). The study had to be terminated prematurely for animal welfare reasons.

The protocol was adjusted and TNBS was administered in different concentrations and a fixed volume of 0.7 ml. TNBS concentrations of 10 mg/ml and 15 mg/ml resulted in only slight endoscopic and histologic inflammation. Mucosal erythema and edema and histologic submucosal inflammation without ulcerations were seen at a TNBS concentration of 20 mg/ml. TNBS at 25–40 mg/ml resulted in mucosal edema and friability. Histologic examination revealed ulcerations and submucosal inflammation. TNBS 30 mg/ml induced a moderate inflammation with MEICS-score 7 and 5 at day 3 and day 7, respectively. The highest TNBS concentration (45 mg/ml) induced severe colitis with general weakening and the rat was therefore euthanized at day 7 (Figure 2).

The protocol optimization demonstrated that 0.7 ml of TNBS (30 mg/ml) induced a moderate colitis that lasted at least 12 days and declined between T7 and T12. However, a small fraction of TNBS tended to leak from the rectum immediately after instillation. The total volume was therefore reduced to 0.6 ml for the subsequent study.

Characterization of moderate TNBS-colitis

Five animals treated with TNBS 30 mg/ml (0.6 ml) developed moderate colitis from the splenic flexure down to the recto-sigmoid junction. The MEICS-score peaked at T3 (5.6 ± 0.9, T3 vs. T12, $p = 0.02$) and T7 (5.0 ± 1.2, T7 vs. T12, $p = 0.11$) (Figure 3A and B). An acute weight loss occurred at T3 (196.7 ± 14.3 g at T0 versus 187.6 ± 17.3 g at T3, mean weight loss 9.3 g, 4.7%, $p = 0.003$). The animal weights recovered to 200.4 ± 24.7 g and 209.4 ± 19.2 g at T7 and T12, respectively. Loose and bloody stools were noticed in two rats. Signs of cryptitis and architectural

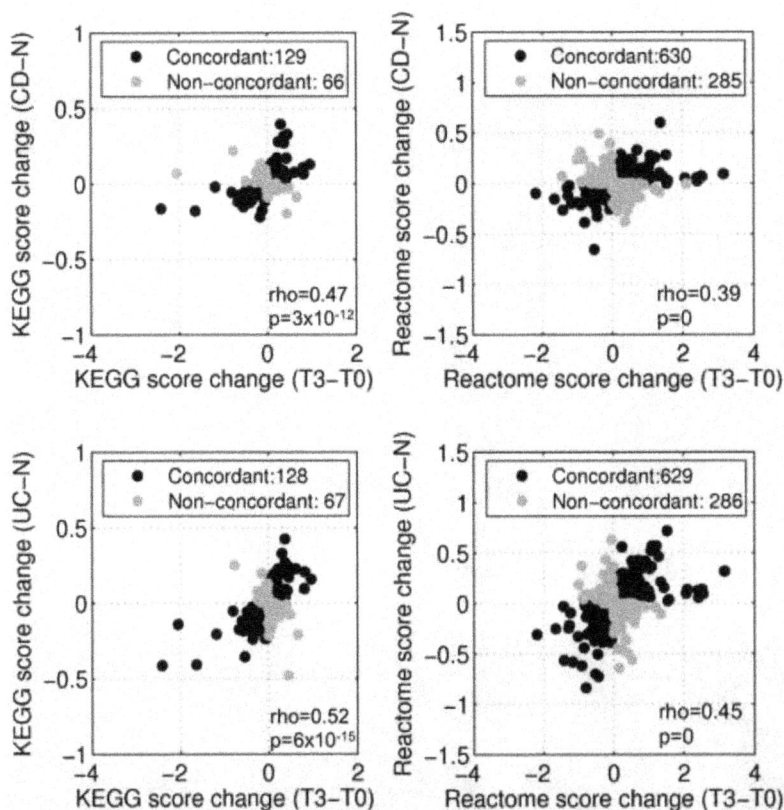

Figure 7. Concordance analysis between TNBS-colitis and IBD transcriptomes at the level of biological pathways. *T3 vs. T0* compared to *CD vs. normal* (top) *and UC vs. normal* (bottom). Left, scatter plots of pathway activity scores of KEGG pathways in TNBS and IBD samples. Right, scatter plots of pathway activity scores of Reactome pathways in TNBS and IBD samples. Rho values correspond to Spearman correlation coefficients with *p*-values representing the level of significance of the correlation. Numbers in the legend correspond to the total number of pathways assigned to each category. A similar figure (Figure S2) for concordant analysis of *T7 vs. T0* and *T12 vs. T0*, compared to *CD vs. normal* and *UC vs. normal* is shown in the supplementary section (KEGG and Reactome score change at the top and bottom, for T7 vs. T0 and T12 vs. T0, respectively).

distortion were seen in endoscopic biopsies, whereas histologic examination of whole colon specimens at T12 demonstrated regenerative changes, ulcerations and transmural inflammation (Figure 4A and B).

Temporal TNBS-colitis gene expression analysis

Gene expression profiling of biopsies collected at time-points T0, T3, T7 and T12 was undertaken. After microarray preprocessing, expression profiles of 8316 genes were reduced to two Principal Components (PCs) to visualize differences in gene expression due to TNBS-induced inflammation (Figure 5A). Colitis induction resulted in distinct gene expression profiles while inter-individual temporal changes due to TNBS were not obvious.

To identify genes with sustained differential expression across all time points, the BETR algorithm was used. Genes with differential expression probabilities >0.99 were called significant. This analysis returned 3414 significantly regulated genes, which were subsequently clustered using the AP algorithm (Figure 5B). Significantly regulated genes were allocated to 13 clusters, with 588 and 63 genes assigned to the largest and smallest clusters, respectively. The full list of gene cluster assignments can be accessed in supplementary Table S1. Functional cluster enrichment for over-represented GO-BP terms identified processes such as *Oxidation reduction* (Clusters 1 and 3), *Cell cycle* (Cluster 2) and *Cell adhesion* (Cluster 4) (Figure 5C).

Comparison of the TNBS and IBD transcriptomes

To quantitate the similarity between the TNBS and IBD transcriptomes, differentially expressed genes at T3, T7 and T12 were compared to differentially expressed genes in CD and UC. Overall, 6142 rat genes could be mapped to human orthologs. The highest concordance was observed between CD and T3 (rho = 0.26, p = 0; $n = 300$ significantly regulated concordant genes) (Figure 6A). Similarly, the most concordance in differential expression was found between UC and T3 (rho = 0.30, p = 0; $n = 765$ significantly regulated concordant genes) (Figure 6D). Up-regulated genes in both TNBS-colitis and human IBD included ADA, PrP^c, and IL-1α, while down-regulated genes consisted of aldehyde dehydrogenase 1 family, member A1 (ALDH1A1), and PPARγ. A full list of comparable gene changes in TNBS–colitis compared to CD and UC is available as supplementary Table S2.

As disruption in single gene expression can affect behavior of molecular pathways [40], concordance between the TNBS model and IBD was also assessed at the level of biological pathways. To ensure that results reflected a real phenomenon rather than a database-specific result, the FCs in gene expression were mapped to their respective identifiers in the KEGG ($n = 195$ pathways) and Reactome ($n = 915$ pathways) pathway databases. The highest concordance between CD and TNBS-colitis was observed at T3 (KEGG: Rho = 0.47, p = 3×10^{-12}, Reactome: Rho = 0.39, p = 0) (Figure 7). Concordant pathways included Reactome pathways

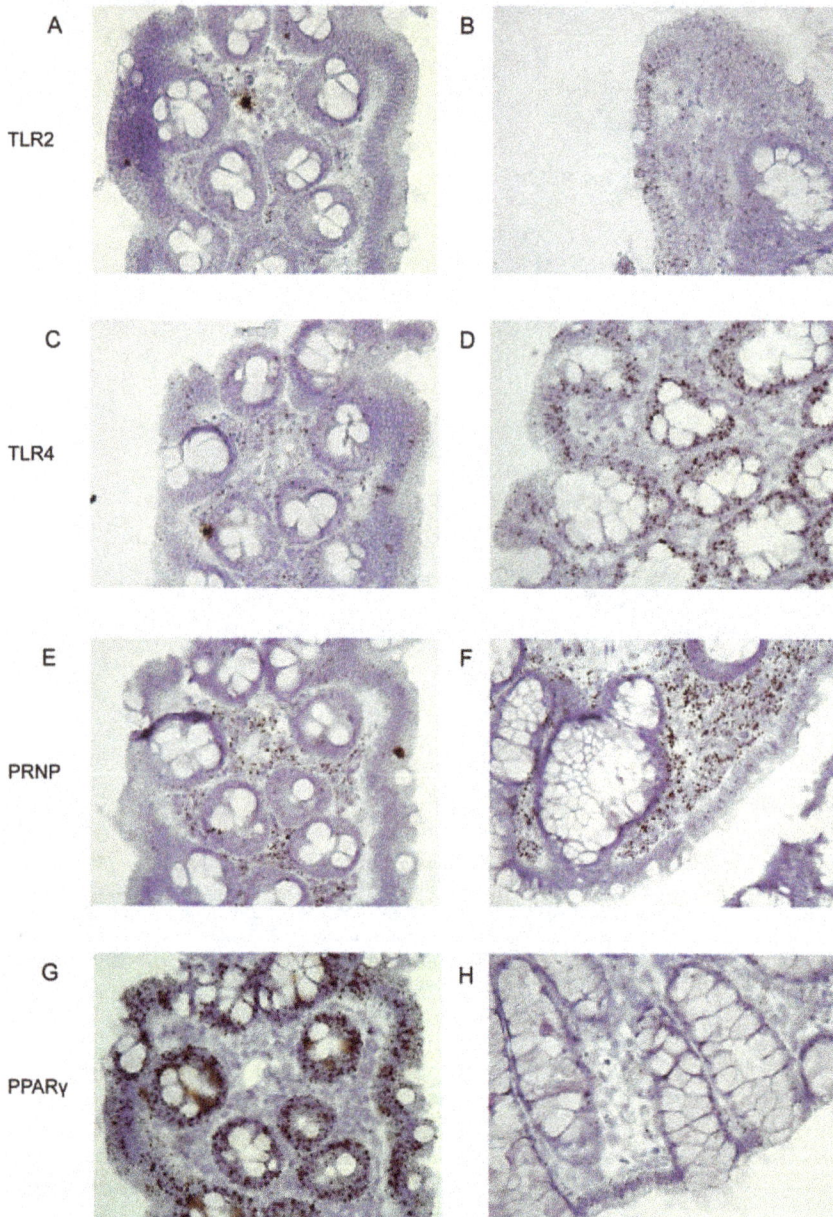

Figure 8. *In situ* **hybridization (ISH) of significantly regulated genes in TNBS colitis mucosal biopsies.** (A and C) The expression of TLR2 and TLR4 is scattered in the epithelium and submucosal immune cells at T0. (B and D) Increased TLR2 and TLR4 expression was noted in the epithelium at T7. (E) PRNP expression in submucosal immune cells at T0. (F) Intense PRNP expressing cells were evident in the submucosa at T12 and also to some degree in the epithelium. (G) Intense clusters of PPARγ expression in epithelial cells at T0. (H) At T12, the expression is almost abolished. Objective x40 in all pictures.

such as *Apoptosis*, *Cell junction organization*, *Interleukin-1 processing*; non-concordant pathways included *GABA-A receptor activation*, *Extrinsic pathways for apoptosis* and *Recycling of bile acids and salts*. Similarly, the most concordance was noted between UC and T3 (KEGG: rho = 0.52, p = 6×10^{-15}, Reactome: rho = 0.45, p = 0) (Figure 7). For example, concordant Reactome pathways included *Nuclear receptor transcription pathway*, *TNF signaling*, and *VEGF ligand-receptor interactions*, while non-concordant Reactome pathways included *Apoptotic execution phase* and *TRAIL signaling*. The full list of regulated pathways in TNBS and IBD is accessible through supplementary Table S3.

In situ hybridization (ISH) of target genes in TNBS-colitis

Markers of mucosal inflammation and selected microarray targets were analyzed using ISH. These included inflammatory cytokines (IL-1α and IL-1β) and TLRs (TLR2 and TLR4), as well as the computationally identified genes PPARγ and PRNP.

An overall increase in gene expression of IL-1α and IL-1β was evident in submucosal inflammatory infiltrates at T3-T12. However, changes in expression varied with the degree of inflammation in individual animals. Colitis induction resulted in increased expression of TLR2 and TLR4 in epithelial cells (Figure 8A, B, C and D). PRNP expression was increased both in submucosal inflammatory cells and to some degree also in

Table 1. P-values and FCs for the target genes at every time point.

Gene	T3		T7		T12	
	FC	P-value	FC	P-value	FC	P-value
IL-1α	8.63	0.008	3.38	0.091	1.58	0.209
IL-1β	6.16	0.063	4.74	0.047	1.94	0.071
TLR2	5.03	0.005	3.46	0.029	1.75	0.027
TLR4	2.09	<0.001	1.36	0.001	1.67	0.005
PRNP	2.13	0.005	2.11	0.005	1.89	0.016
PPARγ	−4.14	<0.001	−3.05	<0.001	−4.63	<0.001

epithelial cells (Figure 8F), while a substantial down-regulation of PPARγ was evident in the epithelium after induction of colitis (Figure 8H). The *in situ* results correlated well with the differential expression noted in the microarray, IL-1α (FC at T3 = 8.6, $p = 0.008$), IL-1β (FC at T7 = 4.7, $p = 0.047$), TLR2 (FC at T3 = 5.03, $p = 0.005$), TLR4 (FC at T3 = 2.09, $p<0.001$), PPARγ (FC at T12 = −4.6, $p<0.001$), and PRNP (FC at T3 = 2.1, $p = 0.005$). P-values and FCs for the target genes at every time point are provided in Table 1.

PCR validation of selected genes

PCR was performed for the following genes: SPINK4, ADA, and FABP1. Mean FCs for SPINK4 were 93.26 for T3 vs. T0, 4.02 for T7 vs. T0 and 1.76 for T12 vs. T0. The corresponding FCs for ADA were 11.93, 16.87 and 13.20 and for FABP1 −199.96, −105.60 and −170.62 which were in accordance with the microarray results (Figure 9).

Discussion

TNBS-colitis is widely used as a model for IBD. However, its resemblance to human disease has not been thoroughly explored. TNBS-colitis in rats was originally described as a model for induction of *long lasting inflammation and ulceration of the rat colon* [12], and the reproducibility was emphasized. The reproducibility and duration/chronicity of inflammation has, however, been subject to debate [14,41]. In the current study, we standardized the protocol for induction of moderate TNBS-colitis in Sprague Dawley rats and evaluated temporal changes in gene expression profiles and biological pathways after the induction of colitis. Importantly, we quantitatively assessed concordance of the TNBS-colitis and IBD transcriptomes.

Doses and concentrations of TNBS used in previous studies differ markedly and no standardized protocol has been generally developed [14,17–20]. We therefore aimed to optimize the method to achieve a reproducible moderate colitis. High concentrations of TNBS (60 mg/ml), administered in small volumes (0.29 and 0.38 ml) induced a localized severe inflammation resulting in deep colonic ulcerations, coprostasis, stenoses and ileus. Milder inflammation and more wide spread inflammation was achieved with lower TNBS concentrations in a larger total volume. A TNBS concentration of 30 mg/ml in a total volume of 0.6 ml resulted in a moderate inflammation involving most of the left colon. However, despite the use of a standardized protocol, a slight inter-individual dissimilarity in the extension and degree of inflammation was seen, reflected by variation in MEICS-score and expression of the pro-inflammatory cytokines IL-1α and IL-1β.

Natural inter-individual variation and factors like anal leakage of TNBS and incomplete bowel emptying prior to the instillation are likely contributors to these observations. To minimize these effects, fecal pellets in the rectum should be eliminated prior to TNBS-instillation.

TNBS induces a hapten-mediated toxic inflammation, and consequently has unavoidable differences compared to IBD [42]. In addition to chemical inflammation, the intestinal microbiota is important in the development of TNBS-colitis [43]. Granulomas have been described in approximately 50% of rats with TNBS-colitis [12]. However, no granulomas were seen in the current study. This may reflect disparities in the microbiota seen in different animal housing facilities.

Endoscopic monitoring of TNBS-colitis with visual assessment has been described. However, in those studies no biopsies were obtained [44,45]. In another study, transcriptomic analysis of TNBS-colitis was performed using whole colon specimens from animals sacrificed at different time points [21]. Consequently, temporal changes in gene expression in individual rats during colitis development has not been investigated. Furthermore, a comparison with a human IBD transcriptome has not been conducted. Our approach thus allows investigators to follow the development of colitis in individual animals visually, and collect biopsies for histologic evaluation and genetic analyses. Endoscopy three days after TNBS instillation allowed for a baseline evaluation of the inflammation. Rats with comparable colitis could therefore be identified prior to study inclusion. A similar approach has been described using MRI to grade the inflammation [14]. In addition, as the animals serve as their own controls it reduces the overall study number.

Computational analysis of longitudinal gene expression profiles in the TNBS-colitis model in this study revealed alterations such as a down-regulation of metabolism and up-regulation of tissue remodeling genes. This suggests that mucosal cells may be deprived of adequate energy sources as well as exposed to pro-fibrotic signaling cascades during the inflammatory response. Similar changes have been reported in IBD patients [46,47] and models of experimental colitis [21]. Additionally, we noted down-regulation of processes including DNA replication and cell cycle, which involved genes such as caspase 1 and 3 (Casp1/3). Casp1 is an enzyme that proteolytically cleaves precursor forms of the inflammatory cytokines IL-1β and IL-18, while Casp3 proteolytically inactivates IL-33, which is a member of the IL-1 superfamily [48]. Interestingly, Casp$^{-/-}$ mice are more susceptible to inflammation-induced tumorigenesis in the colon [49], while IL-33 was recently found to be increased in ulcerative colitis [50,51]. Additionally, previous experimental models have demonstrated that Casp$^{-/-}$ mice are also more susceptible to infections [52] and are more sensitive to DSS-colitis [53]. Taken together, the temporal analysis of TNBS-colitis gene expression profiles revealed biologically relevant changes in key IBD pathways, suggesting that the transcriptome dataset in this study is a useful resource for further biological discovery in this animal model.

Contributions of model organisms to our understanding of generalizable fundamental processes are irrefutable. However, little work has been done to quantitatively assess the concordance between TNBS-colitis and IBD transcriptomes. In our analyses, we noted a divergence between rat and human transcriptomes at the level of single gene loci with only 233–765 (3.8–12.5%) concordant gene loci out of 6142 analyzed. However, several key IBD genes were similarly regulated in the TNBS model and IBD. Genes involved in fibrogenesis and stricture formation [54,55], including collagen type I alpha (COL1A1), matrix metallopeptidase 3 (MMP3) and TIMP metallopeptidase inhibitor 1 and 2

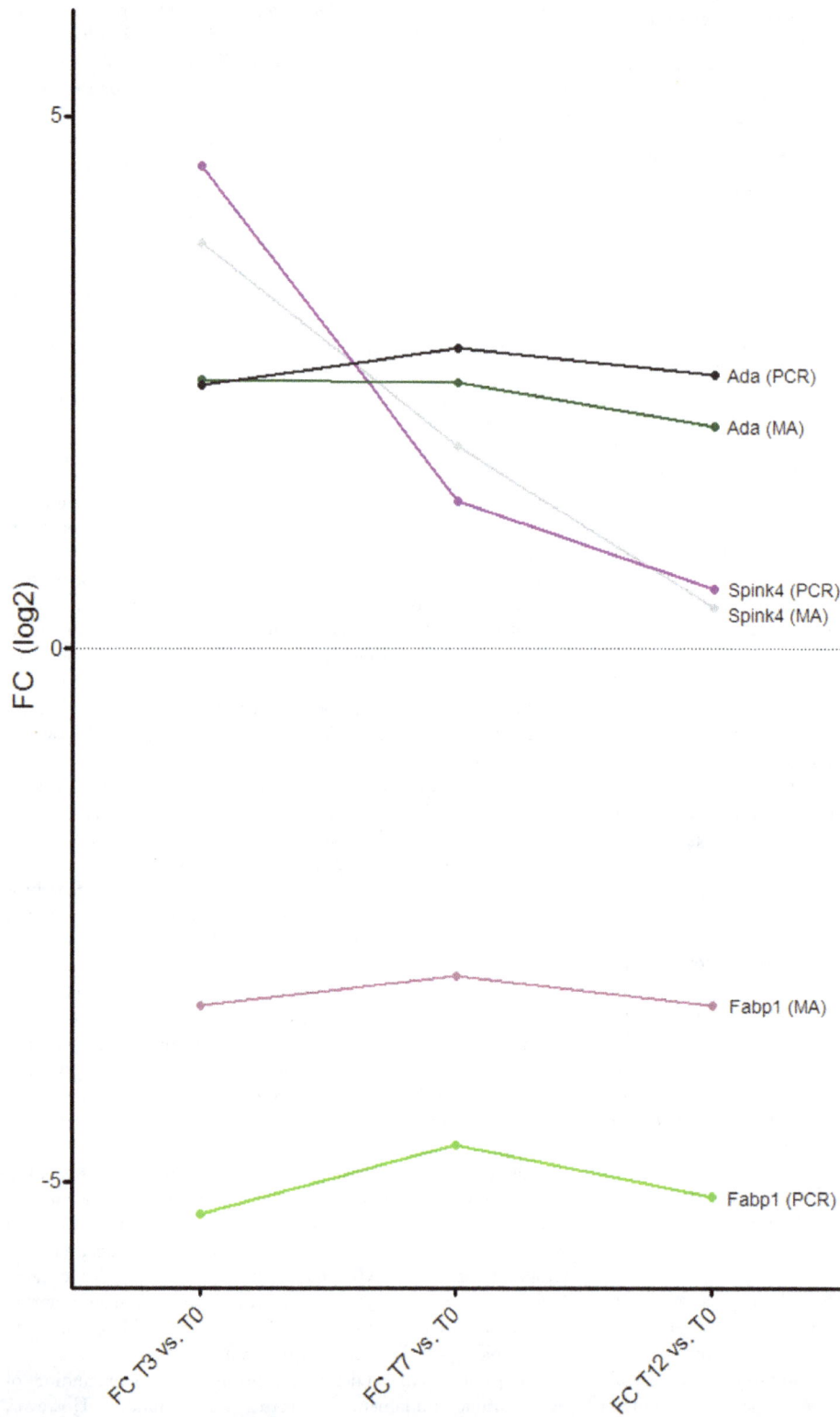

Figure 9. Graph displaying confirmatory PCR. Graph displaying FC for *T3 vs. T0*, *T7 vs. T0* and *T12 vs. T0* for SPINK4, ADA and FABP1 for both microarray (MA) and confirmatory PCR. FC is log2 transformed for illustrative purposes. All p-values are highly significant.

(TIMP1 and TIMP2) are examples thereof. These findings are consistent with other comparative assessments of human disease and animal models [56,57]. Our group has shown that the REG family proteins and CXCL10 are up-regulated in IBD [58,59].

The REG proteins probably play a role in induction of cellular proliferation and induction of apoptosis, thus being of importance for tissue repair and growth. CXCL10 seems to be released from epithelial cells acting as a ligand on CXCLR3+ T-lymphocytes, contributing to the inflammatory response in IBD. In contrast to these results, both REGIV and CXCL10 were down-regulated in the TNBS-model. It is possible that the duration of the TNBS-study was too short to detect a delayed activation of REGIV, however the discrepancy might also reflect the difference between IBD and TNBS-colitis. The discrepancy in regulation of CXCL10 also demonstrates the dissimilarity between human disease and TNBS-colitis. Other chemokines like CXCL1 and CXCL2, have previously been found up-regulated in TNBS-colitis [21] and were up-regulated in our data. We also found CXCL16 to be 1.5 fold elevated at T3. CXCL16 has a role in phagocytosis, mucosal defense and Th1-mediated inflammation, and has been implicated in the pathogenesis of IBD [60–62].

Despite differences at the level of single gene loci, considerably higher homology was noted between TNBS-colitis and IBD at the level of biological pathways. For KEGG-pathways 114–134 (58.5–68.7%) of 195 pathways, while for the Reactome 515–631 (56.3–69.0%) of 915 pathways were concordant. This result was expected, since previous work demonstrates that pathway level analysis is able to uncover subtle biological variability, which may not be captured by gene expression alone [63]. Concordant pathways included *Cell junction organization, Interleukin-1 processing,* and *Dysregulation of fatty acid metabolism.* These pathways represent key elements of IBD pathogenesis. For example, the ability to organize tight junctions, adherent junctions and desmosomes are important protective mechanisms that prevent microorganism invasion, mucosal damage and inflammation [64]. Similarly, aberrant regulation of IL-1α and IL-1β is a contributing mechanism in persistent inflammation in IBD [65,66], while alterations in the expression of genes involved in fatty acid metabolism may contribute to the pathophysiology of ulcerative colitis [46].

Among non-concordant pathways, we identified *TRAIL signaling* as being different between the rat model and IBD. This signaling pathway mediates apoptosis and might be of importance for T-cell death as a therapeutic target in IBD [67].

Overall, these concordance analyses suggests that TNBS-colitis is an appropriate IBD model for the study of specific biological processes such as *Cell junction organization* and *Fatty acid metabolism,* while caution needs to be exercised when analysis is based on a single gene locus.

Other chemically induced colitis models exist. Colitis induced through addition of the polysaccharide dextran sodium sulfate (DSS) in the drinking water or rectal instillation of oxazolone are examples thereof [68]. DSS and TNBS have clinical similarities including bloody diarrhea and weight loss. However, inflammation in DDS seems to be caused by hyperosmotic damage and is confined to the mucosa and lamina propria, in contrast to the TNBS-model where inflammation is hapten-mediated and transmural [69]. Additionally germ free mice develop a lethal colitis when exposed to DSS [70], while a sterile colon seems to be protective against TNBS-colitis [43]. A comparison of genetic expression between DSS, TNBS and CD45RB transfer colitis mice showed that DSS and TNBS had 6 and 18 concordantly up- and down-regulated genes [71]. Another study found 152 and 22 concordantly up- and down-regulated genes between mice with DSS-colitis and UC from a total of 1609 differentially expressed genes [72]. In an analysis of cytokine patterns, closer resemblance was indicated between DSS-colitis and UC, while TNBS-colitis seemed closer to CD [73]. Oxazolone is another example of a rectally administered substance that causes a hapten-mediated colitis in the distal part of the colon with clinically similar symptoms as TNBS-colitis [68,74]. Oxazolon-induced colitis is

mainly driven by Th2 cytokines, while TNBS-colitis is Th1- and Th17-mediated [11,73,74].

Several gene knockout models in mice have been used to study possible pathogenetic mechanisms in IBD. Deletion of the regulatory sequence consisting of adenosine-uracil multimers (AU-rich elements [ARE]) in the 3′-untranslated region of cytokine encoding transcripts in mice (TNF-$^{\Delta ARE/+}$), results in mice with increased transcription of TNF-α; after lipopolysaccharide (LPS)-stimulation these mice develop terminal ileitis and inflammatory arthritis [68,75]. IL-10 knockout mice develop inflammation, mainly localized to the colon [76]. The IL-10 knockout model has highlighted the importance of IL-10 as an anti-inflammatory cytokine. IL-10 is increased in the serum of recovering IBD-patients [77]. IL-10 was not significantly regulated in our TNBS-model which might suggest that IL-10 does not participate in the healing of TNBS colitis.

We sought to validate key changes in the TNBS-colitis transcriptome using ISH. Genes with known roles and of potential importance in IBD were evaluated, namely IL-1α, IL-1β, TLR2, TLR4, PPARγ and PRNP. Gene expression profiling revealed that IL-1α and IL-1β were significantly up-regulated at T3 and T7, compared to T0, while TLR2, TLR4 and PRNP were significantly up-regulated at every time point (T3, T7 and T12) compared to T0. PPARγ was significantly down-regulated at every time point.

ISH confirmed that both IL-1α and IL-1β were weakly expressed in colonic epithelial cells while high expression was found in leukocytes and inflammatory infiltrates. Mediation of inflammation by IL-1α and IL-1β is balanced or counteracted via the IL-1 receptor antagonist (IL-1ra), which was significantly up-regulated at every time point. It has previously been shown in experimental colitis that neutralization of IL-1ra leads to more severe inflammation [78]. In concordance with the TNBS-colitis model, both IL-1α and IL-1β are elevated in IBD. An imbalance between these IL-1s and IL-1ra might contribute to the pathogenesis in IBD [65,79].

The increased TLR2 and TLR4 expression seen in the transcriptome analysis was confirmed by ISH with dense staining in epithelial cells at the luminal surface and in the crypt epithelium. Hitherto, 10 TLRs have been described in humans [6]. TLR1, TLR2, TLR4, TLR5, TLR6, and TLR9 all recognize bacterial products or bacterial components [80]. While TLR2 and TLR4 were up-regulated, TLR5 was significantly down-regulated in our TNBS-colitis model. Intestinal homeostasis between tolerance to intestinal microflora and activation of an inflammatory response appears to be dependent on the type of TLR involved and whether basolateral or apical TLRs are activated [81]. Similar to the TNBS-colitis model, activation of both TLR2 and TLR4 is seen in IBD [5,82,83]. Probiotic treatment also activates TLR2, TLR4 and TLR9 and modulates cytokine production and secretion [84]. Interestingly, IL-10 and TLR4 double knockout mice have an accelerated colitis development compared to IL-10 and TLR9 double knockout and IL-10 single knockout which do not develop colitis [85]. TLR2 and TLR4 up-regulation in epithelial cells in this TNBS-colitis model as well as the cytokine up-regulation indicate bacterial activation of mucosal defense and inflammation [5]. Clearly, the mechanisms of TLR-response are complicated. The mechanisms for the balance of an adequate immune response and adaption of the innate immune system, on one hand, and an inadequate immune response, on the other hand, can partly be explained by tolerance development and polarization differences in TLR-receptor distribution [86,87].

PRNP (PrP^c) mRNA was significantly up-regulated in TNBS-colitis. This was verified by ISH which showed expression in submucosal immune cells and some expression in epithelial cells in animals not yet exposed to TNBS, but expression was more pronounced after colitis induction both in the submucosal immune cells and within the epithelium. PrP^c is expressed in several tissues, including neural tissue, gut-associated lymphoid tissue, enteroendocrine cells and enterocytes [28,88]. Its function is not well known. Expression of PrP^c in the host is thought to be necessary for the propagation and transmission of prion infection [28]. In addition, both pro- and anti-inflammatory roles have been suggested. Reduced inflammatory infiltration has been seen in PrP^c-deficient mice upon stimulation with TLR2 and TLR4 ligands [26]. In contrast, PrP^c over-expressing mice are resistant to colitis induction with DSS while PrP^c deficient mice had significantly higher levels of inflammatory cytokines compared to DSS-treated wild type mice [29]. Increased intestinal barrier permeability has been demonstrated in PrP^c-deficient mice, further supporting a protecting role for PrP^c [89] in colitis and IBD.

PPARγ is one of three identified isoforms of peroxisome proliferator-activated receptors (PPARs) and is expressed in several tissues; expression is high in the colonic epithelial cells [90,91]. It is thought to have an important role in modulation of inflammation. PPARγ suppresses inflammatory cytokines like TNFα, interleukin-6 (IL-6) and IL-1β [24] and maintains defensin production [25]. Gene expression analysis revealed down-regulation of PPARγ after colitis induction. In endoscopic biopsies evaluated by ISH, a high basal expression of PPARγ in non-inflamed colonic epithelium, while a considerable down-regulation in inflamed colon epithelium was identified. This was accompanied by down-regulation of FABP1. FABP1 transcription, in the microarray was confirmed by PCR. The intracellular level of FABP1 positively regulates PPARγ and the two proteins also have a direct protein-protein interaction [92]. Regulation of FABPs is seen in IBD [46], PPARγ is down-regulated in UC [93] and gene polymorphisms of PPARγ have been implicated in the pathogenesis of CD [42,94]. PPARγ-agonists have been shown to ameliorate TNBS-induced colitis [95,96] and the PPARγ ligand *rosiglitazone* has shown efficacy in mild to moderately active IBD [97]. PPARγ might also inhibit tumor growth in colorectal cancer [98]. Alternatively, FABP1 has been suggested as a biomarker of CD because a 10-fold up-regulation was found in one study [99]. Our findings, in contrast, are consistent with loss of PPARγ-mediated anti-inflammatory effects. This supports a potentially important function for PPARγ in the regulation of colonic inflammation and indicates that FABPs could also be a possible target for therapy.

Among the 20 genes with highest FC at all time points were SPINK4; lipopolysaccharide binding protein (LBP), ADA and RETNLB. PCR validation was performed for SPINK4 and ADA. SPINK4 has recently been identified as a risk locus for UC [100] and increased expression is seen in untreated celiac disease [101]. LBP transfers LPS to the LPS-signaling receptor complex (which also contains TLR4), promotes innate immunity against gram negative bacteria, and may serve as a marker of disease activity in CD [102]. ADA deactivates adenosine and thus diminishes the

potentially protective effects of adenosine in mucosal inflammation and hypoxia. A beneficial effect after inhibition of ADA has been demonstrated in experimental colitis [103,104]. RETNLB had a FC of 470 and 253 at T7 and T12, respectively. RETNLB-deficiency in mice increases intestinal permeability and RETNLB seems important to maintain intestinal homeostasis [105].

In conclusion, endoscopy with biopsies in TNBS-colitis models is useful to visually follow temporal changes of inflammation and obtain tissue for histologic and gene expression measurements. TLR and interleukin activation, PPARγ-inhibition and regulation of PRNP (PrP^c), occurs in both TNBS-colitis and IBD. TNBS-colitis is an appropriate IBD-model to study specific biological processes like *TNF signaling*, *Cell junction organization*, and *Interleukin-1 processing*. We conclude that the TNBS-model may be suitable for studying agents targeting these pathways and provide translational information for clinical studies.

Supporting Information

Figure S1 Concordance analysis between TNBS-colitis and IBD transcriptomes at the level of single gene loci. See Figure 6.

Figure S2 Concordance analysis between TNBS-colitis and IBD transcriptomes at the level of biological pathways. See Figure 7.

Table S1 Genes identified with Ensemble IDs, Gene Symbols and Gene Names and their respective cluster assignments (1–13) with involved GO-BPs and KEGG Pathways.

Table S2 Concordant genes identified with Ensemble IDs, Gene Symbols and Gene Names with corresponding FC, *p*-value and False Discovery Rate (FDR) for TNBS, CD and UC, respectively.

Table S3 Homologous pathways (KEGG, Sheet 1) and (Reactome, Sheet 2) in TNBS-colitis compared to CD and UC for different time points of TNBS-colitis (T3, T7 and T12).

Acknowledgments

We want to thank Bjørn Munkvold for laboratory assistance and the staff at the animal facility for their helpfulness and good animal care.

Author Contributions

Conceived and designed the experiments: BG ØB MWF RM. Performed the experiments: ØB MWF BG AvBG RTMZ. Analyzed the data: ØB BG ID AvBG AF AS ISN MK. Contributed reagents/materials/analysis tools: ØB BG ID AvBG AF AS RM. Wrote the paper: ØB MWF ID AvBG AS ISN MK BG.

References

1. Danese S, Fiocchi C (2011) Ulcerative colitis. N Engl J Med 365: 1713–1725.

2. Hammer HF (2011) Gut microbiota and inflammatory bowel disease. Dig Dis 29: 550–553.

3. McGuckin MA, Eri R, Simms LA, Florin TH, Radford-Smith G (2009) Intestinal barrier dysfunction in inflammatory bowel diseases. Inflamm Bowel Dis 15: 100–113.

4. Kleessen B, Kroesen AJ, Buhr HJ, Blaut M (2002) Mucosal and invading bacteria in patients with inflammatory bowel disease compared with controls. Scand J Gastroenterol 37: 1034–1041.

5. Cario E, Podolsky DK (2000) Differential alteration in intestinal epithelial cell expression of toll-like receptor 3 (TLR3) and TLR4 in inflammatory bowel disease. Infect Immun 68: 7010–7017.

6. Cario E (2010) Toll-like receptors in inflammatory bowel diseases: a decade later. Inflamm Bowel Dis 16: 1583–1597.

7. De Jager PL, Franchimont D, Waliszewska A, Bitton A, Cohen A, et al. (2007) The role of the Toll receptor pathway in susceptibility to inflammatory bowel diseases. Genes Immun 8: 387–397.

8. Strober W, Fuss I, Mannon P (2007) The fundamental basis of inflammatory bowel disease. J Clin Invest 117: 514–521.

9. MacDonald TT, Biancheri P, Sarra M, Monteleone G (2012) What's the next best cytokine target in IBD? Inflamm Bowel Dis 18: 2180–2189.

10. Jurjus AR, Khoury NN, Reimund JM (2004) Animal models of inflammatory bowel disease. J Pharmacol Toxicol Methods 50: 81–92.

11. Neurath M, Fuss I, Strober W (2000) TNBS-colitis. Int Rev Immunol 19: 51–62.

12. Morris GP, Beck PL, Herridge MS, Depew WT, Szewczuk MR, et al. (1989) Hapten-induced model of chronic inflammation and ulceration in the rat colon. Gastroenterology 96: 795–803.

13. Wallace JL, Le T, Carter L, Appleyard CB, Beck PL (1995) Hapten-induced chronic colitis in the rat: alternatives to trinitrobenzene sulfonic acid. J Pharmacol Toxicol Methods 33: 237–239.

14. Pohlmann A, Tilling LC, Robinson A, Woolmer O, McCleary S, et al. (2009) Progression and variability of TNBS colitis-associated inflammation in rats assessed by contrast-enhanced and T2-weighted MRI. Inflamm Bowel Dis 15: 534–545.

15. Kim I, Kong H, Lee Y, Hong S, Han J, et al. (2009) Dexamethasone 21-sulfate improves the therapeutic properties of dexamethasone against experimental rat colitis by specifically delivering the steroid to the large intestine. Pharm Res 26: 415–421.

16. Shen C, de Hertogh G, Bullens DM, Van Assche G, Geboes K, et al. (2007) Remission-inducing effect of anti-TNF monoclonal antibody in TNBS colitis: mechanisms beyond neutralization. Inflamm Bowel Dis 13: 308–316.

17. Chen Y, Liu WL, Zhou TH, Cai JT, Du Q, et al. (2009) Therapeutic effects of rectal administration of muscovite on experimental colitis in rats. J Gastroenterol Hepatol 24: 912–919.

18. Akcan A, Kucuk C, Sozuer E, Esel D, Akyildiz H, et al. (2008) Melatonin reduces bacterial translocation and apoptosis in trinitrobenzene sulphonic acid-induced colitis of rats. World J Gastroenterol 14: 918–924.

19. Pan XQ, Gonzalez JA, Chang S, Chacko S, Wein AJ, et al. (2010) Experimental colitis triggers the release of substance P and calcitonin gene-related peptide in the urinary bladder via TRPV1 signaling pathways. Exp Neurol 225: 262–273.

20. Ohta N, Tsujikawa T, Nakamura T, A I (2003) Different-sized triglycerides chains do not influence colitis induced by trinitrobenzene sulfonic acid in rats. Nutr Res 23: 279–286.

21. Martinez-Augustin O, Merlos M, Zarzuelo A, Suarez MD, de Medina FS (2008) Disturbances in metabolic, transport and structural genes in experimental colonic inflammation in the rat: a longitudinal genomic analysis. BMC Genomics 9: 490.

22. Abreu MT (2010) Toll-like receptor signalling in the intestinal epithelium: how bacterial recognition shapes intestinal function. Nat Rev Immunol 10: 131–144.

23. Willson TM, Lambert MH, Kliewer SA (2001) Peroxisome proliferator-activated receptor gamma and metabolic disease. Annu Rev Biochem 70: 341–367.

24. Jiang C, Ting AT, Seed B (1998) PPAR-gamma agonists inhibit production of monocyte inflammatory cytokines. Nature 391: 82–86.

25. Peyrin-Biroulet L, Beisner J, Wang G, Nuding S, Oommen ST, et al. (2010) Peroxisome proliferator-activated receptor gamma activation is required for maintenance of innate antimicrobial immunity in the colon. Proc Natl Acad Sci U S A 107: 8772–8777.

26. Linden R, Martins VR, Prado MA, Cammarota M, Izquierdo I, et al. (2008) Physiology of the prion protein. Physiol Rev 88: 673–728.

27. Marcos Z, Pfieifer K, Bodegas ME, Sesma MP, Guembe L (2004) Cellular prion protein is expressed in a subset of neuroendocrine cells of the rat gastrointestinal tract. J Histochem Cytochem 52: 1357–1365.

28. Ford MJ, Burton LJ, Morris RJ, Hall SM (2002) Selective expression of prion protein in peripheral tissues of the adult mouse. Neuroscience 113: 177–192.

29. Martin GR, Keenan CM, Sharkey KA, Jirik FR (2011) Endogenous prion protein attenuates experimentally induced colitis. Am J Pathol 179: 2290–2301.

30. Becker C, Fantini MC, Wirtz S, Nikolaev A, Kiesslich R, et al. (2005) In vivo imaging of colitis and colon cancer development in mice using high resolution chromoendoscopy. Gut 54: 950–954.

31. Du P, Kibbe WA, Lin SM (2008) lumi: a pipeline for processing Illumina microarray. Bioinformatics 24: 1547–1548.

32. Aryee MJ, Gutierrez-Pabello JA, Kramnik I, Maiti T, Quackenbush J (2009) An improved empirical bayes approach to estimating differential gene expression in microarray time-course data: BETR (Bayesian Estimation of Temporal Regulation). BMC Bioinformatics 10: 409.

33. Birney E, Andrews TD, Bevan P, Caccamo M, Chen Y, et al. (2004) An overview of Ensembl. Genome Res 14: 925–928.

34. Frey BJ, Dueck D (2007) Clustering by passing messages between data points. Science 315: 972–976.

35. Ashburner M, Ball CA, Blake JA, Botstein D, Butler H, et al. (2000) Gene ontology: tool for the unification of biology. The Gene Ontology Consortium. Nature genetics 25: 25–29.

36. Shi Z, Derow CK, Zhang B (2010) Co-expression module analysis reveals biological processes, genomic gain, and regulatory mechanisms associated with breast cancer progression. BMC Syst Biol 4: 74.

37. Drozdov I, Ouzounis CA, Shah AM, Tsoka S (2011) Functional Genomics Assistant (FUGA): a toolbox for the analysis of complex biological networks. BMC research notes 4: 462.

38. Kanehisa M, Goto S, Sato Y, Furumichi M, Tanabe M (2012) KEGG for integration and interpretation of large-scale molecular data sets. Nucleic acids research 40: D109–114.

39. Vastrik I, D'Eustachio P, Schmidt E, Gopinath G, Croft D, et al. (2007) Reactome: a knowledge base of biologic pathways and processes. Genome biology 8: R39.

40. Lee E, Chuang HY, Kim JW, Ideker T, Lee D (2008) Inferring pathway activity toward precise disease classification. PLoS computational biology 4: e1000217.

41. Knollmann FD, Dietrich T, Bleckmann T, Bock J, Maurer J, et al. (2002) Magnetic resonance imaging of inflammatory bowel disease: evaluation in a rabbit model. J Magn Reson Imaging 15: 165–173.

42. Hugot JP (2005) PPAR and Crohn's disease: another piece of the puzzle? Gastroenterology 128: 500–503.

43. Guarner F, Malagelada JR (2003) Role of bacteria in experimental colitis. Best Pract Res Clin Gastroenterol 17: 793–804.

44. Shibata Y, Taruishi M, Ashida T (1993) Experimental ileitis in dogs and colitis in rats with trinitrobenzene sulfonic acid – colonoscopic and histopathologic studies. Gastroenterol Jpn 28: 518–527.

45. Vermeulen W, De Man JG, Nullens S, Pelckmans PA, De Winter BY, et al. (2011) The use of colonoscopy to follow the inflammatory time course of TNBS colitis in rats. Acta Gastroenterol Belg 74: 304–311.

46. Heimerl S, Moehle C, Zahn A, Boettcher A, Stremmel W, et al. (2006) Alterations in intestinal fatty acid metabolism in inflammatory bowel disease. Biochim Biophys Acta 1762: 341–350.

47. Rieder F, Fiocchi C (2008) Intestinal fibrosis in inflammatory bowel disease: progress in basic and clinical science. Current opinion in gastroenterology 24: 462–468.

48. Luthi AU, Cullen SP, McNeela EA, Duriez PJ, Afonina IS, et al. (2009) Suppression of interleukin-33 bioactivity through proteolysis by apoptotic caspases. Immunity 31: 84–98.

49. Hu B, Elinav E, Huber S, Booth CJ, Strowig T, et al. (2010) Inflammation-induced tumorigenesis in the colon is regulated by caspase-1 and NLRC4. Proc Natl Acad Sci U S A 107: 21635–21640.

50. Kobori A, Yagi Y, Imaeda H, Ban H, Bamba S, et al. (2010) Interleukin-33 expression is specifically enhanced in inflamed mucosa of ulcerative colitis. Journal of gastroenterology 45: 999–1007.

51. Seidelin JB, Bjerrum JT, Coskun M, Widjaya B, Vainer B, et al. (2010) IL-33 is upregulated in colonocytes of ulcerative colitis. Immunol Lett 128: 80–85.

52. Brinkman BM, Hildebrand F, Kubica M, Goosens D, Del Favero J, et al. (2011) Caspase deficiency alters the murine gut microbiome. Cell death & disease 2: e220.

53. Dupaul-Chicoine J, Yeretssian G, Doiron K, Bergstrom KS, McIntire CR, et al. (2010) Control of intestinal homeostasis, colitis, and colitis-associated colorectal cancer by the inflammatory caspases. Immunity 32: 367–378.

54. Lawrance IC, Fiocchi C, Chakravarti S (2001) Ulcerative colitis and Crohn's disease: distinctive gene expression profiles and novel susceptibility candidate genes. Hum Mol Genet 10: 445–456.

55. Rieder F, Brenmoehl J, Leeb S, Scholmerich J, Rogler G (2007) Wound healing and fibrosis in intestinal disease. Gut 56: 130–139.

56. Miller JA, Horvath S, Geschwind DH (2010) Divergence of human and mouse brain transcriptome highlights Alzheimer disease pathways. Proc Natl Acad Sci U S A 107: 12698–12703.

57. Gollamudi S, Johri A, Calingasan NY, Yang L, Elemento O, et al. (2012) Concordant signaling pathways produced by pesticide exposure in mice correspond to pathways identified in human Parkinson's disease. PLoS One 7: e36191.

58. Granlund AB, Beisvag V, Torp SH, Flatberg A, Kleveland PM, et al. (2011) Activation of REG family proteins in colitis. Scand J Gastroenterol 46: 1316–1323.

59. Ostvik AE, Vb Granlund A, Bugge M, Nilsen NJ, Torp SH, et al. (2012) Enhanced expression of CXCL10 in inflammatory bowel disease: Potential role of mucosal toll-like receptor 3 stimulation. Inflamm Bowel Dis.

60. Lehrke M, Konrad A, Schachinger V, Tillack C, Seibold F, et al. (2008) CXCL16 is a surrogate marker of inflammatory bowel disease. Scand J Gastroenterol 43: 283–288.

61. Uza N, Nakase H, Yamamoto S, Yoshino T, Takeda Y, et al. (2011) SR-PSOX/CXCL16 plays a critical role in the progression of colonic inflammation. Gut 60: 1494–1505.

62. Olszak T, An D, Zeissig S, Vera MP, Richter J, et al. (2012) Microbial exposure during early life has persistent effects on natural killer T cell function. Science 336: 489–493.

63. Mootha VK, Lindgren CM, Eriksson KF, Subramanian A, Sihag S, et al. (2003) PGC-1alpha-responsive genes involved in oxidative phosphorylation are coordinately downregulated in human diabetes. Nature genetics 34: 267–273.

64. Gassler N, Rohr C, Schneider A, Kartenbeck J, Bach A, et al. (2001) Inflammatory bowel disease is associated with changes of enterocytic junctions. Am J Physiol Gastrointest Liver Physiol 281: G216–228.

65. Casini-Raggi V, Kam L, Chong YJ, Fiocchi C, Pizarro TT, et al. (1995) Mucosal imbalance of IL-1 and IL-1 receptor antagonist in inflammatory bowel disease. A novel mechanism of chronic intestinal inflammation. J Immunol 154: 2434–2440.

66. Cominelli F, Pizarro TT (1996) Interleukin-1 and interleukin-1 receptor antagonist in inflammatory bowel disease. Aliment Pharmacol Ther 10 Suppl 2: 49–53; discussion 54.

67. Mudter J, Neurath MF (2007) Apoptosis of T cells and the control of inflammatory bowel disease: therapeutic implications. Gut 56: 293–303.

68. Mizoguchi A (2012) Animal models of inflammatory bowel disease. Prog Mol Biol Transl Sci 105: 263–320.

69. Gaudio E, Taddei G, Vetuschi A, Sferra R, Frieri G, et al. (1999) Dextran sulfate sodium (DSS) colitis in rats: clinical, structural, and ultrastructural aspects. Dig Dis Sci 44: 1458–1475.

70. Kitajima S, Morimoto M, Sagara E, Shimizu C, Ikeda Y (2001) Dextran sodium sulfate-induced colitis in germ-free IQI/Jic mice. Exp Anim 50: 387–395.

71. te Velde AA, de Kort F, Sterrenburg E, Pronk I, ten Kate FJ, et al. (2007) Comparative analysis of colonic gene expression of three experimental colitis models mimicking inflammatory bowel disease. Inflamm Bowel Dis 13: 325–330.

72. Fang K, Bruce M, Pattillo CB, Zhang S, Stone R, 2nd, et al. (2011) Temporal genomewide expression profiling of DSS colitis reveals novel inflammatory and angiogenesis genes similar to ulcerative colitis. Inflamm Bowel Dis 15: 341–352.

73. Alex P, Zachos NC, Nguyen T, Gonzales L, Chen TE, et al. (2009) Distinct cytokine patterns identified from multiplex profiles of murine DSS and TNBS-induced colitis. Inflamm Bowel Dis 15: 341–352.

74. Wirtz S, Neufert C, Weigmann B, Neurath MF (2007) Chemically induced mouse models of intestinal inflammation. Nat Protoc 2: 541–546.

75. Kontoyiannis D, Pasparakis M, Pizarro TT, Cominelli F, Kollias G (1999) Impaired on/off regulation of TNF biosynthesis in mice lacking TNF AU-rich elements: implications for joint and gut-associated immunopathologies. Immunity 10: 387–398.

76. Rennick DM, Fort MM, Davidson NJ (1997) Studies with IL-10−/− mice: an overview. J Leukoc Biol 61: 389–396.

77. Mitsuyama K, Tomiyasu N, Takaki K, Masuda J, Yamasaki H, et al. (2006) Interleukin-10 in the pathophysiology of inflammatory bowel disease: increased serum concentrations during the recovery phase. Mediators Inflamm 2006: 26875.

78. Ferretti M, Casini-Raggi V, Pizarro TT, Eisenberg SP, Nast CC, et al. (1994) Neutralization of endogenous IL-1 receptor antagonist exacerbates and prolongs inflammation in rabbit immune colitis. J Clin Invest 94: 449–453.

79. Pastorelli L, De Salvo C, Cominelli MA, Vecchi M, Pizarro TT (2011) Novel cytokine signaling pathways in inflammatory bowel disease: insight into the dichotomous functions of IL-33 during chronic intestinal inflammation. Therap Adv Gastroenterol 4: 311–323.

80. Doyle SL, O'Neill LA (2006) Toll-like receptors: from the discovery of NFkappaB to new insights into transcriptional regulations in innate immunity. Biochem Pharmacol 72: 1102–1113.

81. Lee J, Rachmilewitz D, Raz E (2006) Homeostatic effects of TLR9 signaling in experimental colitis. Ann N Y Acad Sci 1072: 351–355.

82. Sturm A, Dignass AU (2008) Epithelial restitution and wound healing in inflammatory bowel disease. World J Gastroenterol 14: 348–353.

83. Frolova L, Drastich P, Rossmann P, Klimesova K, Tlaskalova-Hogenova H (2008) Expression of Toll-like receptor 2 (TLR2), TLR4, and CD14 in biopsy samples of patients with inflammatory bowel diseases: upregulated expression of TLR2 in terminal ileum of patients with ulcerative colitis. J Histochem Cytochem 56: 267–274.

84. Castillo NA, Perdigon G, de Moreno de Leblanc A (2011) Oral administration of a probiotic Lactobacillus modulates cytokine production and TLR expression improving the immune response against Salmonella enterica serovar Typhimurium infection in mice. BMC Microbiol 11: 177.

85. Gonzalez-Navajas JM, Fine S, Law J, Datta SK, Nguyen KP, et al. (2010) TLR4 signaling in effector CD4+ T cells regulates TCR activation and experimental colitis in mice. J Clin Invest 120: 570–581.

86. Lee J, Gonzales-Navajas JM, Raz E (2008) The "polarizing-tolerizing" mechanism of intestinal epithelium: its relevance to colonic homeostasis. Semin Immunopathol 30: 3–9.

87. Otte JM, Cario E, Podolsky DK (2004) Mechanisms of cross hyporesponsiveness to Toll-like receptor bacterial ligands in intestinal epithelial cells. Gastroenterology 126: 1054–1070.

88. Morel E, Fouquet S, Chateau D, Yvernault L, Frobert Y, et al. (2004) The cellular prion protein PrPc is expressed in human enterocytes in cell-cell junctional domains. J Biol Chem 279: 1499–1505.

89. Petit CS, Barreau F, Besnier L, Gandille P, Riveau B, et al. (2012) Requirement of cellular prion protein for intestinal barrier function and mislocalization in patients with inflammatory bowel disease. Gastroenterology 143: 122–132 e115.

90. Fajas L, Auboeuf D, Raspe E, Schoonjans K, Lefebvre AM, et al. (1997) The organization, promoter analysis, and expression of the human PPARgamma gene. J Biol Chem 272: 18779–18789.

91. Su CG, Wen X, Bailey ST, Jiang W, Rangwala SM, et al. (1999) A novel therapy for colitis utilizing PPAR-gamma ligands to inhibit the epithelial inflammatory response. J Clin Invest 104: 383–389.

92. Wolfrum C, Borrmann CM, Borchers T, Spener F (2001) Fatty acids and hypolipidemic drugs regulate peroxisome proliferator-activated receptors alpha – and gamma-mediated gene expression via liver fatty acid binding protein: a signaling path to the nucleus. Proc Natl Acad Sci U S A 98: 2323–2328.

93. Dubuquoy L, Jansson EA, Deeb S, Rakotobe S, Karoui M, et al. (2003) Impaired expression of peroxisome proliferator-activated receptor gamma in ulcerative colitis. Gastroenterology 124: 1265–1276.

94. Sugawara K, Olson TS, Moskaluk CA, Stevens BK, Hoang S, et al. (2005) Linkage to peroxisome proliferator-activated receptor-gamma in SAMP1/YitFc mice and in human Crohn's disease. Gastroenterology 128: 351–360.

95. Sanchez-Hidalgo M, Martin AR, Villegas I, de la Lastra CA (2007) Rosiglitazone, a PPARgamma ligand, modulates signal transduction pathways during the development of acute TNBS-induced colitis in rats. Eur J Pharmacol 562: 247–258.

96. Celinski K, Dworzanski T, Korolczuk A, Slomka M, Radej S, et al. (2011) Activated and inactivated PPARs-gamma modulate experimentally induced colitis in rats. Med Sci Monit 17: BR116–124.

97. Lewis JD, Lichtenstein GR, Deren JJ, Sands BE, Hanauer SB, et al. (2008) Rosiglitazone for active ulcerative colitis: a randomized placebo-controlled trial. Gastroenterology 134: 688–695.

98. Wang D, DuBois RN (2010) Therapeutic potential of peroxisome proliferator-activated receptors in chronic inflammation and colorectal cancer. Gastroenterol Clin North Am 39: 697–707.

99. Dooley TP, Curto EV, Reddy SP, Davis RL, Lambert GW, et al. (2004) Regulation of gene expression in inflammatory bowel disease and correlation with IBD drugs: screening by DNA microarrays. Inflamm Bowel Dis 10: 1–14.

100. Hasler R, Feng Z, Backdahl L, Spehlmann ME, Franke A, et al. (2012) A functional methylome map of ulcerative colitis. Genome Res 22: 2130–2137.

101. Wapenaar MC, Monsuur AJ, Poell J, van 't Slot R, Meijer JW, et al. (2007) The SPINK gene family and celiac disease susceptibility. Immunogenetics 59: 349–357.

102. Lakatos PL, Kiss LS, Palatka K, Altorjay I, Antal-Szalmas P, et al. (2011) Serum lipopolysaccharide-binding protein and soluble CD14 are markers of disease activity in patients with Crohn's disease. Inflamm Bowel Dis 17: 767–777.

103. Antonioli L, Fornai M, Colucci R, Awwad O, Ghisu N, et al. (2010) The blockade of adenosine deaminase ameliorates chronic experimental colitis through the recruitment of adenosine A2A and A3 receptors. J Pharmacol Exp Ther 335: 434–442.

104. Antonioli L, Fornai M, Colucci R, Ghisu N, Da Settimo F, et al. (2007) Inhibition of adenosine deaminase attenuates inflammation in experimental colitis. J Pharmacol Exp Ther 322: 435–442.

105. Hogan SP, Seidu L, Blanchard C, Groschwitz K, Mishra A, et al. (2006) Resistin-like molecule beta regulates innate colonic function: barrier integrity and inflammation susceptibility. J Allergy Clin Immunol 118: 257–268.

13

Dietary α-Eleostearic Acid Ameliorates Experimental Inflammatory Bowel Disease in Mice by Activating Peroxisome Proliferator-Activated Receptor-γ

Stephanie N. Lewis[1,2,3,4]*, Lera Brannan[2], Amir J. Guri[3], Pinyi Lu[1,3,4], Raquel Hontecillas[3,4], Josep Bassaganya-Riera[1,3,4], David R. Bevan[1,2,4]

1 Genetics, Bioinformatics, and Computational Biology Program, Virginia Tech, Blacksburg, Virginia, United States of America, 2 Department of Biochemistry, Virginia Tech, Blacksburg, Virginia, United States of America, 3 Nutritional Immunology and Molecular Medicine Laboratory, Virginia Bioinformatics Institute, Blacksburg, Virginia, United States of America, 4 Center for Modeling Immunology to Enteric Pathogens, Virginia Bioinformatics Institute, Blacksburg, Virginia, United States of America

Abstract

Background: Treatments for inflammatory bowel disease (IBD) are modestly effective and associated with side effects from prolonged use. As there is no known cure for IBD, alternative therapeutic options are needed. Peroxisome proliferator-activated receptor-gamma (PPARγ) has been identified as a potential target for novel therapeutics against IBD. For this project, compounds were screened to identify naturally occurring PPARγ agonists as a means to identify novel anti-inflammatory therapeutics for experimental assessment of efficacy.

Methodology/Principal Findings: Here we provide complementary computational and experimental methods to efficiently screen for PPARγ agonists and demonstrate amelioration of experimental IBD in mice, respectively. Computational docking as part of virtual screening (VS) was used to test binding between a total of eighty-one compounds and PPARγ. The test compounds included known agonists, known inactive compounds, derivatives and stereoisomers of known agonists with unknown activity, and conjugated trienes. The compound identified through VS as possessing the most favorable docked pose was used as the test compound for experimental work. With our combined methods, we have identified α-eleostearic acid (ESA) as a natural PPARγ agonist. Results of ligand-binding assays complemented the screening prediction. In addition, ESA decreased macrophage infiltration and significantly impeded the progression of IBD-related phenotypes through both PPARγ-dependent and –independent mechanisms in mice with experimental IBD.

Conclusions/Significance: This study serves as the first significant step toward a large-scale VS protocol for natural PPARγ agonist screening that includes a massively diverse ligand library and structures that represent multiple known target pharmacophores.

Editor: Jan-Hendrik Niess, Ulm University, Germany

Funding: NIH Biomedical and Behavioral Sciences Research Training Grant R25 GM072767 (Virginia Tech Initiative to Maximize Student Diversity). National Center for Complementary and Alternative Medicine Grant 5R01AT4308. The Genetics, Bioinformatics, and Computational Biology PhD program, Virginia Tech, Blacksburg, VA 24601. The funders had no role in study design, data collection and analysis, decision to publish, or preparation of the manuscript.

Competing Interests: The authors have declared that no competing interests exist.

* E-mail: snl@vt.edu

Introduction

Inflammatory bowel disease (IBD) is a chronic and recurring inflammatory disease with two clinical manifestations: ulcerative colitis (UC) and Crohn's disease (CD). UC and CD affect over 4 million Americans and accrue a significant portion of the estimated $1.7 billion in health care costs for prevalent gastrointestinal diseases (CDC2007). While the etiopathogenesis of IBD remains unclear, it has been suggested that chronic mucosal inflammation characteristic of IBD is associated with a disruption in immune homeostasis [1]. As such, treatments for IBD should correct this immune dysregulation in order to prevent or reduce gut mucosal damage.

There is no cure for IBD, but treatments are available to combat the associated symptoms. One such treatment, 5-aminosalicylic acid, targets the nuclear hormone receptor

peroxisome proliferator-activated receptor-gamma (PPARγ), which is highly expressed in the colonic epithelial and immune cells [2–7]. PPARγ and PPARδ serve as targets for the treatment of inflammatory and immune-mediated diseases because of the role they play in maintaining homeostasis and suppressing inflammation [1,7–9]. PPARγ in particular is known to play a role in transcriptional regulation of anti-inflammatory processes via co-activator recruitment [6,9,10]. Ligand-induced activation of PPARγ can antagonize the activity of pro-inflammatory transcription factors such as nuclear factor kappa-light-chain-enhancer of activated B cells (NF-κB), signal transducer and activator of transcription (STAT), and activator protein (AP)-1 [11]. Other IBD treatments currently available include infliximab, which is an anti-tumor necrosis factor-alpha (TNF-α) antibody [12,13], and corticosteroids, which systemically suppress immunity [14]. These medications are modestly successful for the long-term management of IBD but are associated with significant side effects, including increased risk of infection and cancer [15,16]. Interestingly, the insulin-sensitizing PPARγ agonists used for treating type 2 diabetes, such as rosiglitazone and pioglitazone, have proven useful at ameliorating IBD effects in humans with UC [17]. However, rosiglitazone, and other PPARγ agonists of the thiazolidinediones (TZD) class of anti-diabetic drugs, are unlikely to be adopted by gastroenterologists for the treatment of IBD due to associated side effects [17] including hepatotoxicity, weight gain, fluid retention leading to edema, and congestive heart failure [18]. In this regard, the U.S. Food and Drug Administration (FDA) restricted the use of rosiglitazone in 2010 due to its side effects, whereas the European Medicines Agency completely banned its use in the European market. Natural therapeutics, such as fatty acids that induce PPARγ activation, might be a safer alternative to current treatments and TZDs.

Our group has conducted several preclinical animal model studies to suggest that supplementation of diet with fatty acids, such as conjugated linoleic acid (CLA) [8,19] or agonistic botanicals, is effective at ameliorating colonic inflammation in mouse and pig models of IBD through a PPARγ-dependent mechanism [8,19–21]. In an effort to expedite the drug and natural product therapeutic discovery process, virtual screening (VS) can complement traditional experimental methods for identification of novel PPARγ agonists. VS represents a cost- and time-efficient means of screening thousands of compounds within thematic libraries that justify further experimental assessment [22]. We are undertaking VS to identify novel PPARγ agonists within a collective of large compound databases. As a feasibility test, we screened a small group of known and proposed agonists, with the inclusion of known negative controls. The focus of this small-scale screen was to test our PPARγ structural model, and assess binding of natural compounds, with significant emphasis on conjugated trienes.

Conjugated trienes were selected due in part to their structural similarity to CLA. In addition, conjugated trienes exhibit effectiveness at ameliorating chronic inflammation [23,24]. One such compound, α-eleostearic acid (ESA; 9Z11E13E-18:3), has been found at concentrations of 60–80% in tung and bitter gourd seed oils [25]. ESA has been shown to suppress tumor angiogenesis [26] and MCF-7 breast cancer cell proliferation via PPARγ activation [27], induce apoptosis via lipid peroxidation [28], and induce autophagy-dependent cell death through AKT/mTOR and ERK1/2 signal targeting [29]. Evidence also indicates that punicic acid plays a significant role in increasing lipid peroxidation [30] and inhibiting TNF-α-induced neutrophil hyperactivation to protect against experimentally induced colon inflammation in rats [31]. Our group has found that punicic acid ameliorates type 2 diabetes-induced inflammation by activating PPARγ and PPARα, and repressing TNF-α expression in white adipose tissue and liver [24] and increases peripheral insulin sensitivity [32] without causing any adverse side effects [33]. We have also demonstrated that punicic acid prevents experimental IBD through PPARγ- and PPARδ-dependent mechanisms [34]. Catalpic acid improves abdominal fat deposition, improves glucose homeostasis and up-regulates PPARα expression in adipose tissue of mice [23]. Though these plant-derived conjugated trienes suggest anti-inflammatory efficacy in various disease models, it has been suggested that ESA induces a greater degree of antioxidant activity than punicic acid in mice [35]. Punicic acid ameliorates both diabetes [34] and gut inflammation [24] without causing side effects [33], whereas ESA elicits mainly anti-inflammatory and anti-carcinogenic effects [26–29]. A goal of this study was to test the effectiveness of ESA in an experimental IBD model.

Additionally, small-scale VS was conducted to test the predictability of our VS protocol for identifying PPARγ full agonists in the hopes of finding natural therapeutics and/or prophylactics for treating IBD and other chronic inflammation-related diseases. The computational portion of our study revealed information complementary to the predictions of our *in vitro* analysis, pre-clinical efficacy, and mechanistic testing in mice.

Methods

Docking procedure

AutoDock 4.0 [36] (AD4) was used for structural model testing, while AutoDock Vina [37] (Vina) was used for screening a subset of our in-house ligand database against the selected structural models of PPARγ. AutoDock Tools 1.5.2 (ADT) was used to build the appropriate charged protein and ligand files for docking. Default values for the Lamarckian Genetic Algorithm (LGA) were used for docking with AD4, with the exception of the maximum number of energy evaluations, which was reduced to 250,000. Adjusting this number reduced the screening time without significantly affecting pose prediction. Five iterations of AD4 with 50 poses generated per iteration were conducted for the re-docking step totaling 250 poses per protein structure model. Vina was used for cross-docking and to run the small-scale screening. Three Vina iterations were conducted for each ligand in the cross-docking step, while a single run was conducted for the small-scale screening. As a means to further sample conjugated triene geometry, three AD4 iterations of 50 poses each were run for each compound, which was a total of 150 poses per conjugated triene for each selected protein structure model. Scripts available through the AD4 development site (http://autodock/scripps.edu/) were modified and used to automate the screening process. Modifications to the scripts included exchanging the AD4 executable for the Vina executable and all subsequent necessary changes for Vina functionality.

Structural Model Selection: Re-docking component

Five structures with co-crystallized rosiglitazone were downloaded from the Research Collaboratory for Structural Bioinformatics (RCSB) Protein Data Bank (PDB) [38,39] (http://www.pdb.org). The selected structure IDs were 1FM6 [40], 1ZGY [41], 2PRG [42], 3CS8 [43], and 3DZY [44]. These structures were evaluated to identify a PPARγ structural model that would be appropriate for docking in a full agonist-like pose. Completeness of structure, crystal resolution, and re-docking ability were the factors considered. Re-docking refers to the ability of a docking program to reproduce the co-crystallized binding geometry and orientation of the associated ligand given a rigid macromolecule state. The PDB structures were superimposed and rosiglitazone was isolated from each protein structural model with the UCSF Chimera software package [45].

Re-docking was conducted with both native and non-native initial rosiglitazone conformations. Native refers to use of coordinates for the co-crystallized ligand structure of the respective protein structure model, whereas non-native refers to use of initial coordinates not found in the original PDB file. For the native test, each isolated rosiglitazone was re-docked into its respective protein structure (e.g., five protein models each with a different rosiglitazone coordinate files). For the non-native test, a single rosiglitazone structure was randomly selected for re-docking into all five structure models. Ligand flexibility and random initial geometry for the ligand reduced possible bias associated with use of a native ligand for one test structure, which was non-native for the other four. A comparison of results for the native and non-native ligand re-docking suggested the randomized initial conformation for rosiglitazone does not affect pose prediction as the predicted poses for both test sets were similar (data not shown). The non-native procedure involved docking of a single ligand structure to the protein structures, which is similar to what would be used for large-scale screening. Therefore, data from the non-native re-docking was analyzed and provided here. Both the superimposed positioning and the use of a single rosiglitazone model established a relatively controlled test set: overlaid coordinate space for the test structures, which translated to similar grid areas, with a single ligand coordinate file for testing.

Structural Model Selection: Cross-docking component

Co-crystallized ligands from various PDB files were used for cross-docking to test predictability for other known agonists. Cross-docking refers to docking different ligand structures isolated from multiple PDB structures of the same protein to a single selected model structure. Ligands from 1FM9 [40], 2F4B [46], 2HWQ [47], 2I4J [48], 2I4P [48], 2VSR [49], 2VST [49], 3ET3 [50], 2VV0 [49], 2VV1 [49], 2ZK1 [51], and 2ZK2 [51] were included in the library for this purpose (Table 3).

Small-scale in-house ligand library construction

Our small-scale ligand library included the rosiglitazone structure from re-docking, several of the cross-docking ligands, known PPARγ agonists, and known inactive compounds. Inclusion of the ligands from the re-docking and cross-docking steps served as controls for successful and unsuccessful docking. A search of published literature was conducted to find both naturally and synthetically derived compounds shown experimentally to either activate or not activate PPARγ [52–55]. Structural models for non-crystallized ligands were downloaded from the UCSF ZINC database online (http://zinc.docking.org/). Any structures not available through ZINC were built using the Dundee PRODRG2 server [56] (http://davapc1.bioch.dundee.ac.uk/prodrg/). Structures built with PRODRG2 were examined to ensure conservation of stereochemistry. Charges for all of the ligands in the database and the protein were generated using ADT. Eighty-one compounds total were tested in this study. A complete list of ligands included in the test library can be found in Table S1.

Docking analysis for re-docking and cross-docking

The most energetically favorable pose for each ligand of the re-docking (25 lowest energy poses) and cross-docking (108 lowest energy poses) steps were used for analysis. Reference poses for root mean-squared deviation (RMSD) calculations were taken from crystal structure complexes for each ligand. These protein-ligand complex structures were superimposed onto the test structures to obtain a common coordinate space prior to the RMSD calculation. For re-docking, RMSD values are exact given each PPARγ-rosiglitazone complex was used as the reference for the respective results. However, the reported RMSD values for cross-docking were relative rather than absolute given the co-crystallized reference ligand coordinates are not relative to the protein structure models used for testing. The idea of relative RMSD stems from differences in side chain rotamers between the crystal structures. Side chain position is governed, in part, by ligand binding, which meant differences could be seen in binding cavity residue positions when the rosiglitazone-bound test structures were compared to each additional PPARγ structure model. These differences, which affect intramolecular interactions, resulted in minor deviations of the backbone on some regions for the superimposed structures relative to the test structure. This could

mean the position of each co-crystallized reference ligand relative to the test structures was shifted slightly as well. However, there were areas of the backbone that superimposed without noticeable deviations. As the deviations between backbone positions were not consistent, adjusting for any rotamer-induced shifts in co-crystallized ligand coordinates was not feasible. Therefore, RMSD values for docked poses for each ligand were deemed "relative" as an acknowledgement of these minor variations in coordinates. An average RMSD, population standard deviation, and variance were calculated for each ligand (See Formulas S1). Re-docking and cross-docking results for each ligand relative to each test protein structure were deemed successful if the RMSD was less than 2.0 Å [57].

Docking success versus failure for re-docking and cross-docking was assessed qualitatively as well. Docked poses for rosiglitazone on the surface of the protein or near the opening of the binding cavity were deemed unsuccessful. Poses for which the molecule was not properly oriented, such as the imidizole ring of rosiglitazone positioned near the cavity opening rather than near the rear of the pocket, were deemed unsuccessful as well given such orientations would not match the co-crystallized coordinates. Similar conditions relative to each cross-docking ligand were also identified and assessed.

Docking analysis for small-scale VS

To prepare for analysis of the small-scale VS results, interactions from various crystal structures were identified and cataloged. Reported crystal structure interactions for the five rosiglitazone-containing structures from the re-docking step and six fatty acid-containing structures from the cross-docking step were compiled using RCSB Ligand Explorer [58]. Residue atoms common to more than one interaction list for a specific ligand type were pooled and used as a reference list for analysis after docking. As such, there were two master interaction lists: rosiglitazone-like interactions (Table S2) and fatty acid-like interactions (Table S3). Common interactions between the two lists were also noted (Table S4).

Perl [59] scripts to automate pose distance measurement calculations and pose interaction predictions were also composed and used. The most energetically favorable docked pose for each ligand relative to the macromolecule were pooled for analysis. Only the potential for a ligand to fall into the full agonist category of ligands was assessed in depth for this study. Full agonism has been suggested to require interactions with Ser289, His323, His449, and Tyr473, which are residues positioned in the portion of the binding cavity proximal to the activation function-two (AF-2) region (Figure S1). Interactions in this region govern AF-2 conformational changes necessary for PPARγ activation. Distance measurements between the top docked poses (77 lowest energy poses) were calculated and used to predict interactions. Interactions similar to those seen in the pooled crystal structure data were deemed "successful". Potential hydrogen bonds were assessed based on distances between the donor/acceptor heavy atoms of the test ligand pose and four key residues. Lengths measuring less than 3.3 Å were considered potential hydrogen bond interactions [52,58]. Potential hydrophobic interactions were set to a distance threshold of 3.9 Å between carbon atoms [58]. Predicted interactions for each ligand were counted and a screen for the presence of hydrogen bond interactions with the key residues listed above was conducted to determine docking success.

Ligand Binding Assay

ESA was introduced at various concentrations (0.001–10 μM) to solution containing PPARγ protein complexed with a fluorophore-bound compound (Fluormone™, Invitrogen). This mixture was allowed to incubate for 20 hours. The ability of the test compound, which here was ESA, to displace Fluormone™ was calculated as mean polarization, where a decrease in polarization corresponded to an increase in ligand binding activity as previously described [60].

Transfection of RAW 264.7 cells

RAW 264.7 mouse macrophage precursor cells (ATCC, Manassas, VA) were grown in 24-well plates in DMEM high glucose medium (Invitrogen, Carlsbad, CA) containing 10% fetal bovine serum until 60–70% confluence. Transfected cells were treated with varying concentrations of ESA (0, 1, 5, and 10 μM; Sigma) or rosiglitazone (1 μM; Cayman Chemicals, Ann Arbor, MI) for 24 hours. Other details of the protocol were as previously described [60,61]. Relative luciferase activity was calculated as a ratio between beginning and ending chemiluminescence values for a 10-second time period.

Animal Procedures

The protocol for animal care and genotyping of the mice was described previously [8]. An ESA-supplemented diet was tested against a control (AIN-93G-based) diet in a dextran sodium sulfate (DSS)-induced IBD mouse model. Sixty mice were divided according to diet (ESA versus control), genotype (PPARγ flfl; MMTV-Cre-/PPARγ-floxed versus epithelial cell- and immune cell-specific PPARγ flfl; MMTV-Cre+/PPARγ-null), and DSS-challenge. Ten mice (5 for each genotype) from the control diet group and 9 mice (4 PPARγ-floxed and 5 PPARγ-null) from the ESA diet group were not given DSS-treated water as a control for the disease state. Drinking water with 2.5% DSS was administered to the test mice for a period of seven days. Body weights and disease activity index (DAI) values were recorded each day of the seven-day DSS treatment period. Procedures for assigning DAI values have been previously described [8]. Mice were euthanized on day seven of the DSS challenge by CO_2 asphyxiation followed by secondary thoracotomy. Blood was withdrawn from the heart, after which spleen, mesenteric lymph nodes (MLNs), and colonic samples were examined for gross pathological lesions and isolated from each mouse. Organs were examined to assign scores based on size and macroscopic inflammatory lesions (0–3). Spleen and MLN were crushed to produce single-cell suspensions for flow cytometry, while colon samples were used for mRNA isolation and histological examination. This study was approved by the Virginia Tech Institutional Animal Care and Use Committee (IACUC) on May 15, 2008 under animal welfare assurance number A3208-01.

Histopathology

Experimental design for histopathology was previously described [8,20]. Epithelial erosion, mucosal thickness, and immune cell infiltration were each assessed and scored (0–4) for colon cross-sectional samples stained with hematoxylin and eosin from each mouse.

Immunophenotyping

Whole blood and MLN cells were seeded onto 96-well plates and treated with fluorochrome-conjugated antibodies. Monocyte/macrophage subsets were assessed using anti-F4/80-PE-Cy5 (5 mg/mL, eBioscience) and anti-CD11b-Alexa Fluor 700 (2 mg/mL, eBioscience). The lymphocyte subset was assessed with anti-CD4-Alexa Fluor 700 (2 mg/mL; BD Pharmingen), anti-CD8-PerCp-Cy5.5 (2 mg/mL, eBioscience), anti-CD3 PE-Cy5 (2 mg/mL; BD Pharmingen), anti-FoxP3-PE (2 mg/mL,

eBioscience), and anti-IL10-PE as previously described [62]. Flow results were computed with a BD LSR II flow cytometer and data analysis was performed with the FACS Diva software package (BD).

Quantitative Real-Time RT-PCR

Total RNA was isolated from colonic tissue using procedures previously described [20]. PCR was performed on complementary DNA (cDNA) using Taq DNA polymerase (Invitrogen, Carlsbad, CA) and previously described methods and conditions [8,20]. cDNA concentrations for genes of interest were examined by quantitative real-time PCR using an iCycler IQ System and the iQ SYBR green supermix (Bio-Rad). A standard curve was generated for each gene using methods previously described [20]. In addition, a melting curve analysis was performed for each product using previously described methods [20] in order to determine the number of products synthesized while excluding non-specific products and primer dimers. Real-time PCR was used to quantify the starting amount of nucleic acid of each unknown cDNA sample. Primer sequences, the length of the PCR product, and gene accession numbers have been outlined previously [20,61]. Primers used for this study were the forward and reverse cohorts of VCAM-1, ICAM-1, IL-6, and β-actin [20].

Statistical analysis

Data were analyzed as a completely randomized design with statistical significance assessed using the analysis of variance (ANOVA) method. The general linear model procedure of the Statistical Analysis Software (SAS) package (SAS Institute Inc., Cary, NC) was run for weight, DAI, flow cytometry data, and histopathology scores to determine variance across and significance between treatment groups. Statistical significance was assessed based on a probability value (p) less than or equal to 0.05. Significant models were further assessed using the Fisher's Protected Least Significant Difference multiple comparison method.

Results

Selection of structural model: Re-docking component

Structures with co-crystallized rosiglitazone (example given in Figure S1) were used for re-docking because rosiglitazone was the positive control in the experimental studies, it is a known PPARγ agonist, and the purpose of this docking feasibility test was to find compounds that mimic rosiglitazone-induced activation. The top scoring pose from each of the five 50-pose replicates was selected for further analysis. This selection method was applied for each of the five starting structures, giving a total of 25 poses for comparison.

The RMSD and free energy of binding were averaged for the five poses for each protein structure model (Table 1). Additionally, the population-based standard deviation and variance were calculated. The average pose RMSD values for three structures, 1FM6, 1ZGY, and 2PRG, were within 2.0 Å of the crystal structure position. Of these three, 1ZGY possessed the highest standard deviation and variance values, which suggested that some poses with low and high RMSD values should be present. Examination of the poses for all five structures revealed that the lowest RMSD value (0.99 Å) for all rosiglitazone poses was in the 1ZGY pose group as was the pose with the highest RMSD value (3.05 Å). Thus, we favored the 1ZGY structure for further docking studies because this structure enabled docking at the known rosiglitazone binding position as well as docking at other energetically favorable positions within the binding site, suggesting that it might accommodate ligands of diverse structure. To further confirm this selection, cross-docking with known ligands from other PDB structures was conducted.

Selection of structural model: Cross-docking component

1ZGY, 1FM6, and 2PRG were included in the cross-docking testing as each showed successful re-docking and contained ligand-binding domains without missing loops or sequence segments. Structures 3CS8 and 3DZY were missing the H2'-H3 loop and did not result in accurate pose prediction for rosiglitazone. Rosiglitazone poses for 3CS8 and 3DZY occupied the portion of the binding cavity opening in which the H2'-H3 loop would normally sit (data not shown). This loop proved necessary for successful agonist docking given the poor success rate of re-docking in the absence of this region.

Vina was used for cross-docking instead of AD4 as the former was more time-efficient for the number of ligands used and the number of replicates to be carried out. It has also been reported that Vina better predicts poses for ligands with higher numbers of torsions [63], which was the case for some of the ligands used in cross-docking. Replicates were conducted with Vina for two reasons: to determine if replicates would be necessary in a larger-scale study, and to aid in the protein structure model selection process. Three replicate screens were run and each lowest-energy pose was analyzed (3 protein models × 3 replicates × 12 ligands = 108 lowest energy poses). Analysis of the cross-docking results included a comparison of RMSD values, free energy of binding, and number and identity of known interactions between each ligand and PPARγ based on the crystal structures of the complexes. Results from comparison of RMSD values and free energy of binding are listed in Table 2, with full ligand names listed in Table 3. To simplify the process of cross-docking of several ligands to multiple receptor structures, the initial crystal protein-ligand complexes were superimposed prior to docking. This practice allowed for RMSD values to be easily calculated between the docked ligand poses and crystal reference poses as the structures shared coordinate space.

The results relative to each of the test structure models were not completely consistent across all the models. The lowest overall average RMSD was seen with 1ZGY for the (2S)-ureidofibrate-like derivative. This ligand did not dock as well into 1FM6 and 2PRG. A similar comparative docking pattern was seen for 4-HDHA. Only one ligand, PTG taken from PDB ID 2ZK1 (PTG-1), docked within the 2.0 Å threshold across the three structural models. It should be noted here that the PTG structure taken from PDB ID 2ZK2 possessed different charges than the same compound from 2ZK1. The difference in charge is most likely due to the difference in crystallization states. 2ZK2 had glutathione covalently bound to PTG-1 as part of crystallization, whereas 2ZK1 did not. The

glutathione-PTG-1 compound would therefore have more atoms over which charges would be distributed.

The RMSD, standard deviation, and variance values for farglitazar, 9-HODE, indeglitazar, and PTG-1 showed the most consistency across the three proteins, with PTG-1 showing favorable average RMSD values and negligible variance for each protein structure. For PTG-1, this suggested the ligand docked similarly to all three protein structures. When the replicate poses for the four compounds were assessed visually, the deviations for the 9-HODE poses were due in large part to variation in the placement of the hydrophobic tail portion, the PTG-1 poses docked more similarly to 9-HODE than the PTG-1 reference structure, and the indeglitazar poses occupied the middle portion of the binding cavity rather than the rear activation site. The placement of the indeglitazar and PTG-1 poses appeared to be due to the shape of the binding cavity at the rear of the pocket, which was mentioned previously to be the issue with farglitazar. This hindrance was seen to a lesser degree with PTG-1 as there is sufficient space to allow interactions despite lack of exact congruence to the co-crystallized reference. Indeglitazar and farglitazar poses were consistently unsuccessful due to the binding cavity restriction, whereas PTG-1 occupied a fatty acid-like orientation given the similarity of this compound to the types of ligands that can appropriately fill the allotted molecular space.

All of the poses had negative calculated free energy of binding values given the ligand structures and charge environment of the binding cavity. These values were energetically feasible, but were not an indication of the most favorable conformation for ligands that did not agree with the reference structure geometry. Therefore, RMSD and free energy of binding measurements were not enough to determine successful cross-docking for PPARγ. A visual assessment of poses suggested rosiglitazone and fatty acid compounds dock the best into the selected models. As such, interactions from crystal structures containing these compounds were used to generate a list of favorable interactions that might indicate successful docking. The residues considered are listed in Table S4.

Inclusion of the interaction criteria improved the target structure model selection process. Based on the crystal structure interactions common to rosiglitazone and known fatty acid agonists, the number of possible interactions (Table S5) and instances of key residue hydrogen bonding (Table S6) were counted for all the poses. Both sets of data suggested that 1ZGY was the most appropriate model relative to 1FM6 and 2PRG for the purposes of this study. Poses docked into the 1ZGY model all showed at least one key interaction, whereas the other two models returned poses for some ligands that did not exhibit any known interactions. Additionally, fatty acid and fatty acid-derivatives returned the most favorable poses of all the cross-docking ligand

Table 1. Average RMSD and free energy of binding (kcal/mol) for re-docking of rosiglitazone (N = 5).

| PDB ID | Resolution (Å) | RMSD | | | kcal/mol | | |
		Mean	Standard Deviation	Variance	Mean	Standard Deviation	Variance
1FM6	2.1	1.76	0.561	0.314	−7.58	0.487	0.237
1ZGY	1.8	1.91	0.925	0.856	−7.19	0.247	0.061
2PRG	2.3	1.84	0.357	0.128	−7.66	0.228	0.052
3CS8	2.3	2.81	0.101	0.010	−6.63	0.184	0.034
3DZY	3.1	2.82	0.183	0.034	−7.06	0.133	0.018

Table 2. Average RMSD and free energy of binding from cross-docking for various ligands relative to each listed PDB ID (top row) (N = 3).

	1FM6			1ZGY			2PRG		
	RMSD (Å)								
PDB Ligand ID	**Mean**	**SD[1]**	**Variance**	**Mean**	**SD**	**Variance**	**Mean**	**SD**	**Variance**
243	2.82	0.199	0.040	2.82	0.014	0.000	2.60	0.040	0.002
570	3.19	0.000	0.000	3.08	0.007	0.000	3.13	0.050	0.003
4HD	1.81	0.365	0.134	1.40	0.018	0.000	2.19	0.236	0.056
9HO	1.73	0.184	0.034	1.85	0.270	0.073	1.70	0.162	0.026
DRH	2.74	0.030	0.001	1.55	0.209	0.044	2.17	0.251	0.063
DRJ	1.63	0.807	0.652	1.72	0.417	0.174	2.03	0.175	0.031
DRY	3.23	0.002	0.000	2.26	0.024	0.001	1.89	0.019	0.000
EHA	2.47	0.524	0.275	2.45	0.386	0.149	1.89	0.007	0.000
ET1	2.83	0.001	0.000	2.68	0.003	0.000	2.72	0.001	0.000
HXA	2.49	0.616	0.380	1.99	0.171	0.029	1.85	0.009	0.000
PTG-1	1.78	0.000	0.000	1.78	0.005	0.000	1.65	0.019	0.000
PTG-2	2.68	0.023	0.001	2.53	0.244	0.059	2.53	0.091	0.008
	Free energy of binding (kcal/mol)								
PDB Ligand ID	**Mean**	**SD**	**Variance**	**Mean**	**SD**	**Variance**	**Mean**	**SD**	**Variance**
243	−6.87	0.094	0.009	−6.57	0.047	0.002	−6.47	0.309	0.096
570	−10.43	0.047	0.002	−11.00	0.000	0.000	−10.50	0.082	0.007
4HD	−7.00	0.163	0.027	−7.53	0.170	0.029	−6.97	0.047	0.002
9HO	−6.40	0.082	0.007	−6.70	0.082	0.007	−6.37	0.094	0.009
DRH	−8.23	0.047	0.002	−8.83	0.125	0.016	−8.17	0.047	0.002
DRJ	−8.63	0.094	0.009	−8.80	0.294	0.087	−8.37	0.094	0.009
DRY	−10.03	0.047	0.002	−10.13	0.047	0.002	−10.37	0.047	0.002
EHA	−10.10	0.082	0.007	−10.10	0.082	0.007	−10.60	0.000	0.000
ET1	−8.10	0.000	0.000	−8.50	0.000	0.000	−8.50	0.000	0.000
HXA	−7.00	0.327	0.107	−7.90	0.082	0.007	−7.33	0.047	0.002
PTG-1	−7.00	0.000	0.000	−7.23	0.047	0.002	−7.20	0.082	0.007
PTG-2	−7.17	0.170	0.029	−7.10	0.082	0.007	−7.47	0.094	0.009

[1]SD = Standard Deviation.

types. If interaction analysis is included in the selection process, we see 1ZGY as the predominate candidate for the target structure model in a screen involving rosiglitazone-like and fatty acid compounds.

Conjugated trienes showed association with PPARγ in silico

For the small-scale screen, a library of seventy-seven compounds was selected. These compounds included known active and inactive compounds, with alternate stereochemistry for some structures. This test set allowed for screening of active versus inactive, rosiglitazone-like versus non-TZDs, and molecularly simple versus complex compounds. The interaction data (Tables S7 and S8) reinforced the assumption that the selected target structure model could accommodate rosiglitazone-like and fatty acid compounds. The cross-docking ligands included in the screen docked similarly to what was seen with the cross-docking test. Most of the rosiglitazone-like compounds studied by Markt et al. [55] showed successful docking. These compounds were Chemical Abstracts Service (CAS)# 264908-13-6, CAS# 651724-09-3,

CAS# 853652-40-1, BRL48482, BVT13, CLX-M1, KRP297, and NNC61-4424 (Table S1). Isomers of these compounds with differences in stereochemistry were used as well. Some of these structures did not dock as well, which was expected given it has been suggested from crystal structure studies that chirality can affect agonist activity [48]. We also saw lack of favorable docking for bulkier compounds, which contain multiple ring and aromatic components, and compounds with multiple hydroxyl groups. These ligands included phenolic extracts taken from *Glycyrrhiza glabra* roots isolated by Kuroda et al. [54], α-santonin-derived compounds identified by Tanrikulu et al. [53], and flavonoids screened by Salam et al. [52] (Table S1). The compounds from Kuroda et al. [54] and Tanrikulu et al. [53] compounds were numbered according to extraction fraction and deviation from the original α-santonin scaffold, respectively. The Kuroda et al. subset included compounds that induced low level activation. The Tanrikulu et al. subset contained one highly active compound (Tanrikulu_1), one moderately active compound (Tanrikulu_2), and six inactive compounds (Tanrikulu_3 through Tanrikulu_8). The selected Salam et al. compounds were apigenin, biochanin-A,

Table 3. Full names and structures for compounds listed by ligand ID in Table 2.

PDB Ligand ID	PDB ID	Reference	Ligand Name[1]
243	2VST	[46]	13-hydroxyoctadecadienoic acid (13-HODE)
570	1FM9	[37]	GI262570 (Farglitazar)
4HD	2VV1	[46]	(4S,5E,7Z,10Z,13Z,16Z,19Z)-4-hydroxydocosa-5,7,10,13,16,19-hexaenoic acid (4-HDHA)
9HO	2VSR	[46]	9-hydroxyoctadecadienoic acid (9-HODE)
DRH	2I4P	[45]	(2S)-2-[4-[2-(1,3-benzoxazol-2-yl-heptyl-amino)ethyl]phenoxy]-2-methyl-butanoic acid ((2S)-ureidofibrate-like derivative)
DRJ	2I4J	[45]	(2R)-2-[4-[2-(1,3-benzoxazol-2-yl-heptyl-amino)ethyl]phenoxy]-2-methyl-butanoic acid ((2R)-ureidofibrate-like derivative)
DRY	2HWQ	[44]	[(1-{3-[(6-benzoyl-1-propyl-2-naphthyl)oxy]propyl}-1H-indol-5-yl)oxy]acetic acid (5-substituted indoleoxyacetic acid analogue)
EHA	2F4B	[43]	(5-{3-[(6-benzoyl-1-propyl-2-naphthyl)oxy]propoxy}-1H-indol-1-yl)acetic acid (Indol-1-yl acetic acid)
ET1	3ET3	[47]	3-[5-methoxy-1-(4-methoxyphenyl)sulfonyl-indol-3-yl] propanoic acid (indeglitazar)
HXA	2VV0	[46]	Docosa-4,7,10,13,16,19-hexaenoic acid
PTG	2ZK1 2ZK2	[48]	15-deoxy-delta(12,14)-prostaglandin J2 (PTG)

Ligand IDs from respective PDB files were used. Ligand structures can be found in Table S1.
[1]Abbreviations for ligands mentioned in the text are in parentheses following the full name of the compound.

chrysin, dihydroquercetin, genistein, hesperidin, psi(ψ)-baptigenin, and vitexin. The unsuccessful docking of known active compounds in these groups indicated the receptor structure was not appropriate for docking of these molecule types.

All of the conjugated trienes docked successfully but with similar geometry and energy scores, so a more detailed test for these compounds was conducted to see if a predominant ligand could be identified. AD4 was used to dock jacaric, catalpic, calendic, eleostearic, and punicic acids into the selected structural model, 1ZGY. Three iterations of 50 poses each were run and the lowest energy pose for each run for each fatty acid was selected and compared (15 lowest energy poses). The numbers of potential hydrogen bonds and hydrophobic interactions for each pose were calculated (Table S8). The lowest energy pose with the most potential hydrogen bond interactions was selected for each triene and used for analysis. As there are no crystal structures available with any of these compounds co-crystallized, interactions from PDB structures with fatty acids bound were used to generate an interaction reference list (Table S3). The four key residues that formed hydrogen bonds with rosiglitazone also formed hydrogen bonds with these fatty acids. Therefore, poses that possessed these interactions were deemed successful agonists. Unsuccessful poses were those lacking the agonist interactions and poses with the reactive polar group pointed away from the activation site.

All the conjugated trienes showed favorable docked poses and exhibited interactions with residues associated with PPARγ activation (Table 4). The triene poses occupied a space similar to that seen with rosiglitazone (Figure 1), and exhibited interactions with key residues. Of all the replicate poses for triene docking, the ESA replicates consistently exhibited the most

negative free energy of binding (Table S9). Hydrogen bond interactions with only two of the four key residues were seen; however, it is not clear if interactions with all four residues are absolutely necessary for activation, or if a reduced number of interactions can still induce activation. It is feasible that a reduced number of specific interactions may contribute to the specificity seen with ligand-induced co-activator recruitment for PPARs. A comparison of distance measurements for the interactions showed two Y473-involved interactions for ESA, punicic acid, and jacaric acid. Given the distance measurements, it was proposed that the acid head group straddles Y473, with one oxygen atom closer to one histidine side chain than the other. This was confirmed when the poses were visually assessed. The number of hydrophobic interactions was more consistent for the ESA poses compared to punicic and jacaric acids. As previously mentioned, it is known that punicic acid binds to PPARγ and modulates its activity, while ESA possesses greater antioxidant effects. Given the combination of what was known experimentally about the compounds and the predicted free energy of binding and interactions, ESA was selected as a candidate for validation using a ligand-binding assay and further experimental testing *in vivo*.

ESA bound to and modulated PPARγ in vitro

The results of our molecular docking efforts and various published studies [24,26–31,33,34] indicated that conjugated trienes, specifically ESA, may bind to and modulate PPARγ activity. Ligand-binding and reporter activity assays were conducted to test this assumption. A cell-free ligand-binding assay was implemented to determine if ESA associated with PPARγ *in vitro* and possessed a similar depolarization pattern to rosiglitazone.

Table 4. Distance measurements (in Angstroms [Å]) for docked conjugated triene poses displayed in Figure 1.

Ligand	Color	Residue	Distance (Å)	kcal/mol
eleostearic acid	purple	H323.NE2	3.16	−5.6
		Y473.OH	3.01	
		Y473.OH	3.27	
punicic acid	cyan	H449.NE2	2.84	−4.28
		Y473.OH	3.03	
		Y473.OH	3.07	
calendic acid	orange	H449.NE2	2.81	−4.47
		Y473.OH	3.10	
catalpic acid	gold	S289.OG	3.05	−4.48
		H323.NE2	3.03	
		Y473.OH	3.26	
jacaric acid	green	H449.NE2	2.84	−4.5
		Y473.OH	3.16	
		Y473.OH	3.10	
rosiglitazone	gray mesh	S289.OG	3.02	N/A
		H323.NE2	2.83	
		H449.NE2	3.02	
		Y473.OH	2.85	

Distances were measured between carboxylic oxygen atoms of fatty acids and listed atoms for each residue. Free energy of binding is measured in kilocalories per mole of ligand (kcal/mol). No value is listed for rosiglitazone as this refers to the crystal conformation (denoted "N/A") Residues are labeled as the amino acid designation plus the atom name (e.g., S289.OG refers to the oxygen atom in the gamma position on serine 289).

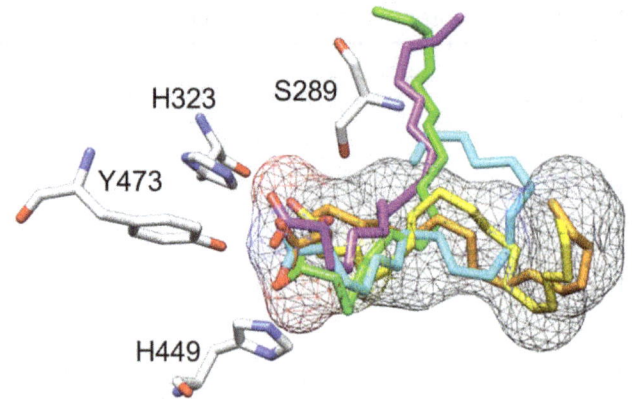

Figure 1. Predicted docked conformations for α-eleostearic (purple), punicic (cyan), calendic (orange), jacaric (green), and catalpic (gold) acids relative to the rosiglitazone-occupied portion of the binding cavity (mesh surface) in the rigid PPARγ structure model. Key residues with which hydrogen bonding occurs are labeled. Atom-specific coloring: red = oxygen; gray = carbon; blue = nitrogen. Table 4 contains distance measurements for each docked pose.

The results suggested the depolarization pattern for ESA was similar to that seen with the rosiglitazone positive control with no significant difference between the two curves (Figure 2A).

An assessment of PPARγ activity modulation was conducted using RAW 264.7 cells and varying ESA concentrations (0–10 μM). Relative luciferase activity was measured to determine ligand-induced activation. The reporter assay suggested ESA does modulate PPARγ activity, but at a concentration 10-fold higher than the rosiglitazone control (Figure 2B), suggesting that there may be a difference in either potency or uptake by the cells between both compounds.

ESA ameliorated clinical signs of IBD

Under our DSS-induced IBD model, ESA significantly ameliorated IBD in mice with the wild phenotype (i.e., PPARγ-floxed). This observation was based on the significant difference between DAI for the last four days of the seven-day challenge (Figure 3). IBD-related disease phenotypes were milder in the ESA-fed PPARγ-expressing group of mice compared to the ESA-fed cell-specific PPARγ-null mice. The control groups (no ESA) for both genotypes showed no improvement in IBD phenotypes over the seven-day time course. Therefore, ESA was effective in ameliorating disease-associated phenotypes in mice with DSS colitis through a PPARγ-dependent mechanism.

Immunophenotypes for harvested tissues

Changes in immune cell subsets due to DSS-induced colitis were assessed in the harvested tissues to investigate the modulation of inflammation by ESA (Figure 4). Flow cytometry was used to characterize the phenotype of macrophages and T cell subsets. DSS augmented the percentages of monocytes or macrophages in the blood and spleen (Figure 4A and 4C). A significant increase in blood monocytes was found in ESA-treated mice. The PPARγ-expressing mice on the ESA diet exhibited a higher percentage of monocytes expressing lymphocyte antigen 6 complex-high (Ly6C^{hi}), which was not seen in the PPARγ-null group (Figure 4B) indicating a PPARγ dependency of this effect. Higher levels of IL-10 were observed in the spleen of the ESA-fed mice for both genotypes although these numerical differences were not statistically significant between the two diets for the PPARγ-expressing genotype (Figure 4D). Lastly, we found a numerical decrease in CD8$^+$ T-cells in the ESA diet group (Figure 4E), where the change was PPARγ-independent.

Histological trends mimicked clinical activity

There was a significant decrease in epithelial erosion (Figure 5A), mucosal thickness (Figure 5B), and immune cell infiltration (Figure 5C) in the ESA-fed PPARγ-expressing mice but not in ESA-fed PPARγ-null mice. This suggested amelioration of experimental IBD phenotypes by ESA is PPARγ-dependent. This agreed with the DAI data and further indicated an ESA-associated PPARγ-dependent improvement in IBD phenotypes.

Gene expression suggested PPARγ-dependent and -independent mechanisms

There was a marked decrease in IL-6 and VCAM-1 mRNA expression between the control- and ESA-fed PPARγ-expressing groups (Figure 6A and 6B). The IL-6 decrease appeared to be PPARγ-independent, while the VCAM-1 decrease was PPARγ-dependent. We also found a decrease in ICAM-1 expression between the control and ESA diet groups, but this decrease also occurred in the PPARγ-null mice suggesting ESA can induce ICAM-1 regulation in a PPARγ-independent manner (Figure 6C).

Discussion

The VS model protein structure and parameters used in this study allowed for prediction of docking conformations for

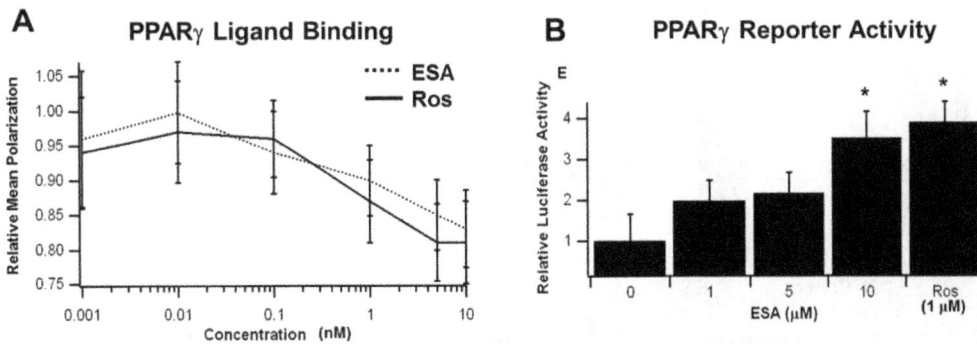

Figure 2. Ligand-binding (A) and reporter assay (B) results for ESA bound to PPARγ with rosiglitazone (Ros) as a positive control. (A) Ligand binding was assessed as a measure of mean polarization for the displaced Fluormone™ molecule versus increasing concentrations of either ligand. (B) Reporter activity was measured as relative luciferase activity for various concentrations of ESA versus 1 μM Ros. Error bars represent standard deviation, while asterisks (*) indicate significance ($p \leq 0.05$) between the data sets.

rosiglitazone-like and fatty acid compounds. The re-docking results for rosiglitazone, cross-docking results for PTG-1 and 9-HODE, and the conjugated triene docking all suggested 1ZGY is appropriate for screening fatty acids and TZD-like compounds. Potential for docking of fatty acid derivative partial agonists, like (2S)-ureidofibrate-like derivative, was also seen, but not fully assessed for this study as full agonism was the binding type of interest. Thus, we have successfully established a VS parameter set appropriate for a large-scale PPARγ full agonist search amongst fatty acids and fatty acid derivatives.

Information regarding interactions known to occur with PPARγ agonists is a suitable means to identify docking success. However, the success rate may be improved by incorporating even more criteria. Such criteria include a more extensive list of key interactions and/or establishment of distinct lists to specify interactions characteristic of each ligand category (e.g., full agonist, partial agonist, and antagonist). Based on the number of interactions and presence of interactions with key residues, we were able to determine which ligand types do and do not fit our selected target structure model. Combining this with RMSD data allowed us to see which types of ligands dock away from the binding cavity given the molecular environment of the selected target structure model. This information regarding ligands that would be excluded in a screen for compounds that interact similarly to what is seen with rosiglitazone can be used to identify one or more additional target structure models to incorporate into a large-scale screen. RMSD data, however, would not be available

from a screen of unknowns, and conclusions would therefore have to be drawn from the interaction and free energy data.

Due to the high degree of precision observed with the cross-docking ligands, it was determined that a single pose for each ligand would be sufficient for the initial analysis step in a large-scale screen. Replicates were necessary for the pre-screening analysis in which parameters and structure models were tested for predictability. Replicates are useful in docking studies to ensure any conclusions are based on consistent interactions. However, running replicates for a library numbering in the thousands is computationally time-consuming and less than practical given replicate poses may possess geometry that is exactly or close to the same. Rather than run replicates on the entire library of compounds, it would be feasible to run more detailed docking with compounds selected as successful binders of interest with the potential for experimental verification.

We observed a complementary relationship between the experimental ESA-IBD study and the computational screening results. In a recent review, we mentioned previous studies in which dual- or pan-agonistic effects have been associated with conjugated trienes [64]. This information, coupled with other published studies regarding synthetic agonists and inactive compounds, provided a means to develop and test computational methods for identifying natural agonists. Our docking analysis suggested ESA possessed a more favorable binding energy compared to the other conjugated trienes. Though comparative relationships have not been established between ESA and all the tested trienes, we do

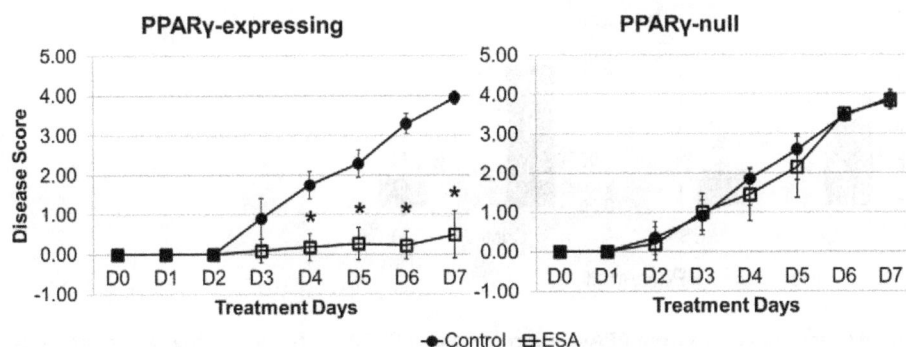

Figure 3. Effect of ESA on disease activity scores for PPARγ-expressing (A) and PPARγ-null (B) mice with experimental IBD. PPARγ-null refers to lack of functional PPARγ product in colon epithelial and immune cells only. Data points represent averaged disease scores for each group with error bars representing standard deviation. Asterisk (*) indicates significance ($p \leq 0.05$).

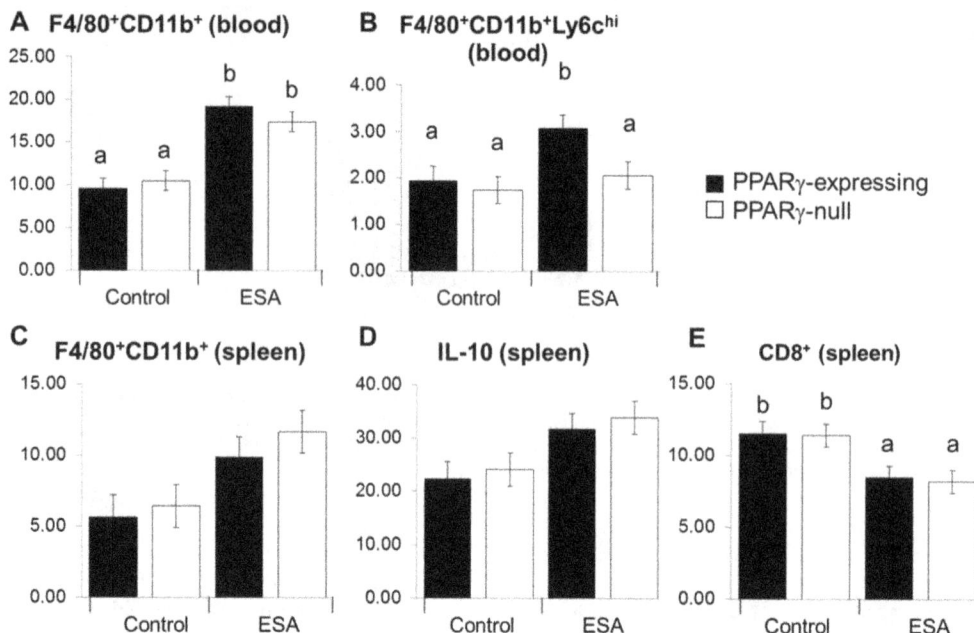

Figure 4. Effect of ESA on immune cell subsets of PPARγ-expression and PPARγ-null mice with experimental IBD. Tissues examined included blood (A and D) and spleen (B, C, and E). Values represent least square means for percentage of gated cells with error bars to indicate standard error. Letters indicate significance ($p \leq 0.05$) where a shared letter indicates groups which are not statistically significantly different.

know that ESA possesses greater antioxidant effects than punicic acid in mice [65]. It is plausible that the differences in efficacy between the compounds is interaction-related, which may result in conformational changes that attenuate co-activator recruitment and subsequent transcriptional regulation. The interaction aspect may have been picked up by our study, but the dynamic significance was not. This second aspect would require further computational testing to see if differences in protein stability and conformation can be detected between the protein-ligand complexes.

The ligand binding and reporter assays verified that ESA binds to and modulates PPARγ. Our docking study suggested fewer interactions occurred in the PPARγ-ESA complex compared to PPARγ-rosiglitazone. It is possible that the absence of interactions with S289 and H449 could result in a different level of ligand-

induced activity attenuation or the interactions with H323 and Y473 may be more important for fatty acid-induced agonism. Given the different levels of agonism, which is ligand-dependent, it is plausible that the specificity toward anti-inflammatory mechanisms observed as PPARγ-dependent in the pre-clinical trial were influenced by some difference in agonism specific to ESA. This notion is further supported by the absence of rosiglitazone-associated phenotypes seen in studies published by other groups [65,66]. Both the Shah et al. and Ramakers et al. studies involved testing rosiglitazone against DSS-induced colitis in mice [65,66]. Ramakers et al. showed weight gain in mice treated with rosiglitazone prior to DSS challenge, followed by significantly greater weight loss compared to the control after DSS challenge [66]. Increases in the severity of colitis-specific colon phenotypes were also seen, but with a decrease in inflammation [66]. The

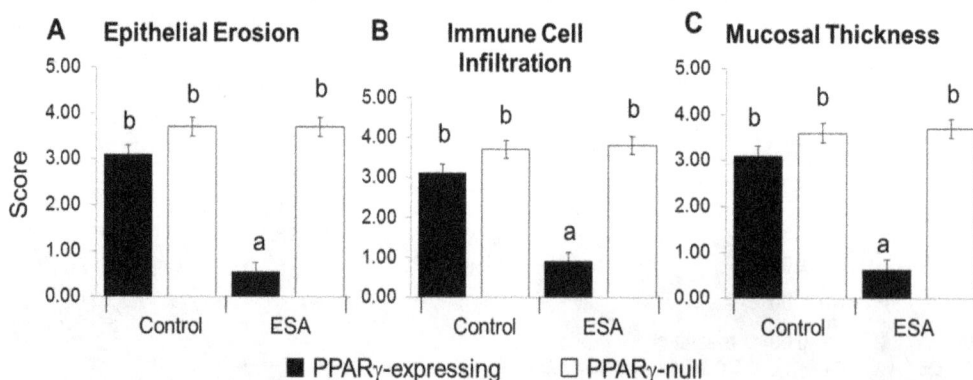

Figure 5. Effect of ESA on histopathological lesions in colons from PPARγ-expressing and PPARγ-null mice with experimental IBD. Epithelial erosion (Erosion) (A), immune cell infiltration (Infiltration) (B), and mucosal thickness (Thickness) (C) were assessed and averaged for all the DSS-treated group of samples. Data are presented as mean score with error bars to indicate standard deviation. Letters indicate significance ($p \leq 0.05$) where a shared letter indicates groups which are not statistically significantly different.

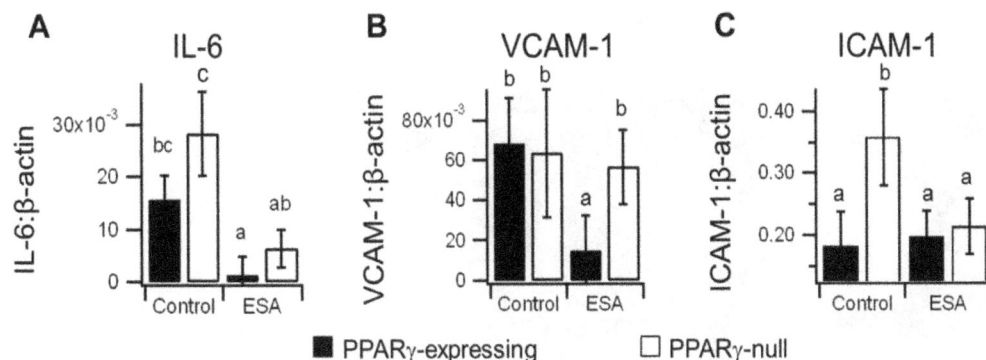

Figure 6. Effect of ESA on colonic concentrations of IL-6 (A), VCAM-1 (B), and ICAM-1 (C) in PPARγ-expressing and PPARγ-null mice with experimental IBD. The mean ratio of expression for each protein relative to constitutively expressed β-actin is shown with error bars to indicate standard deviation. Letters indicate significance ($p \leq 0.05$) where a shared letter indicates groups which are not statistically significantly different.

Shah et al. study indicated a PPARγ-dependent rosiglitazone-induced decrease in macrophage recruitment, but showed no other significant changes to the levels of other cytokines [65].

We have shown that the immune modulatory actions of ESA may be both PPARγ-dependent and PPARγ-independent in mice with experimental IBD, although its effects on disease activity and colonic lesions are dependent on expression of PPARγ by immune and epithelial cells. It is known that PPARγ is highly expressed in immune cells, intestinal epithelial cells (IECs), and adipocytes, with lower expression levels throughout various tissues of the body. Recently, our group published work in which the severity of IBD was tested in a mouse model for IEC-specific PPARγ deletion in a C57BL/6 background [67]. It was determined that the absence of PPARγ from IECs resulted in significantly worse disease scores, greater loss of body weight, and increased inflammation in the colon, spleen, and MLN compared to mice expressing PPARγ [67]. Further, it was concluded that the presence of PPARγ in IEC contributes to anti-inflammatory effects, regulation of immune cell distribution, and gene expression regulation necessary to counteract IBD symptoms [67].

Additionally, there are studies in which PPARγ expression and the effect of ESA on disease pathogenesis have been evaluated in breast cancer cell lines [27,68], pre-adipocytes [69], and colon cancer cell lines [70]. In all cases the fatty acid was capable of significantly ameliorating the disease via PPARγ-dependent responses such as induced apoptosis of cancer cells [27,68,70] and reduced lipid storage during differentiation [69]. Other conjugated trienes, such as punicic acid and catalpic acid [23,24] have shown reduced inflammation responses in cancer, cardiovascular disease [71], and obesity [23,24,71]. All of these studies are strong examples of how PPARγ mediates inflammatory, metabolic, proliferation, signal transduction, and cellular motility processes [67] in various cell types.

It is possible that the presence of other nuclear receptors in the cells play a role in ESA-mediated effects. PPARδ in the colon may play a role in ESA-mediated IBD amelioration given the possibility of dual-agonist and pan-agonist modulation seen with PPARs, and the ability of all three PPARs to accommodate fatty acids. Further computational and experimental tests would be necessary to determine whether ESA mediates both PPARγ and PPARδ transcriptional regulation, which has been previously described for CLA [72]. The anti-inflammatory responses induced by ESA, which appeared to be PPARγ-independent, might also be attributed to other unforeseen targets in the system. For instance,

we previously described the potential of PPARγ agonists to bind to lanthionine synthetase component C-like protein 2 (LANCL2) [60]. Such an association is one proposed molecular mechanism of regulating disease-related inflammatory effects in a PPARγ-independent manner.

Beyond what is seen in IBD, it has been shown that ESA binds to and activates estrogen receptors in breast cancer cell lines [73]. It is also known that hepatocyte nuclear factor-4α (HNF4α), which is essential for maintaining lipid homeostasis via gene regulation and regulating hepatocyte differentiation, is activated by fatty acids [74]. It has been suggested that PPARα ligands can interfere with HNF4α activity [75], but the mechanism by which this occurs is not fully understood. As conjugated trienes like punicic acid activate PPARα in adipocytes [24], and PPARα and fatty acids are present in liver tissue also, it seems feasible that conjugated trienes could come in contact with and bind HNF4α as well. To our knowledge such a study involving HNF4α and ESA or any other conjugated trienes has not been conducted.

The ability of the binding cavity to accommodate many different ligand types represents a major technical obstacle when performing computational docking into PPARγ as a therapeutic target. The issue stems from the dynamic nature of the binding cavity and changes in protein conformation necessary to accommodate different agonists. This dynamic nature is not possible with rigid macromolecule docking techniques, and incorporation of flexibility can be difficult given the number of residues that can possess variable positions and the number of possible rotamers for each residue. The rigidity of crystal structures combined with the variability of residue side chain positions proved an issue for docking non-native ligands to the selected structure model. For example, the docked poses for farglitazar across the three protein structure models examined in the cross-docking step reflected a lack of appropriate molecular volume at the rear of the binding pocket to accommodate the benzyl ketone group on the ligand (Figure 7A). When the three structure models were compared to the 1FM9 crystal structure in which farglitazar was co-crystallized, the space necessary to accommodate the benzyl ketone group of farglitazar was missing given the differences in the side chain positions for Phe282 and Phe363 (Figure 7B). These residues do not pose an issue for rosiglitazone docking, but occupied the portion of the cavity in which farglitazar should have docked, which prevented successful cross-docking of this compound to the selected structure models. As such, selection of a single model to appropriately accommodate

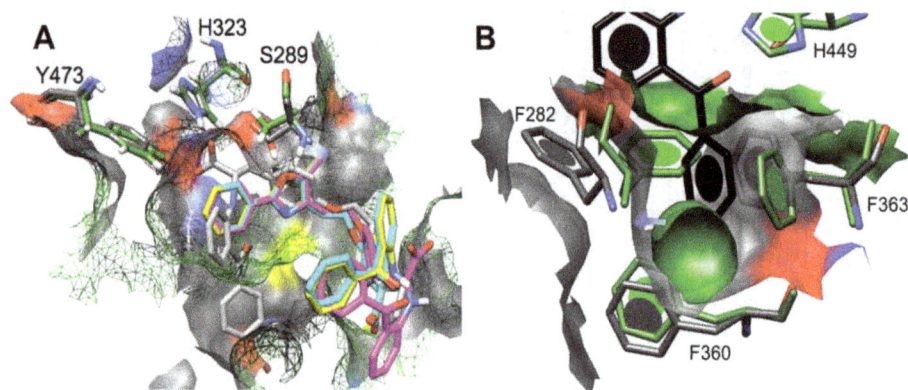

Figure 7. Visual assessments of molecular surface differences that result in unsuccessful docking of specific ligand types to the selected PPARγ structure model. Farglitazar is represented in both panels with atom-specific coloring. (A) 1ZGY and 1FM9 surface representations are green mesh and solid gray, respectively. The three poses predicted for farglitazar relative to 1ZGY are shown in magenta, cyan, and yellow. (B) Side chain rotamers for F282 and F363 are responsible for the differences in cavity surface at the rear of the cavity. Surface colors for 1ZGY and 1FM9 are the same as in (A). Atom-specific coloring: gray/black = carbon, blue = nitrogen, red = oxygen, white = hydrogen, and yellow = sulfur.

a narrow range of ligands and selection of several models to use with a diverse ligand library are two avenues toward identifying PPARγ agonists *in silico*. The first technique is used widely, but the second is not as common due to the amount of time necessary to properly identify target structure models. Given the molecular exclusion of the more hydrophobic compounds in our small-scale screen, the second technique would be ideal for dealing with a diverse library, such as the one we have constructed. Therefore, further testing with additional protein structure models capable of accommodating bulkier and more hydrophobic compounds would be necessary.

An additional technique for improving predictability is molecular dynamics simulation and analysis, which is also extremely time consuming and can prove problematic since parameters for ligands must be developed. Conformational sampling of the PPARγ binding cavity via MD is one means of gleaning useful information in a relatively short amount of time. This technique would provide information about predominant conformations adopted by PPARγ that would aid in the selection of multiple target structure models for docking, and can be easily verified by the large number of available crystal structures.

PPARγ has proven a difficult protein to explore as a drug target given dynamic and specificity issues. The large binding cavity and ability of the protein to accommodate a wide range of compounds presents an issue for rigid docking screening. The ability of the protein to bind compounds of different compound families requires a degree of ligand diversity that is often not employed in conventional VS studies. As a means to improve our method, we are currently testing additional PPARγ crystal structures as docking targets. As a consequence of this study, we have established a need for at least one additional target structure model that can accommodate bulker compounds. An analysis of MD simulations for unbound active, bound active, and unbound inactive forms of PPARγ are ongoing. These simulations, combined with further analysis of available crystal structure models, will allow us to develop additional target structure models. Incorporating conformational variability by screening against multiple protein conformations of the same protein should improve our screening process. We propose matching ligand and protein pharmacophores prior to screening to reduce the incidence of screening ligands against a protein structure into

which the ligands cannot fit or where the charge environment is inappropriate.

The diversity of our compound database is being expanded as well, and will include an extensive list of known PPARγ agonists, decoy compounds that mimic known agonist structure but are inactive toward PPARγ, drugs currently available for treatment of other diseases, and extracts tested experimentally for PPARγ modulation. Such a library would improve enrichment, which is part of the separation of binders from non-binders. Further, inclusion of a weighting system based on the occurrence of known interactions would improve the separation process. With a diverse library in which available therapeutics are included, it may be possible to identify lesser known drug interactions with PPARγ linked to side effects seen with patients taking medications for cancer and neurological diseases. Given the success of our current study and the pending improvements to our method for testing of diverse ligand types, we are making progress toward an extensive and highly effective means to computationally identify feasible PPARγ-targeted drug candidates. Ideally, the established methods could be applied to the other PPARs, other nuclear hormone receptors, and alternate protein family targets where similar considerations must be made.

This study exemplifies how experimental methods can be used to complement and verify computational predictions. We have demonstrated that it is possible to predict ligand association given information known about the binding cavity of the target. We have also established a means to reduce the need for researcher intervention in assessing successful binding by incorporating a search for key interactions. More specifically, we have successfully established a protocol for screening fatty acid compounds against PPARγ for agonism, and were able to predict that ESA and other conjugated trienes would bind to and activate PPARγ using molecular docking. These predictions have been verified through *in vitro* assays both here and in our previous work [24,34]. *In vivo* efficacy was assessed as well to determine if disease-associated benefits could be seen given the activation of PPARγ by ESA. In this regard, ESA did induce both PPARγ-dependent and -independent responses that ameliorated disease activity and intestinal lesions in IBD. The scope of this work implies the techniques described here can aid in streamlining drug discovery and development techniques as the technology develops.

Supporting Information

Figure S1 Colored ribbon representation of PPARγ showing three layers of helical "sandwich", and co-crystallized rosiglitazone (PDB ID 1FM6 [40]). Helices for each layer are colored, with helix H12, which sits at the rear of the binding cavity (AF-2 region), colored in red. Rosiglitazone is colored in green, with oxygen, nitrogen, and sulfur atoms colored red, blue, and yellow, respectively. The insert (upper right) shows a close-up view of the molecular surface of the binding cavity. The thiazolidinedione head group of rosiglitazone sits at the rear of the binding cavity where it can interact with S289, H323, H449, and Y473 in order to change the conformation of the AF-2 region and activate the protein.

Table S1 List of ligands used for virtual screening.

Table S2 List of atoms for key residues common to selected rosiglitazone crystal structures used to assess potential interactions between docked poses and the protein structure model.

Table S3 List of atoms for key residues common to selected fatty acid-bound crystal structures used to assess potential interactions between docked poses and the protein structure model.

Table S4 List of atoms for key residues common to rosiglitazone- and fatty acid-containing PDB structures used to assess potential interactions between docked poses and the protein structure model.

Table S5 Predicted hydrophobic and hydrogen bond interactions for ligands in cross-docking test set relative to a reference list of interactions common to rosiglitazone and selected fatty acids. Poses were taken from docking of each ligand into each of the three listed PPARγ PDB files (top row). Ligand IDs refer to compounds listed in Table 3.

Table S6 Presence or absence of potential hydrogen bond interactions between indicated residues of selected protein structure models and replicate poses of ligands listed by ID. A single "x" indicates one potential interaction for the listed residue was found for the specified ligand, whereas more than one "x" indicates more than one interaction (e.g., "xx" indicates two interactions found). (N = 3)

Table S7 Predicted hydrophobic and hydrogen bond interactions for ligands in small-scale screening test set relative to a reference list of interactions common to rosiglitazone and selected fatty acids (Table S4). Poses were taken from docking of each ligand into each of the three listed PPARγ PDB files (top row). Predicted free energy of binding is listed as kcal/mol.

Table S8 Presence or absence of potential hydrogen bond interactions between indicated residues of selected protein structure models (top row) and ligand poses. A single "x" indicates one potential interaction for the listed residue was found for the specified ligand, whereas more than one "x" indicates more than one interaction (e.g., "xx" indicates two interactions found).

Table S9 Predicted free energy of binding and interaction counts for conjugated trienes. Docking was performed using AD4 with three top-binding replicates for each ligand (150 total conformations). The highest energy conformation with the highest number of hydrogen bonds was used for analysis in Table 4.

Formulas S1

Author Contributions

Conceived and designed the experiments: SNL JB-R RH DRB. Performed the experiments: SNL LB AJG PL. Analyzed the data: SNL AJG RH JB-R DRB. Contributed reagents/materials/analysis tools: SNL JB-R. Wrote the paper: SNL JB-R DRB.

References

1. Wahli W (2008) A gut feeling of the PXR, PPAR, and NF-kB connection. Journal of Internal Medicine 263: 613–619.
2. Dubuquoy L, Rousseaux C, Thuru X, Peyrin-Biroulet L, Romano O, et al. (2006) PPARγ as a new therapeutic target in inflammatory bowel diseases. Gut 55: 1341–1349.
3. Gani OABSM, Sylte I (2009) Molecular recognition of long chain fatty acids by peroxisome proliferator-activated receptor α. Medicinal Chemistry Research 18: 8–19.
4. Guri AJ, Hontecillas R, Ferrer G, Casagran O, Wankhade U, et al. (2008) Loss of PPARγ in immune cells impairs the ability of abscisic acid to improve insulin sensitivity by suppressing monocyte chemoattractant protein-1 expression and macrophage infiltration into white adipose tissue. Journal of Nutritional Biochemistry 19: 216–228.
5. Huang TH-W, Teoh AW, Lin B-L, Lin DS-H, Roufogalis B (2009) The role of herbal PPAR modulators in the treatment of cardiometabolic syndrome. Pharmacological Research 60: 195–206.
6. Reiss AB, Vagell ME (2006) PPARγ Activity in the Vessel Wall: Anti-Atherogenic Properties. Current Medicinal Chemistry 13: 3227–3238.
7. Wu GD (2003) Is There a Role for PPARgamma in IBD? Yes, No, Maybe. Gastroenterology 124: 1538–1542.
8. Bassaganya-Riera J, Reynolds K, Martino-Catt S, Cui Y, Hennighausen L, et al. (2004) Activation of PPARγ and δ by Conjugated Linoleic Acid Mediates Protection From Experimental Inflammatory Bowel Disease. Gastroenterology 127: 777–791.
9. Martin H (2009) Role of PPAR-gamma in inflammataion. Prospects for therapeutic intervention by food components. Mutation Research/Fundamental and Molecular Mechanisms of Mutagenesis 669: 1–7.
10. Tontonoz P, Spiegelman BM (2008) Fat and Beyond: The Diverse Biology of PPARγ. Annual Review of Biochemistry 77: 289–312.
11. Ricote M, Li A, Willson TM, Kelly C, Glass C (1998) The peroxisome proliferator-activated receptor-gamma is a negative regulator of macrophage activation. Nature 391: 79–82.
12. Ljung T, Karlen P, Schmidt D, Hellstrom PM, Lapidus A, et al. (2004) Infliximab in inflammtory bowel disease: clinical outcome in a population based cohort from Stockholm County. Gut 53: 849–853.
13. Hanauer SB, Feagan BG, Lichtenstein GR, Mayer LF, Schreiber S, et al. (2002) Maintenance infliximab for Crohn's disease: the ACCENT I randomised trail. The Lancet 359: 1541–1549.
14. Goldsmith P, McGarity M, Walls AF, Church MK, Millward-Sadler GH, et al. (1990) Corticosteroid treatment reduces mast cell numbers in inflammatory bowel disease. Digestive Diseases and Sciences 35: 1409–1413.
15. Lichtenstein GR, Abreu MT, Cohen R, Tremaine W (2006) American Gastroenterological Association Institute Technical Review on Corticosteroids, Immunomodulators, and Infliximab in Inflammatory Bowel Disease. Gastroenterology 130: 940–987.
16. Compston JE (1995) Review article: osteoporosis, corticosteroids, and inflammatory bowel disease. Alimentary Pharmacology & Therapeutics 9: 237–250.
17. Lewis JD, Lichtenstein GR, Deren JJ, Sands BE, Hanauer SB, et al. (2008) Rosiglitazone for Active Ulcerative Colitis: A Randomized Placebo-Controlled Trial. Gastroenterology 134: 688–659.
18. Nesto RW, Bell D, Bonow RO, Fonseca V, Grundy SM, et al. (2003) Thiazolidinedione Use, Fluid Retention, and Congestive Heart Failure. Circulation 108: 2941–2948.
19. Bassaganya-Riera J, Hontecillas R (2006) CLA and n-3 PUFA differentially modulate clinical activity and colonic PPAR-responsive gene expression in a pig model of experimental IBD. Clinical Nutrition 25: 454–465.
20. Guri AJ, Hontecillas R, Bassaganya-Riera J (2010) Abscisic acid ameliorates experimental IBD by downregulating cellular adhesion molecule expression and suppressing immune cell infiltration. Clinical Nutrition 29: 824–831.
21. Hontecillas R, Wannemeulher M, Zimmerman D, Hutto D, Wilson J, et al. (2002) Nutritional regulation of porcine bacterial-induced colitis by conjugated linoleic acid. Journal of Nutrition 132: 2019–2027.

22. Klebe G (2006) Virtual ligand screening: strategies, perspectives and limitations. Drug Discovery Today 11: 580–594.

23. Hontecillas R, Diguardo M, Duran E, Orpi M, Bassaganya-Riera J (2008) Catalpic acid decreases abdominal fat deposition, improves glucose homeostasis and upregulates PPAR alpha expression in adipose tissue. Clinical Nutrition 27: 764–772.

24. Hontecillas R, O'Shea M, Einerhand A, Diguardo M, Bassaganya-Riera J (2009) Activation of PPAR(gamma) and (alpha) by Punicic Acid Ameliorates Glucose Tolerance and Suppresses Obesity-Related Inflammation. Journal of the American College of Nutrition 28: 184–195.

25. Badami R, Patil K (1980) Structure and occurrence of unusual fatty acids in minor seed oils. Progress in Lipid Research 19: 119–153.

26. Tsuzuki T, Kawakami Y (2008) Tumor angiogenesis suppression by alpha-eleostearic acid, a linoleic acid isomer with a conjugated triene system, via peroxizome proliferator-activated receptor gamma. Carcinogenesis 29: 797–806.

27. Moon H-S, Guo D-D, Lee H-G, Choi Y-J, Kang J-S, et al. (2009) Alpha-eleostearic acid suppresses proliferation of MCF-7 breast cancer cells via activation of PPARγ and inhibition of ERK1/2. Cancer Science 101: 396–402.

28. Tsuzuki T, Tokuyama Y, Igarashi M, Miyazawa T (2004) Tumor growth suppression by α-eleostearic acid, a linoleic acid isomer with a conjugated triene system, via lipid peroxidation. Carcinogenesis 25: 1417–1425.

29. Eom J-M, Seo M-J, Baek J-Y, Chu H, Han SH, et al. (2009) Alpha-eleostearic acid induces autophagy-dependent cell death through targeting AKT/mTOR and ERK1/2 signal together with the generation of reactive oxygen species. Biochemical and Biophysical Research Communications 391: 903–908.

30. Yuan G-F, Wahlqvist ML, Yuan J-Q, Wang Q-M, Li D (2009) Effect of Punicic Acid Naturally Occuring in Food on Lipid Peroxidation in Healthy Young Humans. Journal of the Science of Food and Agriculture 89: 2331–2335.

31. Boussetta T, Raad H, Letteron P, Gougerot-Pocidalo M-A, Marie J-C, et al. (2009) Punicic Acid a Conjugated Linolenic Acid Inhibits TNFα-Induced Neutrophil Hyperactivation and Protects from Experimental Colon Inflammation in Rats. PLoS One 4.

32. Vroegrijk I, van Diepen J, van den Berg S, Westbroek I, Keizer H, et al. (2011) Pomegranate seed oil, punicic acid prevents diet-induced obesity and insulin resistance in mice. Food and Chemical Toxicology;In press.

33. Meerts IA, Verspeek-Rip CM, Buskens CA, Keizer HG, Bassaganya-Riera J, et al. (2009) Toxicology evaluation of pomegranate seed oil. Food and Chemical Toxicology 47: 1085–1092.

34. Bassaganya-Riera J, Diguardo M, Climent M, Vives C, Carbo A, et al. (2011) Activation of PPAR γ and δ by dietary punicic acid ameliorates intestinal inflammation in mice. British Journal of Nutrition;In Press.

35. Saha SS, Ghosh M (2009) Comparative study of antioxidant activity of a-eleostearic acid and punicic acid against oxidative stress generated by sodium arsenite. Food and Chemical Toxicology 47: 2551–2556.

36. Morris GM, Goodsell DS, Halliday RS, Huey R, Hart WE, et al. (1998) Automated docking using a Lamarckian genetic algorithm and an empirical binding free energy function. Journal of Computational Chemistry 19: 1639–1662.

37. Trott O, Olson AJ (2010) AutoDock Vina: Improving the Speed and Accuracy of Docking with a New Scoring Function, Efficient Optimization, and Multithreading. Journal of Computational Chemistry 31: 455–461.

38. Berman HM, Battistuz T, Bhat TN, Bluhm W, Bourne PE, et al. (2002) The Protein Data Bank. Acta Crystallographica Section D: Biological Crystallography D58: 899–907.

39. Berman HM, Westbrook J, Feng Z, Gilliland G, Bhat TN, et al. (2000) The Protein Data Bank. Nucleic Acids Research 28: 235–242.

40. Gampe RT, Montana VG, Lambert MH, Miller AB, Bledsoe RK, et al. (2000) Asymmetry in the PPARg/RXRa Crystal Structure Reveals the Molecular Basis of Heterodimerization among Nuclear Receptors. Molecular Cell 5: 545–555.

41. van der Spoel D, Lindahl E, Hess B, van Buuren AR, Apol E, et al. (2005) Gromacs User Manual version 3.3.

42. Nolte RT, Wisely GB, Westin S, Cobb JE, Lambert MH, et al. (1998) Ligand binding and co-activator assembly of the peroxisome proliferator-activated receptor-γ. Nature 395: 137–143.

43. Li Y, Kovach A, Suino-Powell K, Martynowski D, Xu HE (2008) Structural and biochemical basis for the binding selectivity of peroxisome proliferator-activated receptor gamma to PGC-1alpha. Journal of Biological Chemistry 283: 19132–19139.

44. Chandra V, Huang P, Hamuro Y, Raghuram S, Wang Y, et al. (2008) Structure of the intact PPAR-γ-RXR-α nuclear receptor complex on DNA. Nature 456: 350–357.

45. Pettersen E, Goddard T, Huang C, Couch G, Greenblatt D, et al. (2004) UCSF Chimera—a visualization system for exploratory research and analysis. Journal of Computational Chemistry 25: 1605–1612.

46. Mahindroo N, Wang C-C, Liao C-C, Huang C-F, Lu I-L, et al. (2006) Indol-1-yl Acetic Acids as Peroxisome Proliferator-Activated Receptor Agonists: Design, Synthesis, Structural Biology, and Molecular Docking Studies. Journal of Medicinal Chemistry 49: 1212–1216.

47. Mahindroo N, Peng Y-H, Lin C-H, Tan UK, Prakash E, et al. (2006) Structural basis for the structure-activity relationships of peroxisome proliferator-activated receptor agonists. Journal of Medicinal Chemistry 49: 6421–6424.

48. Pochetti G, Godio C, Mitro N, Caruso D, Galmozzi A, et al. (2007) Insights into the Mechanism of Partial Agonism: Crystal Structures of the Peroxisome Proliferator-Activated Receptor γ Ligand-Binding Domain in the Complex with Two Enantiomeric Ligands. Journal of Biological Chemistry 282: 17314–17324.

49. Itoh T, Louise F, Amin K, Inaba Y, Szanto A, et al. (2008) Structural basis for the activation of PPARγ by oxidized fatty acids. Nature Structural & Molecular Biology 15: 924–931.

50. Artis DR, Lin JJ, Wang W, Mehra U, Perreault M, et al. (2009) Scaffold-based discovery of indeglitazar, a PPAR pan-active anti-diabetic agent. PNAS 106: 262–267.

51. Waku T, Shiraki T, Oyama T, Fujimoto Y, Maebara K, et al. (2009) Structural Insight into PPARγ Activation Through Covalent Modification with Endogenous Fatty Acids. Journal of Molecular Biology 385: 188–199.

52. Salam NK, Huang TH-W, Kota BP, Kim MS, Li Y, et al. (2008) Novel PPAR-gamma Agonists Identified from a Natural Product Library: A Virtual Screening, Induced-Fit Docking and Biological Assay Study. Chemical Biology & Drug Design 71: 57–70.

53. Tanrikulu Y, Rau O, Schwarz O, Proschak E, Siems K, et al. (2009) Structure-Based Pharmacophore Screening for Natural-Product-Derived PPARγ Agonists. ChemBIoChem 10: 75–78.

54. Kuroda M, Mimaki Y, Honda S, Tanaka H, Yokota S, et al. (2010) Phenolics from Glycyrrhiza glabra roots and their PPAR-γ ligand-binding activity. Bioorganic & Medicinal Chemistry 18: 962–970.

55. Markt P, Schuster D, Kirchmair J, Laggner C, Langer T (2007) Pharmacophore modeling and parallel screening for PPAR ligands. Journal of Computer-Aided Molecular Design 21: 575–590.

56. Schuettelkopf A, van Aalten D (2004) PRODRG - a tool for high-throughput crystallography of protein-ligand complexes. Acta Crystallographica D60: 1355–1363.

57. Kellenberger E, Rodrigo J, Muller P, Rognan D (2004) Comparative Evaluation of Eight Docking Tools for Docking and Virtual Screening Accuracy. Proteins 57.

58. Moreland JL, Gramada A, Buzko OV, Zhang Q, Bourne PE (2005) The Molecular Biology Toolkit (MBT): a modular platform for developing molecular visualization applications. BMC Bioinformatics 6: 1–7.

59. Schwartz RL, Phoenix T, Foy BD (2008) Learning Perl. 5th ed ed: O'Reilly Media, Inc.

60. Bassaganya-Riera J, Guri AJ, Lu P, Climent M, Carbo A, et al. (2011) Abscisic Acid Regulates Inflammation via Ligand-Binding Domain-Independent Activation of PPAR gamma. Journal of Biological Chemistry 286: 2504–2516.

61. Guri AJ, Hontecillas R, Si H, Liu D, Bassaganya-Riera J (2007) Dietary abscisic acid ameliorates glucose tolerance and obesity-related inflammation in db/db mice fed high-fat diests. Clinical Nutrition 26: 107–116.

62. Bassaganya-Riera J, Ferrer G, Casagran O, Sanchez S, de Horna A, et al. (2009) F4/80hiCCR2hi macrophage infiltration into the intra-abdominal fat worsens the severity of experimental IBD in obese mice and DSS colitis. e-SPEN, European e-Journal of Clinical Nutrition and Metabolism 4: e90–e97.

63. Chang MW, Ayeni C, Breuer S, Torbett BE (2010) Virtual Screening for HIV Protease Inhibitors: A Comparison of AutoDock 4 and Vina. PLoS One 5: e11955.

64. Bassaganya-Riera J, Guri AJ, Hontecillas R (2011) Treatment of Obesity-Related Complications with Novel Classes of Naturally Occurring PPAR Agonists. Journal of Obesity. pp 1–7.

65. Shah Y, Morimura K, Gonzalez F (2007) Expression of peroxisome proliferator-activated receptor-gamma in macrophage suppresses experimentally induced colitis. American Journal of Physiology, Gastrointestinal and Liver Physiology 292: G657–666.

66. Ramakers JD, Verstege MI, Thuijls G, Te Velde AA, Mensink RP, et al. (2007) The PPARg Agonist Rosiglitazone impairs colonic inflammation in mice with experimental colitis. Journal of Clinical Immunology 27: 275–283.

67. Mohapatra SK, Guri AJ, Climent M, Vives C, Carbo A, et al. (2010) Immunoregulatory Actions of Epithelial Cell PPARγ at the Colonic Mucosa of Mice with Experimental Inflammatory Bowel Disease. PLoS One 5: e10215.

68. Zhang T, Gao Y, Mao Y, Zhang Q, Lin C, et al. (2011) Growth inhibition and apoptotic effect of alpha-eleostearic acid on human breast cancer cells. Journal of Natural Medicines. pp 1–8.

69. Popovich DG, Lee Y, Li L, Zhang W (2011) Momordica charantia Seed Extract Reduced Pre-Adipocyte Viability, Affects Lactate Dehydrogenase Release, and Lipid Accumulation in 3T3-L1 Cells. Journal of Medicinal Food 14: 201–208.

70. Yasui Y, Hosokawa M, Sahara T, Suzuki R, Ohgiya S, et al. (2005) Bitter gourd seed fatty acid rich in 9c, 11t, 13t-conjugated linolenic acid induces apoptosis and up-regulates the GADD45, p53, and PPARγ in human colon cancer Caco-2 cells. Prostaglandins, Leukotrienes, and Essential Fatty Acids 73: 113–119.

71. Hennessy AA, Ross RP, Devery R, Stanton C (2011) The Health Promoting Properties of the Conjugated Isomers of α-Linoleic Acid. Lipids 46: 105–119.

72. Bassaganya-Riera J, Reynolds K, Martino-Catt S, Cui Y, Hennighausen L, et al. (2004) Activation of PPAR gamma and delta by conjugated linoleic acid mediates protection from experimental inflammatory bowel disease. Gastroenterology 127: 777–791.

73. Tran HNA, Bae S-Y, Song B-H, Lee B-H, Bae Y-S, et al. (2010) Pomegranate (Punica granatum) seed linolenic acid isomers: Concentration-dependent modulation of estrogen receptor activity. Endocrin Research 35: 1–16.

74. Hayhurst GP, Lee Y-H, Lambert G, Ward JM, Gonzalez FJ (2001) Hepatocyte Nuclear Factor 4a (Nuclear Receptor 2A1) is Essential for Maintenance of Hepatic Gene Expression and Lipid Homeostasis. Molecular and Cellular Biology 21: 1393–1403.

75. Nagao K, Yanagita T (2008) Bioactive lipids in metabolic syndrome. Progress in Lipid Research 47: 127–146.

14

Immunoregulatory Actions of Epithelial Cell PPAR γ at the Colonic Mucosa of Mice with Experimental Inflammatory Bowel Disease

Saroj K. Mohapatra, Amir J. Guri, Montse Climent, Cristina Vives, Adria Carbo, William T. Horne, Raquel Hontecillas*, Josep Bassaganya-Riera*

Nutritional Immunology and Molecular Nutrition Laboratory, Virginia Bioinformatics Institute, Virginia Polytechnic Institute and State University, Blacksburg, Virginia, United States of America

Abstract

Background: Peroxisome proliferator-activated receptors are nuclear receptors highly expressed in intestinal epithelial cells (IEC) and immune cells within the gut mucosa and are implicated in modulating inflammation and immune responses. The objective of this study was to investigate the effect of targeted deletion of PPAR γ in IEC on progression of experimental inflammatory bowel disease (IBD).

Methodology/Principal Findings: In the first phase, PPAR γ flfl; Villin Cre- (VC-) and PPAR γ flfl; Villin Cre+ (VC+) mice in a mixed FVB/C57BL/6 background were challenged with 2.5% dextran sodium sulfate (DSS) in drinking water for 0, 2, or 7 days. VC+ mice express a transgenic recombinase under the control of the Villin-Cre promoter that causes an IEC-specific deletion of PPAR γ. In the second phase, we generated VC- and VC+ mice in a C57BL/6 background that were challenged with 2.5% DSS. Mice were scored on disease severity both clinically and histopathologically. Flow cytometry was used to phenotypically characterize lymphocyte and macrophage populations in blood, spleen and mesenteric lymph nodes. Global gene expression analysis was profiled using Affymetrix microarrays. The IEC-specific deficiency of PPAR γ in mice with a mixed background worsened colonic inflammatory lesions, but had no effect on disease activity (DAI) or weight loss. In contrast, the IEC-specific PPAR γ null mice in C57BL/6 background exhibited more severe inflammatory lesions, DAI and weight loss in comparison to their littermates expressing PPAR γ in IEC. Global gene expression profiling revealed significantly down-regulated expression of lysosomal pathway genes and flow cytometry results demonstrated suppressed production of IL-10 by CD4+ T cells in mesenteric lymph nodes (MLN) of IEC-specific PPAR γ null mice.

Conclusions/Significance: Our results demonstrate that adequate expression of PPAR γ in IEC is required for the regulation of mucosal immune responses and prevention of experimental IBD, possibly by modulation of lysosomal and antigen presentation pathways.

Editor: Stefan Bereswill, Charité-Universitätsmedizin Berlin, Germany

Funding: This research was funded by a Virginia Bioinformatics Institute exploratory grant. The funders had no role in study design, data collection and analysis, decision to publish, or preparation of the manuscript.

Competing Interests: The authors have declared that no competing interests exist.

* E-mail: rmagarzo@vt.edu (RH); jbassaga@vt.edu (JB-R)

Introduction

Inflammatory bowel disease (IBD), with its two clinical manifestations Crohn's Disease (CD) and Ulcerative Colitis (UC), is a chronic gastrointestinal disorder associated with disruption of the balance between gut commensal bacteria and host responses at the mucosa. The mucosal barrier consists of epithelial tight junctions regulated by cytokines and the underlying immune cell network. Damage to the mucosal barrier is considered sufficient for causing intestinal inflammation. On the other hand, commensal bacteria dampen inflammation via nucleocytoplasmic redistribution of peroxisome proliferator-activated receptor (PPAR) γ and RelA subunit of transcription factor NF-κB [1]. A working model of IBD starts with alterations of the epithelial barrier followed by innate immune responses against the gut microbiota. Later changes involving lymphocytes drive the tissue damage associated with the disease [1].

PPAR γ, a member of the nuclear receptor group of transcription factors, not only regulates lipid and carbohydrate metabolism, but has been recognized as playing an important role in the immune response through its ability to down-modulate the expression of inflammatory cytokines and to direct immune cell differentiation towards anti-inflammatory phenotypes [2,3]. PPAR γ is highly expressed in the intestinal epithelium, immune cells and adipocytes, and regulates a number of genes participating in metabolism, proliferation, signal transduction, and cellular motility [4].

In an experimental model of IBD, activation of PPAR γ by conjugated linoleic acid, abscisic acid or other agonists suppresses gut inflammatory lesions, weight loss and inflammatory mediator expression [4,5,6,7,8]. Most notably, the PPAR γ agonist rosiglitazone showed therapeutic efficacy in humans with UC [9,10]. However, rosiglitazone and other drugs belonging to the thiazolidinedione (TZD) class of anti-diabetic drugs are unlikely to be adopted for the treatment of IBD because of their significant side effects (i.e., fluid retention, hepatotoxicity, weight gain and congestive heart failure) and a U.S. Food and Drug Administration (FDA)-mandated "black box warning" for rosiglitazone and pioglitazone. Thus, understanding the role of PPAR γ in each cell type involved in the pathogenesis of IBD is critical for the informed development of novel, safer and more efficacious therapeutic and prophylactic agents against IBD. We have previously used a cre-lox recombination system to characterize the immune modulatory actions of PPAR γ in mice with a targeted deletion in both immune and epithelial cells (i.e., MMTV-Cre) [3,8] or T cells (i.e., CD4-Cre) [11]. Others have shown that mice lacking PPAR γ in the colonic epithelium displayed increased susceptibility to dextran sodium sulfate (DSS)-induced experimental IBD, histological lesions and elevated levels of the pro-inflammatory cytokines IL-6, IL-1β, TNF-α [12]. The objective of this study was to use a systems approach for investigating the underlying mechanisms by which the deletion of PPAR γ in IEC modulates the severity of experimental IBD, immune cell distribution and global gene expression.

Results

Effect of the deficiency of PPAR γ in IEC and mouse strain on susceptibility to DSS-induced colitis

To examine the affect of IEC-specific PPAR γ deficiency and mouse strain on colitis severity VC+ and VC- mice in a mixed FVB/C57BL/6 background were treated with 2.5% DSS for 0, 2, or 7 days. Figure 1A illustrates the deletion of PPAR γ in the duodenum, jejunum, ileum, cecum and colon of VC+ mice as well as in IEC isolated from these tissues (Figure 1B). The results show that the deletion is more efficient in the large intestine (i.e., cecum and colon), compared to small intestine. Unlike findings reported by Adachi and colleagues, we found no significant differences in disease activity (DAI) or body weight loss between groups (Figure 2A-B). However, the targeted deletion of IEC PPAR γ in mice with a C57BL/6 background resulted in significant weight loss and disease activity in comparison to mice expressing PPAR γ in IEC (Figures 2C-D).

Despite there being no significant differences in either disease activity or body weight between FVB VC- and FVB VC+ mice, there were significant differences observed at the histopathological level. FVB VC+ mice had significantly greater leukocyte infiltration, and erosion of the mucosal epithelium was significantly worsened in comparison to the control VC- mice (Figure 3). VC+ mice with a pure C57BL/6 background showed significantly greater signs of macroscopic inflammation in the spleen, colon, and MLN than VC- mice (Figures 3F-H). In line with the DAI the enhanced inflammation was evident at day 2 and was significantly exacerbated at day 7 of the DSS challenge.

Mice expressing PPAR γ in IEC have greater percentages of CD4+IL10+ T cells in MLN

To assess whether the targeted deficiency of IEC PPAR γinfluences the phenotype of immune cells we performed flow cytometric analyses on cells isolated from the spleen, blood, and MLN. Our analysis indicated that the deficiency of IEC PPAR γ in FVB mice had no significant impact on the percent of CD4+ or CD8+ T cells in any of the tissues analyzed (Figure 4). There was a numerical trend towards increased F4/80+CD11b+

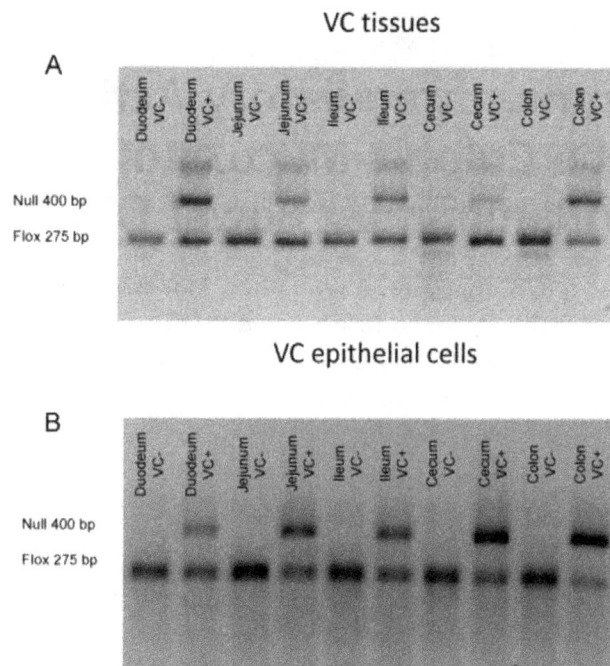

Figure 1. Genotyping of PPAR γ flfl; Villin Cre+ (VC+) and Villin Cre- (VC-) control mice. Conditional deletion of the PPAR γ gene via Villin Cre-mediated recombination was examined in mouse intestine by PCR analysis. The floxed (fl) allele at 275 bp and the null allele at 400 bp. (A) Left to right: depicts fl/fl in homogenized whole duodenum, jejunum, ileum, cecum and colon without recombination (VC-) (lanes 1, 3, 5, 7 and 9) or with recombination (VC+) (lanes 2, 4, 6, 8 and 10). (B) Left to right: depicts fl/fl in epithelial cells isolated from duodenum, jejunum, ileum, cecum and colon without recombination (VC-) (lanes 1, 3, 5, 7 and 9) or with recombination (VC+) (lanes 2, 4, 6, 8 and 10).

macrophages/monocytes in the spleen and blood on days 2 and 7, respectively, though these data were not statistically significant.

In the MLN we also observed no significant differences between FVB VC+ and FVB VC- mice in overall percent of immune cells, but there were some distinct phenotypic differences amongst the CD4+ and F4/80+CD11b+ populations (Figure 5). First, the percentage of IL10-expressing CD4+ T cells was higher in the VC- than the VC+ mice. Second, the percent of macrophages expressing MHC II was significantly elevated in the VC+ mice.

Similar to the mixed FVB strain, there were no significant differences in F4/80+CD11b+, CD4+, or CD8+ immune cell subsets between B6 VC+ and B6 VC- mice (Figure 6). Interestingly, however, macrophages residing in the spleens of B6 VC+ mice expressed significantly more toll-like receptor-4 (TLR-4) on day 7, and expression of CD11c trended to significance. CD4+ T cells from B6 VC+ mice also expressed significantly more IL-4 on day 0, but this difference was absent on days 2 and 7. Also similar to the FVB strain, MHC II expression was up-regulated in MLN-derived F4/80+CD11b+ macrophages in B6 VC+ mice.

Global gene expression analysis in the colonic mucosa of VC- and VC+ mice with DSS colitis

Pairwise comparisons revealed very few genes being modulated in the colonic mucosa after 2 days of DSS challenge. In the VC-mice, 1 gene was differentially expressed in the DSS-treated group

FVB/C57BL/6

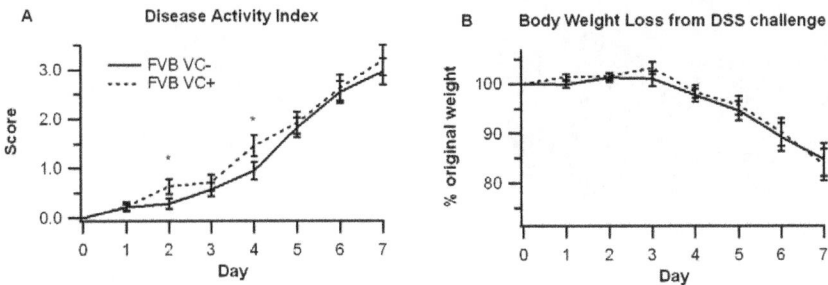

C57BL/6

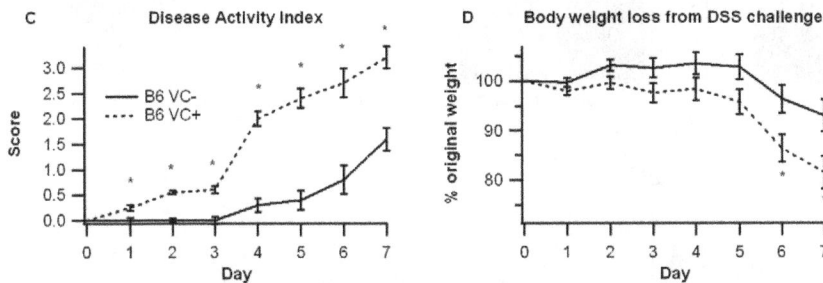

Figure 2. Effect of epithelial cell-specific PPAR γ deletion on disease severity. PPAR γ flfl; Villin Cre+ (VC+) or PPAR γ flfl; Villin Cre- (VC-) mice in a mixed FVB/C57BL/6J (FVB) or C57BL/6J (B6) background were treated with 2.5% dextran sodium sulfate (DSS) or water (no DSS) for 7 days. The disease activity index (DAI), a composite score reflecting clinical signs of the disease (i.e. perianal soiling, rectal bleeding, diarrhea, and piloerection) was assessed daily (A and C) and the average daily loss in body weights (B and D) throughout the 7-day DSS challenge was calculated. Data are represented as mean ± standard error. Points with an asterisk are significantly different ($P<0.05$).

compared to mice that did not receive DSS. For the same comparison in VC+ mice, 5 genes were shown to have a different expression pattern at day 2 compared to day 0 (Figure S1). However DSS changed the expression of a larger set of 1020 genes at the later time point, day 7. Out of these 1020 genes, 877 genes were differentially expressed in VC- mice only; 38 genes in VC+ mice only and 105 genes differentially expressed in both genotypes (Figure S2).

Pathways modulated after DSS challenge

Hypergeometric testing of the 877 genes differentially expressed on day 7 of DSS challenge in VC- mice revealed over-representation of six KEGG pathways: Lysosome, DNA Replication, p53 signaling and metabolic pathways (Tables S1, S2, S3, S4, S5, S6, Figures S3, S4, S5, S6, S7). One pathway (lysosome, KEGG Id: 04142) was found to be significantly associated with effect of DSS. For most of the genes examined, gene expression signals were measured to be higher at day 7 compared to day 0 in VC- mice (positive log-fold change in Table S2). Corresponding log-fold changes for VC+ mice were also recorded for comparison purpose and were found to be smaller in magnitude and statistically non-significant. KEGG pathway lysosome (Id: 04142) was obtained and colored according to fold-change of gene expression in VC- mice. Many genes belonging to this pathway are observed to be up-regulated in this pathway (Figure S3). Gene expression in the DNA replication pathway (KEGG Id: 03030) was found to be significantly down-regulated in VC- mice (Table S3, Figure S4). Metabolic (KEGG Ids: 00520, 00240) and signaling (KEGG Id: 04115) pathways were significantly modulated in VC- mice, with heterogeneity regarding direction of differential expression within the same pathway (Tables S4, S5, S6, Figures S5, S6, S7).

Colonic gene expression by real-time RT-PCR

Adachi et al [12] reported that IEC-specific PPAR γ knock-out mice displayed reduced expression of the PPAR γ target genes Plin2 (ADRP), Fabp2 (FABP) and enhanced expression of pro-inflammatory genes after DSS challenge. We observed the trends in gene expression to be in the same direction as reported by them (Figure 7). Additionally, Fabp2 (FABP) was significantly reduced in VC+ mice compared to VC- mice. Despite showing a significant increase in disease severity, there were no significant differences in the levels of inflammatory proteins IL-1β,IL-6, and IRAK-1, although IRAK-1 expression was numerically down-regulated on day 2 of DSS colitis in IEC-specific PPAR γ null mice (Figure 8).

Discussion

While PPARs have a well-established role in inflammation [13], the specific contribution of intestinal epithelial cell PPAR γ in IBD is actively under investigation. Adachi et al [12] studied DSS induced colitis in mice with a targeted disruption of PPAR γ function in colonic epithelial cells in a mixed FVB/C57BL6 background. They reported that the lack of endogenous epithelial cell PPAR γ expression in colonic epithelial cells results in increased susceptibility to DSS colitis. Our data demonstrate that there are no differences in clinical parameters of disease between IEC-specific PPAR γ-expressing and null mice in the same interbred genetic background. However, we observe an increased susceptibility to DSS colitis in IEC-specific PPAR γ null mice when the experiment was conducted in a C57BL/6 background, indicating strain-specific differences and suggesting that the Th1-[14] and more pro-inflammatory-prone [15] background may accentuate the role of IEC PPAR γ in regulating mucosal inflammation.

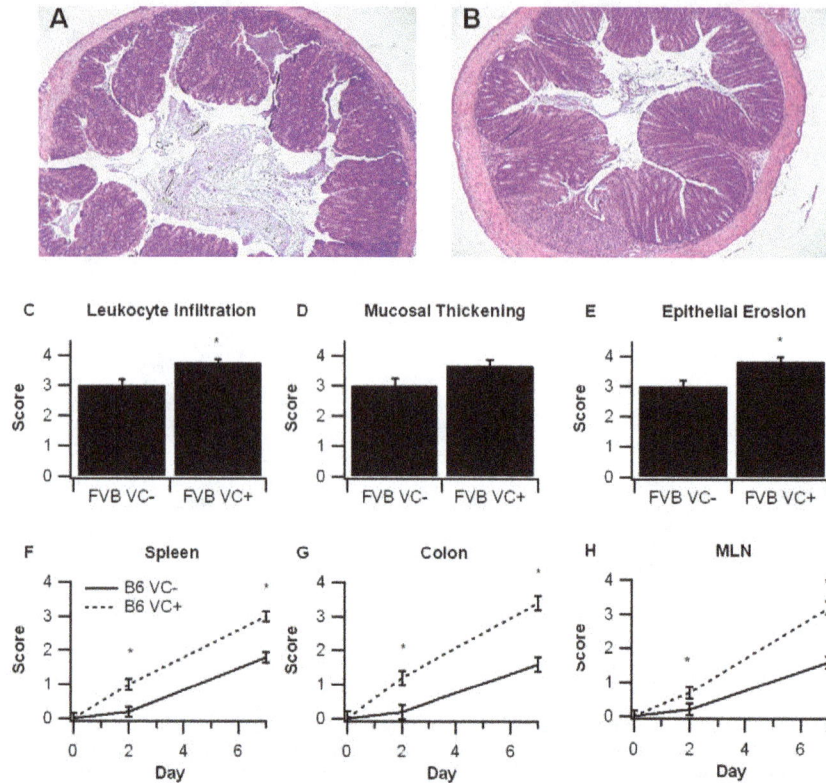

Figure 3. Effect of intestinal epithelial cell-specific PPAR γ deletion on colon histopathology and inflammation. PPAR γ flfl; Villin Cre+ (VC+) or PPAR γ flfl; Villin Cre- (VC-) mice with a mixed FVB/C57BL6/J (FVB) or C57BL6/J (B6) background were treated with 2.5% dextran sodium sulfate (DSS) or water (no DSS) for 7 days. Representative photomicrographs of colonic samples from VC- (A) and VC+ (B) FVB mice with DSS colitis (Original magnification, 40×). Colonic specimens from FVB mice underwent blinded histological examination and were scored (1–4) on leukocyte infiltration (C), and mucosal wall thickening (D), and epithelial erosion (E) on day 7 of the challenge. In B6 mice spleen (F), colon (G), and mesenteric lymph nodes MLN (H) were scored based on macroscopic signs of inflammation on days 2 and 7. Data are represented as mean ± standard error. Points with an asterisk are significantly different ($P<0.05$).

Consistent with the data from Adachi et al. [12], the PPAR γ target Fabp2 (intestinal FABP) is significantly reduced in IEC-specific PPAR γ null mice. The impact of the IEC-specific PPAR γ deletion on pro-inflammatory cytokine gene expression was more modest in our study when compared to Adachi and colleagues. This is also suggested by the lack of clinical (disease activity, body weight) differences between VC- and VC+ mice in a mixed FVB/C57BL/6 background. However, colonic histopathology results reveal significantly greater leukocyte infiltration and epithelial erosion in IEC-specific PPAR γ null mice on day 7 of DSS challenge. After backcrossing the original FVB/C57BL/6 line nine times and generating VC- and VC+ mice in a pure C57BL/6 background the deficiency of PPAR γ in IEC resulted in worsened disease activity, greater weight loss and histological differences, suggesting that the Th1-prone genetic background of C57BL/6 mice is optimal for investigating the contribution of IEC PPAR γ to the pathogenesis of IBD. The mice lacking IEC PPAR γ displayed significantly fewer CD4+IL10+ T cells in the MLN and their macrophages expressed greater amounts of TLR4, the molecular target for LPS, in the spleen. Of note, IL-10-producing CD4+ T cells exert regulatory functions, thereby suggesting that IEC PPAR γ is required for the induction of T cell regulatory responses at the mucosal inductive sites and the prevention of experimental IBD.

While histologically IEC-specific PPAR γ null mice demonstrated characteristic colonic inflammatory lesions after DSS challenge, global transcriptome analysis suggests smaller number of genes being altered in IEC-specific PPAR γ null mice in response to DSS in comparison to T cell-specific PPAR γ null mice [11]. More specifically, inflammatory cytokines, adhesion molecules, genes involved in glucose homeostasis, apoptosis and protein synthesis are down-regulated in the colonic mucosa of mice lacking PPAR γ in T cells [11], whereas the lysosomal gene expression represents the primary pathway modulated in IEC-specific PPAR γ null mice. On day 7 of DSS challenge, pathway analysis reveals six pathways to be characteristically associated with DSS in PPAR γ-expressing mice only. The same analysis applied to IEC-specific PPAR γ null mice does not reveal any characteristic pathway to be altered in this phenotype. Because the pathways were selected from the genes that were significantly different between two genotypes on day 7 of DSS challenge (as shown in the Venn Diagram on Figure S2), these pathways are differentially modulated by DSS on day 7.

Genes of the lysosomal pathway are mostly up-regulated in response to DSS in both VC- and VC+ mice (Figure S3, Table S2), although the magnitude of differential expression (fold-change on day 7 compared day 0) is smaller in VC+ mice. A link between IBD and lysosomal alterations have been suggested earlier [16]. More recently, disruption of PPAR γ in mice resulted in focal hyperplasia, accumulation of lysosomes and dysregulation of pathways related to lysosomal maturation in a prostatic cancer model [17,18]. Cathepsins are lysosomal acid hydrolases whose transcription is enhanced in colonic mucosa in response to dietary DSS. Lysosome associated membrane proteins 1 and 2 (LAMP 1/

Blood

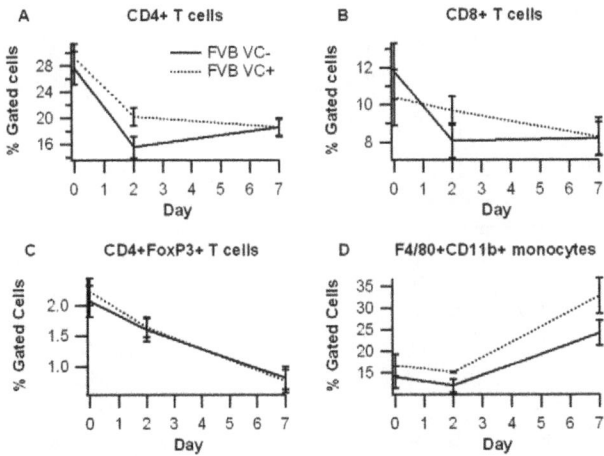

A   CD4+ T cells

B   CD8+ T cells

C   CD4+FoxP3+ T cells

D   F4/80+CD11b+ monocytes

Spleen

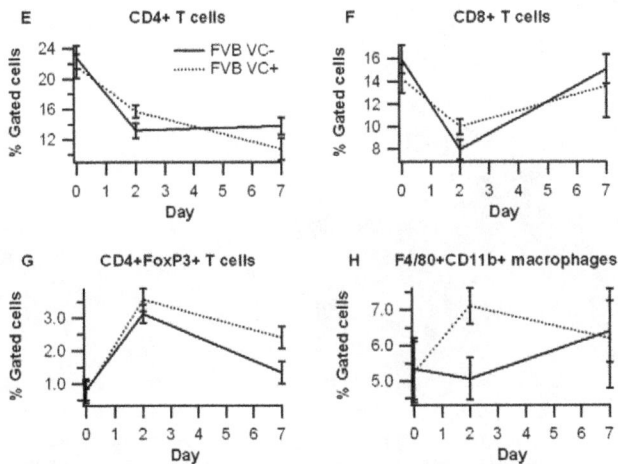

E   CD4+ T cells

F   CD8+ T cells

G   CD4+FoxP3+ T cells

H   F4/80+CD11b+ macrophages

Figure 4. Effect of epithelial cell-specific PPAR γ deletion on immune cell subsets in blood and spleen in FVB/C57BL/6J mice. Blood (A–D) and spleen (E–H) from PPAR γ flfl; Villin Cre+ (VC+) or PPAR γ flfl; Villin Cre- (VC-) mice with a mixed FVB/C57BL/6J background (FVB) were immunophenotyped. Data were collected on days 0, 2, and 7 of DSS challenge and were analyzed with FACS Diva software. Data are represented as mean ± standard error. There were no statically significant differences between groups (P<0.05).

MLN

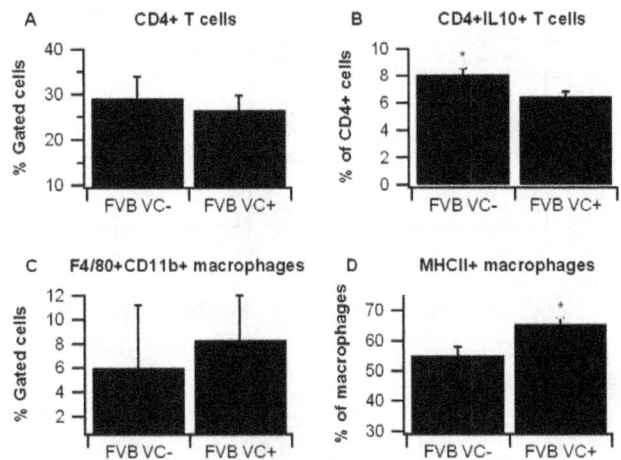

A   CD4+ T cells

B   CD4+IL10+ T cells

C   F4/80+CD11b+ macrophages

D   MHCII+ macrophages

Figure 5. Effect of epithelial cell-specific PPAR γ deletion on immune cell subsets in mesenteric lymph nodes in FVB/C57BL/6J mice. Mesenteric lymph nodes (MLN) from PPAR γ flfl; Villin Cre+ (VC+) or PPAR γ flfl; Villin Cre- (VC-) mice with a mixed FVB/C57BL/6J background (FVB) were immunophenotyped to identify immune cell subsets by flow cytometry. Data were collected on days 0, 2, and 7 of DSS challenge and were analyzed with FACS Diva software. Data are represented as mean ± standard error. Points with an asterisk are significantly different (P<0.05).

processing and presentation [22]. On the other hand IEC PPAR γ serves an important role in suppressing pro-inflammatory cytokine expression and represents a molecular target of anti-inflammatory commensal bacteria [23]. Since lysosomal degradation represents an essential step in antigen presentation via MHC class II, the finding that the targeted disruption of IEC PPAR γ results in altered expression of lysosomal pathway genes may be indicative of a possible role of IEC PPAR γ in the induction of CD4+ T cell regulatory responses by increasing presentation of commensal bacterial antigens.

In summary, by using an IEC-targeted loss-of-function approach we show that expression of IEC PPAR γ is required for preventing colonic inflammatory lesions, up-regulating lysosomal pathway genes and increasing the production of the anti-inflammatory cytokine, IL-10, by CD4+ T cells in the MLN of mice with experimental IBD.

Materials and Methods

Ethics statement

All experimental procedures were approved by the Institutional Animal Care and Use Committee (IACUC) of Virginia Polytechnic Institute and State University (IACUC approval number 08-082-VBI) and met or exceeded requirements of the Public Health Service/National Institutes of Health and the Animal Welfare Act.

Mouse Genotyping

Intestinal tissue specimens and isolated intestinal epithelial cells were obtained from tissue-specific PPAR γ fl/fl; Villin Cre+ (VC+) and Villin Cre- control mice (VC-) kindly provided by Dr. Frank Gonzalez (NCI, Bethesda, MD). Duodenum, jejunum, ileum, cecum and colon were excised. For cell isolation, the different parts of the intestine were washed with PBS, minced and incubated twice in CMF/FBS/EDTA media at 37°C for 15 minutes. The digest was passed through a nylon mesh and

2) are involved in phagosome maturation in which lysosomes fuse with late phagosomes leading to removal of endocytosed microbes [19]. Gene expression of LAMP 1/2 is increased on day 7 of DSS challenge, with the increase being higher in VC- mice and also statistically significant.

The lack of PPAR γ in IEC interferes with lysosomal gene expression in response to DSS, potentially leading to altered antigen presentation. Presentation of microbe-derived peptides along with MHC class II molecules to the T cell receptor is a central event in induction of antigen-specific CD4[+] T cell responses. Analysis of the IBD transcriptome in human subjects [20] revealed up-regulation of genes of immune-response and antigen-presentation, although the mechanism by which classical MHC class II genes exert their influence in IBD is currently unknown [21]. IEC are in contact with intra-epithelial lymphocytes (IELs) and equipped with the machinery for antigen

Spleen

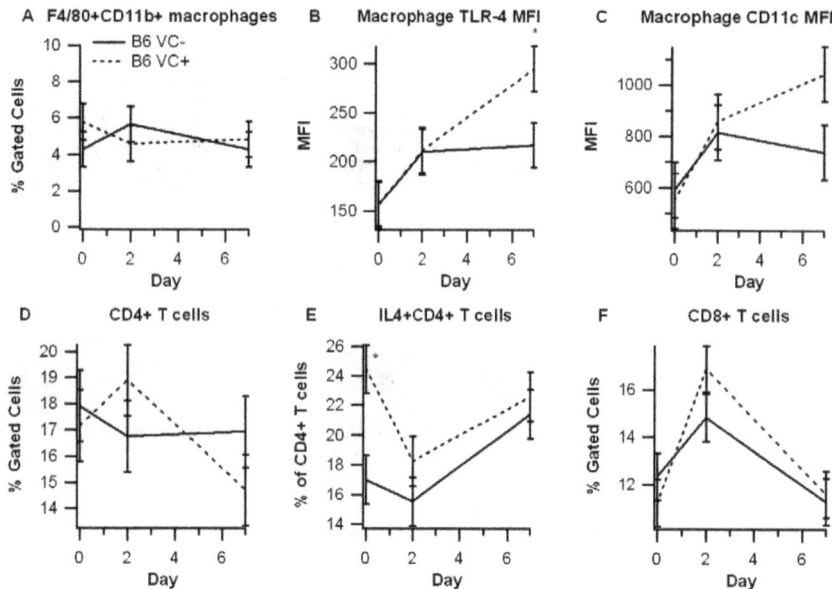

MLN

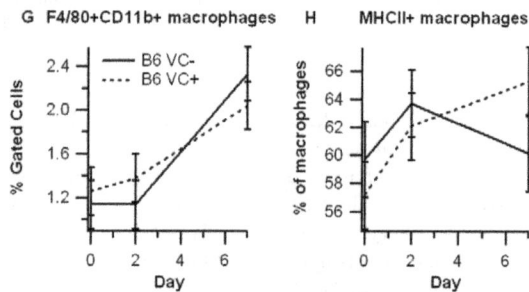

Figure 6. Effect of epithelial cell-specific PPAR γ deletion on immune cell subsets in spleen and mesenteric lymph nodes in C57BL/6J mice. Spleen (A–F) and mesenteric lymph nodes (MLN) (G–H) from PPAR γ flfl; Villin Cre+ (VC+) or PPAR γ flfl; Villin Cre- (VC-) mice with a C57BL/6J background (B6) were immunophenotyped to identify immune cell subsets through flow cytometry. Data were collected on days 0, 2, and 7 of DSS challenge and were analyzed with FACS Diva software. Data are represented as mean ± standard error. Points with an asterisk are significantly different (P<0.05).

supernatants were collected and centrifuged. Cells were washed and resuspended in lysis buffer. DNA was extracted by using the QIAamp DNA Mini Kit, Blood and Body Fluid Spin Protocol (Qiagen). For whole tissue DNA isolation, each part of the intestine was collected and homogenized and then genomic DNA was extracted by QIAamp DNA Mini Kit, Tissue Protocol (Qiagen). PCR was performed as previously described [8,12] and PCR amplifications were resolved through ethidium bromide staining on a 2% agarose gel and run at 120 V for 30 minutes. No differences in the expression of the Villin-Cre recombinase or recombination efficiency were found between the intestines of VC+ mice in a mixed FVB/C57BL/6 and the CB57BL/6 backgrounds (data not shown).

Animal Procedures

PPAR γ flfl; Villin Cre+ (FVB VC+, n = 45) and control PPAR γ flfl; Villin Cre- (FVB VC-, n = 42) mice in a mixed FVB/C57BL/6 background [12] were used for these experiments. These mice express a transgenic recombinase under the control of the Villin-Cre promoter. To facilitate more meaningful comparisons with other mouse knockout strains, we backcrossed these mice nine

times to a C57BL/6 background and generated B6 VC- (n = 15) and B6 VC+ (n = 15) mice in a C57BL/6 background. The mice were housed at the animal facilities at Virginia Polytechnic Institute and State University in a room maintained at 75° F, with a 12:12 h light-dark cycle starting from 6:00 AM. Mice were challenged with 2.5% dextran sodium sulfate (DSS), 36,000–44,000 molecular weight (ICN Biomedicals, Aurora, OH) in the drinking water. DSS damages the epithelial barrier leading to colitis with involvement of macrophages and later, T cells [24]. After the DSS challenge mice were weighed on a daily basis and examined for clinical signs of disease associated with colitis (i.e., perianal soiling, rectal bleeding, diarrhea, and piloerection). For the DSS challenge, the disease activity indices and rectal bleeding scores were calculated using a modification of a previously published compounded clinical score. Briefly, disease activity index consisted of a scoring for diarrhea and lethargy (0–3), whereas rectal bleeding consisted of a visual observation of blood in feces and the perianal area (0–4). Mice in the DSS study were euthanized on days 0, 2, and 7 of the DSS challenge by carbon dioxide narcosis followed by secondary thoracotomy and blood was withdrawn from the heart. Spleen and mesenteric lymph

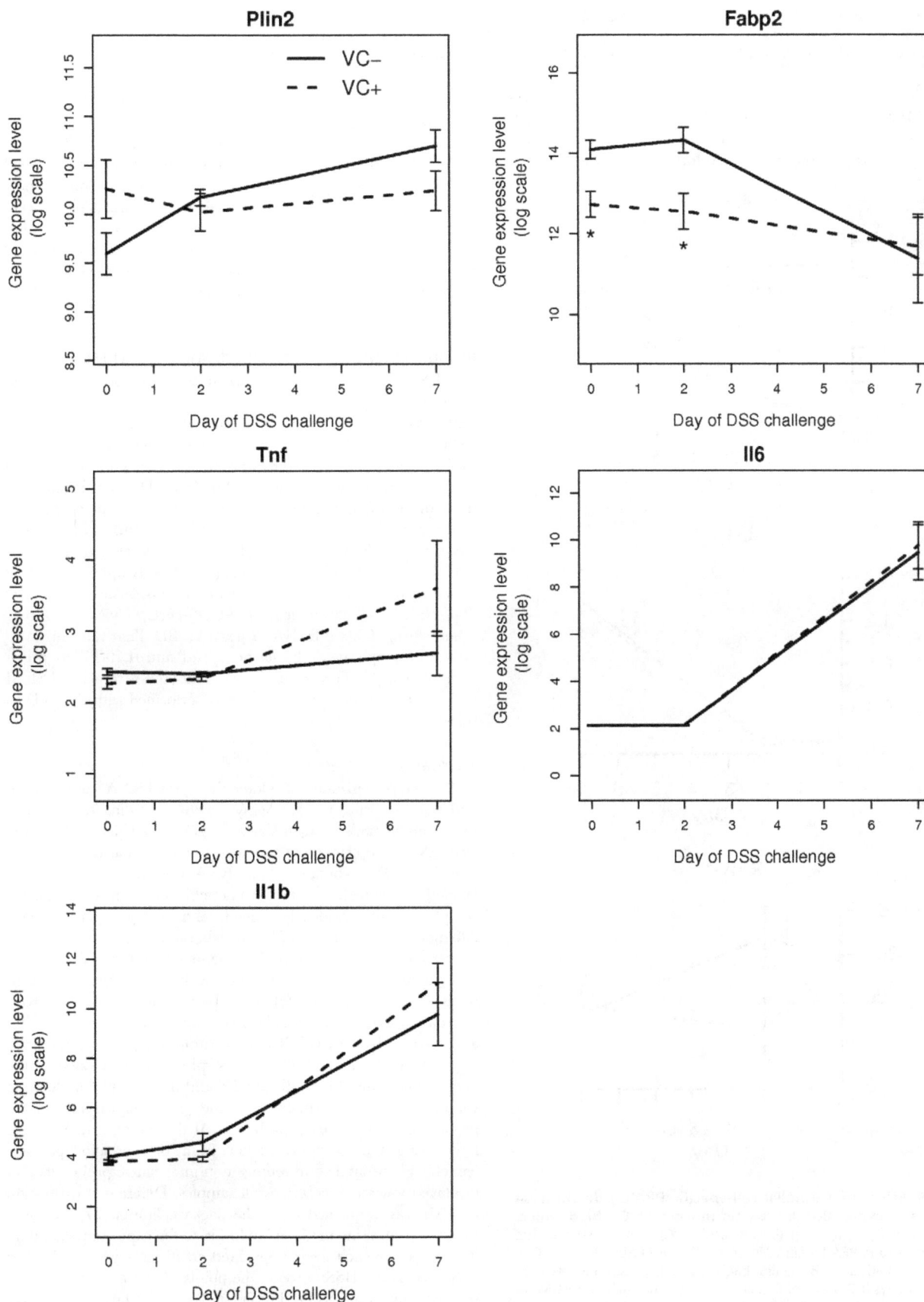

Figure 7. Effect of epithelial cell-specific PPAR γ deletion on target gene expression in colonic mucosa. Expression of PPAR γ targets Plin2 (ADRP), Fabp2 (FABP); and pro-inflammatory genes TNF-α, IL-6 and IL-1β in the colonic mucosa in VC- and VC+ mice at 0, 2 and 7 days after

dextran sodium sulfate (DSS) challenge. Compared to VC- mice, VC+ mice show reduced expression of Plin2 (ADRP) at day 7 of DSS challenge and of Fabp2 (FABP) at earlier time points (days 0 and 2). Expression of pro-inflammatory genes TNF-α, IL-6 and IL-1β are increased in VC+ mice compared to VC- mice after DSS challenge. Statistical significance is indicated by asterisks (P<0.05).

nodes (MLN) were scored based on size and macroscopic inflammatory lesions (0–3), excised, and single-cell suspensions were prepared as previously described for flow cytometry [3].

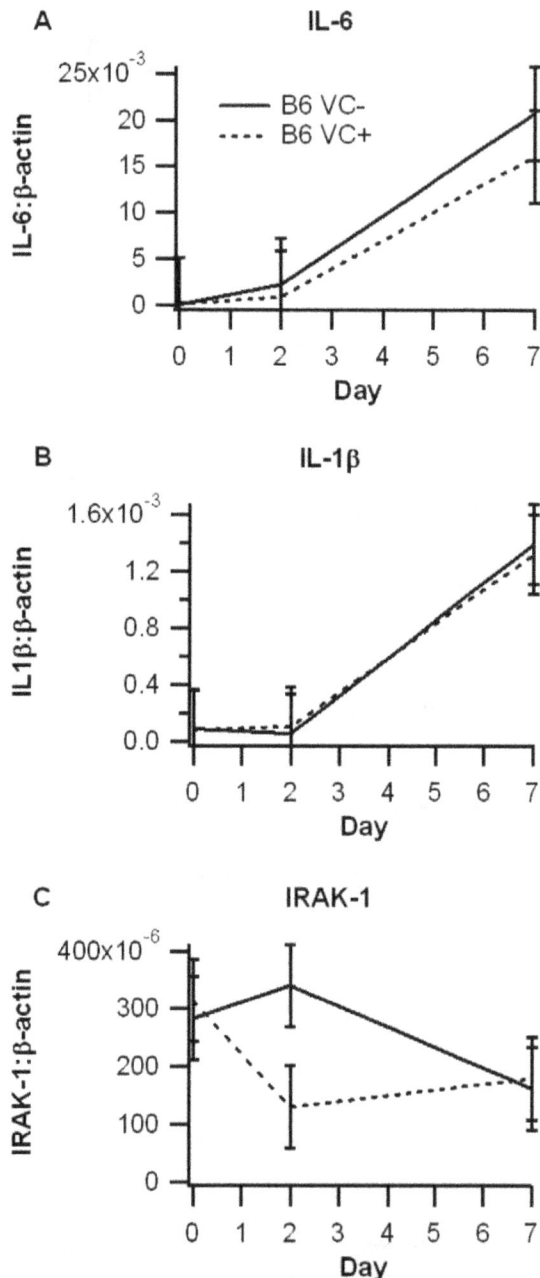

Figure 8. Effect of epithelial cell-specific PPAR γ deletion on target gene expression in colonic mucosa in C57BL/6J mice. Expression of IL-6 (A), IL-1β (B) and IRAK-1 (C) was assessed in the colonic mucosa in PPAR γ flfl; Villin Cre+ (VC+) or PPAR γ flfl; Villin Cre- (VC-) in mice with a C57BL6/J (B6) background. Expression levels were assessed at days 0, 2 and 7 of DSS challenge and normalized relative to the housekeeping gene β-actin. Data are represented as mean ± standard error. There were no statistically significant differences between groups (P<0.05).

Histopathology

Colonic sections were fixed in 10% buffered neutral formalin, later embedded in paraffin, and then sectioned (5 μm) and stained with hematoxylin and eosin (H&E) for examination of microscopic lesions and changes in the mucosal architecture. Colons were graded with a compounded histologic score including the extent of (1) leukocyte infiltration, (2) mucosal thickening, and (3) epithelial cell erosion. The sections were graded with a score of 0–4 for each of the previous categories and data were analyzed as a normalized compounded score.

Immunophenoptying of blood, spleen, and MLN

MLN and spleen-derived cells or whole blood were seeded onto 96-well plates, centrifuged at 4°C at 3000 rpm for 4 minutes, and washed with PBS containing 5% serum and 0.09% sodium azide (FACS buffer). To assess differential monocyte/ macrophage subsets, the cells were then incubated in the dark at 4°C for 20 minutes in FcBlock (20 μg/ml; BD Pharmingen), and then for an additional 20 minutes with fluorochrome-conjugated primary antibodies anti-F4/80-PE-Cy5 (5 μg/mL, ebioscience), anti-CD11b-Alexa Fluor 700 (2 μg/mL, eBioscience) and anti-MHC II-PE (2 μg/mL, eBioscience). For lymphocyte subset assessment, cells were incubated with anti-CD4-Alexa Fluor 700 (2 μg/mL; BD Pharmingen), anti-CD8-PerCp-Cy5.5 (2 μg/mL, eBioscience), CD3 PE-Cy5 (2 μg/mL; BD Pharmingen), anti-FoxP3-PE (2 μg/mL, eBioscience), and anti-IL10-PE as previously shown [3]. Flow results were computed with a BD LSR II flow cytometer and data analyses was performed with FACS Diva software (BD).

Microarray data analysis

After homogenization of colonic tissue, total RNA was extracted and purified using the RNAeasy system according to manufacturer's instructions (Qiagen Valencia, CA). The QIAGEN RNase-free DNase supplement kit was used to ensure that the RNA was free from DNA contamination. RNA was then processed and labeled according to the standard target labeling protocols and the samples were hybridized, stained, and scanned per standard Affymetrix protocols at VBI core laboratory on Mouse 430 2.0 expression arrays (Affymetrix Inc., Santa Clara, CA). All statistical analysis of the data was performed within R statistical environment - Version 2.10.1 [25] using Bioconductor packages. Raw microarray data from CEL files were read with 'affy' package [26] and pre-processed by GC-RMA algorithm that performs the three steps: (i) adjustment of the gene expression signal against the background caused by optical noise and non-specific binding, (ii) robust multi-array normalization, and (iii) summarization of the probes belonging to each probe set. At the outset, a non-specific filter using the function nsFilter from bioconductor package 'genefilter' was applied to remove non-informative probe sets that displayed low variance across all samples. Differential expression analysis was performed using the package limma [27]. A linear model was fit, using the function lmFit, to the expression data (log-intensities) for each gene. The fitted coefficients were compared (DSS versus No DSS; at two time points, day 2 and day 7) using the function contrasts.fit. Empirical Bayes method [28,29] was used to borrow information across genes. This has been shown to make the analysis stable for experiments with small number of arrays. P-values obtained for each gene was corrected for multiple comparisons [30] and a cutoff of 0.05 was applied to identify the genes that are significantly differentially expressed between the conditions. Venn Diagrams were drawn using the function vennDiagram to show the number of genes differentially expressed under different conditions. The microarray data (both raw and normalized) have been submitted at the Gene Expression Omnibus (GEO, http://www.ncbi.nlm.nih.gov/geo/, Series: GSE20621).

Hypergeometric testing for over-represented pathways

All pathways listed at Kyoto Encylopedia for Genes and Genomes (KEGG) were selected for analysis. Genes that were differentially expressed after 7 days of DSS challenge were subjected to hypergemetric testing, with the function hyperGTest from Category package, for discovery of the over-represented KEGG pathways. This procedure used Fisher's exact test to find association between interesting genes (differentially expressed after 7 days of DSS challenge) and membership to a KEGG pathway. Selected KEGG pathways found to be significantly associated with DSS on day 7 were accessed using the bioconductor package KEGGSOAP. Specific gene nodes on each pathway were 'painted' according to the direction of differential expression of that gene on day 7 of DSS treatment: red if up-regulated, green if down-regulated.

Quantitative Real-Time RT-PCR

Total RNA (1 μg) from colons was used to generate a complementary DNA (cDNA) template using the iScript cDNA Synthesis Kit (Bio-Rad, Hercules, CA) using previously described conditions [8]. Each gene amplicon was purified with the MiniElute PCR Purification Kit (Qiagen) and quantitated on an agarose gel by using a DNA mass ladder (Promega). These purified amplicons were used to optimize real-time PCR conditions and to generate standard curves in the real-time PCR assay. Primer concentrations and annealing temperatures were optimized for the iCycler iQ system (Bio-Rad) for each set of primers using the system's gradient protocol. PCR efficiencies were maintained between 92 and 105% and correlation coefficients above 0.98 for each primer set during optimization and also during the real-time PCR of sample DNA.

Complementary DNA (cDNA) concentrations for genes of interest were examined by real-time quantitative PCR using an iCycler IQ System and the iQ SYBR green supermix (Bio-Rad). A standard curve was generated for each gene using 10-fold dilutions of purified amplicons starting at 5 pg of cDNA and used later to calculate the starting amount of target cDNA in the unknown samples. SYBR green I is a general double-stranded DNA intercalating dye and may therefore detect nonspecific products and primer/dimers in addition to the amplicon of interest. In order to determine the number of products synthesized during the real-time PCR, a melting curve analysis was performed on each product. Real-time PCR was used to measure the starting amount of nucleic acid of each unknown sample of cDNA on the same 96-well plate. Genebank accession numbers used for the forward and reverse primers are as follows: β-actin (X03672) forward 5'CCCAGGCATTGCTGACAGG3' and reverse5'TGGAAG-GTGGACAGTGAGGC3' ; IL-6 (NM_031168) forward 5'TT-TCCTCTGGTCTTCTGGAG3' and reverse 5'CTGAAG-GACTCTGGCTTTGT3'; IL-1β (NM_008361) forward GGG-TCGGACTGTTTCTAAGTC3' and reverse 5'CTTGGC-CGAGGACTAAG3'; IRAK-1 (NM_008363) forward 5'CGC-CAAGCACTTCTTGTACGA'3 and reverse 5'GATCAAG-GCCGCGAACT3'.

Statistics

Flow cytometry, disease activity, pathology and real-time RT-PCR data were analyzed as a repeated measures 3×2 factorial arrangement within a completely randomized design. To determine the statistical significance of the model, analysis of variance (ANOVA) was performed using the general linear model procedure of Statistical Analysis Software (SAS), and probability value (P) <0.05 was considered to be significant. When the model was significant, ANOVA was followed by Fisher's Protected Least Significant Difference multiple comparison method.

Supporting Information

Figure S1 Venn diagram showing number of genes differentially expressed on day 2 of Dextran Sodium Sulfate (DSS) challenge. The number inside each circle refers to number of genes differentially expressed on 2nd day of DSS challenge (compared to control, i.e., day 0), for each genotype VC-, VC+. The number inside overlapping region of two circles refers to the number of genes that are common to both genotypes. The number on the bottom right corner corresponds to genes that are not differentially expressed.

Figure S2 Venn diagram showing number of genes differentially expressed on day 7 of Dextran Sodium Sulfate (DSS) challenge. The number inside each circle refers to number of genes differentially expressed on 7th day of DSS challenge (compared to control, i.e., day 0), for each genotype VC-, VC+. The number inside overlapping region of two circles refers to the number of genes that are common to both genotypes. The number on the bottom right corner corresponds to genes that are not differentially expressed.

Figure S3 Lysosomal genes differentially expressed on day 7 of DSS challenge in VC- mice. The pathway diagram from KEGG has been colored according to the direction of change in gene expression. Significantly up-regulated genes are colored in red.

Figure S4 DNA replication (KEGG) genes differentially expressed on day 7 of DSS challenge in VC- mice. The pathway diagram from KEGG has been colored according to the direction of change in gene expression. Significantly down-regulated genes on day 7 in VC- mice are colored in green.

Figure S5 Genes of the KEGG pathway "Aminosugar and nucleotide sugar metabolism" are differentially expressed on day 7 of DSS challenge in VC- mice. The pathway diagram from KEGG has been colored according to the direction of change in gene expression. Significantly up-regulated genes on day 7 in VC- mice are colored in red; down-regulated in green.

Figure S6 Genes of the KEGG pathway "Pyrimidine metabolism" are differentially expressed on day 7 of DSS challenge in VC- mice. The pathway diagram from KEGG has been colored according to the direction of change in gene expression. Significantly down-regulated genes on day 7 in VC- mice are colored in green; up-regulated in red.

Figure S7 Genes of the KEGG "p53 Signaling Pathway" are differentially expressed on day 7 of DSS challenge in VC- mice. The pathway diagram from KEGG has been colored according to the direction of change in gene expression. Significantly up-regulated genes on day 7 in VC- mice are colored in red; down-regulated in green.

Table S1 KEGG pathways modulated on day 7 of DSS challenge in VC- mice. A total of 877 genes, transcriptionally affected on day 7 of VC- (but not VC+) mice, were subjected to hypergeometric testing and revealed enrichment (over-represen-tation) of six KEGG pathways. The first and last columns correspond to the KEGG identifier and name of the pathway, respectively. The second and third columns (Pvalue, OddsRatio) report that there is good association between DSS challenge and the KEGG pathway in VC- mice. The ExpCount records the expected number of genes in the selected gene list to be found at the KEGG pathway, which is exceeded by the actual Count (fifth column). Sixth column (Size) corresponds to the total number of genes in the pathway.

Table S2 Lysosomal genes differentially expressed on day 7 of DSS challenge in VC- mice. Log fold-change in gene expression on day 7 after DSS challenge in VC- and VC+ mice. Degree of differential expression of these genes is statistically significant for VC- mice (suggested by asterisk). Corresponding fold changes in VC+ mice are not statistically significant. Most of the genes are up-regulated in VC- mice.

Table S3 DNA replication (KEGG) genes differentially ex-pressed on day 7 of DSS challenge in VC- mice. Log fold-change in gene expression on day 7 after DSS challenge in VC- and VC+ mice. Degree of differential expression of these genes is statistically significant for VC- mice (suggested by asterisk). Corresponding fold changes in VC+ mice are not statistically significant. The genes are down-regulated in VC- mice.

Table S4 Genes of the KEGG pathway "Aminosugar and nucleotide sugar metabolism" are differentially expressed on day 7 of DSS challenge in VC- mice. Log fold-change in gene expression on day 7 after DSS challenge in VC- and VC+ mice. Degree of differential expression of these genes is statistically significant for VC- mice (suggested by asterisk). Corresponding fold changes in VC+ mice are not statistically significant.

Table S5 Genes of the KEGG pathway "Pyrimidine metabo-lism" are differentially expressed on day 7 of DSS challenge in VC- mice. Log fold-change in gene expression on day 7 after DSS challenge in VC- and VC+ mice. Degree of differential expression of these genes is statistically significant for VC- mice (suggested by asterisk). Corresponding fold changes in VC+ mice are not statistically significant. The genes are mostly down-regulated in VC- mice.

Table S6 Genes of the KEGG "p53 Signaling Pathway" are differentially expressed on day 7 of DSS challenge in VC- mice. Log fold-change in gene expression on day 7 after DSS challenge in VC- and VC+ mice. Degree of differential expression of these genes is statistically significant for VC- mice (suggested by asterisk). Corresponding fold changes in VC+ mice are not statistically significant.

Author Contributions

Conceived and designed the experiments: RH JBR. Performed the experiments: AJG MC CV AC WTH RH JBR. Analyzed the data: SKM AJG MC CV AC WTH RH JBR. Contributed reagents/materials/analysis tools: SKM WTH RH JBR. Wrote the paper: SKM AJG RH JBR.

References

1. Xavier RJ, Podolsky DK (2007) Unravelling the pathogenesis of inflammatory bowel disease. Nature 448: 427–434.
2. Martin H (2009) Role of PPAR-gamma in inflammation. Prospects for therapeutic intervention by food components. Mutat Res 669: 1–7.
3. Hontecillas R, Bassaganya-Riera J (2007) Peroxisome proliferator-activated receptor gamma is required for regulatory CD4+ T cell-mediated protection against colitis. J Immunol 178: 2940–2949.
4. Chen L, Bush CR, Necela BM, Su W, Yanagisawa M, et al. (2006) RS5444, a novel PPARgamma agonist, regulates aspects of the differentiated phenotype in nontransformed intestinal epithelial cells. Mol Cell Endocrinol 251: 17–32.
5. Bassaganya-Riera J, Hontecillas R (2006) CLA and n-3 PUFA differentially modulate clinical activity and colonic PPAR-responsive gene expression in a pig model of experimental IBD. Clin Nutr 25: 454–465.
6. Hontecillas R, Wannemeulher MJ, Zimmerman DR, Hutto DL, Wilson JH, et al. (2002) Nutritional regulation of porcine bacterial-induced colitis by conjugated linoleic acid. J Nutr 132: 2019–2027.
7. Guri AJ, Hontecillas R, Bassaganya-Riera J (2010) Abscisic acid ameliorates experimental IBD by downregulating cellular adhesion molecule expression and suppressing immune cell infiltration. Clinical Nutrition In Press.
8. Bassaganya-Riera J, Reynolds K, Martino-Catt S, Cui Y, Hennighausen L, et al. (2004) Activation of PPAR gamma and delta by conjugated linoleic acid mediates protection from experimental inflammatory bowel disease. Gastroen-terology 127: 777–791.
9. Lewis JD, Lichtenstein GR, Deren JJ, Sands BE, Hanauer SB, et al. (2008) Rosiglitazone for active ulcerative colitis: a randomized placebo-controlled trial. Gastroenterology 134: 688–695.
10. Lewis JD, Lichtenstein GR, Stein RB, Deren JJ, Judge TA, et al. (2001) An open-label trial of the PPAR-gamma ligand rosiglitazone for active ulcerative colitis. Am J Gastroenterol 96: 3323–3328.
11. Guri AJ, Mohapatra SK, Horne WT, Hontecillas R, Bassaganya-Riera J (2010) Immunoregulatory actions of T cell PPAR gamma at the colonic mucosa in mice with experimental IBD. BMC Gastroenterology. In Revision.
12. Adachi M, Kurotani R, Morimura K, Shah Y, Sanford M, et al. (2006) Peroxisome proliferator activated receptor gamma in colonic epithelial cells protects against experimental inflammatory bowel disease. Gut 55: 1104–1113.
13. Clark RB (2002) The role of PPARs in inflammation and immunity. J Leukoc Biol 71: 388–400.
14. Zhang WW, Mendez S, Ghosh A, Myler P, Ivens A, et al. (2003) Comparison of the A2 gene locus in Leishmania donovani and Leishmania major and its control over cutaneous infection. J Biol Chem 278: 35508–35515.
15. Matsutani T, Anantha Samy TS, Kang SC, Bland KI, Chaudry IH (2005) Mouse genetic background influences severity of immune responses following trauma-hemorrhage. Cytokine 30: 168–176.
16. O'Morain C, Smethurst P, Levi AJ, Peters TJ (1984) Organelle pathology in ulcerative and Crohn's colitis with special reference to the lysosomal alterations. Gut 25: 455–459.
17. Jiang M, Fernandez S, Jerome WG, He Y, Yu X, et al. (2009) Disruption of PPARgamma signaling results in mouse prostatic intraepithelial neoplasia involving active autophagy. Cell Death Differ 17: 469–481.
18. Jiang M, Jerome WG, Hayward SW (2010) Autophagy in nuclear receptor PPARgamma-deficient mouse prostatic carcinogenesis. Autophagy 6: 175–176.
19. Huynh KK, Eskelinen EL, Scott CC, Malevanets A, Saftig P, et al. (2007) LAMP proteins are required for fusion of lysosomes with phagosomes. EMBO J 26: 313–324.
20. Costello CM, Mah N, Hasler R, Rosenstiel P, Waetzig GH, et al. (2005) Dissection of the inflammatory bowel disease transcriptome using genome-wide cDNA microarrays. PLoS Med 2: e199.
21. Yamamoto-Furusho JK (2007) Genetic factors associated with the development of inflammatory bowel disease. World J Gastroenterol 13: 5594–5597.

22. Hershberg RM, Mayer LF (2000) Antigen processing and presentation by intestinal epithelial cells - polarity and complexity. Immunol Today 21: 123–128.

23. Kelly D, Campbell JI, King TP, Grant G, Jansson EA, et al. (2004) Commensal anaerobic gut bacteria attenuate inflammation by regulating nuclear-cytoplasmic shuttling of PPAR-gamma and RelA. Nat Immunol 5: 104–112.

24. Strober W, Fuss IJ, Blumberg RS (2002) The immunology of mucosal models of inflammation. Annu Rev Immunol 20: 495–549.

25. R_Development_Core_Team (2009) R: A langauge and environment for statistical computing. ViennaAustria: R Foundation for Statistical Computing.

26. Gautier L, Cope L, Bolstad BM, Irizarry RA (2004) affy—analysis of Affymetrix GeneChip data at the probe level. Bioinformatics 20: 307–315.

27. Smyth GK (2005) Limma: linear models for microarray data. In: Gentleman R, Carey VJ, Dudoit S, Irizarry R, Huber W, eds. Bioinformatics and computational biology solutions using R and Bioconductor. New York: Springer. pp 397–420.

28. Loennstedt I, Speed TP (2002) Replicated microarray data. Statistica Sinica 12: 31–46.

29. Smyth GK (2004) Linear models and empirical bayes methods for assessing differential expression in microarray experiments. Stat Appl Genet Mol Biol 3: Article3.

30. Benjamini Y, Hochberg Y (1995) Controlling the false discovery rate: a practical and powerful approach to multiple testing. Journal of the Royal Statistical Society Series B 57: 289–300.

15

Dirichlet Multinomial Mixtures: Generative Models for Microbial Metagenomics

Ian Holmes[1], Keith Harris[2], Christopher Quince[2]*

1 Department of Bioengineering, University of California, Berkeley, California, United States of America, **2** School of Engineering, University of Glasgow, Glasgow, United Kingdom

Abstract

We introduce Dirichlet multinomial mixtures (DMM) for the probabilistic modelling of microbial metagenomics data. This data can be represented as a frequency matrix giving the number of times each taxa is observed in each sample. The samples have different size, and the matrix is sparse, as communities are diverse and skewed to rare taxa. Most methods used previously to classify or cluster samples have ignored these features. We describe each community by a vector of taxa probabilities. These vectors are generated from one of a finite number of Dirichlet mixture components each with different hyperparameters. Observed samples are generated through multinomial sampling. The mixture components cluster communities into distinct 'metacommunities', and, hence, determine envirotypes or enterotypes, groups of communities with a similar composition. The model can also deduce the impact of a treatment and be used for classification. We wrote software for the fitting of DMM models using the 'evidence framework' (http://code.google.com/p/microbedmm/). This includes the Laplace approximation of the model evidence. We applied the DMM model to human gut microbe genera frequencies from Obese and Lean twins. From the model evidence four clusters fit this data best. Two clusters were dominated by Bacteroides and were homogenous; two had a more variable community composition. We could not find a significant impact of body mass on community structure. However, Obese twins were more likely to derive from the high variance clusters. We propose that obesity is not associated with a distinct microbiota but increases the chance that an individual derives from a disturbed enterotype. This is an example of the 'Anna Karenina principle (AKP)' applied to microbial communities: disturbed states having many more configurations than undisturbed. We verify this by showing that in a study of inflammatory bowel disease (IBD) phenotypes, ileal Crohn's disease (ICD) is associated with a more variable community.

Editor: Jack Anthony Gilbert, Argonne National Laboratory, United States of America

Funding: CQ is funded by an EPSRC Career Acceleration Fellowship EP/H003851/1. KH by a Unilever directly funded research grant to the University of Glasgow. IH was supported by NIH/NIGMS grant R01-GM076705. The funders had no role in study design, data collection and analysis, decision to publish, or preparation of the manuscript.

Competing Interests: KH is directly funded through a Unilever research grant to develop bioinformatics tools. All tools developed under this grant are being released open source.

* E-mail: christopher.quince@glasgow.ac.uk

Introduction

Next generation sequencing, applied to microbial metagenomics, has transformed the study of microbial diversity. Microbial metagenomics, or sequencing of DNA extracted from microbial communities, provides a means to determine what organisms are present without the need for isolation and culturing, which can access less than 1% of the species in a typical environment [1]. Prior to next generation sequencing individual DNA fragments from a sample were cloned and then Sanger sequenced [2] – a procedure that is slow and expensive when done on a per read basis. Direct next generation sequencing, for example 454 pyrosequencing [3] or Illumina [4], is cheaper and faster, which has allowed much larger studies of microbial diversity, with more reads in total, and with more communities sampled. However, the development of statistics to extract ecologically meaningful information from these data sets has not developed as quickly as the experimental methodology. In particular, tools that can account for the discrete nature, sparsity, and variable size of these data sets are lacking. We propose the Dirichlet multinomial mixture as a generative modelling framework that addresses this need.

Broadly, microbial metagenomics data can be of two types: either amplicons or shotgun metagenomics. Amplicons are generated by PCR amplification of a specific marker gene region – typically a variable region from the 16S rRNA gene – prior to sequencing, so that the data consists of reads from homologous genes in different organisms. In shotgun metagenomics DNA is fragmented in some way and those fragments sequenced, generating reads from throughout the genome of the different community members. For both amplicons and shotgun reads it is possible to classify sequence reads against known taxa, and determine a list of those organisms that are present and the read frequency associated with them [5]. For the majority of environments, many organisms will not have been taxonomically classified and sequenced before, in which case the list of taxa may have to be generated at a low resolution phylogenetic level, e.g. phylum, to achieve a reasonable proportion of classified reads. Alternatively, an unsupervised strategy can be used to identify proxies to traditional taxonomic units by clustering sequences, so called Operational Taxonomic Units (OTUs) [6]. This is commonly performed in the case of homologous marker genes from amplicons but can also be applied to shotgun metagenomics data [7]. Whether supervised or unsupervised approaches are used the end result is the same: a community is represented by a list of types, either taxa or OTUs, and their frequency. For shotgun metagenomics data much more analysis is possible, utilising information about the function of genes that are sequenced, but here we will focus on the analysis of community structure generated by microbial metagenomics. Typically, this will be generated as amplicons, which typically will be 454 pyrosequenced, but we would emphasise that the approach can be applied to any list of taxa or OTUs with discrete abundances.

Early studies of microbial communities focussed on cataloguing diversity in individual samples, asking: how many different taxa or OTUs were present [8,9]? A striking result was that the observed diversity was very high, and that most species were observed with low abundance; this phenomenon has been termed the 'rare biosphere' [8]. These early studies ignored the impact of sequencing and PCR errors which can inflate OTU diversities [10], but even after the application of algorithms capable of removing those errors [11], observed diversities remain high in most environments and abundances are still skewed to low abundances in almost all [10,12]. The consequence of this is that even with very large read numbers we will have only sampled a fraction of the true diversity [13].

The natural extension to examining the diversity in an individual sample is to look at patterns across samples from similar environments. Barcoding allows multiple samples to be sequenced in a single run but difficulties quantifying DNA concentration means that the number of reads from each sample will usually vary substantially [14]. Sub-sampling can be used to reduce all samples to the same size but that inevitably throws away large amounts of meaningful data. The majority of studies have used exploratory statistics to search for natural patterns in the data, unsupervised learning again. A common strategy is to use multivariate ordination techniques, where samples are positioned in a space of reduced dimensionality so as to preserve the distances between them in the original higher dimensional space; often two or three dimensional ordinations are used and then it is possible to look for patterns by eye. A classic example of an ordination method is principal components analysis (PCA), which generates new dimensions that are linear combinations of the original, chosen so as to preserve the Euclidean distance between samples [15]. Euclidean distances are not very appropriate for microbial community analysis, much better is to use measures that incorporate the phylogentic divergence between types, e.g. Unifrac [16]. Ordination can be performed with arbitrary distance metrics using multidimensional scaling methods, these can be either metric in that they preserve distances or non-metric in that they preserve the ranking of the distances. An example of a metric multidimensional scaling is principal coordinates analysis which has proven a useful and popular tool when coupled with Unifrac for exploratory data analysis [17].

Clustering is another means of exploratory data analysis which searches for natural groups or partitions in the samples. Hierarchical clustering, where a tree of relationships is generated without explicitly grouping samples unless an arbitrary cut-off is chosen, is quite commonly used in microbial community analyses, partitional clustering where the samples are divided into groups has traditionally been less popular. This may be because of the need to decide a priori how many clusters are present. Generally variants of the k-means algorithm have been used together with heuristics to decide how good a clustering is. To date there has been no model based clustering of microbial community data. This question of the natural number of types of communities has received particular attention recently in the context of the human gut, for which it has been suggested that three microbial community types, known as envirotypes (or, in the context of the gut, enterotypes) are to be found [18]. Classification, or supervised learning, is closely related to clustering, except here the problem is not to find natural groups in the data but to predict the group of a new sample, given a labelling of samples in a training data set. Two studies applying classification methods to microbial communities have appeared recently [19,20]. Most of the algorithms used were, as for the unsupervised approaches, developed for continuous data with the notable exception of the multinomial naive Bayes (MNB) model in Knights et al. (2001) [20].

There are, however, problems inherent in using standard multivariate techniques for the analysis of microbial metagenomics data. The data, even if normalised into relative abundances, is fundamentally discrete and can only be approximately modelled by continuous variables. In addition, the high diversity (relative to sampling effort) results in very sparse data sets; most taxa appear in only a few samples at low abundance. Finally, the samples vary in read number: a small sample will inherently be more noisy than a larger one. All these issues can be addressed using an explicit sampling scheme. Instead of viewing the sample as representing the community, we view it as having being generated by sampling from the community. The most natural assumption to make is sampling with replacement, so that the likelihood of an observed sample is a multinomial distribution with a parameter vector where a given entry represents the probability that a read is from a given taxa. These probabilities in the limit of very large community sizes will become the relative frequencies of the taxa. This provides a discrete model, that accounts for different sample sizes, and can model sparse data.

We will show how this multinomial sampling can be used as a starting point for a generative modelling framework, one that explicitly describes a model for generating the observed data [21]. This provides model-based alternatives for both clustering and classification of microbial communities. The natural prior for the parameters of the multinomial distribution is the Dirichlet. This is a probability distribution over probability vectors. In the context of microbial communities we can view it as describing a metacommunity from which communities can be sampled. Its parameters then describe both the mean expected community and the variance in the communities. As we will show, one of the major advantages of the Dirichlet prior is that the community parameter vectors which are unobserved can be integrated out or marginalised to give an analytic solution to the *evidence*: the probability that the data was generated by the model. By extending the Dirichlet prior to a mixture of Dirichlets [22–24], so that the data set is generated not by a single metacommunity but a mixture of multiple metacommunities, we obtain both a more flexible model for our data and a means to cluster communities. To perform the clustering, we simply impute for each sample the component which is most likely to have generated it. This separates samples into groups according to the metacommunity it has the highest probability of deriving from. The advantage of this approach over simple k-means type strategies is twofold: (1) the clusters can be of different sizes depending on the variability of the metacommunity, and more importantly (2) because we now have an explicit probabilistic model that is appropriate to the data, then we can use the evidence together with methods to penalise model complexity to provide a rigorous means of determining optimal cluster number.

Multinomial sampling has been used previously in the study of microbial communities [20], and it has been coupled with a

Dirichlet prior [25], but the extension of that prior to a mixture of Dirichlet components in this context is completely novel, as is the explicit association of each Dirichlet component with a different metacommunity. The major challenge for our framework is how to fit the Dirichlet mixture given the very large dimensionality of microbial metagenomics data sets. This will make Gibbs sampling to obtain posterior distributions for the Dirichlet parameters challenging, at least for OTU based data sets. Instead, we utilise the analytic form for the evidence and fit the Dirichlet parameters by maximising this, given a gamma hyperprior distribution for those parameters, this is an example of the 'evidence framework' [26]. In practice, this is achieved by coupling an Expectation-Maximisation (EM) algorithm for the Dirichlet mixture parameters with multi-dimensional optimisation of each component's parameters. To answer the crucial question of model fit, we use a Laplace approximation to integrate out the hyperparameters, and estimate the evidence of the complete model. In contrast, the extension to a classifier is relatively simple. We simply fit the model to the different classes, estimate priors as the frequencies of the classes in the training data, and then use Bayes' theorem to calculate the probability that a sample to be classified was generated from each of the classes. We now explain in more detail the model framework and illustrate its utility by application to two example data sets of human gut microbiota [27,28].

Materials and Methods

Multinomial sampling

Our starting point is a matrix of occupancies $\mathbf{X}$ with elements X_{ij} that give the observed abundance of taxa j in community sample i where j runs from 1 to the total number of taxa S, and i from 1 to the total number of communities N. We will denote the rows of this matrix that give the occupancies in each individual community sample by the N vectors $\bar{X}_i$. We assume that each community sample is generated from a multinomial distribution with parameter vector $\bar{p}_i$. The elements of $\bar{p}_i$, p_{ij}, are the probabilities that an individual read taken from community i belongs to species j. The multinomial distribution corresponds to sampling with replacement from the community. This gives a likelihood for observing each community sample:

$$L_i(\bar{X}_i|\bar{p}_i) = J_i! \prod_{j=1}^{S} \frac{p_{ij}^{X_{ij}}}{X_{ij}!}, \qquad (1)$$

where the $J_i = \sum_{j=1}^{S} X_{ij}$ are the total number of reads from each community i. The total likelihood is the product of the community sample likelihoods:

$$L(\mathbf{X}|\bar{p}_1, \ldots, \bar{p}_N) = \prod_{i=1}^{N} L_i(\bar{X}_i|\bar{p}_i).$$

Dirichlet mixture priors

In a Bayesian approach we now need to define a prior distribution for the multinomial parameter probability vectors $\bar{p}_i$. We will refer to these as 'communities' since they reflect the underlying structure of the community i that is sampled. A prior based on the Dirichlet distribution is natural, as it is conjugate to the multinomial and (as we will discuss) has a number of convenient properties. The Dirichlet is a probability distribution over distributions:

$$\mathrm{Dir}(\bar{p}_i|\bar{\alpha} \equiv \theta\bar{m}) = \Gamma(\theta) \prod_{j=1}^{S} \frac{p_{ij}^{\theta m_j - 1}}{\Gamma(\theta m_j)} \delta\left(\sum_{j=1}^{S} p_{ij} - 1\right). \qquad (2)$$

This distribution has S parameters which we can represent as a vector $\bar{\alpha}$ that is a measure i.e. all elements are strictly positive, $\alpha_i > 0 \; \forall \; i$. We can express $\bar{\alpha} = \theta\bar{m}$, where $\theta = \sum_{j=1}^{S} \alpha_j$ and $\bar{m}$ is a normalised measure with $\sum_{j=1}^{S} m_j = 1$. The elements m_j then give the mean p_{ij} values and the value θ acts like a precision, determining how close the values lie to that mean: a large θ gives little variance about the mean values, while a small θ leads to widely distributed samples. Conceptually we view these parameters as describing a 'metacommunity', from which different communities can be sampled. The Dirac delta function ensures normalisation, i.e. $\sum_j p_{ij} = 1$.

To provide a more flexible modelling framework and to allow clustering we extend this single Dirichlet prior to a mixture of K Dirichlets, indexed $k = 1, \ldots, K$, each with parameters $\bar{\alpha}_k$ and weight π_k [22,23]. Each community vector $\bar{p}_i$ is assumed to derive from a single metacommunity. For each sample i, we represent this using a K-dimensional indicator vector $\bar{z}_i$ that consists of zeros except for the entry corresponding to the metacommunity that sample i derives from which is equal to one. The prior probabilities for the vectors $\bar{z}_i$ are then just the mixture weights, so:

$$P(\bar{z}_i) = \prod_{k=1}^{K} \pi_k^{z_{ik}} \qquad (3)$$

and the complete mixture prior is:

$$P(\bar{p}_i|Q) = \sum_{k=1}^{K} \mathrm{Dir}(\bar{p}_i|\bar{\alpha}_k)\pi_k, \qquad (4)$$

where the Dirichlet distribution is given by Equation 2 , and the mixture prior hyperparameters are $Q = (K, \bar{\alpha}_1, \ldots, \bar{\alpha}_K, \pi_1, \ldots, \pi_K)$.

The numerical behaviour of the model can be improved by placing independent and identically distributed Gamma hyperpriors on the Dirichlet parameters α_{jk}, i.e., $\alpha_{jk} \sim \Gamma(\eta, \nu)$. Thus,

$$p(\bar{\alpha}_1, \ldots, \bar{\alpha}_K) = \prod_{j=1}^{S} \prod_{k=1}^{K} \frac{\nu^\eta \alpha_{jk}^{\eta-1} e^{-\nu\alpha_{jk}}}{\Gamma(\eta)} =$$
$$\Gamma(\eta)^{-KS} \nu^{\eta KS} \exp\left\{-\nu \sum_{j=1}^{S} \sum_{k=1}^{K} \alpha_{jk}\right\} \prod_{j=1}^{S} \prod_{k=1}^{K} \alpha_{jk}^{\eta-1}, \qquad (5)$$

as we will later use the following reparameterisation: $\lambda_{jk} = \log \alpha_{jk}$, the change of variables formula for probability density functions was used to convert the prior for α_{jk} into one for λ_{jk}, which yields the result that:

$$p(\bar{\lambda}_1, \ldots, \bar{\lambda}_K) = \Gamma(\eta)^{-KS} \nu^{\eta KS} \exp\left\{-\nu \sum_{j=1}^{S} \sum_{k=1}^{K} \alpha_{jk}\right\} \prod_{j=1}^{S} \prod_{k=1}^{K} \alpha_{jk}^{\eta}. (6)$$

Posterior distribution of the multinomial parameters

The posterior distribution of the community parameters is obtained by multiplying the Dirichlet mixture prior by the multinomial likelihood (Equation 1) and appropriately normalising to give for community i:

$$P(\bar{p}_i|\bar{X}_i,Q) = \frac{\sum_{k=1}^{K} L_i(\bar{X}_i|\bar{p}_i)\,\mathrm{Dir}(\bar{p}_i|\bar{\alpha}_k)\pi_k}{\sum_{k=1}^{K} P(\bar{X}_i|\bar{\alpha}_k)\pi_k}. \tag{7}$$

The Dirichlet is a conjugate prior for the multinomial: for a single Dirichlet the posterior is itself a Dirichlet with parameters obtained by summing the observed counts and the Dirichlet parameters, $\bar{\alpha} + \bar{X}_i$. For the Dirichlet mixture this conjugacy is maintained and Equation 7 can also be written as a Dirichlet mixture:

$$P(\bar{p}_i|\bar{X}_i,Q) = \sum_{k=1}^{K} \mathrm{Dir}(\bar{p}_i|\bar{\alpha}_k + \bar{X}_i)P(z_{ik}=1|\bar{X}_i,Q). \tag{8}$$

We will discuss the calculation of the posterior probabilities, $P(z_{ik}=1|\bar{X}_i,Q)$, for a sample deriving from a metacommunity below.

Marginalising the multinomial parameters

The denominator of Equation 7 is equivalent to $P(\bar{X}_i|Q)$, the evidence for community sample i. This is obtained by integrating the numerator, i.e. the mixture prior $P(\bar{p}_i|Q)$ multiplied by the likelihood $L_i(\bar{X}_i|\bar{p}_i)$, over all possible community priors. It is the complete probability of observing this data marginalising out the unseen vector of probabilities $\bar{p}_i$. One of the useful properties of the Dirichlet prior is that this evidence has a closed form. So focussing on just a single mixture component k:

$$P(\bar{X}_i|\bar{\alpha}_k) = \int L_i(\bar{X}_i|\bar{p}_i)\,\mathrm{Dir}(\bar{p}_i|\bar{\alpha}_k)d\bar{p}_i$$

$$= \frac{B(\bar{\alpha}_k + \bar{X}_i)}{B(\bar{\alpha}_k)} J_i! \prod_{j=1}^{S} \frac{1}{X_{ij}!},$$

where the function B is the multinomial Beta function and can be expressed in terms of Gamma functions as:

$$B(\bar{\alpha}) = \frac{\Pi_{j=1}^{S} \Gamma(\alpha_j)}{\Gamma(\sum_{j=1}^{S} \alpha_j)}.$$

So far we have considered the posterior and evidence for just a single community sample i. The evidence over all samples is just the product of the evidences for each sample:

$$P(\mathbf{X}|Q) = \prod_{i=1}^{N} \left(\sum_{k=1}^{K} \frac{B(\bar{\alpha}_k + \bar{X}_i)}{B(\bar{\alpha}_k)} J_i! \prod_{j=1}^{S} \frac{1}{X_{ij}!} \pi_k \right). \tag{9}$$

EM algorithm for fitting the mixture of Dirichlets prior

Our strategy for fitting the mixture of Dirichlets is to maximise the evidence given the gamma hyperpriors. The strictly Bayesian approach would be to sample from the unobserved hyperparameters, Q, and latent variables $\bar{z}_i$, given the hyperpriors, using Markov chain Monte Carlo (MCMC), and then marginalise.

This would be computationally challenging for the high dimensional $\bar{\alpha}_k$ vectors that are encountered in microbiomics data. Maximising the evidence allows us to obtain a single parameter vector that will correspond to the most likely set of parameters given the gamma hyperpriors. The technique is well established and is known as the 'evidence framework' [21,26]. The posterior distribution of the hyperparameters is given by the product of the evidence (Equation 9) and the hyperprior for the $\bar{\alpha}_k$ given by Equation 5. Strictly, to distinguish this from the posterior of the multinomial parameters we should refer to this as the marginal posterior distribution but our meaning should be clear from the context used. We are also implicitly assuming uniform hyperpriors for the other components of Q, the mixing coefficients $\bar{\pi}$. Maximising the posterior of the hyperparameters is equivalent to maximising the log posterior of the hyperparameters, $F(Q) \equiv \log P(Q|\mathbf{X})$. Thus:

$$\hat{Q} = \mathrm{argmax}_Q P(Q|\mathbf{X})$$
$$= \mathrm{argmax}_Q P(\mathbf{X}|Q)P(Q)$$
$$= \mathrm{argmax}_Q F(Q),$$

where

$$F(Q) \propto \log P(\mathbf{X}|Q) + \log P(Q)$$

$$\propto \sum_{i=1}^{N} \log \left(\sum_{k=1}^{K} \pi_k \frac{B(\bar{\alpha}_k + \bar{X}_i)}{B(\bar{\alpha}_k)} \right) - v \sum_{j=1}^{S} \sum_{k=1}^{K} \alpha_{jk} + \eta \sum_{j=1}^{S} \sum_{k=1}^{K} \log \alpha_{jk}. \tag{10}$$

We now use a binary latent variable matrix $\mathbf{Z}$ with elements z_{ik} that are 1 if the ith community sample belongs to the kth metacommunity and 0 otherwise. The rows of this matrix are the $\bar{z}_i$ vectors introduced above. This allows us to maximise the log posterior distribution using the popular expectation-maximisation (EM) algorithm [21]. Augmenting the data with these latent variables, the evidence and log posterior distribution, respectively, become:

$$P(\mathbf{X},\mathbf{Z}|Q) = \prod_{i=1}^{N} \prod_{k=1}^{K} \left(\frac{B(\bar{\alpha}_k + \bar{X}_i)}{B(\bar{\alpha}_k)} J_i! \prod_{j=1}^{S} \frac{1}{X_{ij}!} \pi_k \right)^{z_{ik}},$$

$$F(Q,\mathbf{Z}) \propto \sum_{i=1}^{N} \sum_{k=1}^{K} z_{ik} \{ \log \pi_k + \log B(\bar{\alpha}_k + \bar{X}_i) - \log B(\bar{\alpha}_k) \}$$

$$- v \sum_{j=1}^{S} \sum_{k=1}^{K} \alpha_{jk} + \eta \sum_{j=1}^{S} \sum_{k=1}^{K} \log \alpha_{jk}.$$

Using Jensen's inequality we obtain a lower bound for the expected log posterior distribution:

$$E_{\mathbf{Z}}[F(Q,\mathbf{Z})] \geq \sum_{i=1}^{N} \sum_{k=1}^{K} E[z_{ik}] \{ \log \pi_k + \log B(\bar{\alpha}_k + \bar{X}_i) - \log B(\bar{\alpha}_k) \}$$

$$- v \sum_{j=1}^{S} \sum_{k=1}^{K} \alpha_{jk} + \eta \sum_{j=1}^{S} \sum_{k=1}^{K} \log \alpha_{jk} + \text{terms independent of } Q. \tag{11}$$

We can calculate $E[z_{ik}]$ as follows:

$$E[z_{ik}] = P(z_{ik} = 1 | \bar{X}_i)$$

$$= \frac{P(z_{ik} = 1)P(\bar{X}_i | z_{ik} = 1)}{\sum_{k'} P(z_{ik'} = 1)P(\bar{X}_i | z_{ik'} = 1)}$$

$$= \frac{\pi_k \dfrac{B(\bar{\alpha}_k + \bar{X}_i)}{B(\bar{\alpha}_k)}}{\sum_{k'} \pi_{k'} \dfrac{B(\bar{\alpha}_{k'} + \bar{X}_i)}{B(\bar{\alpha}_{k'})}}, \tag{12}$$

where we have used Bayes' theorem and $P(\bar{X}_i | z_{ik} = 1) = P(\bar{X}_i | \bar{\alpha}_k)$.

Following Sjölander et al (1996) [22], we now reparameterise and optimise the expected log posterior distribution with respect to these new parameters: to keep the α_{jk}'s positive, we set $\alpha_{jk} = e^{\lambda_{jk}}$, and to keep the π_k's normalised, we set $\pi_k = \mu_k / \sum_{k'} \mu_{k'}$. Optimising $E_{\mathbf{Z}}[F(Q, \mathbf{Z})]$ with respect to μ_k is equivalent to solving the following equation:

$$\frac{\partial E_{\mathbf{Z}}[F(Q, \mathbf{Z})]}{\partial \mu_k} = \frac{1}{\mu_k} \sum_{i=1}^{N} E[z_{ik}] - \frac{N}{\sum_{k'} \mu_{k'}} = 0.$$

Rearranging this equation we obtain:

$$\frac{\mu_k}{\sum_{k'} \mu_{k'}} = \frac{1}{N} \sum_{i=1}^{N} E[z_{ik}],$$

and thus:

$$\pi_k = \frac{1}{N} \sum_{i=1}^{N} E[z_{ik}]. \tag{13}$$

Our EM algorithm to find $\hat{Q}$ thus alternates between updating the responsibilities $E[z_{ik}]$, the mixing coefficients $\bar{\pi}$ and the Dirichlet parameters $\bar{\alpha}_k$, $k = 1, \ldots K$:

- Calculate $E[z_{ik}]$ using Equation 12.
- Update λ_{jk} by finding parameters that minimise the negative of Equation 11. In practice we used the Broyden-Fletcher-Goldfarb-Shanno (BFGS) algorithm as implemented in the Gnu Science Library [29].
- Calculate π_k using Equation 13.
- Repeat until convergence of $E_{\mathbf{Z}}[F(Q, \mathbf{Z})]$, which can be calculated from Equation 11.

We will refer to the hyperparameter values obtained by this method as the maximum posterior estimates (MPE).

Model comparison through Laplace approximation. We need to determine the number of components K in the Dirichlet mixture. We cannot simply choose the one with the largest log posterior, $F(Q)$, as this takes no account of model complexity: as the number of components is increased, $F(Q)$ must increase. We could use a heuristic like the Aikaike Information Criterion (AIC) or Bayesian Information Criterion (BIC) to penalise the model parameters but these can give misleading results [21]. Better is to take a fully Bayesian approach to model comparison where probabilities are used to represent uncertainty in the choice of model. Applying Bayes' theorem, the posterior probability of the K component model H_K given the data matrix $\mathbf{X}$ is:

$$p(\mathcal{H}_K | \mathbf{X}) \propto p(\mathcal{H}_K) p(\mathbf{X} | \mathcal{H}_K),$$

where $p(\mathcal{H}_K)$ is the prior probability for the K component model, which allows us to express a preference for different models, and $p(\mathbf{X} | \mathcal{H}_K)$ is the model evidence, which expresses the preference of the data for different models. In our case, the model evidence is given by:

$$p(\mathbf{X} | \mathcal{H}_K) = \int p(\mathbf{X} | Q, \mathcal{H}_K) p(Q | \mathcal{H}_K) dQ.$$

This integral cannot be calculated analytically, but it can be estimated using the Laplace approximation:

$$\log p(\mathbf{X} | \mathcal{H}_K) \approx \log p(\mathbf{X} | \hat{Q}, \mathcal{H}_K) + \log p(\hat{Q} | \mathcal{H}_K) + \frac{M}{2} \log(2\pi) - \frac{1}{2} \log |H|, \tag{14}$$

where M is the number of parameters in Q, $\hat{Q}$ are the parameters maximising the posterior distribution, and H is the Hessian matrix of second derivatives of the negative log posterior evaluated at $\hat{Q}$:

$$H = -\nabla\nabla \log p(\mathbf{X} | \hat{Q}, \mathcal{H}_K) p(\hat{Q} | \mathcal{H}_K) = -\nabla\nabla \log p(\hat{Q} | \mathbf{X}). \tag{15}$$

Thus,

$$H = -\nabla\nabla \log p(\mathbf{X} | \hat{Q}, \mathcal{H}_K) - \nabla\nabla \log p(\hat{Q} | \mathcal{H}_K).$$

The nonzero elements of the Hessian matrix are given below:

$$-\frac{\partial^2 E_{\mathbf{Z}}[F(Q, \mathbf{Z})]}{\partial \lambda_{jk}^2} =$$

$$-\alpha_{jk} \sum_{i=1}^{N} E[z_{ik}] \left(-\Psi(\alpha_{jk}) + \Psi(A_k) + \Psi(c_{jk}) - \Psi(C_k) \right)$$

$$-\alpha_{jk}^2 \sum_{i=1}^{N} E[z_{ik}] \left(-\Psi_1(\alpha_{jk}) + \Psi_1(A_k) + \Psi_1(c_{jk}) - \Psi_1(C_k) \right) + \nu\alpha_{jk},$$

$$-\frac{\partial^2 E_{\mathbf{Z}}[F(Q, \mathbf{Z})]}{\partial \lambda_{j'k} \partial \lambda_{jk}} = -\alpha_{jk}\alpha_{j'k} \sum_{i=1}^{N} E[z_{ik}](\Psi_1(A_k) - \Psi_1(C_k)),$$

and

$$-\frac{\partial^2 E_{\mathbf{Z}}[F(Q, \mathbf{Z})]}{\partial \pi_k^2} = \frac{1}{\pi_k^2} \sum_{i=1}^{N} E[z_{ik}],$$

where $A_k = \sum_{j=1}^{S} \alpha_{jk}$, $c_{jk} = \alpha_{jk} + X_{ij}$, $C_k = \sum_{j=1}^{S} c_{jk}$, $\Psi(z) = \frac{\Gamma'(z)}{\Gamma(z)}$ and $\Psi_1(z) = \frac{d}{dz}\Psi(z)$. In the results we will give the negative of Equation 14 so that a better fit corresponds to a smaller value. The Hessian also allows us to calculate uncertainties in the parameter estimates of Q, through computing the inverse, then the diagonal elements give the variance of the corresponding parameter.

Data Sets

Twins. To illustrate the application of these ideas to a real data set we reanalysed a study of the gut microbiomes of twins and

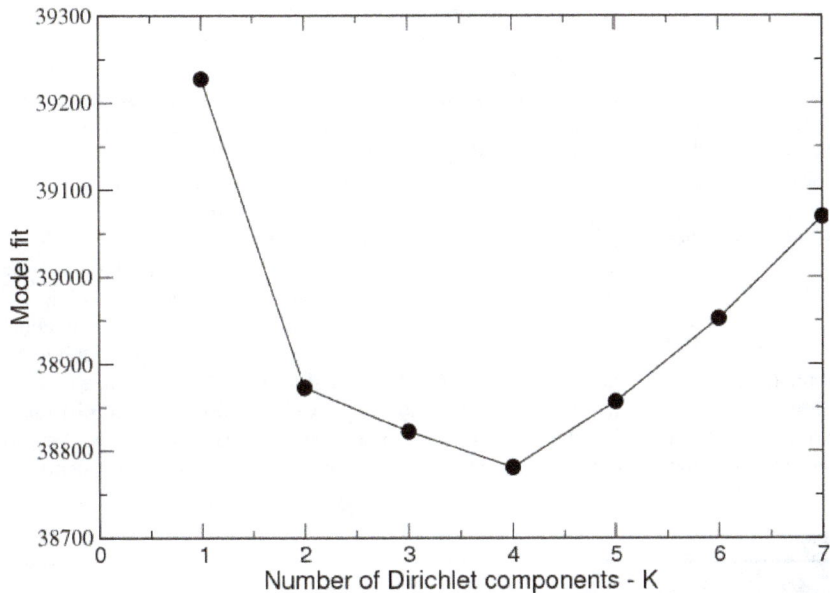

Figure 1. Model fit for mixture of Dirichlets prior to Twins dataset. Evaluates model fit for increasing number of Dirichlet mixture components K using the Laplace approximation to the negative log model evidence.

their mothers [27]. These comprised faecal samples from 154 different individuals characterised by family and body mass index – 'Lean', 'Obese' and 'Overweight'. Each individual was sampled at two time points approximately two months apart. The V2 hypervariable region of the 16S rRNA gene was amplified by PCR and then sequenced using 454. We reanalysed this data set filtering the reads, denoising and removing chimeras using the AmpliconNoise pipeline [10,11]. Denoised reads were then classified to the genus level using the RDP stand-alone classifier [5]. This gave a total of 570,851 reads split over 278 samples since

of the 308 possible some failed to possess any reads following filtering. The size of individual samples varied from just 53 to 10,585 with a median of 1,599. A total of 129 different genera were observed with a genera diversity per sample that varied from just 12 to 50 with a median of 28. One extra category 'Unknown' was used for those reads that failed to be classified with greater than 50% bootstrap certainty. We will refer to this as the 'Twins' data set.

IBD. We also include a brief analysis of microbiome data from a study of inflammatory bowel diseases (IBDs) [28]. This

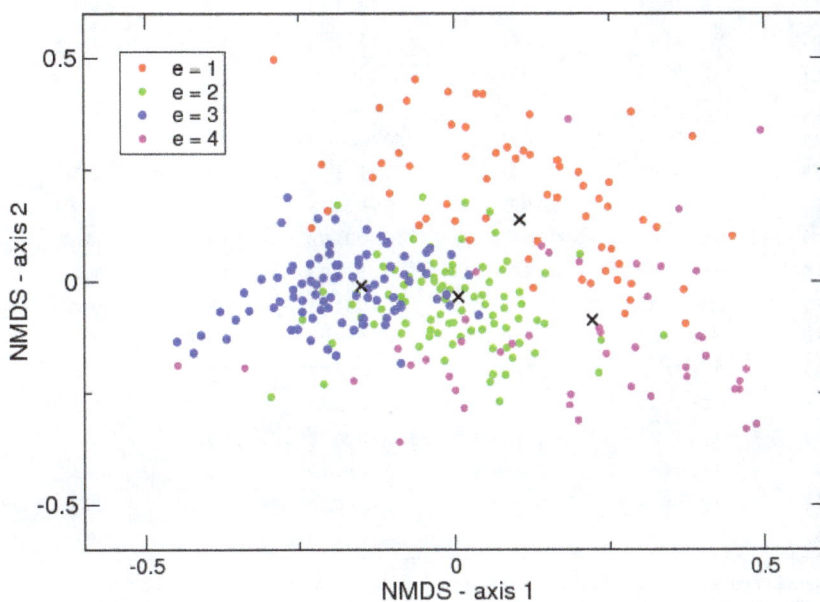

Figure 2. NMDS plot of Twins dataset with hierarchical cluster labellings. Samples arising from each of the four components are shown in red, green, blue and magenta, respectively. The black crosses indicate the Dirichlet means of each component.

comprised faecal samples from 78 individuals where the V5-6 region of the 16S rRNA gene was pyrosequenced using 454. 35 samples were from healthy individuals, 12 from individuals with colonic Crohn's disease (CCD), 15 from individuals exhibiting ileal Crohn's disease (ICD), and 16 from individuals with ulcerative colitis (UC). We processed the data as above. This gave a total of 134,276 reads with individual samples varying in size from 394 to 3,258 with a median of 1,710 reads. 93 separate genera were observed in these samples with a genera diversity per sample that varied from 8 to 33 with a median of 22.

Results

Clustering Twins data at the metacommunity level

The mixture of Dirichlets prior can be used to cluster samples at the metacommunity level. Assuming each sample represents a unique community, we can try to infer which metacommunity that

community is most likely to have originated from. This is the component for which the posterior probability of each membership is the highest, i.e. the value of k that maximizes $P(z_{ik} = 1 | \bar{X}_i, \hat{Q})$ for a particular sample i. We will denote this value as e. These posterior probabilities will be the equilibrium values of the $E[z_{ik}]$ calculated by the EM fitting algorithm.

To use the mixture of Dirichlets prior for clustering at the metacommunity level we first need to determine what the number of clusters or mixture components K should be. To do this we fitted Dirichlet mixtures by minimising the negative log posterior as described above. To calculate model fit accounting for complexity we then used the Laplace approximation to the model evidence. We did this for increasing values of K starting with just a single component $K = 1$. The results are shown in Figure 1 where we see a minimum for $K = 4$ suggesting, firstly, that a mixture of Dirichlets is more appropriate than a single Dirichlet prior for this data set and that, secondly, the mixture has four components.

Table 1. Genera frequencies in the Twins Clusters.

Rank	Genus	m_{0j}	m_{1j}	m_{2j}	m_{3j}	m_{4j}	Diff.	C. Diff.
1	Bacteroides	17.5	5-6.8-8	21-22.6-25	35-38.8-43	7-8.3-11	46.3	29.2
2	Unknown	30.8	26-29.1-33	31-33.6-37	20-22.4-25	39-45.2-53	27.2	46.4
3	Faecalibacter.	10.0	12-13.8-16	8-8.8-10	12-13.8-16	3-4.0-5	14.9	55.8
4	Prevotella	0.60	4.2-5.18-6.3	0.2-0.22-0.3	0.1-0.14-0.2	0.2-0.40-0.7	5.6	59.4
5	Alistipes	2.33	1.5-1.86-2.4	3.5-4.02-4.7	1.4-1.66-2.0	0.7-0.99-1.4	4.2	62.0
6	Dorea	2.71	2.7-3.32-4.1	1.2-1.49-1.8	1.4-1.73-2.1	3.1-4.05-5.3	4.1	64.6
7	Ruminococcus	2.05	1.9-2.36-3.0	3.1-3.57-4.2	0.8-0.95-1.2	0.6-0.92-1.4	4.1	67.2
8	Oscillibacter	2.56	2.3-2.84-3.5	3.4-3.96-4.6	1.3-1.59-1.9	0.9-1.20-1.7	4.0	69.7
9	Roseburia	4.13	3.0-3.63-4.5	2.0-2.32-2.8	3.9-4.47-5.2	4.2-5.40-6.9	3.9	72.2
10	Subdoligran.	2.84	2.8-3.40-4.2	2.6-3.04-3.6	1.6-1.91-2.3	1.2-1.62-2.3	2.9	74.0
11	Collinsella	1.37	1.8-2.32-2.9	0.5-0.66-0.8	0.5-0.67-0.9	1.3-1.76-2.5	2.7	75.8
12	Eubacterium	1.03	1.9-2.47-3.1	0.3-0.40-0.5	0.4-0.52-0.7	0.8-1.16-1.6	2.7	77.5
13	Hespellia	1.04	0.4-0.54-0.8	0.5-0.65-0.8	0.5-0.69-0.9	1.4-1.95-2.6	2.1	78.8
14	Coprococcus	2.37	2.3-2.84-3.5	1.6-1.90-2.3	1.1-1.32-1.6	1.7-2.31-3.1	2.1	80.1
15	Streptococcus	1.12	0.9-1.21-1.6	0.4-0.57-0.7	0.5-0.62-0.8	1.2-1.65-2.2	1.7	81.2
16	Coprobacillus	1.13	0.6-0.77-1.1	0.8-0.95-1.2	0.5-0.59-0.8	1.1-1.58-2.2	1.5	82.2
17	Catenibacterium	0.35	0.8-1.09-1.5	0.1-0.09-0.2	0.1-0.15-0.2	0.2-0.30-0.6	1.2	82.9
18	Eggerthella	0.47	0.1-0.24-0.4	0.2-0.30-0.4	0.2-0.22-0.3	0.7-1.00-1.4	1.2	83.7
19	Clostridium	0.74	0.5-0.68-0.9	0.3-0.42-0.6	0.3-0.39-0.5	0.7-1.03-1.5	1.0	84.3
20	Anaerotruncus	1.02	0.8-1.07-1.4	0.7-0.85-1.1	0.4-0.52-0.7	0.5-0.76-1.1	1.0	84.9
21	Odoribacter	0.67	0.6-0.77-1.0	0.5-0.62-0.8	0.2-0.32-0.4	0.1-0.21-0.4	1.0	85.6
22	Barnesiella	0.56	0.5-0.71-1.0	0.5-0.60-0.8	0.2-0.22-0.3	0.1-0.13-0.3	1.0	86.2
23	Megasphaera	0.38	0.5-0.68-1.0	0.1-0.11-0.2	0.1-0.20-0.3	0.3-0.54-0.9	0.9	86.7
24	Paraprevotella	0.29	0.5-0.71-1.0	0.1-0.11-0.2	0.1-0.10-0.2	0.1-0.18-0.4	0.9	87.3
25	Lactobacillus	0.29	0.4-0.60-0.9	0.1-0.12-0.2	0.0-0.08-0.1	0.2-0.40-0.7	0.8	87.8
26	Butyricimonas	0.42	0.4-0.58-0.8	0.2-0.30-0.4	0.1-0.20-0.3	0.1-0.13-0.3	0.8	88.3
27	Butyricicoccus	0.87	0.6-0.79-1.1	0.4-0.47-0.6	0.5-0.60-0.8	0.6-0.84-1.2	0.8	88.8
28	Lactonifactor	0.63	0.5-0.65-0.9	0.3-0.35-0.5	0.3-0.34-0.5	0.6-0.81-1.2	0.8	89.3
29	Parabacteroides	0.77	0.4-0.59-0.8	0.5-0.64-0.8	0.3-0.40-0.5	0.5-0.68-1.0	0.8	89.8
30	Dialister	0.57	0.3-0.49-0.7	0.2-0.27-0.4	0.3-0.42-0.6	0.5-0.78-1.2	0.7	90.2

Percentage relative abundance of the first 30 out of 131 genera in the estimate of the mean of the reference single Dirichlet component, $\bar{m}_0$, and the four Dirichlet mixture components, $\bar{m}_1, \ldots, \bar{m}_4$ fitted to the Twins data. For the mixture components the upper and lower 95% credible intervals are also given in the format (lower-MPE-upper). These are calculated as the maximum posterior estimate minus/plus two standard deviations as calculated from the inverse Hessian. Genera are ranked in order of their contribution to the total mean difference of 158%, split 34%, 26%, 51% and 47% across components, and the cumulative fraction of this difference accounted for given in the last column in the table.

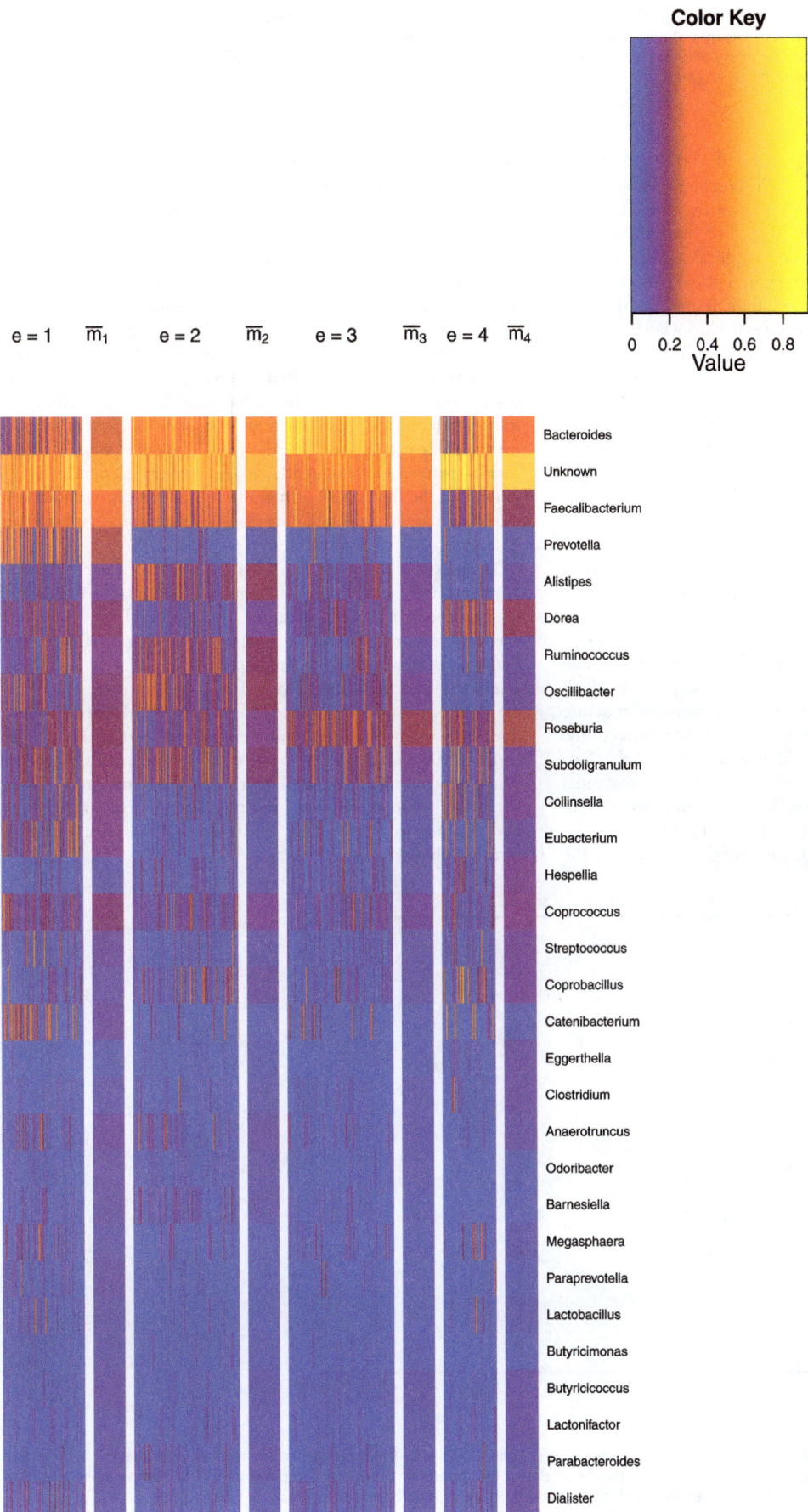

Figure 3. Heat map of the Twins data and hierarchical clustering. Heat map showing the Twins data with samples grouped according to the cluster most likely to have generated them. Only 30 out of 131 genera are shown, those with the greatest variability across clusters, see Table 1. To the right of each cluster the mean of the Dirichlet component for that mixture is shown. The data is square root transformed and therefore to convert the scale to relative abundance, values must be squared.

The four components have weights $\bar{\pi} = (0.22, 0.31, 0.30, 0.17)$. They differ also in how variable their communities are with $\bar{\theta} = (30.2, 52.0, 53.3, 18.7)$. Therefore we have two less abundant highly variable clusters 1 and 4 and two more abundant homogeneous clusters 2 and 3. To graphically illustrate this optimal clustering in Figure 2 we used non-metric multidimensional scaling (NMDS) to generate two-dimensional positions for each community sample, and the mean vectors associated with the four Dirichlet components $\bar{m}_1, \ldots, \bar{m}_4$, that reflect their Bray-Curtis distances using the isoMDS function of R [30]. From this the higher variability in the first and fourth clusters is readily apparent. Another striking observation is that communities are not necessarily associated with the closest cluster mean. Partially this may reflect imperfect mapping to the two-dimensional space but it will also likely reflect properly accounting for sampling through the multinomial-Dirichlet structure.

To explore the component composition we use the Dirichlet parameter vector obtained by fitting a single mixture to the data set as a reference, which we will denote $\bar{\alpha}_0 = \theta_0 \bar{m}_0$. For interest $\theta_0 = 24.4$ a value that is intermediate to that of the four components. We can get a sense of how different the components are by calculating the sum of their posterior mean absolute differences to the reference $\sum_{j=1}^{S} |m_{kj} - m_{0j}|$. A quantity which will vary between 0 and 200% for metacommunities that are identical and completely dissimilar to the reference respectively. Calculating this gives 34%, 26%, 51% and 47% for the four components, and a total of 158%, indicating substantial differences in community structures for each component from the reference. How the different OTUs contribute to these differences is shown in Table 1. Comparing the means of the

posterior distributions for the four components we find that 30 out of 131 genera account for over 90% of this difference. The Bacteroides alone account for 29% of this difference. This genera is substantially over represented in the third cluster comprising nearly 39% of the community, close to the reference at 23% in the second cluster and observed at much lower proportions in the first and fourth clusters at around 7% and 8%, respectively. The next most significantly different category is actually 'Unknown' with nearly 15% more sequences failing to be classified with sufficient confidence in the fourth component, and 8% less in the third component than the reference. Faecilibacterium are substantially under-represented in the fourth component whereas Prevotella is mostly found in the first. The other genera exhibit various patterns but frequently we see over representation in one of or both the first and fourth clusters and little representation in the second and third e.g. Colinsella, Eubacterium, Streptococcus, et cetera.

These patterns are also illustrated graphically in the 'heat map' of relative frequencies shown in Figure 3. The relative frequencies of the 30 genera accounting for the most difference between clusters are shown for all the samples. The samples are grouped into the cluster that they had the highest probability of being generated from, as defined above. The cluster means are plotted to the right of the samples mapped to that cluster. Roughly we have that the two low variance clusters are dominated by Bacteroides and Faecilibacterium, albeit to a greater extent in the third cluster. The high variance, first and fourth clusters, contain a greater variety of genera but with substantially more Prevotella and Faecilibacterium in the first, rather than the fourth, where no genus really dominates.

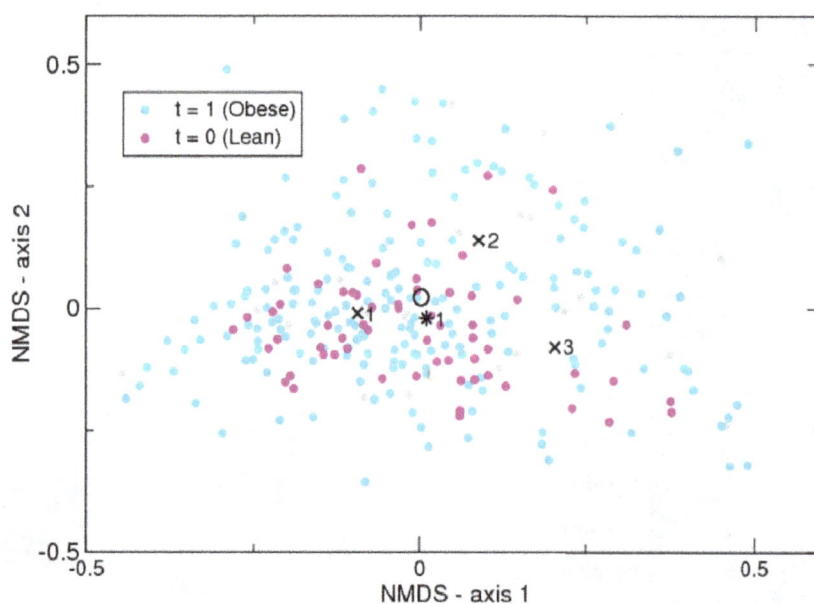

Figure 4. NMDS plot of Twins dataset with class labels. Samples from Lean ($t = 0$) individuals are shown in magenta and Obese ($t = 1$) in Cyan. Overweight are grey. The black crosses indicate the Dirichlet means of each component of the three components for the Obese class, the black asterisk the single component for the Lean class. We also show the posterior mean of the entire Obese class as a black circle.

Table 2. Confusion matrices for classification of Twins data.

Predicted	Random forests		Dirichlet multinomial	
Actual	**Lean**	**Obese**	**Lean**	**Obese**
Lean	19	42	33	28
Obese	5	188	29	164

The two rows give the number of 'Lean' and 'Obese' individuals predicted to be 'Lean' and 'Obese' by the random forests and Dirichlet multinomial classifiers following leave-one-out validation. A classification threshold of 0.5 was used for both algorithms.

Generative classifier for Twins data

The Dirichlet-multinomial framework can also be used for classification. This is a supervised learning approach as opposed to the unsupervised approach used in the previous section. Here, we will consider the case of binary classes but any number of classes is a simple extension. Given a training data set of N samples $\bar{X}_i$ then we denote class membership with the N dimensional vector $\bar{t}$ with elements t_i which are either 0 or 1. The classification problem is to deduce the class $c = \{0,1\}$ of a new sample $\bar{Y}$. To do this we associate a separate Dirichlet multinomial mixture model with each class. We denote the hyperparameters of these mixtures by $Q_0 = (K, \alpha_1, \ldots, \alpha_K)$ and $Q_1 = (K', \alpha_1', \ldots, \alpha_{K'}')$, respectively. Then we can marginalise over the multinomial parameters of the sample to be classified so that:

$$P(c=1|\bar{Y}) = \frac{P(\bar{Y}|Q_1)P(c=1)}{P(\bar{Y}|Q_0)P(c=0) + P(\bar{Y}|Q_1)P(c=1)} \quad (16)$$

is the probability of the sample belonging to the second class and $P(c=0|\bar{Y}) = 1 - P(c=1|\bar{Y})$. The prior class probabilities are estimated as the observed class frequencies so that

$P(c=0) = 1 - \frac{\sum_{i=1}^N t_i}{N}$ and $P(c=1) = \frac{\sum_{i=1}^N t_i}{N}$. The class mixture themselves are determined just as before but with data points restricted to those class members. We can also determine if the fit is significant by comparing the sum of model fits of the classes with the model fit ignoring the class variables. This is our generative classification scheme.

We will apply this to the Twins data denoting individuals with 'Lean' BMI by $t_i = 0$ and 'Obese' as $t_i = 1$. We will ignore the 'Overweight' category to avoid ambiguity. In Figure 4 we replot the NMDS plot of Figure 2 with these class labels. There is no dramatic separation of points according to class labels. We found that for the Lean $t_i = 0$ class a single component Dirichlet mixture was optimal but that for the Obese $t_i = 1$ class three components minimised the Laplace approximation to the model evidence. The means of each of the three Obese components were quite different but the posterior mean for the entire prior sampling from all three according to their weights (black circle in Figure 4) is close to the single component from the Lean class (black asterisk Figure 4). In fact, accounting for uncertainty in both the Dirichlet priors and the sampling from those, then only one low frequency genera, Megasphaera, was significantly differently expressed between classes, having a 97% probability of being more abundant in Obese people. In addition, fitting to the two classes separately did not give a significantly better fit than fitting to the whole data set, 35640 vs. 35385. It is also apparent from comparing Figure 2 and Figure 4 that each of the class components map onto one of the components from the clustering of the whole data set, this was confirmed by comparing the Bray-Curtis distances between the two sets of mean vectors, the component from the Lean class maps onto the second of the four from the whole data set, and the three components from the Obese class map onto the third, first and fourth, respectively. In summary, it appears that the difference between Lean and Obese classes lies not at the level of mean community composition but that the Obese individuals contain a

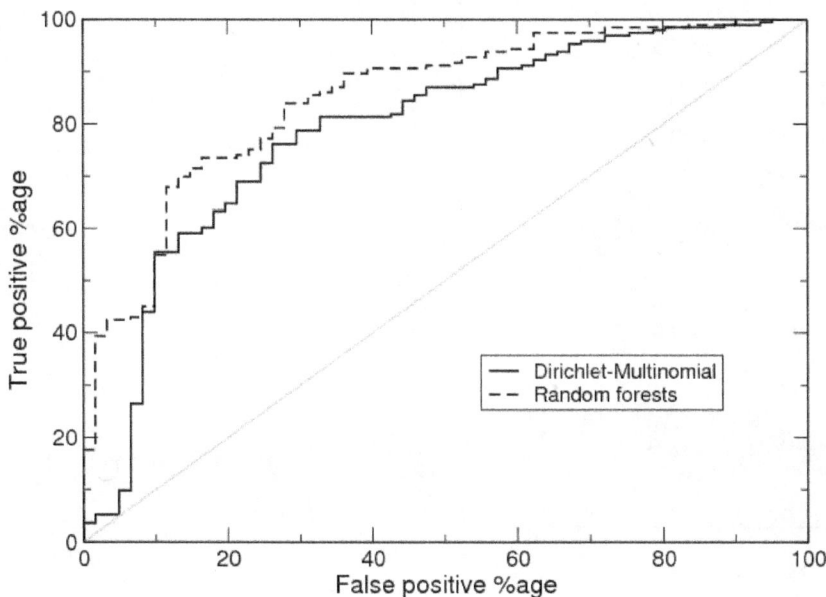

Figure 5. Receiver operating characteristic (ROC) curves for the Twins Dirichlet multinomial and random forests classifiers. Gives true positive percentage on the y-axis i.e. Obese individuals correctly identified vs false positive percentage i.e Lean individuals flagged as Obese.

greater variety of community structures including three out of the four components found in the complete data set.

In a recent evaluation of classification algorithms applied to microbial community data the random forests algorithm was found to perform best [20], substantially outperforming elastic nets, support vector machines, and multinomial naive Bayes (MNB). The random forests algorithm is an example of ensemble learning where many classifiers are generated and their predictions are aggregated. In particular, it is an extension of the machine learning technique known as bootstrap aggregating or bagging for short. The bagging approach constructs decision trees from bootstrap samples of the data and makes class predictions via majority vote. Random forests adds an extra layer of randomness to bagging by changing how the decision trees are constructed. Instead of splitting each node using the best split amongst all the variables, the best split amongst a subset of randomly chosen predictors is used. Moreover, the random forests algorithm also gives a measure of the importance of a variable by calculating how much prediction error increases when data for that variable is permuted. Random forests therefore seemed like an appropriate benchmark to compare the performance of our generative classifier to. Following Knights et al. (2011) [20], we implemented the random forests algorithm using the randomForest package in R, though we tuned the parameters of the algorithm (the number of variables in the random subset at each node and the number of trees in the forest) according to the heuristics suggested by Liaw and Wiener (2002) [31].

To compare the two classification methods we performed leave-one-out validation. We removed each sample in turn from the data set, trained the classifier, and classified the missing data point. Assigning the data point as Obese if the predicted probability was greater than or equal to 0.5. We obtained a slightly lower error rate, i.e. fraction of samples misclassified, for the random forests algorithm (18.5%) as opposed to the Dirichlet multinomial generative classifier (22.4%). Examining the 'confusion matrix'

for each classifier, Table 2, that is the number of individuals from each true class classified into the two classes, reveals that the generative classifier does have a better distribution of errors across classes. We then generated receiver-operating characteristic (ROC) curves for each classifier. These are shown in Figure 5. They are generated by ordering samples by decreasing likelihood of being Obese: for the generative classifier that is simply the probability of being Obese i.e. $P(c = 1)$; for random forests this is the weighted vote. We then lower a threshold from 1.0 to 0.0 with intervals defined by the sample probabilities. All samples with probability greater than or equal to a given threshold are classified as Obese, all other samples as Lean. Based on these classifications, the false positive percentage (i.e. Lean classified as Obese) and true positive rate (Obese classified as Obese) are calculated and plotted against each other. This is repeated for all thresholds. It is a means of summarising the performance of a classifier over all decision thresholds. Both classifiers do substantially better than random but at lower thresholds random forests outperforms the generative classifier with fewer false positives. A summary statistic is the area under the ROC curve, for random forests this was 85%; for the Dirichlet-Multinomial 79% was obtained.

Analysis of IBD phenotypes

We conclude with a brief analysis of the inflammatory bowel disease (IBD) phenotypes. In Figure 6 we show an NMDS plot with samples coloured according to phenotype for this data set generated as described above. It is apparent from this that the Healthy (H) individuals, and those exhibiting colonic Crohn's disease (CCD) and ulcerative colitis (UC), have similar, fairly homogeneous community structures whereas the individuals with ileal Crohn's disease (ICD) have a much larger variation in community structure. We can use the DMM model to quantify this, we fitted single component models, to all the samples together, and then each phenotype separately. The θ values obtained were 15.7 for the whole data set and (H) 22.2, (CCD)

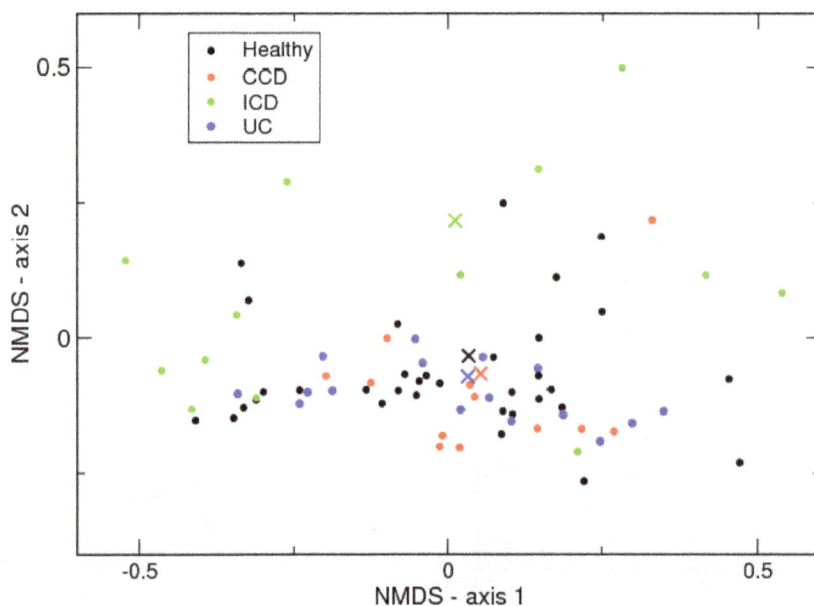

Figure 6. NMDS plot of IBD dataset with class labels. Samples from Healthy individuals (black), and three IBD phenotypes, (red) colonic Crohn's disease (CCD), (green) ileal Crohn's disease (ICD), and (blue) ulcerative colitis (UC) are shown. The Dirichlet means of single component fits to each type are shown by the corresponding coloured cross.

Table 3. Genera frequencies in the IBD phenotypes.

Rank	Genus	m_{0j}	h_j	c_j	i_j	u_j	Diff.	C. Diff.
1	Unknown	27.8	24-28.4-34	26-33.4-44	14-21.1-33	27-34.7-44	19.8	18.9
2	Bacteroides	27.2	24-28.7-35	22-28.7-38	12-19.6-31	26-32.5-41	15.9	34.1
3	Faecalibacter.	3.61	3.3-4.36-5.8	3.6-5.39-8.0	0.7-1.52-3.4	3.1-4.46-6.4	5.5	39.4
4	Escherichia/Shigella	0.93	0.3-0.58-1.0	0.2-0.50-1.1	2.1-3.85-7.0	0.2-0.41-0.8	4.2	43.4
5	Parabacteroides	3.49	2.3-3.19-4.3	1.9-3.07-4.9	2.6-4.77-8.6	1.5-2.31-3.6	3.2	46.5
6	Sutterella	1.00	0.6-0.95-1.5	0.2-0.49-1.1	1.3-2.63-5.3	0.1-0.30-0.7	2.9	49.2
7	Alistipes	3.61	3.3-4.41-5.9	2.4-3.79-6.0	1.3-2.56-5.1	1.9-2.92-4.4	2.7	51.8
8	Prevotella	0.77	0.5-0.79-1.3	0.0-0.15-0.6	0.9-1.98-4.4	0.2-0.36-0.8	2.3	54.0
9	Dorea	1.98	1.2-1.65-2.3	0.9-1.48-2.5	1.4-2.70-5.2	0.8-1.29-2.1	2.2	56.2
10	Klebsiella	0.47	0.2-0.34-0.6	0.1-0.21-0.7	0.9-1.95-4.4	0.1-0.16-0.5	2.2	58.2
11	Bifidobacterium	1.91	1.1-1.59-2.3	1.5-2.48-4.1	1.2-2.32-4.7	0.7-1.14-1.9	2.1	60.2
12	Barnesiella	1.65	1.3-1.88-2.7	0.8-1.47-2.6	0.1-0.49-1.9	0.8-1.30-2.2	1.9	62.1
13	Oscillibacter	2.49	2.0-2.75-3.8	1.4-2.31-3.8	0.7-1.60-3.6	1.3-1.97-3.1	1.9	63.9
14	Streptococcus	0.67	0.3-0.44-0.8	0.2-0.44-1.0	0.8-1.76-3.7	0.2-0.37-0.8	1.8	65.6
15	Coprococcus	1.73	0.9-1.37-2.0	0.7-1.20-2.1	1.2-2.41-4.7	0.9-1.46-2.4	1.8	67.4
16	Veillonella	0.17	0.0-0.03-0.2	0.0-0.00-0.0	0.7-1.59-3.6	0.0-0.09-0.4	1.8	69.1
17	Subdoligranulum	2.33	1.8-2.47-3.4	1.2-1.93-3.2	0.7-1.62-3.6	1.2-1.86-3.0	1.7	70.7
18	Paraprevotella	0.55	0.4-0.60-1.0	0.0-0.14-0.5	0.6-1.36-3.3	0.1-0.21-0.6	1.6	72.3
19	Acidaminococcus	0.19	0.0-0.06-0.3	0.0-0.07-0.5	0.6-1.35-3.3	0.0-0.09-0.4	1.5	73.7
20	Lactobacillus	0.20	0.0-0.13-0.3	0.0-0.13-0.5	0.5-1.27-3.1	0.0-0.00-0.0	1.4	75.1
21	Ruminococcus	1.47	1.0-1.40-2.0	0.7-1.29-2.3	0.4-1.01-2.7	0.5-0.94-1.6	1.2	76.3
22	Lactonifactor	0.11	0.0-0.06-0.2	0.0-0.00-0.0	0.4-1.01-2.7	0.0-0.00-0.0	1.2	77.4
23	Odoribacter	1.11	0.7-1.04-1.5	0.4-0.73-1.4	0.3-0.93-2.5	0.4-0.69-1.2	1.0	78.4
24	Butyricicoccus	1.01	0.6-0.92-1.4	0.3-0.53-1.1	0.3-0.93-2.5	0.4-0.66-1.1	1.0	79.3
25	Fusobacterium	0.09	0.0-0.06-0.3	0.0-0.00-0.0	0.3-0.80-2.5	0.0-0.00-0.0	0.9	80.2

Percentage relative abundance of the first 25 out of 95 genera in the estimate of the mean of the reference single Dirichlet component, $\bar{m}_0$, fitted to all IBD individuals, and the four single component Dirichlet models, fitted to healthy ($\bar{h}$), colonic Crohn's disease (CCD - $\bar{c}$), ileal Crohn's disease (ICD - $\bar{i}$), and ulcerative colitis (UC - $\bar{u}$) phenotypes. For the mixture components the upper and lower 95% credible intervals are also given in the format (lower-MPE-upper). These are calculated as the maximum log posterior estimate minus/plus two standard deviations as calculated from the inverse Hessian. Genera are ranked in order of their contribution to the total difference of 104% to the reference split 9%, 20%, 48%, 27% across phenotypes, and the cumulative fraction of this difference accounted for given in the last column in the table.

39.4, (ICD) 5.1, (UC) 38.5 for the phenotypes. Remembering, that θ is related to the inverse of the variance, then this confirms that the ICD phenotype is associated with an increase in metacommunity variability. We also show the metacommunity means in Figure 6 as crosses: H, CCD and UC have a similar location whereas the ICD mean is displaced. Exactly how the different OTUs contribute to the differences in the ICD samples is shown in Table 3 and graphically in Figure 7. The proportion of the Unknown, Bacteroides, and Faecalibacterium genera are reduced whereas numerous other genera for example the Escherichia/ Shigella, Sutterella, and Prevotella are increased.

Discussion

We have demonstrated that the Dirichlet multinomial mixture is a powerful framework for the generative modelling of microbial community data. It operates at several levels, it allows read numbers and hence sampling noise to be naturally accounted for, and the Dirichlet parameters are easily interpretable in terms of the mean and variance of the communities generated from each component. Used for 'unsupervised learning' or clustering it

provides a means to determine clusters of communities or envirotypes, a highly topical problem in the analysis of microbial community data. Since it is a probabilistic model, we can harness rigorous statistical theory for determining how well the data is explained by a given cluster number.

We illustrated this approach with the Twins data set. Using our models, the most probable estimate for the number of envirotypes present in this sample (or 'enterotypes' as they are known in the context of gut microbiota samples) is four. Our measure of model fit, the negative logarithm of the approximate model evidence, was 41 less than the next best cluster number, three. Thus, in the context of our model the probability that there are four rather than three or five clusters is practically a 100%. However, a direct implication of the Bayesian approach is that any point estimate of the number of envirotypes represents a summary (in our case, the mode) of the posterior distribution over the number of clusters. For other data sets the predicted cluster number may be more uncertain. This uncertainty can be naturally incorporated by our approach.

Our analysis, and its statistical implications, may be contrasted with a previous analysis of this same Twins dataset, which used a

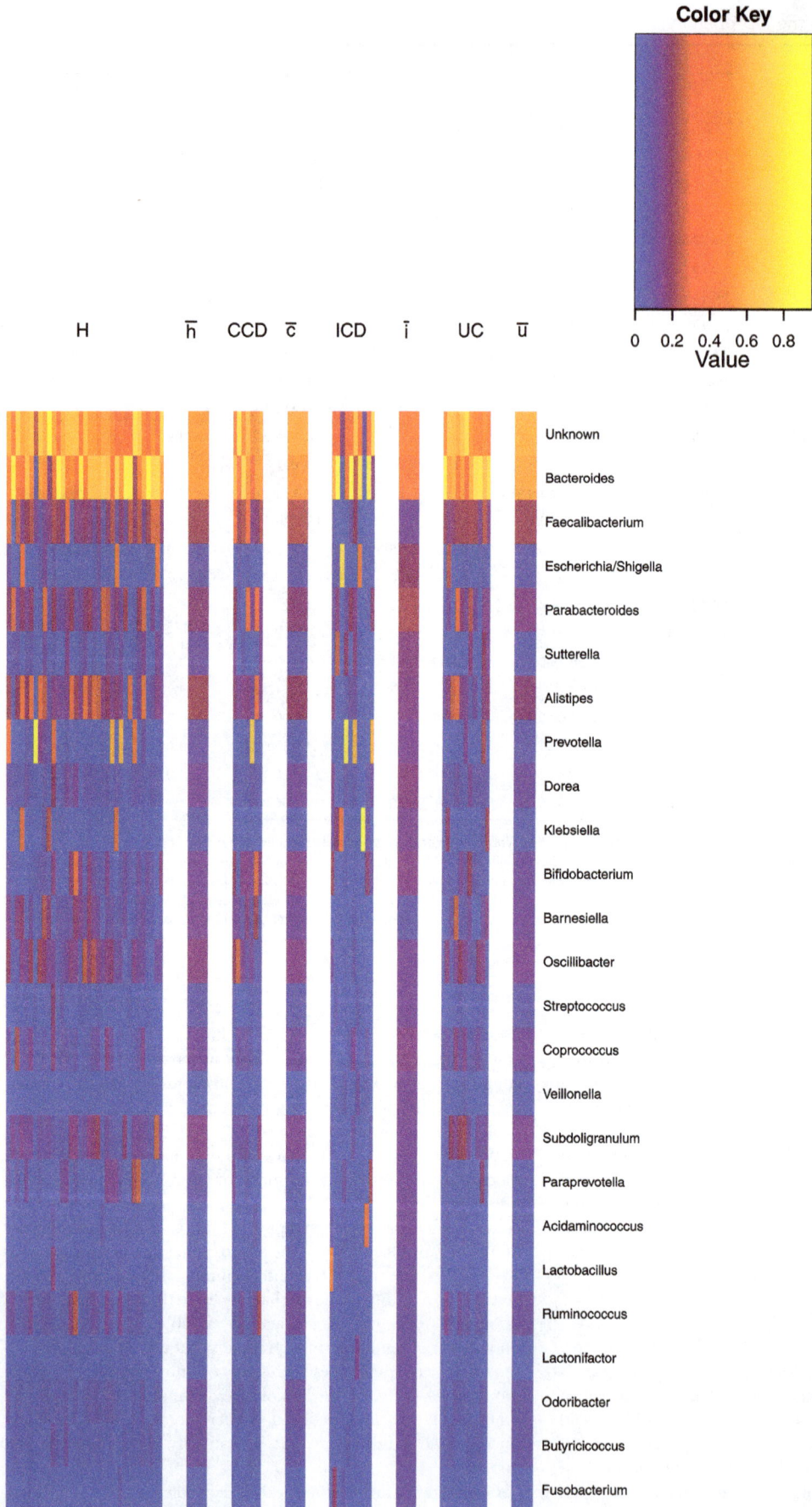

Figure 7. Heat map of the IBD data divided by phenotype together with phenotype means. Heat map showing the IBD data with samples grouped according to the IBD pheonotype. The means of the four single component Dirichlet models, fitted to healthy ($\bar{h}$), colonic Crohn's disease (CCD - $\bar{c}$), ileal Crohn's disease (ICD - $\bar{i}$), and ulcerative colitis (UC - $\bar{u}$) phenotypes are also shown. Only 25 out of 95 genera are shown, those with the greatest variability across phenotypes, see Table 3. The data is square root transformed and therefore to convert the scale to relative abundance, values must be squared.

partitioning around medoid (PAM) clustering coupled with the heuristic Calinski-Harabasz (CH) index [18]. The CH approach makes no acknowledgment of the fact that there is inherent uncertainty in the number of clusters, and thus may potentially be misread as offering an unambiguous and definitive assessment of the number of clusters. Furthermore, the PAM clustering algorithm does not allow clusters to be of variable spread. This may be the reason why they found three rather than four clusters. The extra flexibility of the DMM model could better represent the true patterns in the data. This, to us, supports the promise of a probabilistic model with the flexibility to model clusters of different size and a Bayesian approach to determining the cluster number.

Used for 'supervised learning' the Dirichlet multinomial mixture provides an effective classifier. Absolute classification power as summarised by the area under the ROC curve is less than for the best performing of previously tested algorithms - random forests. However, using the standard classification threshold of 0.5 it had a better distribution of errors across classes, outperforming random forests on the smaller 'Lean' class. In general, we would expect discriminative classifiers, which only model the conditional probability of the class label given the data, to outperform generative models, which fit the actual class distributions. On the other hand, the generative approach allows much easier interpretation of the fitted models, which is often more important than accuracy *per se*. The fitted Dirichlet parameters describe both the composition of the communities, and critically variance in composition associated with the classes. The probabilistic framework that we present also allows the hypothesis of whether two classes do differ in community composition to be rigorously tested. Or equivalently whether a discrete experimental treatment significantly impacts community structure.

Generative models provide a framework for both clustering and classification but their full power derives from their ability to combine the two. We will illustrate this for the Twins data. In Table 4 we give the proportion of samples from each BMI category, i.e. Lean, Obese and Overweight, that fell into our four enterotypes. For this data set we did not see a significant difference in mean community composition between Lean and Obese individuals. However, it is clear that the two classes do differ significantly in their probability of deriving from each of the clusters. Lean individuals are much less likely to derive from the first and fourth clusters than Obese individuals. They are much more likely to derive from the second and somewhat less likely from the third. This suggests a novel explanation for the differences in taxa frequency that have been previously reported

between Lean and Obese individuals from this data. BMI itself is not correlated with changes in community structure rather it influences the likelihood of deriving from the four enterotypes.

This raises the intriguing possibility that the first and fourth enterotypes may be associated with a disturbed possibly unhealthy gut microbiota – 'dysbiosis'. This implies that obesity does not guarantee a disturbed microflora but increases its likelihood. Finally, we return to the observation that the first and fourth enterotypes have a higher variance in community structure than the second and third. We suggest that this is an example of the 'Anna Karenina principle' as applied to microbial communities. This principle popularised by Jared Diamond [32] derives from the first line of Tolstoy's novel: "Happy families are all alike; every unhappy family is unhappy in its own way" [33]. We propose that the same thing may apply to microbial communities in human health, there are many more configurations associated with dysbiosis than are possible for a healthy community which is relatively predictable and homogeneous as it requires certain key components. This is not to suggest that the first and fourth enterotypes are associated with higher genera level diversity in individual samples, the median diversities are not significantly different between the enterotypes, it is the diversity in community compositions that increases. Our observations are also consistent, therefore, with the conclusion of the original study that the major impact of obesity was a reduction in OTU diversity [27].

This interpretation of the Twins data is obviously speculative and will require further studies with more meta-data on host health to corroborate. The analysis of the IBD phenotype data represents a first step in this direction. There we did find a much more variable microbiota associated with one of the disease phenotypes, ileal Crohn's disease, but not colonic Crohn's or ulcerative colitis. This is, therefore partial support for the AKP. However, it is possible that the latter two diseases are not strongly associated with gut dysbiosis. Certainly, at the genera level we were unable to discriminate their community compositions from healthy individuals. The number of samples in each of the disease phenotypes was also quite small. We hope that future large-scale sequencing projects will allow us to investigate this question further. The 'Human Microbiome Project' is restricted to healthy individuals but that will allow us to verify the existence of the two enterotypes that we propose are associated with a healthy microbiota [34].

The software for fitting the Dirichlet multinomial mixture is available for download from the Google Code project MicrobeDMM (http://code.google.com/p/microbedmm/).

Table 4. Comparison of BMI and cluster or 'Enterotype'.

BMI	e = 1	e = 2	e = 3	e = 4
Lean	6.6%	60.7%	24.6%	8.2%
Obese	25.9%	21.2%	33.2%	19.7%
Overweight	29.2%	33.3%	25.0%	12.5%

Proportion of samples with a given BMI deriving from the four enterotypes $e=1$, $e=2$, $e=3$, and $e=4$.

Acknowledgments

We wish to thank Jose Carlos Clemente, Alan Walker and three anonymous reviewers for comments on an earlier draft of this manuscript, Peter Turnbaugh for providing the Twins data, and Ben Willing, Johan Dicksved and Anders Andersson for providing the IBD data set.

Author Contributions

Conceived and designed the experiments: IH KH CQ. Performed the experiments: IH KH CQ. Analyzed the data: IH KH CQ. Contributed reagents/materials/analysis tools: IH KH CQ. Wrote the paper: IH KH CQ.

References

1. Streit W, Schmitz R (2004) Metagenomics - the key to the uncultured microbes. Curr Opin Microbiol 7: 492–498.

2. Dorigo U, Volatier L, Humbert JF (2005) Molecular approaches to the assessment of biodiversity in aquatic microbial communities. Water Res 39: 2207–2218.

3. Margulies M, Egholm M, Altman W, Attiya S, Bader J, et al. (2005) Genome sequencing in microfabricated high-density picolitre reactors. Nature 437: 376–380.

4. Caporaso JG, Lauber CL, Walters WA, Berg-Lyons D, Lozupone CA, et al. (2011) Global patterns of 16S rRNA diversity at a depth of millions of sequences per sample. Proc Natl Acad Sci USA;e-pub ahead of print doi: 10.1073/pnas.1000080107.

5. Wang Q, Garrity GM, Tiedje JM, Cole JR (2007) Naive Bayesian classifier for rapid assignment of rRNA sequences into the new bacterial taxonomy. Appl Environ Microbiol 73: 5261–5267.

6. Schloss P, Handelsman J (2005) Introducing DOTUR, a computer program for defining operational taxonomic units and estimating species richness. Appl Environ Microbiol 71: 1501–1506.

7. Schloss PD, Handelsman J (2008) A statistical toolbox for metagenomics: assessing functional diversity in microbial communities. BMC Bioinf 9.

8. Sogin ML, Morrison HG, Huber JA, Mark Welch D, Huse SM, et al. (2006) Microbial diversity in the deep sea and the underexplored "rare biosphere". Proc Natl Acad Sci USA 103: 12115–12120.

9. Huber JA, Mark Welch D, Morrison HG, Huse SM, Neal PR, et al. (2007) Microbial population structures in the deep marine biosphere. Science 318: 97–100.

10. Quince C, Lanzen A, Curtis TP, Davenport RJ, Hall N, et al. (2009) Accurate determination of microbial diversity from 454 pyrosequencing data. Nat Methods 6: 639–641.

11. Quince C, Lanzen A, Davenport RJ, Turnbaugh PJ (2011) Removing noise from pyrosequenced amplicons. BMC Bioinf 12.

12. Turnbaugh PJ, Quince C, Faith JJ, McHardy AC, Yatsunenko T, et al. (2010) Organismal, genetic, and transcriptional variation in the deeply sequenced gut microbiomes of identical twins. Proc Natl Acad Sci USA 107: 7503–7508.

13. Quince C, Curtis TP, Sloan WT (2008) The rational exploration of microbial diversity. ISME J 2: 997–1006.

14. Hamady M, Walker JJ, Harris JK, Gold NJ, Knight R (2008) Error-correcting barcoded primersfor pyrosequencing hundreds of samples in multiplex. Nat Methods 5: 235–237.

15. Ramette A (2007) Multivariate analyses in microbial ecology. FEMS Microbiol Ecol 62: 142–160.

16. Lozupone C, Knight R (2005) UniFrac: a new phylogenetic method for comparing microbial communities. Appl Environ Microbiol 71: 8228–8235.

17. Caporaso JG, Kuczynski J, Stombaugh J, Bittinger K, Bushman FD, et al. (2010) QIIME allows analysis of high-throughput community sequencing data. Nat Methods 7: 335–336.

18. Arumugam M, Raes J, Pelletier E, Le Paslier D, Yamada T, et al. (2011) Enterotypes of the human gut microbiome. Nature 473: 174–180.

19. Sun Y, Cai Y, Mai V, Farmerie W, Yu F, et al. (2010) Advanced computational algorithms for microbial community analysis using massive 16S rRNA sequence data. Nucleic Acids Res 38.

20. Knights D, Costello E, Knight R (2011) Supervised classification of human microbiota. FEMS Microbiol Rev 35: 343–359.

21. Bishop CM (2006) Pattern Recognition and Machine Learning Springer: Yale University Press.

22. Sjolander K, Karplus K, Brown M, Hughey R, Krogh A, et al. (1996) Dirichlet mixtures: A method for improved detection of weak but significant protein sequence homology. Comput Appl Biosci 12: 327–345.

23. X Y, Yu YK, Altschul SF (2010) Compositional adjustment of Dirichlet mixture priors. J Comput Biol 17: 1607–1620.

24. Bouguila N (2011) Count data modeling and classification using finite mixtures of distributions. IEEE Trans Neural Netw 22: 186–198.

25. D K, Kuczynski J, Charlson ES, Zaneveld J, Mozer MC, et al. (2011) Bayesian community-wide culture-independent microbial source tracking. Nat Methods 8: 761–763.

26. Mackay DJ (1992) Bayesian interpolation. Neural Comput 4: 415–417.

27. Turnbaugh PJ, Hamady M, Yatsunenko T, Cantarel BL, Duncan A, et al. (2009) A core gut microbiome in obese and lean twins. Nature 457: 480–484.

28. Willing BP, Dicksved J, Halfvarson J, Andersson AF, Lucio M, et al. (2010) A Pyrosequencing Study in Twins Shows That Gastrointestinal Microbial Profiles Vary With Inflammatory Bowel Disease Phenotypes. Gastroenterology 139: 1844–U105.

29. Galassi M (2009) GNU Scientific Library Reference Manual. URL http://www.gnu.org/software/gsl/. ISBN 0-954612-07-8.

30. R Development Core Team (2010) R: A Language and Environment for Statistical Computing. R Foundation for Statistical Computing, Vienna, Austria. URL http://www.R-project.org. ISBN 3-900051-07-0.

31. Liaw A, Wiener M (2002) Classification and regression by randomforest. R news 2: 18–22.

32. Diamond J (1997) Guns, Germs, and Steel. New York, New York: W. W. Norton.

33. Tolstoy L (1877) Anna Karenina. Moscow, Russia: The Russian Messenger.

34. Peterson J, Garges S, Giovanni M, McInnes P, Wang L, et al. (2009) The NIH Human Microbiome Project. Genome Res 19: 2317–2323.

16

Expression of Human Beta-Defensins in Children with Chronic Inflammatory Bowel Disease

Matthias Zilbauer[1,2]*, **Andreas Jenke[1]**, **Gundula Wenzel[1]**, **Jan Postberg[1]**, **Andreas Heusch[1]**, **Alan D. Phillips[3]**, **Gabriele Noble-Jamieson[2]**, **Franco Torrente[2]**, **Camilla Salvestrini[2]**, **Robert Heuschkel[2]**, **Stefan Wirth[1]**

1 Department of Paediatrics, HELIOS Klinikum Wuppertal, Germany, **2** Department of Paediatric Gastroenterology, Addenbrooke's Hospital, Cambridge, United Kingdom, **3** Centre for Paediatric Gastroenterology, Royal Free Hospital, London, United Kingdom

Abstract

Background: Human beta-defensins (hBDs) are antimicrobial peptides known to play a major role in intestinal innate host defence. Altered mucosal expression of hBDs has been suggested to be implicated in chronic inflammatory bowel disease pathogenesis. However, little is known about expression of these peptides in children.

Methods: Intestinal biopsies were obtained from the duodenum (n = 88), terminal ileum (n = 90) and ascending colon (n = 105) of children with Crohn's disease (n = 26), ulcerative colitis (n = 11) and healthy controls (n = 16). Quantitative real-time (RT) PCR was performed and absolute mRNA copy numbers analyzed for hBD1-3 as well as inflammatory cytokines IL-8 and TNF-alpha.

Results: Significant induction of hBD2 and hBD3 was observed in the inflamed terminal ileum and ascending colon of IBD children. In the ascending colon induction of hBD2 was found to be significantly lower in children with Crohn's disease compared to ulcerative colitis. A strong correlation was found between inducible defensins hBD2 and 3 and the inflammatory cytokines IL-8 and TNF-alpha, both in the terminal ileum and ascending colon.

Conclusion: Our study demonstrates distinct changes in hBD expression throughout the intestinal tract of children with IBD, lending further support for their potential role in disease pathogenesis.

Editor: Stefan Bereswill, Charité-Universitätsmedizin Berlin, Germany

Funding: This study was funded by the German society of Paediatric Gastroenterology (GPGE), Witten/Herdecke University, the Crohn's in Childhood Research Association (CICRA) and the Crohn's and Colitis in Childhood (3Cs) charity. The funders had no role in study design, data collection and analysis, decision to publish, or preparation of the manuscript.

Competing Interests: The authors have declared that no competing interests exist.

* E-mail: mz304@medschl.cam.ac.uk

Introduction

Human beta-defensins (hBDs) are a group of evolutionarily conserved antimicrobial peptides (AMPs) known to play a major role in innate host defence at various mucosal surfaces including the gastrointestinal (GI) tract. Three of the most extensively studied members are hBD1, -2 and -3. Under physiological conditions, hBD1 is expressed constitutively by intestinal epithelial cells while hBD2 and -3 are induced during infection and inflammation [1,2]. In addition to their potent antimicrobial properties against commensal and pathogenic bacteria [3,4], beta-defensins have been shown to function as multieffector molecules capable of enhancing host defence by recruiting various innate as well as adaptive immune cells to the site of infection, induction of neovasculogenesis and enhancing wound closure [5,6,7]. Given these versatile functions it is not surprising that impaired expression and/or function of these peptides has been implicated in the development of several diseases, including chronic inflammatory bowel disease (IBD). The two major entities are Crohn's disease (CD) and ulcerative colitis (UC), which differ in disease distribution as well as histological changes of the affected bowel segment. While CD causes transmural inflammation throughout the entire GI mucosa, changes in UC are restricted to the colonic mucosa. IBD disease pathogenesis is highly complex and remains incompletely understood. However, increasing evidence suggests that impaired or altered innate host defence mechanism(s) are likely to play a major role as highlighted by the association of NOD2 mutations and CD [8].

Several studies have reported on modulated hBD expression in the mucosa of IBD patients. For example, both constitutively expressed hBD1 as well as inducible defensins hBD-2 and -3 were found to be markedly up-regulated in the inflamed colonic mucosa of adults with IBD [9,10,11]. Moreover, induction seemed to be less pronounced in CD compared to UC [9]. In addition to mucosal hBD expression, reduced gene copy numbers for hBD1 and hBD2 have been shown to predispose to the development of CD - further highlighting the likely involvement of these peptides in IBD disease pathogenesis [12,13]. However, studies published to date have been performed almost exclusively on adult patients with longstanding disease, and very little is known about hBD expression in paediatric IBD.

The aim of this study was to investigate expression of hBD1-3 in small and large bowel biopsies of children with IBD and healthy controls. Furthermore, the potential impact of mucosal inflammation on hBD expression was analysed by assessing histological changes and mucosal expression of the inflammatory cytokines IL-8 and TNF-alpha.

Results

Intestinal human beta-defensin expression in healthy children

First we analysed expression of hBD1-3 throughout the intestinal tract of healthy children. hBD1 was expressed constitutively in small and large bowel biopsies with levels being significantly higher in the colon compared to duodenum and TI (Figure 1a). In contrast to hBD1, inducible defensins hBD2 and -3 were infrequently expressed, with low copy numbers and no significant differences between bowel segments (Figure 1a and b). In addition to beta-defensins we also analysed mucosal expression of inflammatory cytokines IL-8 and TNF-alpha. As shown in Figure 1d and e, significantly higher levels for both IL-8 (P = 0.0222) and TNF-alpha (P = 0.0014) were found in the healthy TI compared to duodenum and ascending colon.

Intestinal hBD1 expression in children with IBD and healthy controls

Next we investigated expression of hBD1 in our patient cohort. Comparing hBD1 levels in children with UC and healthy controls, no difference was found in any of the bowel segments tested (Figure 2a–c). In contrast, significantly higher mRNA copy numbers were observed in duodenal and TI biopsies obtained from CD children compared to controls. Despite higher hBD1 levels in colonic biopsies of CD patients, this did not reach statistical significance (Figure 1c). However, subdividing IBD biopsies further into histologically inflamed (I) and non-inflamed (NI), revealed significantly higher hBD1 levels in the non-inflamed ascending colon and TI (Figure 2d and e).

Expression of inducible beta-defensins and inflammatory cytokines in paediatric small bowel biopsies

As shown in Figure 1 expression levels of hBD2 and hBD3 are low in the healthy mucosa. However, up-regulation has been shown to occur during infection and inflammation. We therefore analysed expression of hBD2 and -3 as well as inflammatory cytokines IL-8 and TNF-alpha in small bowel biopsies of our patient cohort. As shown in Figure 3a-d, significant up-regulation of both inducible beta-defensins was found in the duodenum of CD children. However, interestingly, this was despite the absence of significant inflammation as assessed by histological examination and expression of inflammatory cytokines IL-8 and TNF-alpha (Figure 3c and d). In contrast to the duodenum, significantly increased levels of both hBD2 and hBD3 were found exclusively in the inflamed mucosa of CD patients, which also expressed high levels of IL-8 and TNF-alpha.

Colonic expression of inducible beta-defensins and inflammatory cytokines in paediatric IBD

In addition to the small bowel, we also analysed beta-defensin expression in colonic biopsies of IBD patients. Similar to our findings in the TI, expression of hBD2 and -3 was significantly induced in the inflamed mucosa of children with CD and UC (Figure 4a and b). Interestingly, induction of hBD2 was found to be significantly less pronounced in CD compared to UC biopsies

despite equal levels of inflammatory cytokines IL-8 and TNF-alpha (Figure 4c and d). In contrast to hBD2, no difference was found in hBD3 levels comparing inflamed colonic mucosa of both patient groups. Significant induction of IL-8 and TNF-alpha in the histologically inflamed (I) colonic mucosa was observed. Moreover, increased levels of both inflammatory cytokines were also noted in histologically non-inflamed (NI) colonic biopsies of CD children (Figure 4c and d).

Correlation of intestinal beta-defensin and inflammatory cytokine expression

Having noted significant changes of both constitutively and inducible beta-defensins in the inflamed GI mucosa if children with IBD, we analysed the correlation between inducible defensins hBD2 and hBD3 and the inflammatory cytokines within each bowel segment. For these calculations, both results of all children with IBD (inflamed and non-infloamed) and those of healthy control biopsies were included. As shown in Table 1, a highly significant correlation of hBD2 and hBD3 with IL-8 as well as TNF-alpha was found in TI and AC biopsies. In contrast, correlation analysis in the non-inflamed duodenum were largely non significant.

Discussion

Human beta-defensins have been shown to play a key role in intestinal innate host defence [14]. It is therefore not surprising that altered expression and/or function of these peptides has been implicated in IBD disease pathogenesis. However, little is known about the role and regulation of hBDs in paediatric patients. In this study we have investigated beta-defensin gene expression in over 250 intestinal biopsies obtained from children with IBD and healthy controls.

First we analysed expression of hBD1-3 and the inflammatory cytokines TNF-alpha and IL-8 in the mucosa of healthy children. We were able to confirm previously reported data showing constitutive expression of hBD1 throughout the GI tract while hBD2 and -3 were either not detected or present in low mRNA copy numbers [1]. Following this we investigated hBD expression in children with IBD. Here we observed significant induction of hBD2 and hBD3 in the inflamed TI and AC of children with CD as well as UC. Moreover, hBD2 induction in the inflamed colonic mucosa of CD children was found to be significantly less prominent compared to UC despite equal levels of IL-8 and TNF-alpha. This data is consistent with previously published findings on adult populations [9,15], however it seems that hBD2 expression is less impaired in paediatric compared to adult CD, perhaps suggesting that further regulation occurs in long standing disease. In contrast to hBD2, no significant difference in TI or colonic hBD3 induction was observed between patient groups. This is again in contrast to previously published data on adult patients [9].

With regards to expression of hBD1, we found mRNA levels to be increased in the small and large bowel of CD patients only, whereas levels in UC biopsies did not differ from healthy control samples, further highlighting distinct differences between CD and UC. Interestingly, sub-dividing biopsies into inflamed and non-inflamed samples revealed that hBD1 up-regulation was mainly found in the non-inflamed mucosa of CD children. This however has to be interpreted with caution since it could simply signify a degree of epithelial cell loss within the inflamed tissue.

Given the fact that changes of hBD expression were particularly prominent in the inflamed small and large bowel, we analysed correlation of hBDs with inflammatory cytokines IL-8 and TNF-

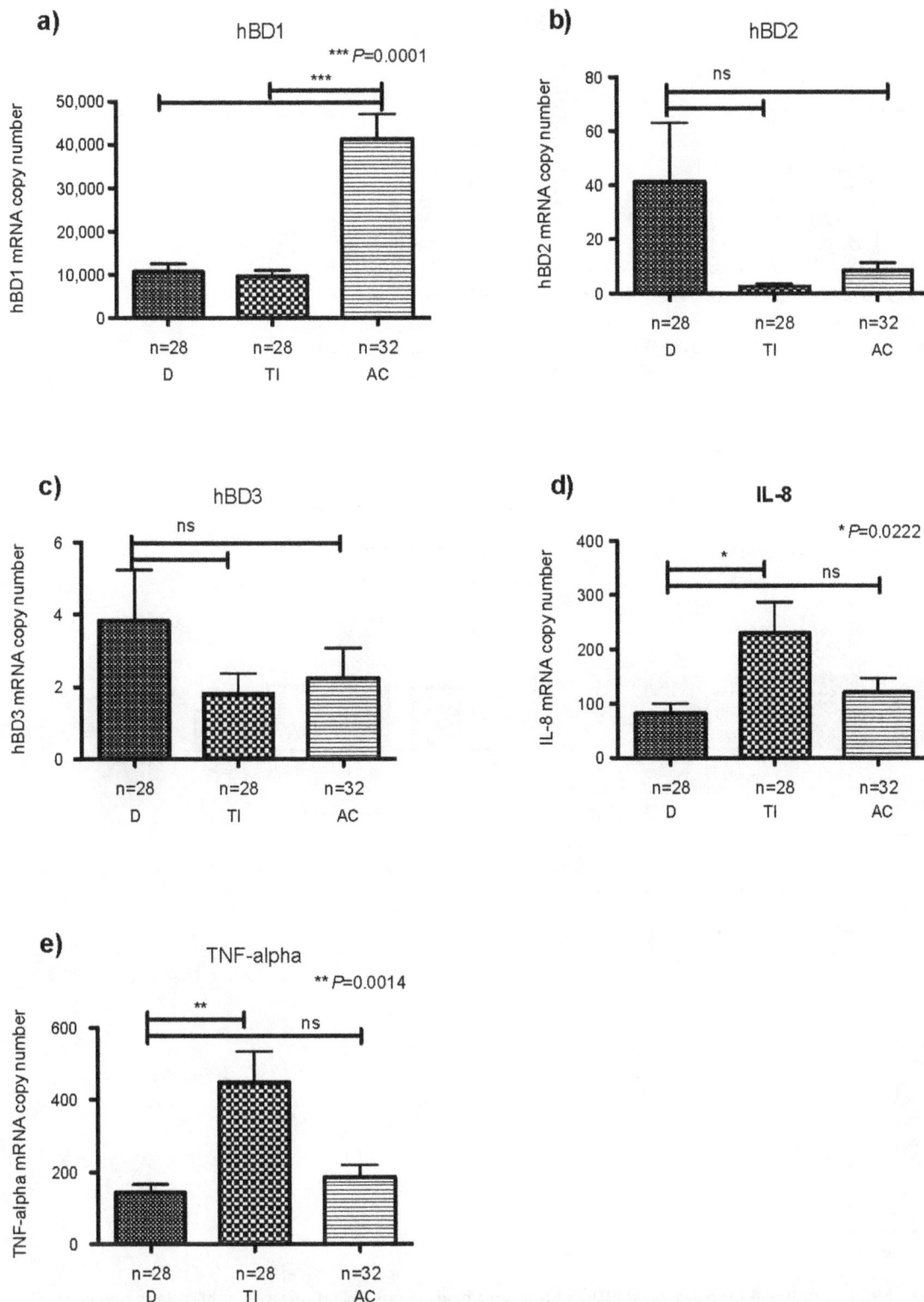

Figure 1. Expression of hBDs and inflammatory cytokines in the intestinal mucosa of healthy children. Biopsies were obtained from duodenum (D), terminal ileum (TI) and ascending colon (AC). Absolute mRNA copy number for hBD1-3 (a-c), IL-8 (d) and TNF-alpha (e) in each biopsy were quantified by real-time PCR using the standard curve method. Expression levels were normalized against the geometrical mean of two selected housekeeping genes (GPDH and β-actin). Data is expressed as the mean ± standard error of mean (SEM). The number of biopsies analysed for each patient group is stated (n). Values for $P<0.05$ were considered to be statistically significant.

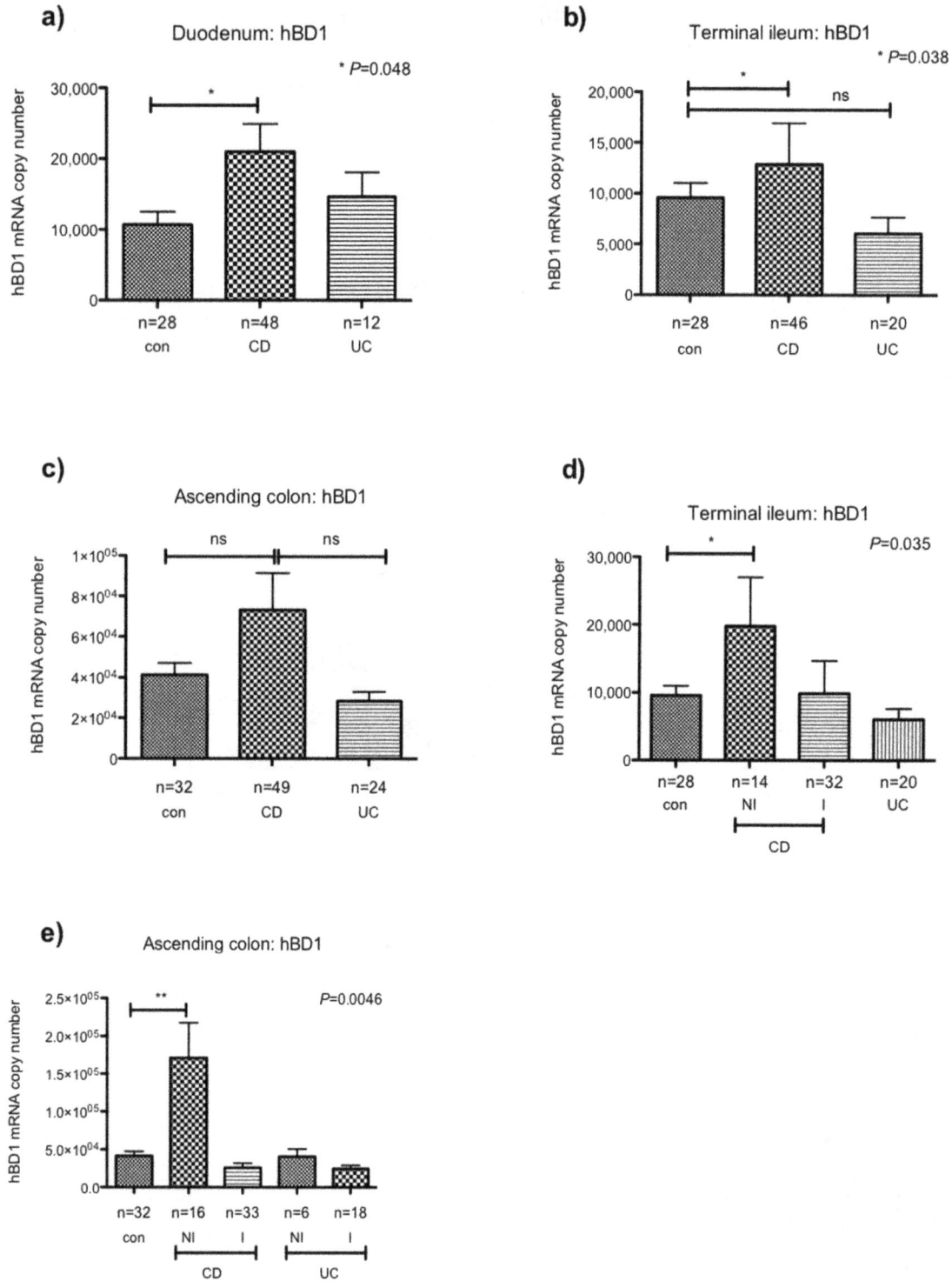

Figure 2. Expression of hBD1 in mucosal biopsies from IBD children and healthy controls. Expression of hBD1 in the duodenum (a), terminal ileum (b) and ascending colon (c) was analysed in children with Crohn's disease (CD), ulcerative colitis (UC) and healthy controls (con). For the TI (d) and AC (e), biopsy samples from CD patients were subdivided into histologically non-inflamed (NI) and inflamed (I). Data is expressed as the mean ± standard error of mean (SEM) of absolute mRNA copy numbers. The number of biopsies analysed for each patient group is stated (n). Values for $P<0.05$ were considered to be statistically significant.

alpha. As expected, we found a strong positive correlation between the inducible defensins hBD2 and hBD3 and both inflammatory cytokines in the TI and AC confirming previous reports [16]. In contrast, analysis in the non-inflamed duodenum proved to be largely non-significant, suggesting regulatory mechanisms may vary between bowel segments.

Overall our data suggests differential regulation of hBDs in the mucosa of children with IBD, depending both on disease type

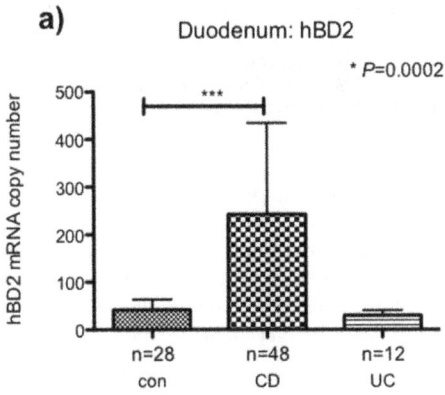

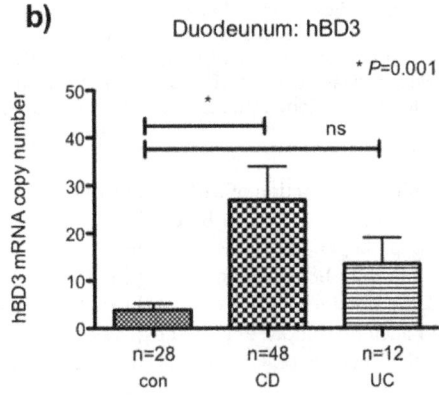

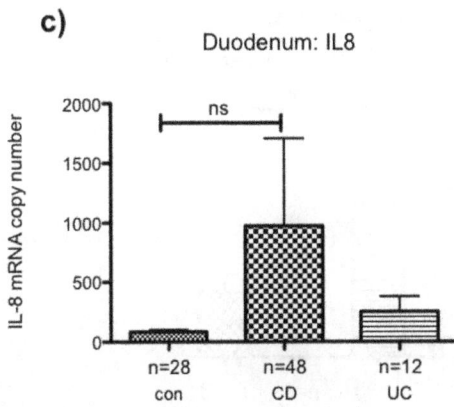

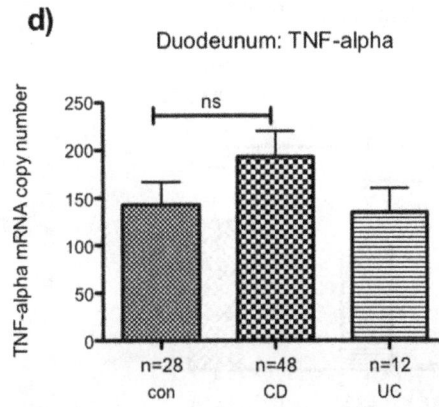

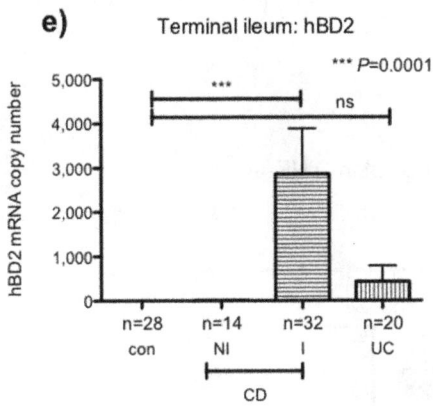

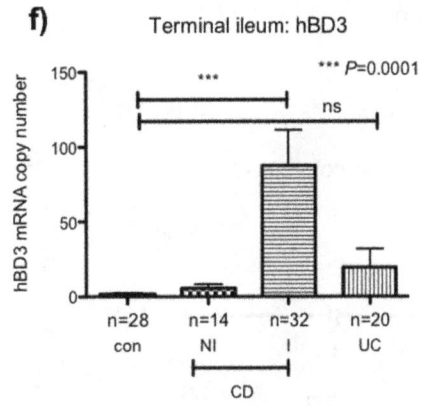

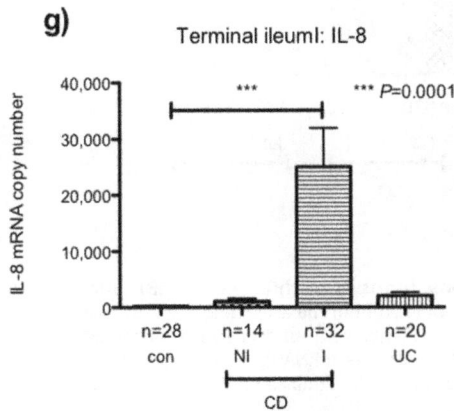

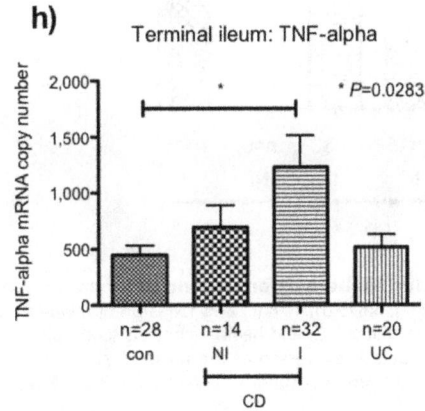

Figure 3. Expression of inducible beta defensins and inflammatory cytokines in small bowel biopsies of IBD children and healthy controls. Expression of hBD2 (a and e), hBD3 (b and f), IL-8 (c and g) and TNF-alpha (d and h) was analysed in the duodenum (a–d) and TI (e–h) of children with Crohn's disease (CD), ulcerative colitis (UC) and healthy controls (con). For the TI, biopsy samples from CD patients were subdivided into histologically non-inflamed (NI) and inflamed (I). Data is expressed as the mean ± standard error of mean (SEM) of absolute mRNA copy numbers. The number of biopsies analysed for each patient group is stated (n). Values for $P<0.05$ were considered to be statistically significant.

and region of the gut. Specifically, induction of hBD2 and hBD3 in the inflamed TI and AC mucosa is likely to be of biological relevance for IBD disease pathogenesis. However, the exact mechanism(s) involved remain to be elucidated. Despite the observed reduction in hBD2 induction in CD compared to UC, one should be cautious to conclude that an impaired expression of hBDs is a main causative feature of CD. Importantly, in addition to the well-documented antimicrobial properties of hBDs, evidence is rapidly increasing on their role as potent immune modulators capable of enhancing inflammatory processes and hence potentially contributing to the onset and/or persistence of chronic intestinal inflammation [7]. Functional studies are required to shed further light on these important questions.

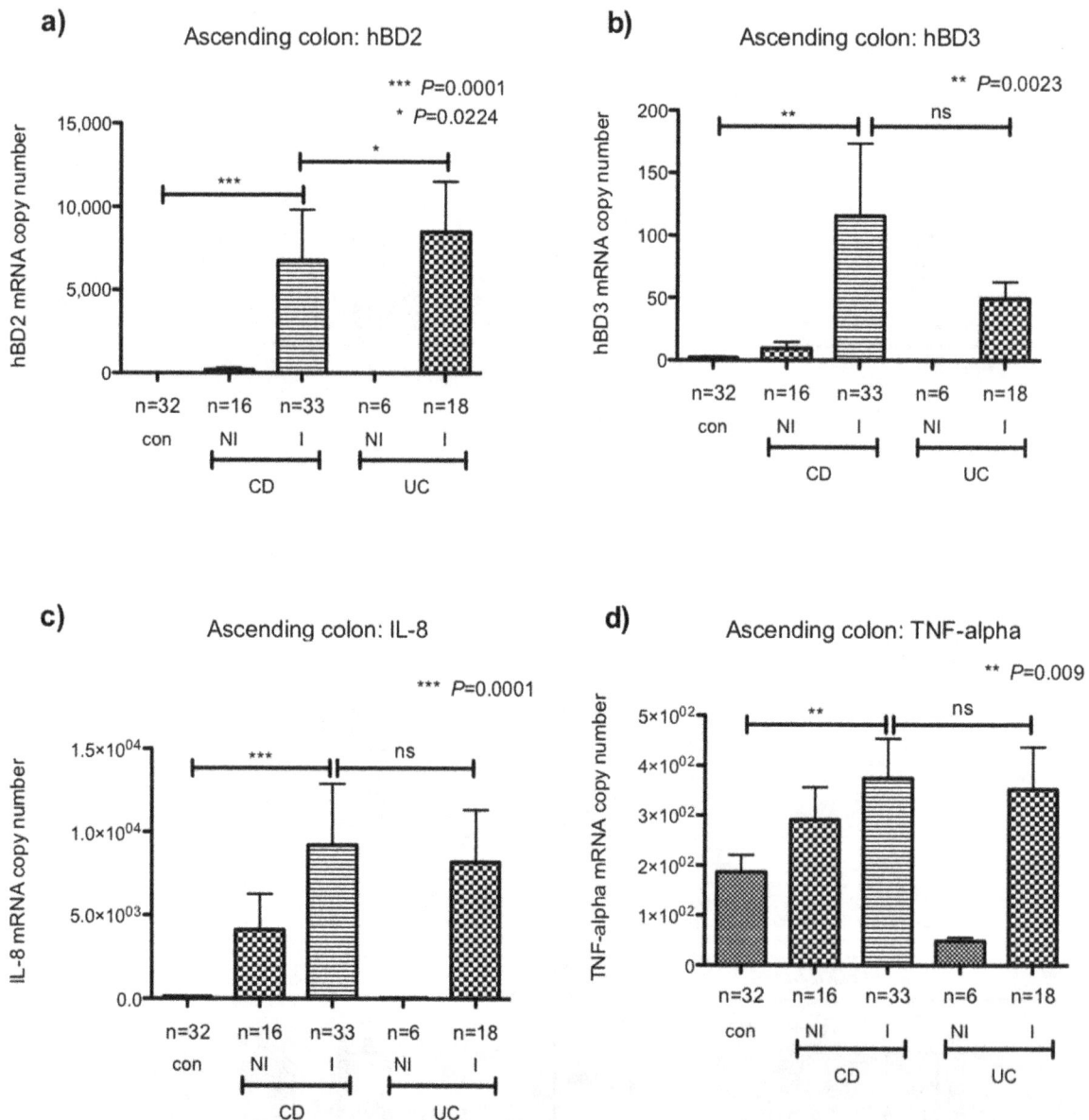

Figure 4. Expression of inducible beta defensins and inflammatory cytokines in colonic biopsies of children with IBD and healthy controls. Expression of hBD2 (a), hBD3 (b), IL-8 (c) and TNF-alpha (d) was analysed in biopsies obtained from the ascending colon of children with Crohn's disease (CD), ulcerative colitis (UC) and healthy controls (con). Biopsies from CD and UC patients were subdivided into histologically non-inflamed (NI) and inflamed (I). Data is expressed as the mean ± standard error of mean (SEM) of absolute mRNA copy numbers. The number of biopsies analysed for each patient group is stated (n). Values for $P<0.05$ were considered to be statistically significant.

Table 1. Correlation of intestinal beta-defensin and inflammatory cytokine mRNA expression levels.

Duodenum (n = 88)	TNF-alpha	IL-8
hBD2	ns	*
	P = 0.389	P = 0.047
	r = 0.09295	r = 0.2124
hBD3	ns	ns
	P = 0.1982	P = 0.2295
	r = −0.1385	r = 0.129
Terminal Ileum (n = 94)	TNF-alpha	IL-8
hBD2	*	***
	P = 0.0143	P<0.0001
	r = 0.2519	r = 0.6101
hBD3	*	***
	P = 0.0269	P<0.0001
	r = 0.2283	r = 0.5951
Ascending Colon (n = 105)	TNF-alpha	IL-8
hBD2	***	***
	P<0.0001	P<0.0001
	r = 0.393	r = 0.6556
hBD3	**	***
	P = 0.0011	P<0.0001
	r = 0.3145	r = 0.5738

Correlation of gene expression between beta-defensins (hBD2 and hBD3) and inflammatory cytokines (IL-8 and TNF-alpha) in the duodenum, terminal ileum and ascending colon was tested by calculating Spearman's rank correlation coefficient (r). The number of biopsies included into calculations is stated (n). Values for P<0.05 were considered to be statistically significant.

Materials and Methods

Patient cohort and sample collection

Patients for this study were recruited over a period of 18 months (08/2008 to 02/2010) from 3 paediatric gastroenterology centres in the UK (London and Cambridge) and Germany (Wuppertal). A total number of 53 children were included consisting of 26 CD (mean age 12.6 years, 15 female), 11 UC (mean age 11.2 years, 4 female) and 16 healthy controls (age mean 12.1 years, 9 female). Diagnosis of CD and UC was based on standard criteria using clinical, radiological, endoscopic, and histopathological findings in accordance with Porto criteria [13]. As healthy control group, children with macroscopically and histologically normal mucosa as well as no evidence of any underlying GI condition were recruited. Endoscopy was performed by experienced paediatric gastroenterologists, who collected 1–2 additional biopsies within close proximity of the area in which biopsies were taken for routine histology. Biopsies were collected from the duodenum (D; n = 88), terminal ileum (TI; n = 90) and ascending colon (AC; n = 105).

Ethical approval for this study was obtained for all participating hospitals and fully informed written consent was taken from legal guardians and children where appropriate.

Histological scoring and tissue storage

Biopsies taken for routine histological examination were evaluated by two experienced paediatric histopathologists and the presence of inflammation recorded. Tissue specimens were classified as inflamed if any of the following features were present:

significant infiltration of inflammatory cells, ulceration, cryptitis or crypt abscesses. In the absence of these findings, tissue was classified as non-inflamed. Biopsy samples for real-time (RT) analysis were directly transferred into RNAlater (QIAGEN) and stored at −80°C until further processing.

RNA extraction and reverse transcription PCR

RNA was extracted from biopsies using QIAGEN RNeasy extraction kit according to the manufacturer's instructions. Integrity of extracted RNA was analyzed by agarose gel electrophoresis and quantified using spectrophotometric absorbance at 260 nm. Following, 500 ng of RNA were reverse transcribed using QIAGEN QuantiFast kit, which included DNAse treatment to eliminate any residual genomic DNA.

Real-Time (RT)-PCR and absolute quantification of mRNA copy numbers

Real Time (RT)-PCR analysis was performed on a Rotor Gene 6000 real time rotary analyzer (Corbett Life Science) using SYBR green methodology. Briefly, reverse transcribed cDNA corresponding to 12.5 ng of RNA were used in a 20 μl PCR reaction containing 10 μl QuantiFast SYBR green master mix (QIAGEN), 2 μl gene specific primers (100 nM of each primer) and 8 μl cDNA in H_2O. Primer sequences used were as follows: hBD1: forward5′-acc ttc tgc tgt tta ctc tct gct-3′ reverse 5′-gac att gcc ctc cac tgc t-3′ hBD2: forward 5′-cca gcc atc agc cat gag ggt-3′ reverse 5′-gga gcc ctt tct gaa tcc gca-3′ hBD3 forward 5′-agc cta gca gct atg agg atc-3′, reverse 5′-ctt cgg cag cat ttt cgg cca-3′ TNF-alpha forward 5′-ccc agg gac ctc tct cta atc a-3′ reverse 5′-gct aca ggc ttg tca ctc gg-3′ IL-8 forward 5′-atg act tcc aag ctg gcc gtg gc-3′ reverse 5′tct cag ccc tct tca aaa act tc-3′. Cycling conditions were as follows: 10 min 95°C, followed by 40 cycles at 95°C for 20 sec and 60°C for 40 sec. At the end of each run melting point analysis was performed to validate specificity of PCR transcripts. All samples were analyzed in triplicate. Absolute quantification was performed using the standard curve method. Briefly, for each gene tested, reference plasmids containing the target sequence were produced (by cloning into p-drive Vector) and the amount of plasmid measured using a Nano-drop Spectrophotometer (ND-1000, Labtech International). Copy numbers were calculated using Avogadro's formula and standard curves generated by performing serial dilutions of plasmid samples ranging from 10^7 to 10^2 copies. In each PCR run a reference standard was included and the primer specific standard curve imported using software provided by Corbett Life Science.

All samples were normalized against the geometric mean of two reference genes (GAPDH and β-actin), which were chosen after testing a group of 7 commonly used reference genes using geNorm Visual Basic application for Microsoft Excel as described previously [17].

Statistical analysis

Mean expression levels of all genes tested were obtained from triplicate real time PCR measurements. Data are presented as the mean +/− standard error of mean (SEM). Testing for significant differences between groups was performed using an unpaired t-test for values with Gaussian distribution and the Mann-Whitney test for values without Gaussian distribution. The Kolmogorov-Smirnov test was utilised to determine Gaussian distribution. For correlation analysis Spearman's rank coefficient was calculated. Values for P<0.05 were considered statistically significant. All analysis were performed using Graphpad Prism version 5 (Graphpad Software, San Diego, CA).

Acknowledgments

The authors would like to thank C. Foerster (Hepatitis laboratory, HELIOS Children's Hospital, Wuppertal, Germany) for excellent technical support. We also thank Dr. Liz Hook and Dr. Flora Jessop (Department of Histopathology, Addenbrooke's Hospital, Cambridge) for expert histological scoring of biopsies and Paul Rolfe for support in taking research samples by providing outstanding anaesthetic support.

References

1. Dhaliwal W, Bajaj-Elliott M, Kelly P (2003) Intestinal defensin gene expression in human populations. Mol Immunol 40: 469–475.
2. Lehrer RI (2004) Primate defensins. Nat Rev Microbiol 2: 727–738.
3. Zilbauer M, Dorrell N, Boughan PK, Harris A, Wren BW, et al. (2005) Intestinal innate immunity to Campylobacter jejuni results in induction of bactericidal human beta-defensins 2 and 3. Infect Immun 73: 7281–7289.
4. Eckmann L (2005) Defence molecules in intestinal innate immunity against bacterial infections. Curr Opin Gastroenterol 21: 147–151.
5. Selsted ME, Ouellette AJ (2005) Mammalian defensins in the antimicrobial immune response. Nat Immunol 6: 551–557.
6. Otte JM, Werner I, Brand S, Chromik AM, Schmitz F, et al. (2008) Human beta defensin 2 promotes intestinal wound healing in vitro. J Cell Biochem 104: 2286–2297.
7. Bowdish DM, Davidson DJ, Hancock RE (2006) Immunomodulatory properties of defensins and cathelicidins. Curr Top Microbiol Immunol 306: 27–66.
8. Ogura Y, Bonen DK, Inohara N, Nicolae DL, Chen FF, et al. (2001) A frameshift mutation in NOD2 associated with susceptibility to Crohn's disease. Nature 411: 603–606.
9. Wehkamp J, Harder J, Weichenthal M, Mueller O, Herrlinger KR, et al. (2003) Inducible and constitutive beta-defensins are differentially expressed in Crohn's disease and ulcerative colitis. Inflamm Bowel Dis 9: 215–223.
10. Fahlgren A, Hammarstrom S, Danielsson A, Hammarstrom ML (2003) Increased expression of antimicrobial peptides and lysozyme in colonic epithelial cells of patients with ulcerative colitis. Clin Exp Immunol 131: 90–101.
11. Fahlgren A, Hammarstrom S, Danielsson A, Hammarstrom ML (2004) beta-Defensin-3 and -4 in intestinal epithelial cells display increased mRNA expression in ulcerative colitis. Clin Exp Immunol 137: 379–385.
12. Fellermann K, Stange DE, Schaeffeler E, Schmalzl H, Wehkamp J, et al. (2006) A chromosome 8 gene-cluster polymorphism with low human beta-defensin 2 gene copy number predisposes to Crohn disease of the colon. Am J Hum Genet 79: 439–448.
13. Kocsis AK, Lakatos PL, Somogyvari F, Fuszek P, Papp J, et al. (2008) Association of beta-defensin 1 single nucleotide polymorphisms with Crohn's disease. Scand J Gastroenterol 43: 299–307.
14. Doss M, White MR, Tecle T, Hartshorn KL (2010) Human defensins and LL-37 in mucosal immunity. J Leukoc Biol 87: 79–92.
15. Wehkamp J, Fellermann K, Herrlinger KR, Baxmann S, Schmidt K, et al. (2002) Human beta-defensin 2 but not beta-defensin 1 is expressed preferentially in colonic mucosa of inflammatory bowel disease. Eur J Gastroenterol Hepatol 14: 745–752.
16. Chang YY, Ouyang Q (2008) [Expression and significance of mucosal beta-defensin-2, TNFalpha and IL-1beta in ulcerative colitis]. Zhonghua Nei Ke Za Zhi 47: 11–14.
17. Vandesompele J, De Preter K, Pattyn F, Poppe B, Van Roy N, et al. (2002) Accurate normalization of real-time quantitative RT-PCR data by geometric averaging of multiple internal control genes. Genome Biol 3: RESEARCH0034.

Author Contributions

Conceived and designed the experiments: MZ AJ RH SW. Performed the experiments: MZ GW. Analyzed the data: MZ AJ RH SW. Manuscript preparation and discussion: MZ AJ JP AH AP RH SW. Patient recruitment, endoscopy and biopsy taking: MZ GNJ FT CS RH SW.

17

Smoking Cessation Induces Profound Changes in the Composition of the Intestinal Microbiota in Humans

Luc Biedermann[1], Jonas Zeitz[2], Jessica Mwinyi[1,3], Eveline Sutter-Minder[4], Ateequr Rehman[5¤], Stephan J. Ott[5,6], Claudia Steurer-Stey[7,8], Anja Frei[7,8], Pascal Frei[1], Michael Scharl[1], Martin J. Loessner[4], Stephan R. Vavricka[1,9], Michael Fried[1], Stefan Schreiber[5,6], Markus Schuppler[4], Gerhard Rogler[1]*

1 Division of Gastroenterology and Hepatology, University Hospital Zurich, Zurich, Switzerland, 2 Division of Internal Medicine, University Hospital Zurich, Zurich, Switzerland, 3 Division of Clinical Pharmacology and Toxicology, University Hospital Zurich, Zurich, Switzerland, 4 Institute of Food, Nutrition and Health, ETH Zurich, Zurich, Switzerland, 5 Institute of Clinical Molecular Biology, Christian Albrechts University of Kiel, Kiel, Germany, 6 Division of General Internal Medicine, University Hospital Schleswig-Holstein, Kiel, Germany, 7 Institute of General Practice, University of Zurich, Zurich, Switzerland, 8 Smoking Consulting Programme, University Hospital Zurich, Zurich, Switzerland, 9 Division of Gastroenterology and Hepatology, Hospital Triemli, Zurich, Switzerland

Abstract

Background: The human intestinal microbiota is a crucial factor in the pathogenesis of various diseases, such as metabolic syndrome or inflammatory bowel disease (IBD). Yet, knowledge about the role of environmental factors such as smoking (which is known to influence theses aforementioned disease states) on the complex microbial composition is sparse. We aimed to investigate the role of smoking cessation on intestinal microbial composition in 10 healthy smoking subjects undergoing controlled smoking cessation.

Methods: During the observational period of 9 weeks repetitive stool samples were collected. Based on abundance of 16S rRNA genes bacterial composition was analysed and compared to 10 control subjects (5 continuing smokers and 5 non-smokers) by means of Terminal Restriction Fragment Length Polymorphism analysis and high-throughput sequencing.

Results: Profound shifts in the microbial composition after smoking cessation were observed with an increase of *Firmicutes* and *Actinobacteria* and a lower proportion of *Bacteroidetes* and *Proteobacteria* on the phylum level. In addition, after smoking cessation there was an increase in microbial diversity.

Conclusions: These results indicate that smoking is an environmental factor modulating the composition of human gut microbiota. The observed changes after smoking cessation revealed to be similar to the previously reported differences in obese compared to lean humans and mice respectively, suggesting a potential pathogenetic link between weight gain and smoking cessation. In addition they give rise to a potential association of smoking status and the course of IBD.

Editor: Markus M. Heimesaat, Charité, Campus Benjamin Franklin, Germany

Funding: This research was supported by research grants from the Swiss National Science Foundation to SRV (Grant No 320000-114009/1), to GR (Grant No. 310030-120312) and the Swiss IBD Cohort (Grant No. 3347CO-108792), and by the Zurich Centre for Integrative Human Physiology of the University of Zurich. The funders had no role in study design, data collection and analysis, decision to publish, or preparation of the manuscript.

Competing Interests: The authors have declared that no competing interests exist.

* E-mail: gerhard.rogler@usz.ch

¤ Current address: Department of Environmental Health, Sciences, University Medical Center, Freiburg, Germany

Introduction

The human intestinal microbiota has important influences on the development of innate immunity [1,2], regulation of epithelial development and nutrition [3,4]. The gut microbiota and alterations in its complex composition have been identified as an contributing factor in the pathogenesis of various diseases, such as inflammatory bowel disease (IBD) [5,6] or irritable bowel syndrome [7–9]. Cigarette smoking is considered to be one of the most important environmental risk factors in IBD pathogenesis [10–13]. In the two main subtypes of IBD, Crohn's disease (CD) and ulcerative colitis (UC), there is a known divergent effect of smoking on the disease course. While smoking is clearly detrimental in CD [14,15] (in many [16] but not all [14] studies this seems especially to be the case with regard to ileal CD) it has a well-known protective effect in UC with a lower incidence of the disease in smokers [11] and a more severe disease course after smoking cessation [17]. In addition, the gut microbiota seems to play a crucial role in the pathogenesis of obesity and the metabolic syndrome [18,19], characterized by distinctive shifts in the relative abundance of mayor phyla in obese vs. lean humans [20,21] and mice [22], respectively. Around 80% of individuals who cease smoking gain weight to an average of 7–8 kg [23], interestingly even despite stable [24] or even decreased [25] total caloric intake. Furthermore an alteration of the oropharyngeal and tracheal microbiota in smokers compared to non-smokers has been shown recently [26].

In the last few years considerable progress has been achieved in the comprehension of the enormous diversity of the intestinal microbiota, its component genes (microbiome) and host genetic factors influencing its development after birth with the spread of culture independent methods [27]. Nevertheless, the precise role of environmental factors, such as nutrition, medication use or smoking on the composition of the gut microbiota is largely unknown. Accordingly, and in view of the above mentioned microbial discoveries with regard to the pathogenesis of obesity and IBD we aimed to investigate the development of human intestinal microbial composition during controlled smoking cessation. Microbiota analyses of repetitive stool samples were performed in the course of a controlled prospective study with 10 healthy smoking subjects undergoing smoking cessation (intervention group) and 10 healthy control subjects, 5 continuous smoking (control group smokers) and 5 non-smoking (control group non-smokers) subjects. Our hypothesis at the beginning of the study was, that smoking may influence the composition of the intestinal microbiota and accordingly, that smoking cessation may also alter intestinal microbial composition. We further hypothesized, that the weight change after smoking cessation migt be associated with a shift to a microbiota pattern harbouring similarities to the recently characterized found in the "obese microbiota" in humans or animal models and that these microbial shifts might indicate a pattern associated with a pro-inflammatory situation.

Materials and Methods

Study design

The study was fully approved by the local Ethics Committee. Observation period was 9 weeks (1 week before and 8 weeks after cessation of smoking) including 5 study visits, among them t1 (Screening), t2 and t3 (4 and 8 weeks respectively after smoking cessation). All 5 study visits took place in facilities of the smoking consulting program of the University Hospital Zurich, Switzerland. At screening visit (S = t1) written informed consent was obtained. Inclusion (age $\geq$18 and $\leq$60 years; written consent; smoker (defined as daily cigarette consumption of $\geq$10); readiness to quit smoking) and exclusion criteria (intercurrent bacterial or viral disease of the colon; pregnancy, lactation; patients with more than 40 mg prednisone per day (or equivalent); diabetes mellitus; severe comorbid disease (making a participation at the study not possible according to opinion of the test physician); justified doubt about the co-operation of the patient; patients with active infection or systemic antibiotic, antiviral, or antifungal treatment in the last 3 weeks before the screening investigation; patients with alcohol or drug misuse in the last year; patients with short bowel syndrome; patients with parenteral nutrition; severe comorbid conditions) were checked. Full medical record, medication use, alcohol intake and smoking habits were assessed and a physical examination including body height and weight was performed. During the whole study period intensive counseling was provided by both, physicians and psychologists with special experience in consultation in smoking cessation. Subjects were instructed to keep on smoking according to their regular smoking habits up to baseline (T0; 7–10 days after screening). Baseline was prespecified as the date of complete smoking cessation.

At the baseline study visit and the subsequent control visits 1 week (T1), 4 weeks (T4) and 8 weeks (T8) after smoking cessation physical examination including body weight and assessment of medication intake was re-performed. Mandatory strict adherence to complete smoking cessation was verified by a breath carbon monoxide monitor (piCO+TM Smokerlyzer®; Bedfont Scientific Ltd & decode.uk). Measuring was done in concordance to the guidance of the manufacturer, always performed under direct observation of a study physician. A cut-off level of >6 ppm was chosen to define current smoking [28]; a single level above 6 ppm or self-declaration of on-going smoking after T0 led to study drop out. Supplemental nicotine administration or use of smoking cessation medications was not allowed. Stool samples, which have been shown to be representative of inter-individual differences in microbial composition [29], were collected at every study visit. Samples of 3 time points were used for further analyses; at screening (one week prior to smoking cessation, t1), 4 and 8 weeks after smoking cessation (t2, t3) corresponding to week 0, 5 and 9 in the continuing smoking and non-smoking subjects. Study subjects had to complete a daily food-frequency protocol three times over a period of 7 consecutive days (one week before t1, t2, and t3), allowing assessment of food patterns in a qualitative and approximated quantitative manner.

Microbiota analyses

Stool samples were collected in conventional fecal samples storage tubes containing phosphate buffered saline (PBS)/Ethanol, the latter leading to an immediate denaturation of bacterial cell wall. Methods for T-RFLP are depicted in the SI Materials and Methods. For pyrosequencing genomic DNA from fecal pellets was extracted and quantified. We amplified variable region V1–V2 of the 16S rRNA gene using forward and reverse primer, the latter containing a unique 10 base multiplex identifier (MIDs designated as XXXXXXXXXX) to tag each Polymerase Chain Reaction (PCR) product. Replicate PCRs were performed for each sample and negative controls. The amplified product was run on agarose gel and the specific band was excised and amplicons were purified. Equal amount of PCR products were mixed in a single tube and sequenced using Roche® 454 titanium chemistry. Replicate PCRs were performed for each sample as well as negative controls (water). All sequence reads were screened and filtered for quality and length; chimeric sequences were removed as were sequences failing quality criteria (further details in the SI Materials and Methods). Taxonomy was assigned by comparison against the Ribosomal Database Project (RDP) release 10 [30]. The complete raw sequencing data of this study is accessible via the European Nucleotide Archive in the Sequence Read Archive (SRA) under the study accession number ERP002222 (available at the URL http://www.ebi.ac.uk/ena/data/view/ERP002222; Samples accessions: ERS212677).

Statistical Analysis

Paired Student's t-test was used for a comparison of average daily calorie intake (and respective fraction of calories attributable to carbohydrates, proteins, fat, fibres and alcohol). Analyses of the T-RFLP data was performed using T-Rex (T-RFLP analysis Expedited) [31]. A doubly centred Principal Component Analyses (PCA), also known as the Additive Main Effects and Multiplicative Interaction Model (AMMI) with 9 environments (intervention group, control group smokers, control group non-smokers; each at t1, t2 and t3) was performed. For the sequences obtained by pyrosequencing paired Student's t-test was used for taxonomy based comparison of between group changes. Beforehand skewness of value distribution was ruled out with StatView™. Cd-hit [32] was used to identify and cluster similar sequences for phylogenetic analyses and to define OTUs with the commonly applied sequence identity cut-off of 0.97. Sequence alignment was performed using NAST from the Greengenes server [33] including all sequences with a minimum length of 150 bases. A phylogenetic tree was constructed using FastTree 2. To perform a phylogeny-based analyses of beta diversity we used Fast UniFrac [34], a bioinformatic software tool that can be used to characterize variations in bacterial community membership over time in dependency of external influences, such as nutrition or space in a large numbers of samples and sequences. Analyses in Fast UniFrac can be performed either by considering only the absolute abundance of sequences in every sample (unweighted) or by taking the relative abundance of bacterial species into account (here, the branches of certain bacterial lineages are weighted according to their quantitative occurrence). A normalization step can be performed (each sample treated equally instead of each unit of branch as in the non-normalized mode; for normalization the UniFrac value is divided by the distance scale factor, which is the average distance from the root of each sequence). Initially, sequences were processed by identifying and selecting the occurring OTU and a phylogenetic tree was built. A sample distance matrix was constructed, showing the overall phylogenetic distance between each pair of sequences. This matrix provides the basis to conduct PCA and hierarchical clustering using the UPGMA (Unweighted Pair Group Method with Arithmetic Mean) algorithm.

Bonferroni correction was applied in case of multiple testing. As a resampling method bootstrapping was performed including 75% of available sequences in each run in altogether 1000 permutations using the software tool QIIME [35] (Quantitative Insights Into Microbial Ecology).

The term phylogenetic diversity was coined by Faith [36] and characterizes the amount of biodiversity in a given sample by summarizing the total length of all branches leading to the investigated set of taxa in a phylogenetic tree, i.e. a quantification of the phylogenetic heritage of organisms in a given set of species. Alpha diversity was calculated using the Phylogenetic Diversity Analyser (PDA) [37]. Rarefaction curves were constructed using QIIME.

Results

Calorie intake and body weight in the course of smoking cessation

During the observational period there was a mean 2.2 kg increase in body weight in the 10 subjects undergoing smoking cessation (mean body weight at screening 71.8 kg, corresponding to a mean BMI of 24.1 kg/m^2; mean body weight at T8 74.0 kg, corresponding to a mean BMI of 24.8 kg/m^2; Table S1). However, neither a significant alteration of total average daily calorie intake, nor the fraction of nutritional components (carbohydrates, proteins, fat, fiber and alcohol) was identified based on the weekly food-frequency-protocols as indicated in Figure S1 and Tables S2, S3 (as a sole exception a slight but significant increase in calorie intake from alcohol between t2 and t3 was observed).

Alteration in the microbial composition, indicated by T-RFLP analysis

As a first step we conducted a universal terminal-restriction fragment length polymorphisms (T-RFLP) analysis. Doubly centered Principal Component Analyses (PCA) of the resulting data with 9 environments (intervention group, control group smokers, control group non-smokers; each at t1, t2 and t3) indicated a clear shift in the intervention group between samples from t1 and t2, as well as t2 and t3. The observed shift was most pronounced along the first principal component axis, representing the major part of the observed difference (58.5%; Figure S2). No such shift was observed in the non-smoking control group, where a close clustering was maintained over the different time points. In

the smoking control group a somewhat wider separation was detected, however almost exclusively along the second principal component axis. The latter represents substantial less difference in species composition (37.7%) as compared to the first principal component axis (Figure S2, Table S4).

Differences in the abundance of sequences before and after smoking cessation

For a more comprehensive analysis of the microbial diversity harbored by the stool samples we next performed a 454 pyrosequencing approach to analyze the variable regions V1–V2 of the 16S rRNA gene. After applying an initial cleaning step on the generated raw sequence data as described in the methods section we generated a total of 335'902 sequences. The vast majority of sequences (97.3%) could be assigned to four phyla: *Firmicutes* (51.9%), *Proteobacteria* (33%), *Bacteroidetes* (7.1%) and *Actinobacteria* (5.4%) (Further identified bacteria included members of the phyla *Verrucomicrobia, Lentisphaerae, Tenericutes, Cyanobacteria, Synergistetes, Fusobacteria, Deinococcus-Thermus, TM7, Acidobacteria* and *OD1*, whereas 0.9% of sequences could not be classified (Figure S3)).

We found an increase of sequences from *Firmicutes* and *Actinobacteria* and a simultaneous decrease of the *Proteobacteria* and *Bacteroidetes* fractions after smoking cessation (Figure 1a). These changes were exclusively observed in the intervention group and a substantial part of the shift occurred between t1 and t2. The increase of *Firmicutes* and *Actinobacteria* as well as the decrease of *Proteobacteria* between t1 and t2 in the intervention group was significant in the paired Student's T-Test (0.027, 0.014 and 0.041 respectively), while the decrease in the fraction of *Bacteroidetes* did not reach statistical significance (0.109). Although the detected changes between t1 and t2 seemed to be further accentuated 8 weeks after smoking cessation in t3 (except for the *Proteobacteria*) the composition of phyla between t2 and t3 remained strikingly similar with the exception of *Bacteroidetes*, pointing to both a relatively brisk (within 4 weeks) and durable (8-week interval) effect of smoking cessation on microbial composition. In contrast, the composition of phyla in both control groups remained relatively stable. Here not one single change in the composition of phyla reached statistical significance (Figure 1b). However, the observed changes in the control groups were not exclusively restricted to the phylum level. Significant changes were also detected on the genus level (Figure S5). We did not observe any per individual correlation between changes in body weight and microbial composition.

Differences in microbiota composition indicated by phylogenetic microbial analyses

PCA including 9 environments revealed a clear separation of bacterial community composition in the intervention group, most pronounced between t1 and t2, whereas the control groups clustered closely together (Figure 2 and Figure S6 for unweighted and weighted analyses, respectively). UniFrac distance serves as a measure of difference in the phylogenetic lineages between different environments. The highest UniFrac distance was determined in subjects undergoing smoking cessation, comparing the time points prior to and after the intervention (I1 to I2 versus N1 to N2 and S1 to S2: p = 0.045; I1 to I3 versus N1 to N3 and S1 to S3: p = 0.026). In contrast no significant differences between the samples from the intervention and control groups were observed after the intervention (I2 to I3 versus N2 to N3 and S2 to S3: p = 0.244, not significant). These findings illustrate that the samples prior to and after smoking cessation were more different

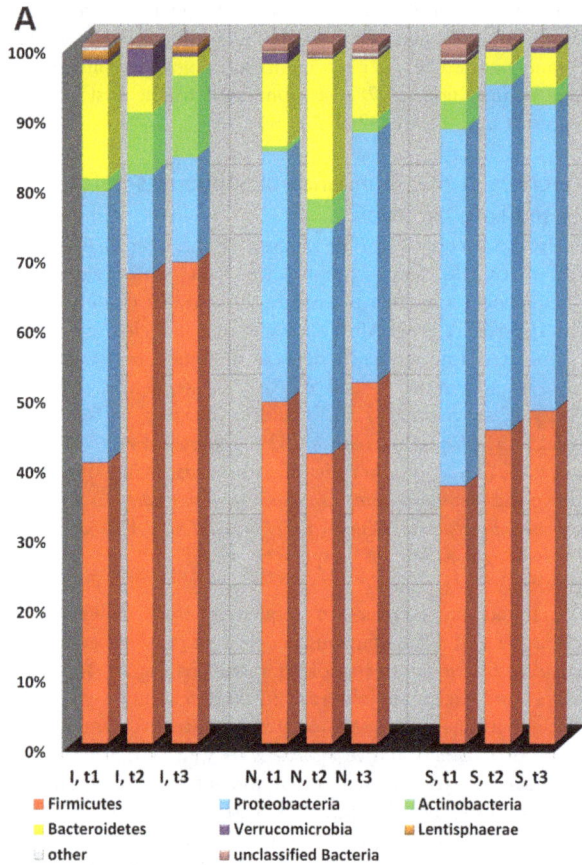

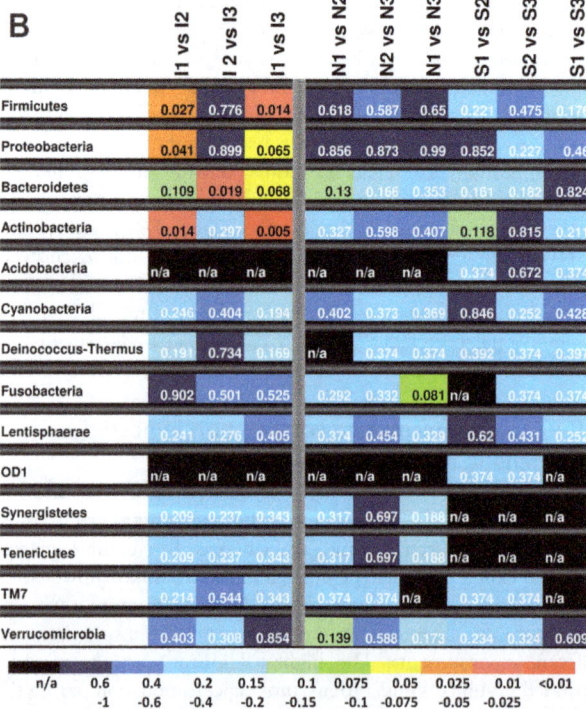

Figure 1. Comparison of the major phyla of the gut microbiota before and after smoking cessation. (A) Phyla Composition. The results for the intervention group (I) and the control groups (non-smoking = N; smoking = S) are given for samples taken one week prior to smoking cessation (t1) as well as four weeks (t2) and eight weeks (t3) thereafter. Whereas the intervention group revealed a significant

increase in fractions of *Firmicutes* and *Actinobacteria* and a decrease in fractions of *Proteobacteria* and *Bacteroidetes*, the microbiota of the control groups remained rather stable. The phyla *Tenericutes, Verrucomicrobia, Synergistetes, Fusobacteria, Deinococcus-Thermus, TM7, Acidobacteria* and *OD1* are summarized under "other". (B) Heat Map. The result of paired Student's t-test is shown on the phylum level with a color coded heat map. Significance levels are shown in different colors (shades of red, significant shifts in bacteria composition; shades of yellow, green and blue, non-significant shifts) and are indicated by the exact significance values within the colored squares of the graph. The major changes in the microbiota in the intervention group were observed between the time points before (t1) and after (t2, t3) smoking cessation. In contrast no significant changes were detected in the control groups and – with the exception of *Bacteroidetes* – after smoking cessation between t2 and t3 in the intervention group (an extended version of the heat map including all identified genera is shown in Figure S5, n/a = not applicable).

to each other (Figure 3a). In addition, clustering the samples based on the distance matrix the separation of bacterial lineages at t1 and t2 in the intervention group occurred significantly closer to the root (i.e. higher UniFrac distance units) of the constructed tree compared to any other separation process observed within intervention and control groups. Weighted UniFrac Significance reflected a significant difference between t1 and t2 (non-normalized UniFrac Significance 0.036, with Bonferroni correction applied). After normalizing, significance was additionally observed for t1 to t3, exclusively in the intervention group (<0.001 for both, t1 to t2 and t1 to t3, Bonferroni correction applied). Jackknife analysis used as a statistical technique of repetitive resampling (bootstrapping) revealed perfect reproducibility underlining robustness of our results (Figure S7).

Microbial diversity analyses (α-diversity)

Both Phylogenetic Diversity and endemic Phylogenetic Diversity [38] (the sum of all branch lengths of species exclusively found in the respective environment) as measures for α-diversity were shown to be substantially higher 4 weeks after smoking cessation compared to the samples obtained whilst smoking. After 8 weeks there was still a trend towards increased diversity levels compared to baseline. In the control groups both diversity indices were relatively stable during the whole observation period (Figure S8). Rarefaction curves, a means of correction for number of sequences obtained per sample, underlined the increased microbial diversity after smoking cessation (Figure 3b, Figure S9).

Discussion

The results of our controlled trial suggest that smoking is to be included in the growing list of known factors influencing the composition of the intestinal microbiota. We found evidence with two independent methodological approaches that smoking cessation induces a substantial modification of the intestinal microbial composition with no indication of any concomitant alteration in nutrition. A variety of different analyses of the high-throughput sequencing data indicated differences before and after smoking cessation, suggestive for profound and robust microbial shifts. On the phylum level strikingly even alterations regarding the major four phyla were identified in the individuals undergoing smoking cessation (Figure 1, Figure S4). On the level of OTUs quantitative changes (relative abundance of some bacterial lineages in the complex microbial mixture) are indicated by alterations in the weighted UniFrac mode, while the similar findings in the unweighted analyses in addition point to qualitative changes (i.e. occurrence of new OTUs after smoking cessation and disappearance of former OTUs prior to the intervention).

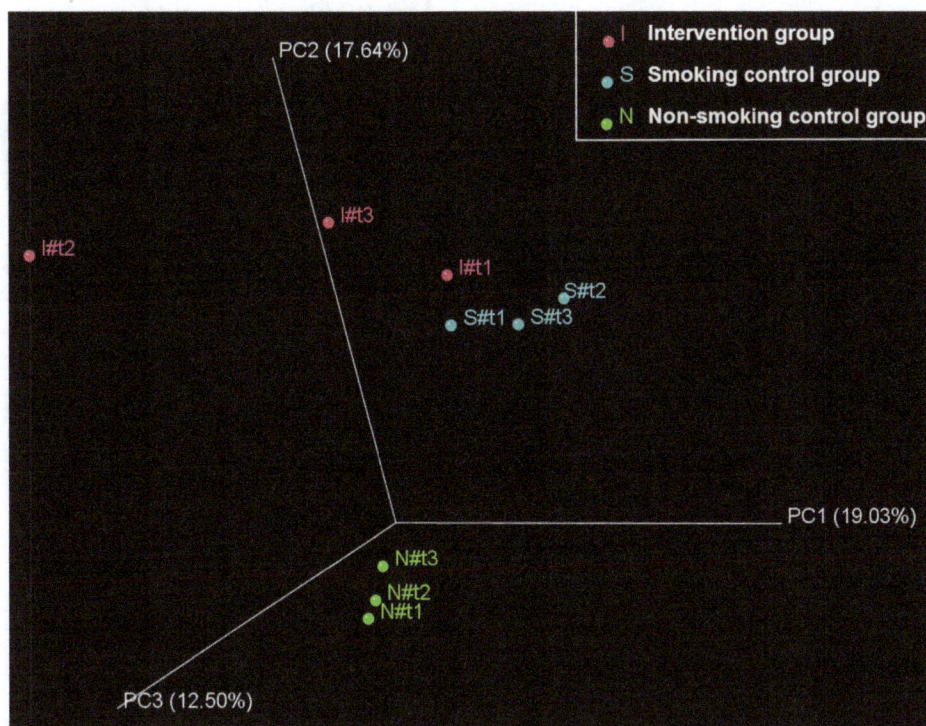

Figure 2. Phylogeny-based Principal Component Analysis. Bacterial communities of the three different treatment groups were clustered using PCA and the unweighted UniFrac distance matrix as an input (weighted PCA is shown in Figure S6). With PCA, a multivariate statistical analyses, axes that reflect the largest part of sample variation are identified (Percentage values at the axes reflect the level of variation explained by each principal coordinate; the first axis indicates the largest fraction of difference). Separation of the different sample collectives in 3 dimensions is visualized. A separation of the samples from the intervention group (I), that is most predominant 4 weeks after smoking cessation, was revealed. In contrast, the samples from the non-smoking (N) and smoking (S) control groups clustered together closely, thus reflecting their overall similar microbial composition.

Furthermore, aside from pure microbial shifts an increase in microbial plurality is suggested by the increase in α-diversity after smoking cessation (Figure 3b, Figure S9). However, due to the limited observation period after smoking cessation, it is not possible to draw any conclusions on a potential sustained long-term increase of α-diversity due to smoking cessation. A long-term effect towards an increased microbial richness rather appears doubtful, as the initial increase in diversity somewhat mitigated after 8 weeks in all our analyses of α-diversity. Also, there were no substantial differences in α-diversity between smokers and non-smokers in the control groups. Interestingly, in contrast to our findings, oropharyngeal microbial diversity was found to be increased in smokers compared to non-smokers [26]. Thus, to clarify this issue further studies on the long-term effect of smoking on α-diversity of the intestinal microbiota are necessary.

We observed similar shifts in microbial composition on the phylum level after smoking cessation as described in obese versus lean humans [21,20] and mice [22] (a lower proportion of *Bacteroidetes* and a higher proportion of *Firmicutes* and *Actinobacteria*), while a concomitant average weight gain of 2.2 kg during the whole observational period occurred. However, neither a change in total daily calorie intake nor nutritional components was suggested owing to analyses of the food-frequency questionnaires. Thus, the common perception that a change in dietary habits is the key factor for weight gain after smoking cessation is challenged. Our findings may suggest a potential role of an altered composition of the intestinal microbiome and hence metabolome with subsequent modifications in gut microbiota's metabolic

function in the pathogenesis of weight gain after smoking cessation.

The above mentioned disordered oropharyngeal and tracheal microbial communities in smokers [26] appears to be intuitively plausible due to the direct contact of cigarette smoke with the respiratory epithelial cells and mucus harboring the local microbiota. Possible pathophysiologic links explaining the influence of smoking and smoking cessation on the intestinal microbial composition are much less evident. However, our study was not designed to investigate potential causative mechanisms. In addition, due to the study design it was not possible to investigate whether there are any loco-regional differences such as for instance between the terminal ileum and recto-sigmoid. This would be of interest with regard to the discrepancy of smoking between UC and CD.

Another limitation of our study is that despite the controlled study setup to largely rule out external influences such as for instance medication intake (e.g. antibiotics or supportive drugs for smoking cessation) or non-adherence to strict smoking cessation, we cannot completely ascertain lack of confounding effects such as exercise or subtle changes in dietary habits unrecognized by analysis of food-frequency protocols. However, the following considerations argue against a major contributing role of hidden dietary alterations. First, the assumption that an alteration of diet and increase of calorie intake would explain the observed weight gain is not based on robust evidence, as indications that increased calorie intake is the principal explanation for weight gain after smoking cessation are at best conflicting. In contrast, there are

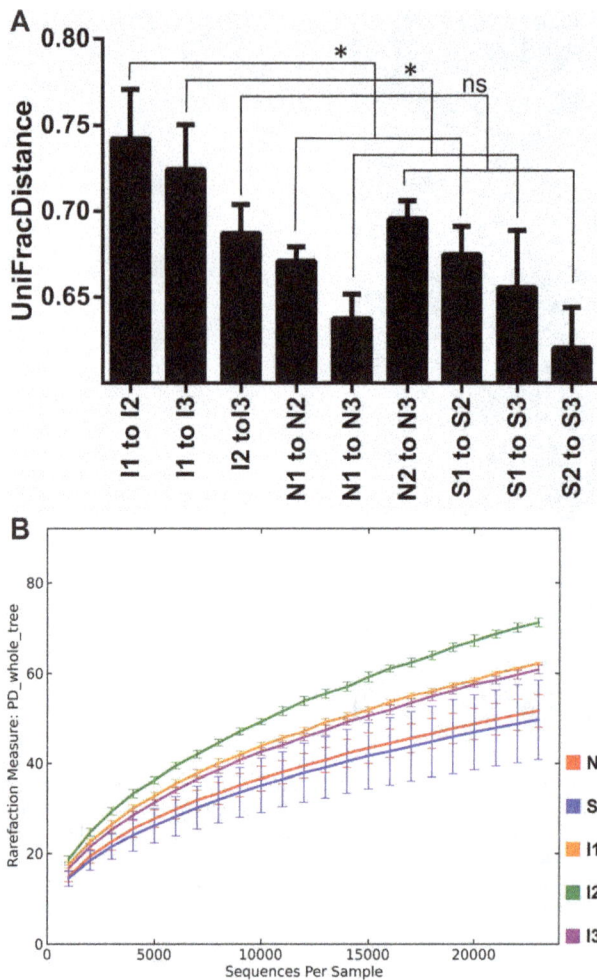

Figure 3. UniFrac distance between samples and rarefaction curve of phylogenetic diversity. (A) Unweighted UniFrac distance. The higher a UniFrac distance value between two samples the more different the bacterial composition. The highest distance values were determined for subjects undergoing smoking cessation between t1 and t2 as well as between t1 and t3. All other distance values were substantially smaller (error bars indicate SEM; *: p<0.05; ns: not significant). (B) Rarefaction curves. These curves express the accumulation of phylogenetic richness that would be obtained with continuous sampling effort and hence minimize potential differences that would be a result of the variable number of sequences obtained per sample. For the control groups the three sampling time points were combined in a single curve, while for the intervention group separated curves for t1, t2 and t3 were depicted to visualize the increased phlyogenetic diversity (PD) in the samples 4 weeks after smoking cessation (I2) compared to I1 and I3 (additional indices of α-diversity are depicted in Figure S9).

important studies suggesting alternative mechanisms for weight gain, such as a decreased metabolic resting rate [39] or changes in metabolic properties in the adipose tissue, in specific an increase of the lipoprotein lipase activity [40]. While a smaller study found no increase in calorie intake after smoking cessation in subjects gaining weight [24], an indicator for alternative mechanisms for the well-known effect of weight gain [23] are the results of the multiple risk factor intervention trial [25]; one of the largest studies ever performed in this field. This trial included more than 11000 men with an observational period of 6 years, thoroughly investigating weight gain and calorie intake in nonsmokers, quitters,

recidivists, and continued smokers in a usual care group in comparison to a special intervention group with specific counseling. Interestingly, despite a reduced calorie intake and a generally healthier diet after counseling compared to baseline, and an even bigger reduction in calories compared to continuing smokers, men who ceased smoking gained weight. This was strikingly in contradiction to nonsmokers, continuing smokers, and even recidivists, who all lost weight. Second, although alterations in intestinal microbiota composition due to diet are well known, profound shifts seem to necessitate a longer time period as a recent human study found significant changes on the phylum level to occur predominantly after 12 weeks [21]. In contrast no stable switches between enterotype groups occurred in the short-term, despite a controlled and randomized short-term feeding experiment using two extremely divergent diets (high-fat/low-fiber versus low-fat/high-fiber) [41]. Third, a uniform shift in the phyla composition such as the one observed in our patients undergoing smoking cessation (Figure S4) indeed might be assumed to occur in interventions with prespecified and standardized major changes of diet. But this would less likely to be expected in individually different and uncontrolled slight dietary changes undetected by food-frequency protocols.

Although we identified continuous microbial shifts 8 weeks after smoking cessation, this relatively short observational period does not permit conclusions about a long-term alteration. Nevertheless, the continuing increase in body mass observed in subsequent 4 years [23] after the first year after smoking cessation (where the major part of the weight gain occurs) points to a potential sustained microbial alteration. Larger prospective long-term studies are needed to address this issue.

Although the role of cigarette smoking as one of the most important environmental risk factor in the pathogenesis of IBD is well established [10–13], the numerous epidemiological reports on smoking status and course of IBD are in sharp contrast with the very limited mechanistic explorations of the effect of smoking cigarettes on the gut and intestinal inflammation. The molecular and cellular mechanisms by which smoking interferes with the pathogenesis of CD and UC are only poorly understood. While several potential mechanisms, such as modulation of mucosal immune responses, alterations in intestinal cytokine and eicosanoid levels or modifications in gut permeability have been proposed, none of these hypotheses could hitherto offer a satisfying explanation [42]. As the importance of the intestinal microbiota in the pathogenesis of IBD is well established, the profound shifts in the composition of the intestinal microbiota observed in our study may shed some light to a potential pathogenetic link of cigarette smoking, smoking cessation, and course of disease in IBD, including the discrepancy in CD and UC. However, as we did not investigate the intestinal microbial evolution during smoking cessation specifically in patients with IBD, this potential pathogenetic link largely remains a speculative deduction and our findings need to be confirmed in CD and UC patients. We nevertheless believe, that the results of our observational study, demonstrating intestinal microbial shifts after smoking cessation for the first time, point to a potential interaction of disease-modifying factors in IBD. This may give us a further piece of information with regard to an enormously complex interplay, where we clearly are just at the beginning of our understanding – the interplay of the intestinal microbiota, chronic inflammatory bowel disease, systemic metabolic interactions and environmental factors (such as smoking).

In conclusion, smoking cessation induces profound changes in intestinal microbial composition. Interestingly, these changes appear to occur in a comparable manner both microbiologically and clinically (weight gain) as those induced by transplantation of an 'obese microbiota' into lean mice [20]. These alterations in conjunction with weight gain point to further evidence for the assumed role of the intestinal microbiota and its metabolic properties derived to the host in the pathogenesis of obesity and the metabolic syndrome. Our findings invite confirmatory larger and long-term studies as well as further research on the effect of environmental factors on intestinal microbial composition.

Supporting Information

Figure S1 Average daily calorie intake. No significant changes in total calorie intake or nutritional components were observed before (t1) and after smoking cessation (t2, t3), except for a modest increase in average daily alcohol consumption between t2 and t3 (error bars indicating SEM; Carb: carbohydrate; da: daily average). Further details on the individual caloric intake are given Table S2 and S3.

Figure S2 PCA with 9 environments. Separation of the samples from the intervention group (E7 = I, t1; E8 = I, t2; E9 = I, t3) alongside the first principal component axis (IPCA1) reflecting the largest difference, 58.5% (as outlined in Table D, Table S4.). There is a close association of samples from the non-smoking control group (E1 = N, t1; E2 = N, t2; E3 = N, t3). A wider separation is to be seen in the smoking control group (E4 = S, t1; E5 = S, t2; E6 = S, t3), however almost exclusively alongside the second principal component axis (IPCA2), reflecting a substantially smaller difference (37.7%).

Figure S3 Distribution of phyla in all samples in percentages. The fraction other (0.1% of all sequences) in the right pie chart consists of *Synergistetes*, *Fusobacteria*, *Deinococcus-Thermus*, *TM7*, *Acidobacteria* and *OD1*.

Figure S4 Composition of phyla per individual. The fractions of the four most abundant phyla and changes over time are depicted. Individuals within a group are aligned based on abundance of *Firmicutes*. While there is an relatively stable composition per individual in the non-smoking (N1-5) and smoking (S1-5) control groups, obvious shifts in the subjects from the intervention group (I1-10) can be detected between the time points before (t1) and after (t2, t3) smoking cessation.

Figure S5 Heat map with color-coded significance levels. The results of paired Student's T-Test is depicted on the level of phylum (analogs to Main Figure 1b) including separate analysis for all genera constituting each phylum.

Figure S6 Weighted PCA. Analog to Main Figure 2. Findings are similar to the unweighted analysis. Again a clear separation of samples of the intervention group is obvious. Although there is some variation in the non-smoking Control group (N) as well, the difference is notably smaller (smoking control group = S).

Figure S7 Jackknife analysis. In this statistical approach to test for reproducibility of results, resampling is done several times with a number of sequences (in general sample size of around 75% of the number of sequences in the sample with the lowest count is recommended (runs were performed with sample size 18000). To increase statistical power we set number of permutations to 1000. QIIME constructs a color coded bootstrapped tree (red = 75–100% support, yellow = 50–75%, green = 25–50% and blue for <25%; unweighted (A) and weighted (B) tree). The number besides the nodes indicates the percentage of how many times the node was reproduced during resampling. A perfectly high reproducibility can be seen.

Figure S8 PD and PD-Endemism. There are substantially higher values in the intervention group after smoking cessation. PD-Endemism refers to the amount of branch length that is uniquely represented by a certain environment while PD is indicative of the total phylogenetic branch length, that is spanned by all species included in the environment.

Figure S9 Rarefaction curves (analog to main Figure 3b; curves express the accumulation of phylogenetic richness that would be obtained with continuous sampling effort and hence minimize potential differences that would be a result of the variable number of sequences obtained per sample). In addition to the phylogeny-based PD whole tree (phylogenetic tree is needed for calculation of this α-diversity measure) (A), two further indices of α-diversity, chao1 (B) and observed species (C) are depicted. The latter two indices reveal a significantly increased α-diversity also 8 weeks after smoking cessation. For the control groups the three sampling time points were combined in a single curve, while for the intervention group separated curves for t1, t2 and t3 were depicted to visualize the increased microbial diversity (PD) in the samples 4 weeks after smoking cessation (I2) compared to I1 and I3.

Table S1 Evolution of body weight and BMI in the 10 subjects undergoing smoking cessation.

Table S2 Overview of individual calorie intake in the 10 subjects undergoing smoking cessation.

Table S3 Paired T-Test (Comparison of total calories as well as fraction of carbohydrates, proteins, fat fibers and alcohol between t1, t2 and t3). With the exception of calories from alcohol between t2 and t3 no significant changes are detected.

Table S4 Summary of additive main effects and multiplicative interaction model (AMMI) results. Table **A** shows the results of the analysis of variance (ANOVA) with a two-way data matrix (df = degrees of freedom, SS = sum of squares and MS = mean square). Table **B** shows the interaction sums of squares (SS), giving an estimate of the contribution of idiosyncratic noise to the observed pattern, which in this case is regarded as meaningful. However, the value for the interaction pattern is clearly positive (a negative value would occur if the estimated interaction noise is more meaningful than the interaction total). Table **C** shows the per cent of variation from each source in AMMI (while main effects variation reflects variation from T-RFs and Environments, replicated data interaction effects reflects interaction pattern and interaction noise; variation due to Interaction Effects reflect dissimilarity of the investigated microbial communities). Table **D** shows how much of the predicted interaction signal variation is captured in the first IPCAs (in the table the first four IPCAs are depicted; here complete capture is already achieved with 3 axes.

(TIF)

Text S1

Acknowledgments

We acknowledge the following colleagues: M. Herensperger (technical support in fecal sample collection and performance of T-RFLP analyses), B. Lang (endorsement in the recruitment of study subjects), R. Knight and C. Lozupne (Fast UniFrac) as well as R. Bukowski (T-Rex) and T. Hughes (phylo3D, walrus) (support with their bioinformatic software tools), R. Speich (for providing L.B. with the opportunity to start this research) as well as the subjects participating in this study.

Author Contributions

Critical revision of the manuscript: GR M. Schuppler JM ESM AR M. Scharl JZ PF CCS ML MF SRV. Conceived and designed the experiments: GR SRV LB M. Schuppler MF ML CSS. Performed the experiments: LB ESM M. Schuppler JZ AF MF M. Scharl PF SO SS. Analyzed the data: LB JM GR AR SO SS ESM. Contributed reagents/materials/analysis tools: LB JZ AR SO CSS AF ML M. Scharl. Wrote the paper: LB GR.

References

1. Lee YK, Mazmanian SK (2010) Has the microbiota played a critical role in the evolution of the adaptive immune system. Science 330 (6012): 1768–1773.
2. Mazmanian SK, Liu CH, Tzianabos AO, Kasper DL (2005) An immunomodulatory molecule of symbiotic bacteria directs maturation of the host immune system. Cell 122 (1): 107–118.
3. Gill SR, Pop M, Deboy RT, Eckburg PB, Turnbaugh PJ, et al. (2006) Metagenomic analysis of the human distal gut microbiome. Science 312 (5778): 1355–1359.
4. Sonnenburg JL, Xu J, Leip DD, Chen C, Westover BP, et al. (2005) Glycan foraging in vivo by an intestine-adapted bacterial symbiont. Science 307 (5717): 1955–1959.
5. Seksik P, Nion-Larmurier I, Sokol H, Beaugerie L, Cosnes J (2009) Effects of light smoking consumption on the clinical course of Crohn's disease. Inflamm. Bowel Dis. 15 (5): 734–741.
6. Frank DN, St. Amand AL, Feldman RA, Boedeker EC, Harpaz N, et al. (2007) Molecular-phylogenetic characterization of microbial community imbalances in human inflammatory bowel diseases. Proceedings of the National Academy of Sciences 104 (34): 13780–13785.
7. Rajilić–Stojanović M, Biagi E, Heilig HGHJ, Kajander K, Kekkonen RA, et al. (2011) Global and Deep Molecular Analysis of Microbiota Signatures in Fecal Samples From Patients With Irritable Bowel Syndrome. Gastroenterology 141 (5): 1792–1801.
8. Codling C, O'Mahony L, Shanahan F, Quigley EMM, Marchesi JR (2010) A molecular analysis of fecal and mucosal bacterial communities in irritable bowel syndrome. Dig. Dis. Sci 55 (2): 392–397.
9. Kassinen A, Krogius-Kurikka L, Mäkivuokko H, Rinttilä T, Paulin L, et al. (2007) The fecal microbiota of irritable bowel syndrome patients differs significantly from that of healthy subjects. Gastroenterology 133 (1): 24–33.
10. Nos P, Domènech E (2011) Management of Crohn's disease in smokers: is an alternative approach necessary. World J. Gastroenterol. 17 (31): 3567–3574.
11. Mahid SS, Minor KS, Soto RE, Hornung CA, Galandiuk S (2006) Smoking and inflammatory bowel disease: a meta-analysis. Mayo Clin. Proc. 81 (11): 1462–1471.
12. Danese S, Sans M, Fiocchi C (2004) Inflammatory bowel disease: the role of environmental factors. Autoimmun Rev 3 (5): 394–400.
13. Cosnes J, Seksik P (2006) Facteurs environnementaux dans la maladie de Crohn. Acta Endoscopica 36 (5): 679–688.
14. Cosnes J, Carbonnel F, Beaugerie L, Le Quintrec Y, Gendre JP (1996) Effects of cigarette smoking on the long-term course of Crohn's disease. Gastroenterology 110 (2): 424–431.
15. Holdstock G, Savage D, Harman M, Wright R (1984) Should patients with inflammatory bowel disease smoke? Br Med J (Clin Res Ed) 288 (6414): 362.
16. Lindberg E, Järnerot G, Huitfeldt B (1992) Smoking in Crohn's disease: effect on localisation and clinical course. Gut 33 (6): 779–782.
17. Beaugerie L, Massot N, Carbonnel F, Cattan S, Gendre JP, et al. (2001) Impact of cessation of smoking on the course of ulcerative colitis. Am. J. Gastroenterol. 96 (7): 2113–2116.
18. Backhed F, Ding H, Wang T, Hooper LV, Koh GY, et al. (2004) The gut microbiota as an environmental factor that regulates fat storage. Proc Natl Acad Sci U S A 101 (44): 15718–15723.
19. Vijay-Kumar M, Aitken JD, Carvalho FA, Cullender TC, Mwangi S, et al. (2010) Metabolic syndrome and altered gut microbiota in mice lacking Toll-like receptor 5. Science 328 (5975): 228–231.
20. Turnbaugh PJ, Ley RE, Mahowald MA, Magrini V, Mardis ER, et al. (2006) An obesity-associated gut microbiome with increased capacity for energy harvest. Nature 444 (7122): 1027–1031.
21. Ley RE, Turnbaugh PJ, Klein S, Gordon JI (2006) Microbial ecology: human gut microbes associated with obesity. Nature 444 (7122): 1022–1023.
22. Ley RE, Bäckhed F, Turnbaugh P, Lozupone CA, Knight RD, et al. (2005) Obesity alters gut microbial ecology. Proc. Natl. Acad. Sci. U.S.A. 102 (31): 11070–11075.
23. O'Hara P, Connett JE, Lee WW, Nides M, Murray R, et al. (1998) Early and late weight gain following smoking cessation in the Lung Health Study. Am. J. Epidemiol 148 (9): 821–830.
24. Rodin J (1987) Weight change following smoking cessation: the role of food intake and exercise. Addict Behav 12 (4): 303–317.
25. Stamler J, Rains-Clearman D, Lenz-Litzow K, Tillotson JL, Grandits GA (1997) Relation of smoking at baseline and during trial years 1–6 to food and nutrient intakes and weight in the special intervention and usual care groups in the Multiple Risk Factor Intervention Trial. Am. J. Clin. Nutr 65 (1 Suppl): 374S–402S.
26. Charlson ES, Chen J, Custers-Allen R, Bittinger K, Li H, et al. (2010) Disordered Microbial Communities in the Upper Respiratory Tract of Cigarette Smokers. PLoS ONE 5 (12): e15216.
27. Pace NR (1997) A molecular view of microbial diversity and the biosphere. Science 276 (5313): 734–740.
28. Middleton ET, Morice AH (2000) Breath Carbon Monoxide as an Indication of Smoking Habit*. Chest 117 (3): 758–763.
29. Eckburg PB, Bik EM, Bernstein CN, Purdom E, Dethlefsen L, et al. (2005) Diversity of the human intestinal microbial flora. Science 308 (5728): 1635–1638.
30. Cole JR, Wang Q, Cardenas E, Fish J, Chai B, et al. (2009) The Ribosomal Database Project: improved alignments and new tools for rRNA analysis. Nucleic Acids Research 37 (Database): D141.
31. Culman SW, Gauch HG, Blackwood CB, Thies JE (2008) Analysis of T-RFLP data using analysis of variance and ordination methods: A comparative study. Journal of Microbiological Methods 75 (1): 55–63.
32. Huang Y, Niu B, Gao Y, Fu L, Li W (2010) CD-HIT Suite: a web server for clustering and comparing biological sequences. Bioinformatics 26 (5): 680–682.
33. DeSantis TZ, Hugenholtz P, Keller K, Brodie EL, Larsen N, et al. (2006) NAST: a multiple sequence alignment server for comparative analysis of 16S rRNA genes. Nucleic Acids Research 34 (Web Server): W394.
34. Hamady M, Lozupone C, Knight R (2009) Fast UniFrac: facilitating high-throughput phylogenetic analyses of microbial communities including analysis of pyrosequencing and PhyloChip data. ISME J 4 (1): 17–27.
35. Caporaso JG, Kuczynski J, Stombaugh J, Bittinger K, Bushman FD, et al. (2010) QIIME allows analysis of high-throughput community sequencing data. Nat Meth 7 (5): 335–336.
36. Faith DP (1992) Conservation evaluation and phylogenetic diversity. Biological Conservation 61 (1): 1–10.
37. Minh B, Klaere S, Haeseler A (2006) Phylogenetic Diversity within Seconds. Systematic Biology 55 (5): 769–773.
38. Faith DP, Reid CAM, Hunter J (2004) Integrating Phylogenetic Diversity, Complementarity, and Endemism for Conservation Assessment. Conservation Biology 18 (1): 255–261.
39. Dallosso HM, James WP (1984) The role of smoking in the regulation of energy balance. Int J Obes 8 (4): 365–375.
40. Ferrara CM, Kumar M, Nicklas B, McCrone S, Goldberg AP (2001) Weight gain and adipose tissue metabolism after smoking cessation in women. Int. J. Obes. Relat. Metab. Disord 25 (9): 1322–1326.
41. Wu GD, Chen J, Hoffmann C, Bittinger K, Chen Y, et al. (2011) Linking Long-Term Dietary Patterns with Gut Microbial Enterotypes. Science.
42. Birrenbach T, Böcker U (2004) Inflammatory bowel disease and smoking: a review of epidemiology, pathophysiology, and therapeutic implications. Inflamm. Bowel Dis. 10 (6): 848–859.

18

Telmisartan Attenuates Colon Inflammation, Oxidative Perturbations and Apoptosis in a Rat Model of Experimental Inflammatory Bowel Disease

Hany H. Arab[1]*, Muhammad Y. Al-Shorbagy[2], Dalaal M. Abdallah[2], Noha N. Nassar[2]

1 Department of Biochemistry, Faculty of Pharmacy, Cairo University, Cairo, Egypt, 2 Department of Pharmacology and Toxicology, Faculty of Pharmacy, Cairo University, Cairo, Egypt

Abstract

Accumulating evidence has indicated the implication of angiotensin II in the pathogenesis of inflammatory bowel diseases (IBD) via its proinflammatory features. Telmisartan (TLM) is an angiotensin II receptor antagonist with marked anti-inflammatory and antioxidant actions that mediated its cardio-, reno- and hepatoprotective actions. However, its impact on IBD has not been previously explored. Thus, we aimed to investigate the potential alleviating effects of TLM in tri-nitrobenezene sulphonic acid (TNBS)-induced colitis in rats. Pretreatment with TLM (10 mg/kg p.o.) attenuated the severity of colitis as evidenced by decrease of disease activity index (DAI), colon weight/length ratio, macroscopic damage, histopathological findings and leukocyte migration. TLM suppressed the inflammatory response via attenuation of tumor necrosis factor-α (TNF-α), prostaglandin E_2 (PGE$_2$) and myeloperoxidase (MPO) activity as a marker of neutrophil infiltration besides restoration of interleukin-10 (IL-10). TLM also suppressed mRNA and protein expression of nuclear factor kappa B (NF-κB) p65 and mRNA of cyclo-oxygenase-2 (COX-2) and inducible nitric oxide synthase (iNOS) proinflammatory genes with concomitant upregulation of PPAR-γ. The alleviation of TLM to colon injury was also associated with inhibition of oxidative stress as evidenced by suppression of lipid peroxides and nitric oxide (NO) besides boosting glutathione (GSH), total anti-oxidant capacity (TAC) and the activities of superoxide dismutase (SOD) and glutathione peroxidase (GPx). With respect to apoptosis, TLM downregulated the increased mRNA, protein expression and activity of caspase-3. It also suppressed the elevation of cytochrome c and Bax mRNA besides the upregulation of Bcl-2. Together, these findings highlight evidences for the beneficial effects of TLM in IBD which are mediated through modulation of colonic inflammation, oxidative stress and apoptosis.

Editor: Rupesh Chaturvedi, Vanderbilt University School of Medicine, United States of America

Funding: The authors have no support or funding to report.

Competing Interests: The authors have declared that no competing interests exist.

* E-mail: hany.arab@pharma.cu.edu.eg

Introduction

Inflammatory bowel diseases (IBD), including ulcerative colitis (UC) and Crohn's disease (CD), are chronic, relapsing, immuno-logically mediated inflammatory disorders of the gastrointestinal tract that jeopardize the quality of life of patients suffering from these disorders [1]. During the progression of IBD, disruption of intestinal epithelial barrier is regarded as the central event in IBD pathogenesis which is followed by robust immune responses towards intestinal flora in a context of genetic predisposition [2]. Activation of intestinal immune system is associated with excessive generation of inflammatory cytokines such as tumor necrosis factor-α (TNF-α) which amplifies the inflammatory cascade by triggering the generation of other proinflammatory cytokines and enhancing the recruitment of macrophages and neutrophils [1,2]. The infiltration of neutrophils generates excessive amounts of reactive oxygen species (ROS), nitric oxide (NO) and prostaglan-din E_2 (PGE$_2$) which ultimately provoke mucosal disruption [1]. Excessive generation of ROS and cytokines has been reported to activate several transcription factors that upregulate the inflammatory response. Among them, the nuclear factor kappa B (NF-κB) induces transcription of proinflammatory genes including cyclo-oxygenase-2 (COX-2) and inducible nitric oxide synthase (iNOS) [3]. Increased levels of interleukin-10 (IL-10) have been reported in IBD patients [4] and experimental animals [5,6] where they attenuate the exaggerated inflammatory response [2]. The pathogenesis of IBD also involves increased frequency of apoptosis with consequent loss of intestinal epithelial cells [7].

Angiotensin II (Ang II), the main effector peptide of the rennin-angiotensin system (RAS), has potent proinflammatory features linked with the pathogenesis of several chronic inflammatory disorders including IBD [8]. Via its actions on angiotensin II type 1 (AT1) receptors, angiotensin II promotes tissue inflammation through upregulation of adhesion molecules, increasing vascular permeability, and thus, enhancing neutrophil infiltration, which contributes to gut ulceration [9]. It also increases the release of proinflammatory cytokines such as TNF-α, probably, through activation of NF-κB. Additionally, Ang II triggers oxidative stress via activation of NADH/NADPH oxidase with consequent generation of superoxide anions [8].

Accumulating evidence has indicated the efficacy of members of Ang II receptor blockers (ARBs) such as valsartan and olmesartan in the attenuation of colon injury in experimental colitis [10,11].

Among several candidates of ARBs, telmisartan (TLM) has unique anti-inflammatory and antioxidant features owing to the blockade of Ang II AT1 receptors besides its partial agonist actions on peroxisome proliferator activated receptor-gamma (PPAR-γ) [12]. Previously, PPAR-γ agonists such as rosiglitazone have displayed marked protective effects in experimental colitis [13]. Interestingly, TLM has exerted versatile beneficial effects against atherosclerosis and myocardial infarction [14,15]. TLM also exhibits favorable actions in vascular dysfunction [16], cardiac remodeling [17], renal injury [18], hepatic fibrosis [19], stroke [20] and testicular injury [21]. Additional advantages of TLM include excellent toxicity profile, the longest half-life among all ARBs, and its cost-effective price [12]. Together, these findings encouraged us to investigate the potential alleviating effects of TLM and the underlying mechanisms in tri-nitrobenezene sulphonic acid (TNBS)-induced colitis, an experimental model of human IBD.

In the current study, colon inflammation was assessed by disease activity index (DAI), colon weight/length ratio, macroscopic damage, histopathological assessment and leukocyte invasion as indicated by myeloperoxidase (MPO) activity. To delineate the underlying mechanisms of TLM, we investigated its effects on the inflammatory status by assessing the mRNA/protein expression of NF-κB together with the mRNA expression of COX-2, iNOS and PPAR-γ. Besides, the colonic levels of TNF-α, IL-10 and PGE$_2$ were investigated. The redox status was monitored by assessing the levels of lipid peroxides, NO, reduced glutathione (GSH) and total antioxidant capacity (TAC) along with superoxide dismutase (SOD) and glutathione peroxidase (GPx) antioxidant enzymes. Additionally, we investigated the colonic apoptosis via estimating the mRNA expression of cytochrome c, Bcl-2 associated x protein (Bax) and B cell lymphoma-2 (Bcl-2) in addition to the mRNA, protein expression and the activity of caspase-3. To the best of our knowledge, this is the first report that describes the ameliorative effects of TLM in TNBS-induced colitis via its anti-inflammatory, anti-oxidant and anti-apoptotic actions.

Materials and Methods

Ethics Statement

This study was carried out in strict accordance with the recommendations in the Guide for the Care and Use of Laboratory Animals published by the US National Institute of Health (NIH publication No. 85-23, revised 1996). The protocol was approved by the Committee of Animal Care and Use of Faculty of Pharmacy, Cairo University. All efforts were made to minimize animal suffering.

Animals

Adult male Wistar rats weighing 200±20 g were purchased from the National Institute for Research, Cairo, Egypt. The animals were kept at controlled environmental conditions in terms of constant temperature (23±1 °C), humidity (60±10%), and a 12/12 h light/dark cycle. They were acclimatized for one week before any experimental procedures and were allowed standard rat chow and water *ad libitum*.

Chemicals

Telmisartan (Micardis) was obtained from Boehringer Ingelheim, Germany. TNBS was purchased from Sigma-Aldrich (St. Louis, MD, USA). All Other chemicals were of highest purity and analytical grade. ELISA kits for determination of TNF-α, IL-10 and PGE$_2$ along with caspase-3 colorimetric kit were purchased from R &D systems, MN, USA while the TAC kit was provided by Cayman Chemical Company, Ann arbor, MI, USA.

Experimental design and treatment protocol

In the current study, animals were randomly divided into four groups (8 rats per group). Group I (Control gp): received physiological saline rectally + oral vehicle. Group II (Control + TLM gp): received saline rectally + oral TLM. Group III (TNBS gp): received rectal TNBS instillation (50 mg/kg) + oral vehicle. Group IV (TNBS + TLM): received TNBS rectally + oral TLM. TLM was suspended in 0.5% carboxymethyl cellulose vehicle and was administered (10 mg/kg/day) by oral gavage starting 1 week before the induction of TNBS colitis and was continued till the 4th day post TNBS instillation. The animals were euthanized using an overdose of anesthesia on the 5th day of TNBS induction. The selected dose of TLM was based on its previously displayed anti-inflammatory actions in animal models of autoimmune myocarditis [22], cardiac ischemic reperfusion injury [23], myocardial infarction [15] and hepatic fibrosis [19]. The chosen regimen is consistent with previous reports investigating the effects of olmesartan and valsartan in experimental colitis [10,11] and the PPAR-γ agonist rosiglitazone in TNBS colitis [13].

Induction of colitis

TNBS colitis was induced according to the procedures described by Morris et al. [24] with modifications [25]. Briefly, animals were fasted for 24 hours with free access to water. Animals were anaesthetized with chloral hydrate (300 mg/kg i.p.) and a medial grade polyurethane catheter with 2 mm external diameter was inserted into the anus and its tip was advanced in the descending colon to 8 cm from the anus verge. Rats were kept in a vertical head-down position and TNBS (50 mg/kg) in 50% ethanol was rectally instilled slowly within 1 min and the catheter was kept in place for another min, and gently removed. Then, TNBS-treated rats were left in the head-down position for 1 min to avoid leakage of the intracolonic instillate and then kept on warm bedding till regain of consciousness. The control group received physiological saline rectally instead of TNBS solution.

Tissue collection and preparation

On the 5th day post TNBS-instillation, rats were euthanized under deep ether anesthesia and laparatomy was immediately performed. The distal 8 cm portion of the colon was excised, freed of adherent adipose tissue, longitudinally split and washed with ice-cold saline to remove fecal residues. Then it was blotted dry, weighed and macroscopic assessment of colitis was performed. Sections of the distal colon were utilized for histopathological, immunohistochemical and biochemical investigations.

Measured parameters

1. Disease activity index (DAI). The scores of DAI ranging from 0 (healthy) to 12 (severe colitis) were calculated as previously described [26]. The sum of scores for the % loss of body weight (score 0-4), stool consistency (score 0-4) and rectal bleeding (scores 0-4) were calculated (Table 1). Diarrhea was manifested by presence of mucus on animal feces sticking to fur while rectal bleeding ranged from occult blood to gross bleeding on the fecal matter.

2. Assessment of colon damage by macroscopic scoring. The severity of colitis was evaluated by an independent observer blinded to the identity of treatments. The colon damage was scored on a 0–10 scale according to the criteria described by Tsune et al. [27]: 0 = no macroscopic changes; 1 = focal hyperemia, no ulcers; 2 = ulcer without significant inflammation (hyperemia and bowel wall thickening); 3 = ulceration with inflammation at one site; 4 = two or more sites of ulceration/

Table 1. Scoring of disease activity index (DAI).

Weight loss	Stool consistency	Rectal bleeding
0 = < 1%	0 = normal	0 = negative
1 = 1-5%	2 = loose stool	2 = positive
2 = 5-10%	4 = diarrhea	4 = gross bleeding
3 = 10-15%		
4 = >15%		

inflammation; 5 = major sites of damage extending > 1cm along colon length; 6 – 8 = when the area of damage exceeds 2 cm along the colon, the score was increased by one for each additional 1 cm. Besides, the adhesion scores were added according to the criteria of Bobin-Dubigeon et al. [28]: 0 = no adhesion; 1 = minor adhesion; 2 = major adhesion.

3. Histopathological examination and microscopic scoring. Full thickness colon biopsy specimens were fixed in 10% buffered formol saline for 24 h. The specimens were washed, dehydrated by alcohol, cleared in xylene and embedded in paraffin at 56°C in hot air oven for another 24 h. Sections of 3 μm thickness were stained with hematoxylin and eosin (H&E) and examined under the light microscope (Leica Microsystems, Germany). All histopathologic processing and assessment of specimens were performed by an experienced observer blinded to the identity of the sample being examined to avoid any bias.

The colon microscopic damage was scored on a 0–5 scale as described by Galvez et al. [29] as follows: 0 = normal colonic tissue; 1 = inflammation or focal ulceration limited to the mucosa; 2 = focal or extensive ulceration and inflammation limited to the mucosa and the submucosa; 3, focal or extensive ulceration and inflammation with involvement of muscularis ; 4 = focal or extensive ulceration and inflammation with involvement of the serosa; and 5, extensive ulceration and transmural inflammation with involvement of the serosa.

4. Immunohistochemical detection of NF-κB p65 and caspase-3. Paraffin embedded tissue sections of 3 μm thickness were rehydrated in xylene and then in graded ethanol solutions and heated in citrate buffer (pH 6) for 5 min. The slides were blocked with 5% bovine serum albumin (BSA) in Tris buffered saline (TBS) for 2 h. The sections were then immunostained with primary polyclonal rabbit anti-NF-κBp65 (Santa Cruz Biotechnology Inc, CA, USA) or caspase-3 (Thermo Scientific, IL, USA) at a concentration of 1 μg/ml in 5% BSA in TBS and were incubated overnight at 4 °C. Following primary antibody incubation step, the slides were washed with TBS and were then incubated with goat anti-rabbit secondary antibody. Finally, the sections were washed with TBS and incubated for 5–10 min in a solution of 0.02% diaminobenzidine (DAB) containing 0.01% H_2O_2. Counter staining was performed using hematoxylin and the slides were visualized under light microscope (Leica Microsystems, Germany).

5. Colon MPO activity. Activity of MPO, a marker for neutrophil infiltration, was estimated according to the method of Krawisz et al. [30] with slight modifications. One unit of MPO activity is defined as the amount of enzyme converting 1 μmol of H_2O_2 to water in 1 min at 25°C. The colon homogenates were subjected to 3 cycles of freezing/thawing, 30 sec of sonication and centrifuged at 20,000×g for 20 min at 4°C. O-dianisidine hydrochloride (0.167%) and H_2O_2 (0.0005%) in potassium

phosphate buffer (50 mmol/L, pH 6) were added to the supernatant and the absorbance rate was monitored at 460 nm for 4 min.

6. Inflammatory cytokines (TNF-α and IL-10). The levels of TNF-α and IL-10 in colon homogenate supernatants were measured using ELISA kits (R &D systems incorporation, USA). All the procedures were performed according to the manufacturer's instructions. The assays of these cytokines employ the quantitative sandwich enzyme immunoassay technique and the optical densities were measured at 450 nm using microplate reader (Biochrom Asys, UK). The intensity of the color was proportional to the amount of the corresponding cytokine bound in the initial step. The corresponding levels were expressed as pg/g tissue.

7. PGE₂ concentration. The levels of colon PGE₂ were determined using an ELISA kit (R &D systems incorporation, USA), according to the manufacturer's instructions and the colonic levels were presented as pg/ mg tissue.

8. Lipid peroxides concentration. Determination of lipid peroxide levels, expressed as malondialdehyde (MDA), was carried out according to the thiobarbituric acid assay of Buege and Aust [31]. The absorbance was recorded at 535 nm and the results were expressed as nmol/g tissue.

9. Nitric oxide concentration. Total NO was determined by measuring its stable metabolites, particularly, nitrite (NO_2^-) and nitrate (NO_3^-) based on the method of Miranda et al. [32] with the modification of replacing zinc sulfate instead of ethanol for the precipitation of proteins in the supernatant of colon homogenates. Absorbance was measured at 540 nm and the results were expressed as nmol/g tissue.

10. Reduced glutathione. Colon GSH levels were determined as previously described by Beutler et al. [33], using 5,5'-dithiobis 2-nitrobenzoic acid (DTNB) reagent. The optical density for the colored product was read at 412 nm and results were expressed as nmol/g tissue.

11. Determination of TAC. TAC was determined using Cayman total antioxidant assay kit according to the manufacturer's instructions. The assay relies on the ability of antioxidants in the supernatants of colon homogenates to inhibit the oxidation of ABTS (2,2-azino-di-[3-ethylbenzthiazoline sulphonate]) by metmyoglobin. The amount of the oxidized product was estimated by reading absorbance at 405 nm. The capacity of the antioxidants in the sample to prevent ABTS oxidation was compared to that of Trolox, a water-soluble tocopherol analogue and the results were quantified as μmol of Trolox equivalent/g tissue.

12. Superoxide dismutase activity. SOD activity was assayed according to the method of Marklund and Marklund [34] which assesses the ability of colonic SOD to prevent auto-oxidation of pyrogallol. The change in absorbance at 420 nm was obtained at 1 min interval for 3 min. One unit of SOD is defined as the amount of enzyme that affords 50% inhibition of pyrogallol auto-oxidation in 1 min. Results were expressed as U/mg protein.

The protein content of colonic homogenate was determined using the method of Lowry et al. [35].

13. Glutathione peroxidase activity. GPx activity was determined according to the method of Paglia and Valentine [36], that resides on the ability of the enzyme to oxidize GSH which was monitored via recording the decrease in absorbance of NADPH at 340 nm. One unit of enzyme is defined as the amount of enzyme that oxidizes 1 μmol NADPH /min at 25°C.

14. Quantitative real-time RT-PCR. Total RNA was extracted from colon tissues using RNeasy Mini kit (Qiagen, CA, USA) and the purity of obtained RNA was verified spectrophotometrically at 260/280 nm. Equal amounts of RNA (2 μg) were reverse transcribed into cDNA using Superscript Choice systems (Life Technolgies, USA) according to the manufacturer's instructions. To assess the expression of inflammation and apoptosis-associated target genes, quantitative real-time PCR was performed using SYBR green PCR Master mix (Applied Biosystems, CA, USA) as described by the manufacturer. Briefly, in a 25 μl reaction volume, 5 μl of cDNA was added to 12.5 μl of 2× SYBR green Master mix and 200 ng of each primer. The sequences of primers are described in Table 2. PCR reactions included 10 min at 95°C for activation of AmpliTaq Gold DNA polymerase, followed by 40 cycles at 95°C for 15 sec (denaturing) and 60°C for 1 min (annealing/extension). The expression level was calculated from the PCR cycle number (C_T) where the increased fluorescence curve passes across a threshold value. The relative expression of target genes was obtained using comparative C_T ($\Delta\Delta C_T$) method. The ΔC_T was calculated by subtracting GAPDH C_T from that of target gene whereas $\Delta\Delta C_T$ was obtained by subtracting the ΔC_T of calibrator sample (control gp) from that of test sample (control+ TLM, TNBS or TNBS+ TLM gp). The relative expression was calculated from the $2^{-\Delta\Delta CT}$ formula [37].

15. Caspase-3 activity. Caspase-3 activity was colorimetrically assayed using R &D systems kit as described by the manufacturer. Briefly, an aliquot of the homogenate supernatant was incubated with the labeled substrate DEVD-pNA (acetyl-Asp-Glu-Val-Asp p-nitroanilide). The cleavage of the peptide by the caspase releases the chromophore pNA, which was read at 405 nm using Biochrom Asys microplate reader, UK. According to the manufacturer's instructions, the results were expressed as fold change of caspase-3 activity.

Statistical analysis

Parametric data were expressed as mean ± SEM, and statistical comparisons were carried out using one-way analysis of variance (ANOVA), followed by Tukey-Kramer post hoc test which was used for multiple comparisons between groups. Non-parametric values were expressed as median and the statistical differences among groups were identified using Kruskal-Wallis analysis of variance followed by the rank-based Mann–Whitney U-test for group comparisons. Statistical analysis was performed using SPSS program, version 17. The minimal level of significance was identified at $p < 0.05$.

Results

Telmisartan ameliorates the severity of TNBS-induced injury in rats

We assessed the efficacy of TLM in alleviating colon injury using TNBS-induced colitis, an experimental model of human IBD [38]. To investigate the severity of colitis, its clinical signs including body weight loss, diarrhea and rectal bleeding were explored. Rats challenged with TNBS suffered marked weight loss (>10%) as a result of colonic inflammation compared with vehicle-treated control group (Figure 1A). The animals also displayed high DAI scores associated with incidence of diarrhea and rectal bleeding in addition to increased colon weight/length ratio, a reliable marker of colon inflammation [10], (Figure 1B, C). These data were confirmed by the macroscopic examination of colon that revealed severe colonic injury characterized by mucosal

Table 2. Primer sequences used for real-time PCR.

mRNA species	Accession no.	Primer sequence
PPAR-γ	NM_013124	Forward 5'- AGACCACTCCCACTCCTTTG -3'
		Reverse 5'-AGGTCATACTTG TAATCTGC-3'
NF-κB p65	NM_199267	Forward 5'-GTCATCAGGAAGAGGTTTGGCT-3'
		Reverse 5'-TGATAAGCTTAGCCCTTGCAGC-3'
COX-2	NM_017232	Forward 5'-GCTCAGCC ATACAGCAAATCC-3'
		Reverse 5'-GGGAGTCGGGCAAT CATCAG-3'
iNOS	NM_ 012611	Forward 5'-ACCTTCCGGGCAGCCTGTGA-3'
		Reverse 5'-CAAGGAGGGTGGTGCGGCTG-3'
Cytochrome C	NM_012839	Forward 5'-TTTGAATTCCTCATTAGTAGCTTTTTTGG-3'
		Reverse 5'-CCATCCCTACGCATCCTTTAC-3'
Bax	NM_017059	Forward 5'-CAAGAAGCTGAGCGAGTGTCT-3'
		Reverse 5'-CAATCATCCTCTGCAGCTCCATATT-3'
Bcl-2	NM_016993	Forward 5'-TGCGCTCAGCCCTGTG-3'
		Reverse 5'-GGTAGCGACGAGAGAAGTCATC-3'
Caspase-3	NM_012922	Forward 5'-GCAGCTAACCTCAGAGAGACATTC-3'
		Reverse 5'-ACGAGTAAGGTCATTTTTATTCCTGACTT-3'
GAPDH	NM_017008	Forward 5'-TGCTGGTGCTGAGTATGTCG-3'
		Reverse 5'-TTGAGAGCAATGCCAGCC-3'

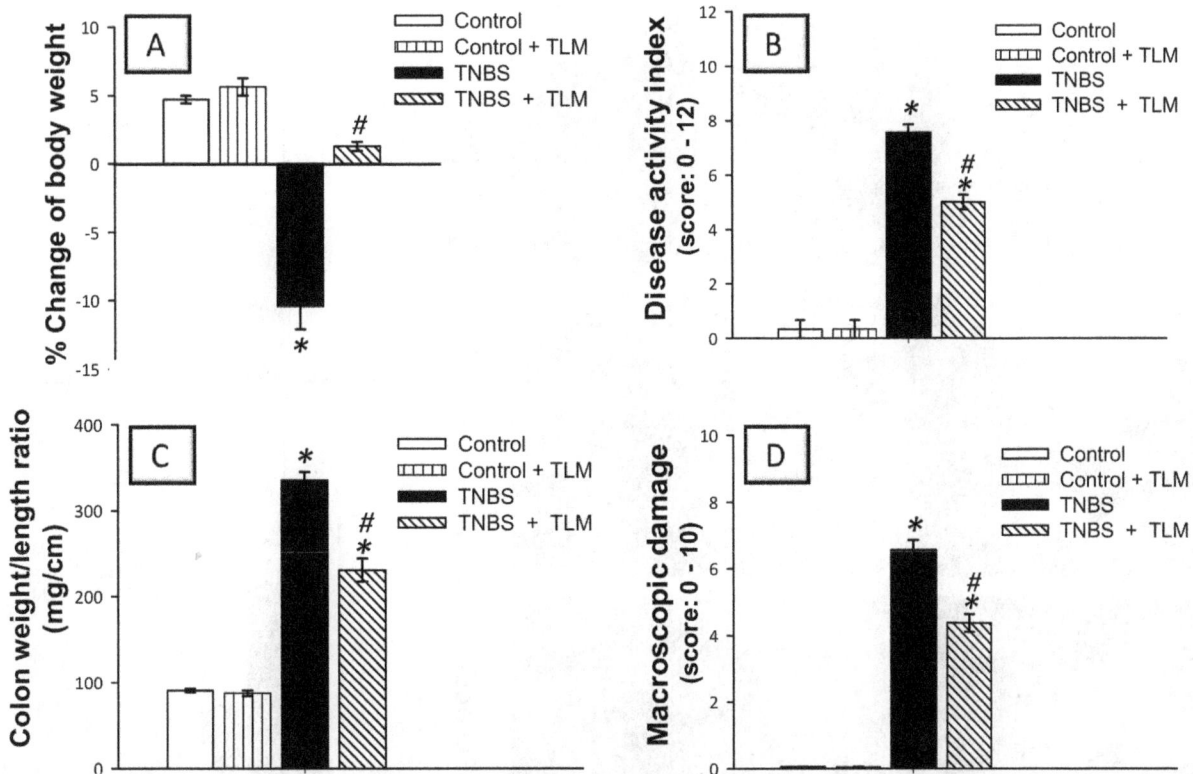

Figure 1. Effect of telmisartan on the severity of TNBS-induced colitis in rats. (A) Change of Body weight (%) (B) Disease activity index. (C) Colon weight/length ratio. (D) Colon macroscopic damage. Colon injury was induced by a single intrarectal instillation of TNBS (50 mg/kg) in 50% ethanol solution whereas the control group received the same volume of physiological saline solution rectally. Telmisartan was orally administered (10 mg/kg/day), starting 1 week before TNBS instillation and was continued till the 4th day post TNBS insult. On the 5th day, rats were euthanized and the colons were immediately excised. Values of body weight changes and colon weight/length ratio (parametric data) are expressed as mean ± SEM (n = 8) while the scores of disease activity index and macroscopic damage (non-parametric) are expressed as median; n = 8. *Significant difference from control gp at $p<0.05$, # Significant difference from TNBS colitis gp at $p<0.05$. TLM; telmisartan, TNBS; tri-nitrobenzene sulfonic acid.

damage, thickening of bowel wall, hyperemia, edema and ulcerations (Figure 1D). Interestingly, TLM mitigated these changes and diminished the severity of colonic injury as compared to TNBS colitis group. Thus, these data suggest that TLM attenuated the development of TNBS colitis.

Telmisartan mitigates colonic histopathological changes and recruitment of immuno-inflammatory cells

We next assessed whether TLM has protective effects against the histopathological damage in colons of rats with TNBS colitis. Colon sections from control and control+TLM groups revealed an intact architecture of colon tissues (Figure 2A, B). On the other hand, colons of TNBS group revealed significant tissue injury with high scores of microscopic damage indicating focal necrosis of mucosa and submucosal and ulceration of the colonic mucosa with loss of lining epithelium. Diffuse leukocyte infiltration, mainly as neutrophils, was detected in the mucosa including the lamina propria, in addition to submucosa, muscularis. In addition, diffuse edema was observed in the submucosal layer (Figure 2C–E). TLM protected against these alterations and reduced the histopathological scores revealing attenuated inflammatory cell infiltration and preservation of colon cytoarchitecture while edema was still detected (Figure 2F, G).

Leukocyte invasion to colonic tissues was confirmed by a 7.4-fold increase of MPO activity, a biochemical index for neutrophil influx [39], as compared to the control group (Figure 2H). TLM

administration afforded a 53% reduction of MPO activity as compared to TNBS group. Together, these data indicate that TLM attenuated mucosal damage and leukocyte invasion in TNBS-induced colitis.

Telmisartan modulates colon inflammatory cytokines and PGE$_2$

To gain an insight into the inflammatory milieu of colons, we investigated the levels of TNF-α & IL-10 cytokines along with PGE$_2$. Instillation of TNBS resulted in severe inflammatory response as indicated by remarkable increases in colonic levels of the proinflammatory TNF-α (380%) and PGE$_2$ (412%) as compared to the control group (Figure 3A, C). Meanwhile, the anti-inflammatory IL-10 levels were also elevated (295% of control group). Administration of TLM lowered TNF-α, PGE$_2$ and IL-10 by 49%, 39% and 51% respectively, as compared to TNBS colitis group. These observations indicate that TLM can modulate the inflammatory cytokines and PGE$_2$ to mitigate TNBS colitis.

Telmisartan abrogates the mRNA expression of NF-κB, COX-2 and iNOS genes

Since the beneficial effects of TLM are partly ascribed to its PPAR-γ partial agonist properties [12], we verified its impact on the mRNA expression of PPAR-γ in colonic tissues. As depicted in Figure 4A, TNBS administration suppressed PPAR-γ (41% of the control levels) whereas TLM upregulated its levels in colonic

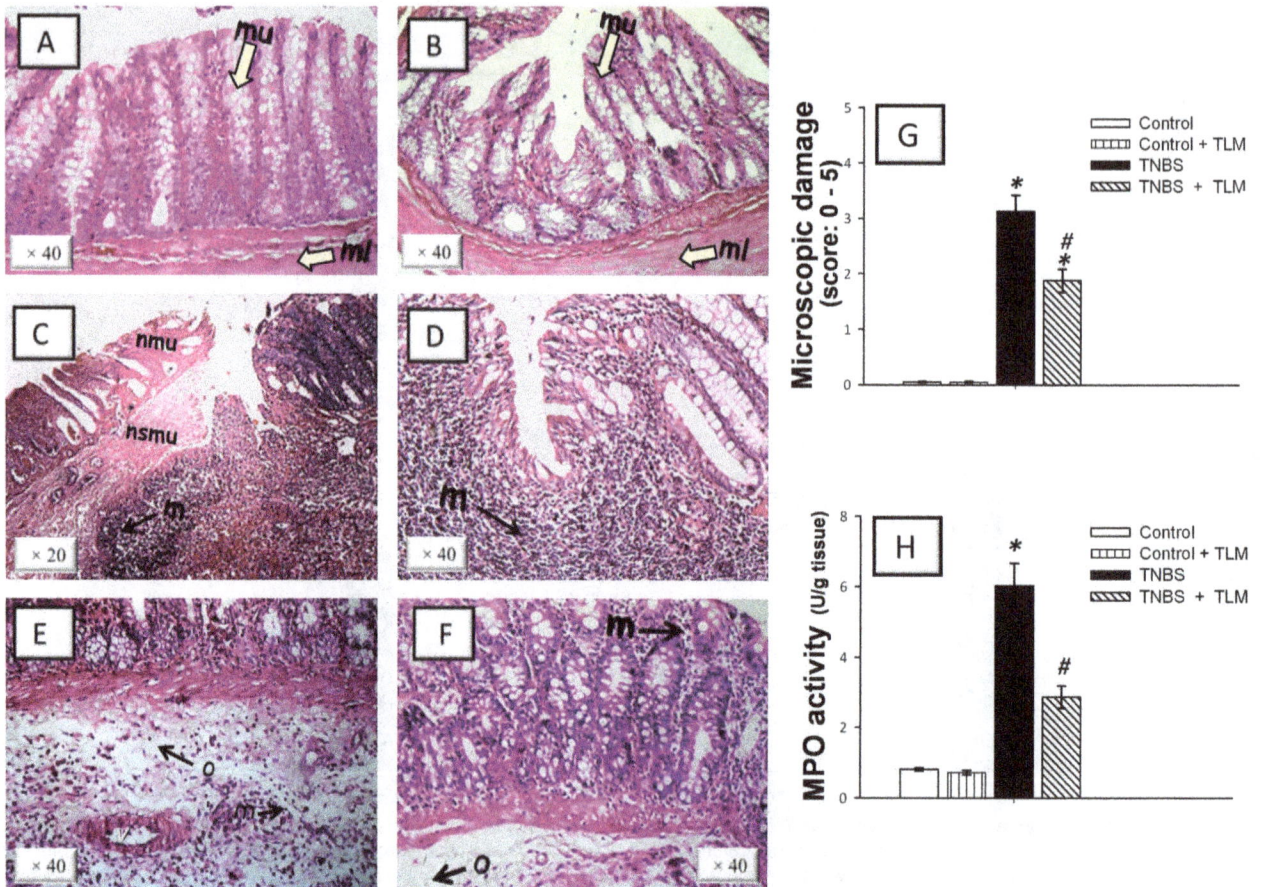

Figure 2. Telmisartan ameliorates histopathological damage and myeloperoxidase activity in colonic tissues of rats with TNBS colitis. Representative photomicrographs of sections from colonic samples taken on the 5th day post TNBS-rectal instillation. (A) Control rats receiving saline rectally showed normal architecture of mucosa (mu) with intact epithelial surface, submucosa and muscularis (ml) layer (open arrows). (B) Control rats receiving saline rectally + TLM (10 mg/kg/day p.o.) displayed no histological modifications. (C-E) TNBS-treated group (50 mg/kg) was characterized by focal necrosis of mucosa (nmu) and submucosa (nsmu) and diffuse infiltration of leukocytes (m) and edema (o) in the submucosal layer. (F) TNBS + TLM administration (10 mg/kg/day p.o.) revealed mucosal preservation, diminished inflammatory cell invasion and edema. Hematoxylin and eosin staining. (G) Microscopic damage scores (expressed as median; n = 8). (H) TLM inhibits colon myeloperoxidase (MPO) activity (mean ± SEM; n = 8). Histological analysis was performed 5 days post TNBS instillation and TLM was administered for 12 days starting 1 week before colitis induction. *Significant difference from control gp at $p < 0.05$, # Significant difference from TNBS colitis gp at $p < 0.05$. TLM; telmisartan, TNBS; tri-nitrobenzene sulfonic acid.

tissues indicating a possible role of PPAR-γ in attenuation of colon inflammation. We further extended our investigation to assess the mRNA expression of NF-κB, COX-2 and iNOS which play crucial proinflammatory roles during the pathogenesis of IBD [40]. In animals with TNBS colitis, data revealed significant increase in the colonic expression of activated NF-κB p65 subunit at the mRNA level (12.5 fold) which was also confirmed by immunohistochemistry that demonstrated extensive NF-κB p65 expression (Figure 4B, C). In the same context, the mRNA expression of COX-2 and iNOS, downstream targets of NF-κB, was elevated by 14.7- and 19.8-fold increases, respectively, as compared to control rats (Figure 5). Interestingly, TLM significantly decreased the mRNA/protein expression of NF-κB p65 and the mRNA of COX-2 and iNOS, indicating that TLM downregulation of these proinflammatory genes is implicated in its beneficial protective effects against colitis.

Telmisartan inhibits oxidative stress and enhances colon antioxidant defenses

During the development of IBD, the inflammatory process provokes oxidative stress and diminishes cellular antioxidant capacity [3]. Instillation of TNBS resulted in a marked oxidative stress as indicated by increased levels of MDA (308%) and NO (231%) along with diminished levels of GSH (25%) and TAC (51%) and activities of SOD (59%) and GPx (56%), as compared to control group (Figures 6 and 7). Administration of TLM afforded significant protection against oxidative stress as evidenced by decrease of MDA & NO levels in addition to reinstatement of GSH & TAC levels and SOD & GPx activities, as compared to TNBS colitis group. These effects suggest that TLM attenuation of oxidative perturbations and boosting of colonic enzymatic and non-enzymatic antioxidant defenses play a role in attenuation of TNBS colitis.

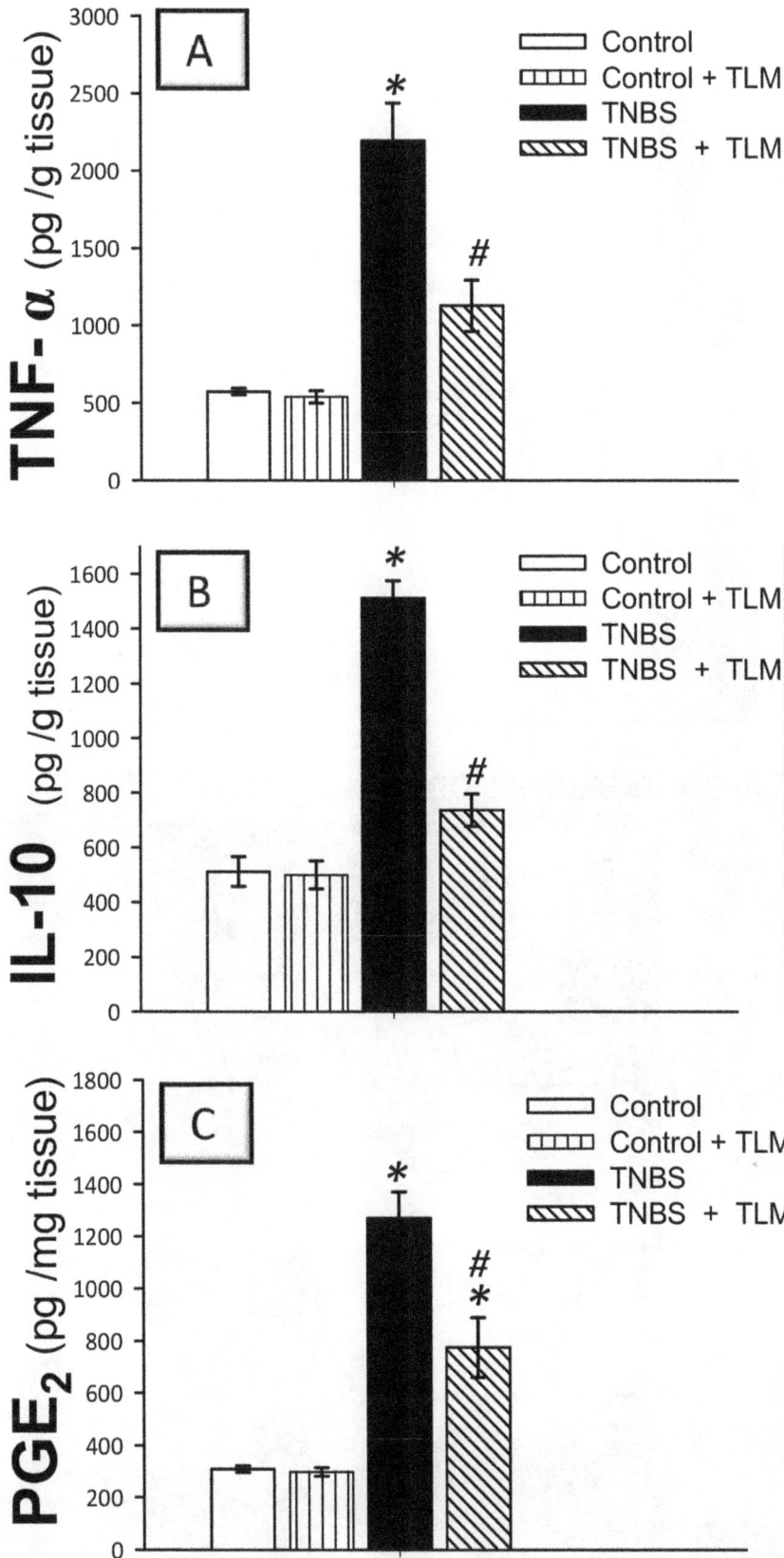

Figure 3. Telmisartan modulates inflammatory cytokines and PGE$_2$.in colon of rats with TNBS colitis. Levels of tumor necrosis factor-α; TNF-α (A), interleukin-10; IL-10 (B) and prostaglandin E$_2$; PGE$_2$ (C) were determined by ELISA. Measurements were performed 5 days post TNBS instillation and TLM was administered for 12 days starting 1 week before colitis induction. Data are expressed as mean $\pm$ SEM (n = 8) *Significant difference from control gp at $p < 0.05$, # Significant difference from TNBS colitis gp at $p < 0.05$. TLM; telmisartan, TNBS; tri-nitrobenzene sulfonic acid.

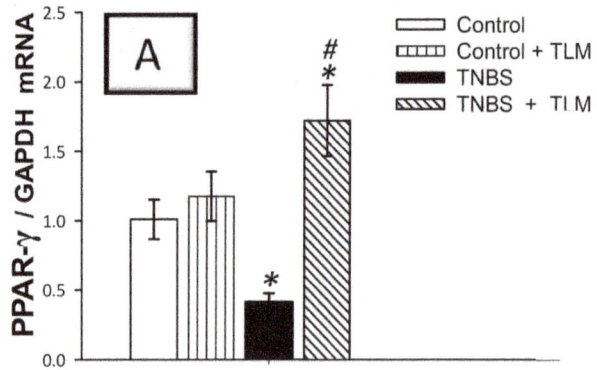

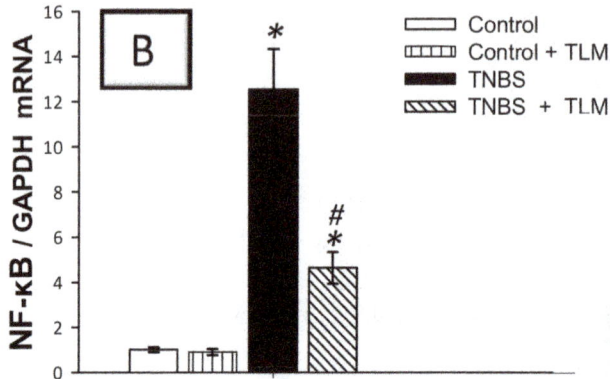

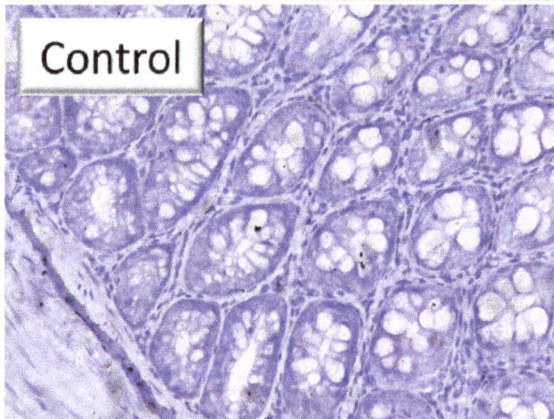
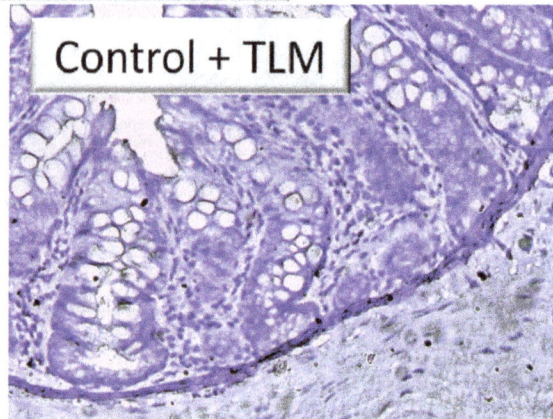
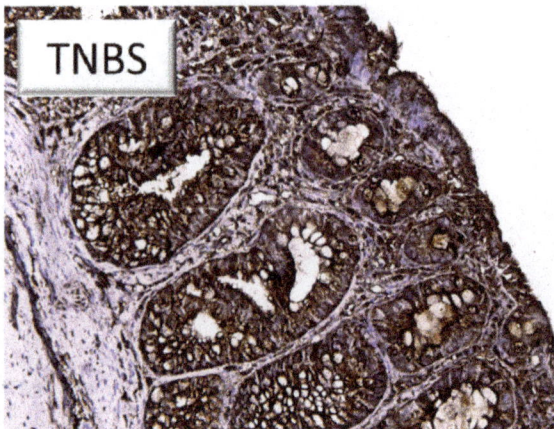
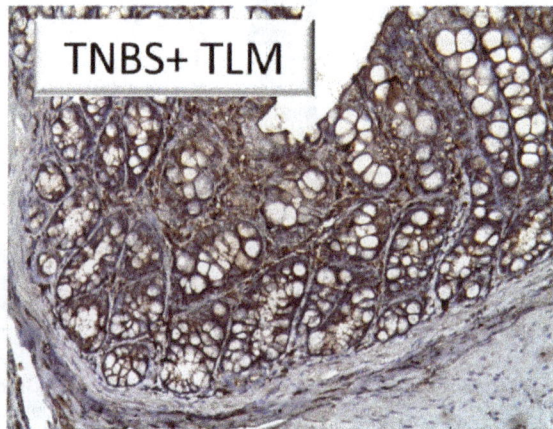

Figure 4. Effect of telmisartan on the mRNA expression of PPAR-γ and mRNA/ protein expression of NF-κB in the colon of rats with TNBS colitis. (A) mRNA expression of peroxisome proliferator activated receptor-gamma; PPAR-γ. (B) mRNA expression of nuclear factor kappa B; NF-κB. The mRNA expression was detected by quantitative real-time RT-PCR. Measurements were performed 5 days post TNBS instillation and TLM was administered for 12 days starting 1 week before colitis induction. Data are expressed as mean ± SD (n = 6). *Significant difference from control gp at p<0.05, # Significant difference from TNBS colitis gp at p<0.05. (C) Immunohistochemical detection of NF-κB p65 expression. Representative images for the detection of NF-κBp65 expression from colon samples harvested on the 5th day post TNBS (magnification: × 200). Control and control + TLM gps: minimal expression; TNBS gp: extensive expression (brown color); TNBS+ TLM gp: attenuated expression. TLM; telmisartan, TNBS; tri-nitrobenzene sulfonic acid.

Telmisartan downregulates the mRNA expression of apoptotic genes

During the pathogenesis of IBD, exposure of intestinal mucosa to intracellular stressors such as ROS under inflammatory stimuli triggers intestinal epithelial cell apoptosis [7,41]. Thus, we investigated whether TLM can suppress apoptosis in colonic mucosa to protect against TNBS colitis. This was addressed via assessing the mRNA expression of cytochrome c, Bax, Bcl-2 and

caspase-3. As observed in Figure 8A, instillation of TNBS triggered apoptosis of inflamed colon as indicated by a 2.7 fold increase of caspase-3 mRNA expression, a reliable indicator for apoptosis [7]. This finding was further augmented by the increased activity as well as protein expression of caspase-3 (Figure 8B, C) in TNBS colitis group. In the same context, increased mRNA expression of the pro-apoptotic cytochrome c (3.7 fold) and Bax (5.9 fold) together with downregulation of Bcl-2, an anti-apoptotic

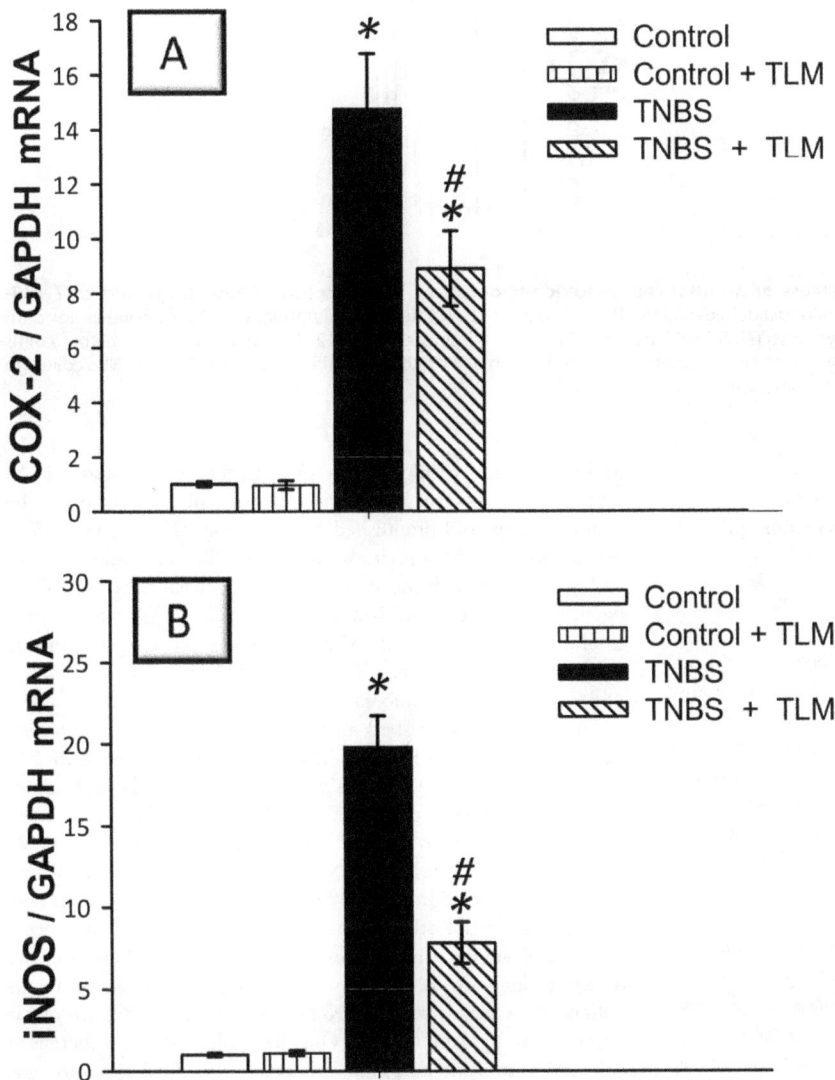

Figure 5. Effect of telmisartan on the mRNA expression of COX-2 and iNOS proinflammatory genes in colon of rats with TNBS colitis. (A) Cyclo-oxygenase-2; COX-2. (B) Inducible nitric oxide synthase; iNOS. The mRNA expression was detected by quantitative real-time RT-PCR. Measurements were performed 5 days post TNBS instillation and TLM was administered for 12 days starting 1 week before colitis induction. Data are expressed as mean ± SD (n=6). *Significant difference from control gp at p<0.05, # Significant difference from TNBS colitis gp at p<0.05. TLM; telmisartan, TNBS; tri-nitrobenzene sulfonic acid.

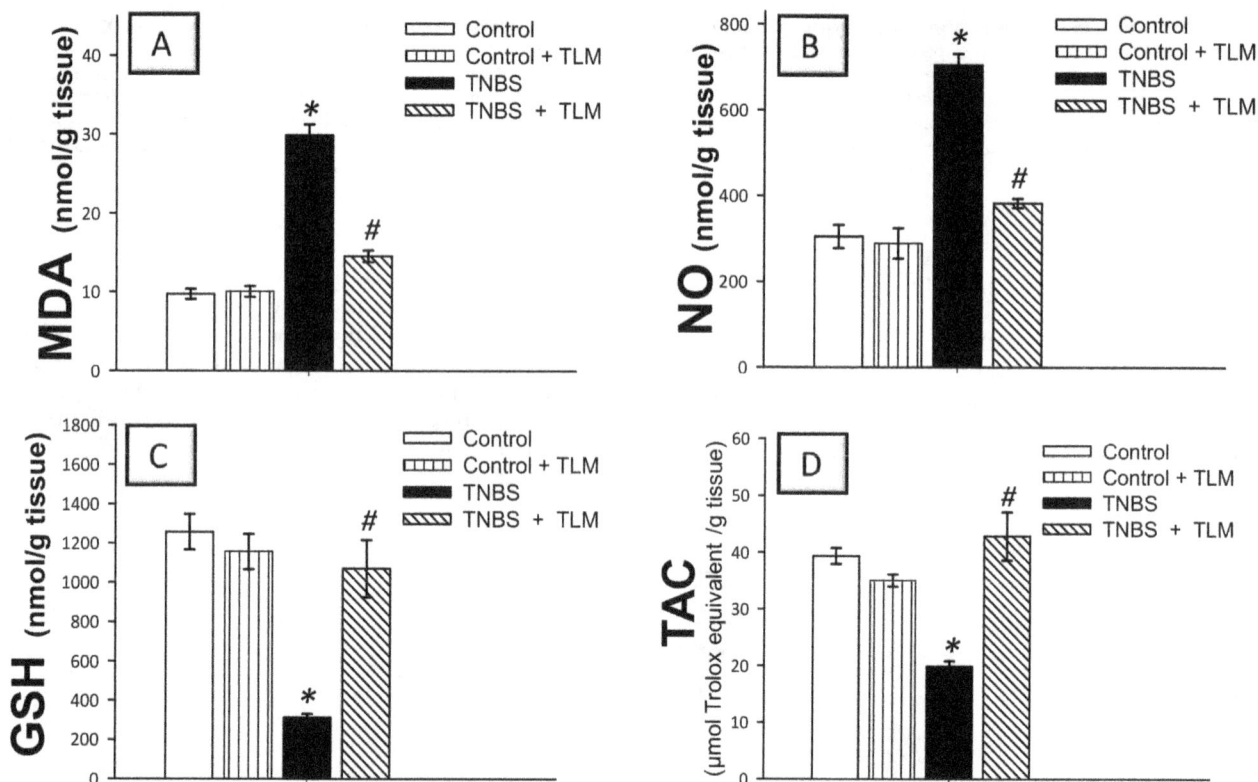

Figure 6. Telmisartan ameliorates oxidative stress and enhances antioxidant defenses in the colon of rats subjected to TNBS-induced colitis. (A) Lipid peroxides expressed as malondialdehyde; MDA. (B) Nitric oxide; NO. (C) Reduced glutathione; GSH. (D) Total antioxidant capacity; TAC. Measurements were performed 5 days post TNBS instillation and TLM was administered for 12 days starting 1 week before colitis induction. Data are expressed as mean ± SEM (n = 8) *Significant difference from control gp at $p<0.05$, # Significant difference from TNBS colitis gp at $p<0.05$. TLM; telmisartan, TNBS; tri-nitrobenzene sulfonic acid.

gene, were observed (Figure 9). Interestingly, administration of TLM counteracted these changes in favor of cell survival suggesting that TLM protects the colonic mucosa from apoptosis in TNBS-induced colitis.

Discussion

The current study highlights the alleviating effects of TLM, an Ang II AT-1 receptor antagonist with PPAR-γ partial agonist features, in TNBS-induced colitis, an experimental model of human IBD. These beneficial effects were associated with modulation of colonic PPAR-γ, NF-κB and its downstream COX-2, iNOS and inflammatory cytokines. TLM attenuated oxidative stress and boosted the antioxidant defenses. It also downregulated colonic pro-apoptotic signals with concomitant upregulation of the anti-apoptotic Bcl-2 (Figure 10).

Besides its classical role in the regulation of blood pressure and fluid homoeostasis, novel activities of RAS have been identified including immune cell modulation with proinflammatory actions [8]. RAS has been implicated in the pathogenesis of IBD via upregulation of Ang II AT1 receptors throughout the colon [1,8]. Ang II is involved in several key steps of the inflammatory cascade that ultimately provoke intestinal injury and ulceration including polymorphonuclear leukocyte (PMN) infiltration, probably, via upregulation of adhesion molecules [8,42].

TNBS-induced colitis mimics human IBD with respect to several histological alterations including mucosal invasion of PMN cells as indicated by MPO which also generates hypochlorous acid

and contributes to colon injury [39]. In the current study, TLM attenuated leukocyte influx to inflamed colon as revealed by histopathology and diminished MPO activity. These observations are in accord with previous studies [15,23]. The mitigation of leukocyte influx may account for the beneficial effects of TLM against colon injury and is most likely mediated via the observed inhibition of TNF-α and oxidative stress since they trigger the expression of P-selectin, ICAM-1 and MAdCAM-1 adhesion molecules in colonic mucosa [42].

Our data also described an upregulation of the inflammatory status with increased levels of TNF-α and PGE₂ along with NF-κB, COX-2 and iNOS in rats with TNBS colitis. These findings are consistent with previous reports [3,10,43,44]. Ang II has been previously reported to increase the generation of TNF-α probably via activation of NF-κB [8]. TNF-α is a pleiotropic cytokine which has been implicated in IBD pathogenesis via activation of immune cells, generation of other proinflammatory cytokines and overexpression of angiotensinogen and Ang II [2,8]. Furthermore, the observed increase in colonic PGE₂ can be attributed to its enhanced synthesis via COX-2 enzyme whose expression is upregulated by Ang II [8]. Our data also revealed increased colonic levels of the anti-inflammatory IL-10. Previously, upregulation of IL-10 has been reported in plasma of patients with IBD [4] and colons of rats with TNBS- and dextran sulfate-induced colitis [5,6]. Increased circulating levels of IL-10 can be envisioned as a compensatory mechanism against colonic injury and is thought to play a role in limiting mucosal inflammation since IL-10 downregulates MHC class II antigen presentation and

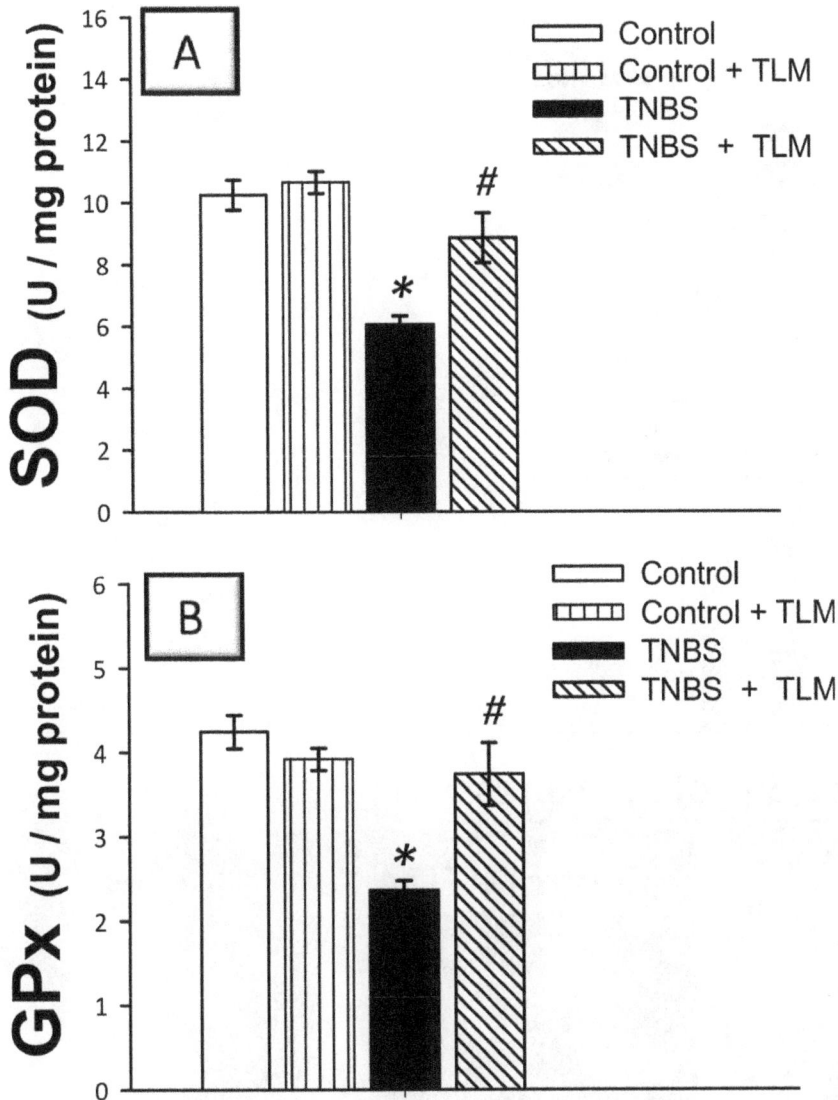

Figure 7. Telmisartan enhances activites of superoxide dismutase; SOD (A) and glutathione peroxidase; GPx (B) antioxidant enzymes in colon of rats with TNBS colitis. Measurements were performed 5 days post TNBS instillation and TLM was administered for 12 days starting 1 week before colitis induction. Data are expressed as mean $\pm$ SEM (n = 8) *Significant difference from control gp at $p<0.05$, # Significant difference from TNBS colitis gp at $p<0.05$. TLM; telmisartan, TNBS; tri-nitrobenzene sulfonic acid.

subsequent release of pro-inflammatory cytokines [45]. However, the increased IL-10 levels might not be adequate to fully control colon inflammation due to low IL-10 bioavailability [46].

Ang II has been reported to activate several nuclear transcription factors including NF-κB which is also driven by ROS and inflammatory cytokines [3,8]. The NF-κB regulates the expression of several proinflammatory genes including TNF-α, COX-2 and iNOS that play key roles in IBD and TNBS colitis [8]. NF-κB, a heterodimer of p65 and p50 subunits of Rel protein family, is retained in inactive state via association with the inhibitory protein IκBα in the cytosol. Upon exposure of cells to stress conditions, activation of NF-κB is triggered via phosphorylation and proteasomal degradation of IκBα which liberates NF-κB that translocates to the nucleus to control the expression of target genes [40]. In the current study, the mRNA and the protein expression of activated NF-κB p65 subunit were elevated in rats with TNBS colitis. This finding is in agreement with previous studies [40,47]. Our data also revealed enhanced levels of COX-2 and iNOS

which are downstream targets of NF-κB. COX-2 generates an arsenal of PGE$_2$ and TXB$_2$ which provokes intestinal hyperemia and edema whereas iNOS activation releases a surplus of NO which undermines colon integrity via synthesis of peroxynitrite, a potent oxidizing agent which is formed via reaction of NO with superoxide anion [48].

Interestingly, TLM increased the levels of PPAR-γ with concomitant suppression of colon NF-κBp65, COX-2, and iNOS along with TNF-α, PGE$_2$ and NO. Similar findings have been reported for TLM in autoimmune myocarditis [49], stroke [20] and renal oxidative damage [50]. Upregulation of TLM to PPAR-γ has been reported to suppress the production of inflammatory mediators, at least partly, via inhibition of NF-κB [21]. The observed inhibition of NF-κB together with its downstream effectors as COX-2, iNOS and TNF-α is regarded as an advantage in the management of IBD [47]. Since the promoter regions of COX-2, iNOS and TNF-α contain consensus binding motifs for NF-κB, it would be conceivable to understand that

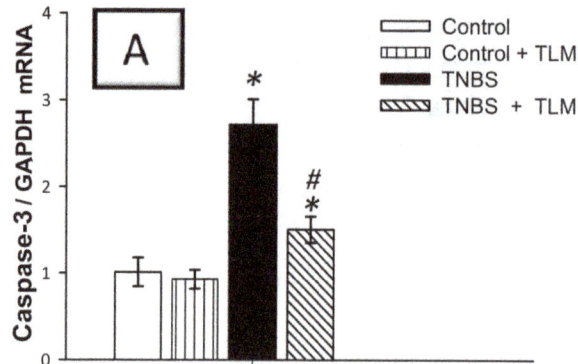

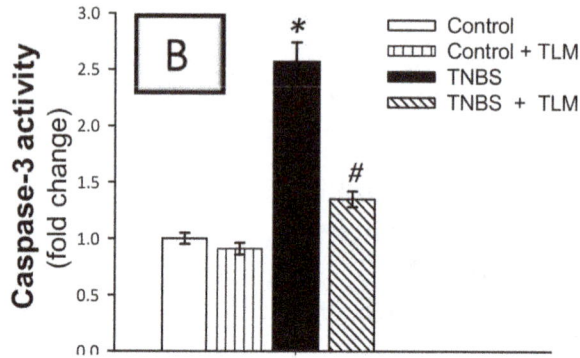

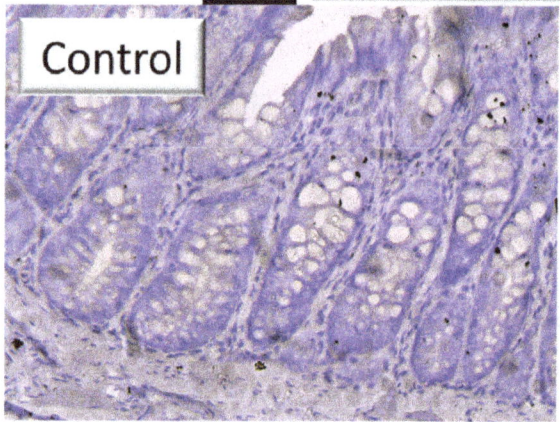

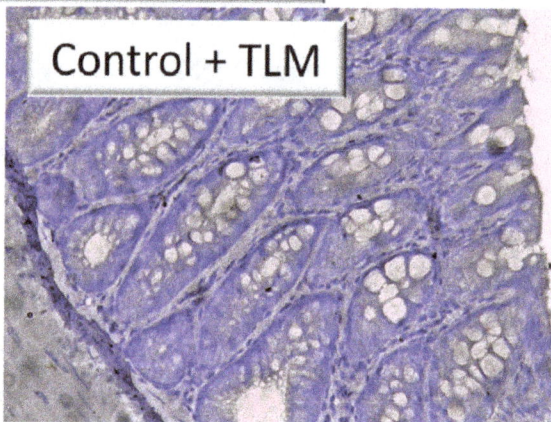

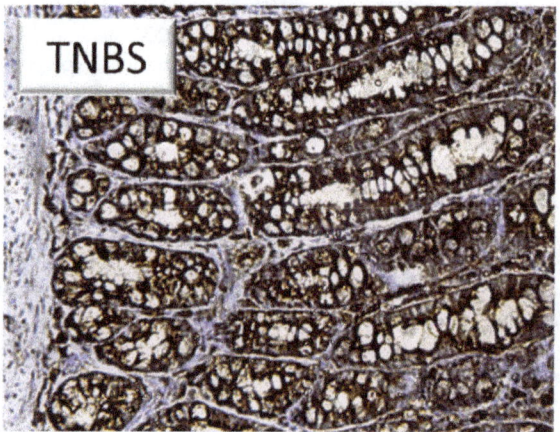

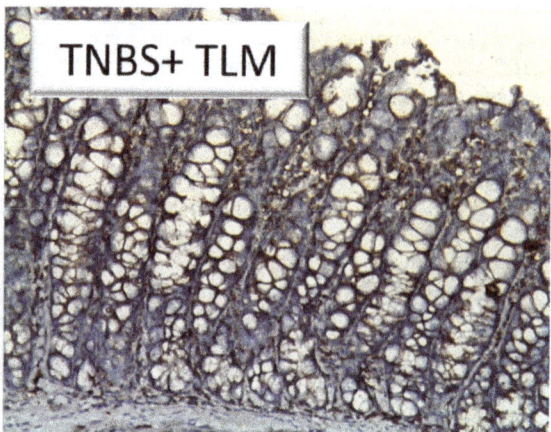

Figure 8. Effect of telmisartan on the mRNA expression, activity and protein expression of caspase-3 in the colon of rats with TNBS colitis. (A) Caspase-3 mRNA expression. (B) Caspase-3 activity. Measurements were performed 5 days post TNBS instillation and TLM was administered for 12 days starting 1 week before colitis induction. Caspase-3 mRNA expression was detected by quantitative real-time RT-PCR (data are expressed as mean ± SD; n = 6) and the activity was measured using ELISA (results are expressed as mean ± SEM; n = 8). *Significant difference from control gp at $p<0.05$, # Significant difference from TNBS colitis gp at $p<0.05$. (C) Immunohistochemical detection of caspase-3 protein expression. Representative images of caspase-3 expression from colon samples harvested on the 5th day post TNBS (magnification: × 200). Control and control + TLM gps: minimal expression; TNBS gp: extensive expression (brown color); TNBS+ TLM gp: attenuated expression. TLM; telmisartan, TNBS; tri-nitrobenzene sulfonic acid.

downregulation of these targets is secondary to NF-κB inhibition by TLM [49]. TLM also attenuated PGE$_2$ and NO levels, an effect probably linked to inhibition of COX-2 and iNOS enzymes, respectively [3]. The observed restoration of IL-10 by TLM probably reflects improvement of the inflammatory status which was associated with suppression of proinflammatory signals. In this context, the observed TLM lowering of TNF-α may be implicated in the mitigation of colonic IL-10 levels, since the release of IL-10 is driven by elevated levels of proinflammatory cytokines [45]. Thus, the current data reinforce the alleviating actions of TLM in TNBS colitis owing to its pleiotropic anti-inflammatory actions.

The implication of oxidative stress in the pathogenesis of IBD has been highlighted by several clinical [51] and experimental studies [1] where the surge of ROS and NO generated by activated neutrophils and macrophages inflicts intestinal injury. Ang II has been reported to trigger oxidative stress with generation of superoxide anions via NADH/NADPH oxidase in addition to hydrogen peroxide and hydroxyl radicals [8,52]. In the current study, enhanced oxidative stress was verified by increase in lipid peroxides & NO with concomitant decrease of GSH & TAC levels and SOD & GPx activities in TNBS-induced colitis. These observations are in line with previous studies [3,10,43,44].

In the current study, TLM combated oxidative stress and boosted the antioxidant status in animals with TNBS colitis as evidenced by reduction of MDA and NO levels in addition to reinstatement of GSH &TAC levels and SOD & GPx activities. These findings are in agreement with previous studies and they reinforce the premise that the antioxidant properties of TLM are implicated in alleviation of TNBS colitis [15,23,43,49]. The antioxidant features of TLM have been ascribed to scavenging hydroxyl radicals via its benzimidazolic and benzoic moieties [53] in addition to downregulation of NADPH oxidase subunits [14,23]. Interestingly, Fujita et al. [50] demonstrated that TLM inhibited renal oxidative stress in diabetic mice via upregulation of Nrf2 and SOD. The observed preservation of GSH, TAC and SOD & GPx antioxidant enzymes signifies the role of TLM in boosting colonic antioxidant defenses and correlates well with the reported preservation of endogenous antioxidants in experimental myocardial infarction [15].

Our results also described an *in vivo* activation of apoptosis in colonic tissues as indicated by upregulation of cytochrome c, Bax and caspase-3 pro-apoptotic genes along with downregulation of the anti-apoptotic Bcl-2. These data are in concert with previous literature [47,54]. Evidence has highlighted the pro-apoptotic effects of Ang II which were totally abolished by Ang II neutralizing antibodies and ARBs [55]. The increased apoptosis of epithelial cells likely results in alteration of the epithelial barrier, thereby contributing to intestinal injury [7]. Elevated rate of colonic apoptosis has been reported in patients with UC and TNBS colitis [54,56]. It has been reported that the oxidative stress triggers the expression of several genes responsible for cellular death by apoptosis [54]. Apoptosis is regulated, in part, by the Bcl-2 family including Bcl-2 and Bax. Bcl-2 is regarded as a prosurvival signal whereas Bax is a pro-apoptotic member since it binds and antagonizes the effects of Bcl-2 [7]. Increased Bax/

Bcl-2 ratio enhances the release of cytochrome c from mitochondria to cytosol, which activates caspase-9 and ultimately caspase-3, the major executioner caspase [7,54].

Our data revealed that TLM upregulated Bcl-2 with downregulation of the pro-apoptotic cytochrome c, Bax and caspase-3, indicating attenuation of colonic apoptosis. These findings are consistent with previous reports that described the inhibition of TLM to apoptosis in autoimmune myocarditis [49] and testis of diabetic rats [21]. The attenuation of colonic apoptosis can be ascribed to the observed inhibition of oxidative stress since excessive exposure of intestinal mucosa to ROS under inflammatory stimuli enhances epithelial apoptosis [41]. Besides, the observed elevation of PPAR-γ is likely engaged in apoptosis suppression as suggested by previous studies for TLM [15,23] and for PPAR-γ agonists such as rosiglitazone [57].

During colonic inflammation, several proinflammatory cytokines such as INF-γ, IL-1β and IL-8 besides anti-inflammatory cytokines as IL-4 play a major role in the pathogenesis of IBD and, thus, their investigation can delineate molecular aspects of TLM protective actions [58]. Our future studies will focus on investigating these targets in order to precisely elucidate the underlying molecular mechanisms for TLM in IBD. In our experiments, while several molecular aspects of inflammation and apoptosis were examined at the level of mRNA, some of these parameters were confirmed by the protein expression as in case of NF-κB p65 and caspase-3 that also revealed good correlation with the mRNA data. Additionally, at both mRNA and protein expression levels, elevation of COX-2 and iNOS along with suppression of PPAR-γ have been previously reported in experimental IBD models [59,60]. In these studies, the effective treatment mitigated the expression of these genes at both mRNA and protein levels [59,60]. Previously, decrease in the mRNA levels of proinflammatory genes have been regarded as an early sign of suppressed inflammatory signaling [60]. Yet, the mRNA and protein expression are differently expressed, probably due to post-translational modification of mRNA [61]. Thus, upcoming investigation of the molecular events at both mRNA and protein levels will precisely delineate the underlying mechanisms for TLM actions in experimental IBD.

Conclusions

In conclusion, the current study highlights evidences for the promising protective effects of TLM in TNBS-induced colitis, an experimental model of IBD. These favorable actions were linked with modulation of PPAR-γ, NF-κB and its downstream COX-2, iNOS and inflammatory cytokines. TLM mitigated oxidative perturbations and boosted enzymatic/non-enzymatic antioxidant defenses. Besides, it downregulated colonic pro-apoptotic genes with concomitant upregulation of Bcl-2. Among available ARBs, TLM displays the strongest binding to AT1 receptors, the longest half-life and high lipophilicity besides its partial PPAR-γ agonist properties [12]. Together, the current study suggests the beneficial effects of TLM in experimental IBD. Further studies are warranted to investigate the potential therapeutic efficacy of

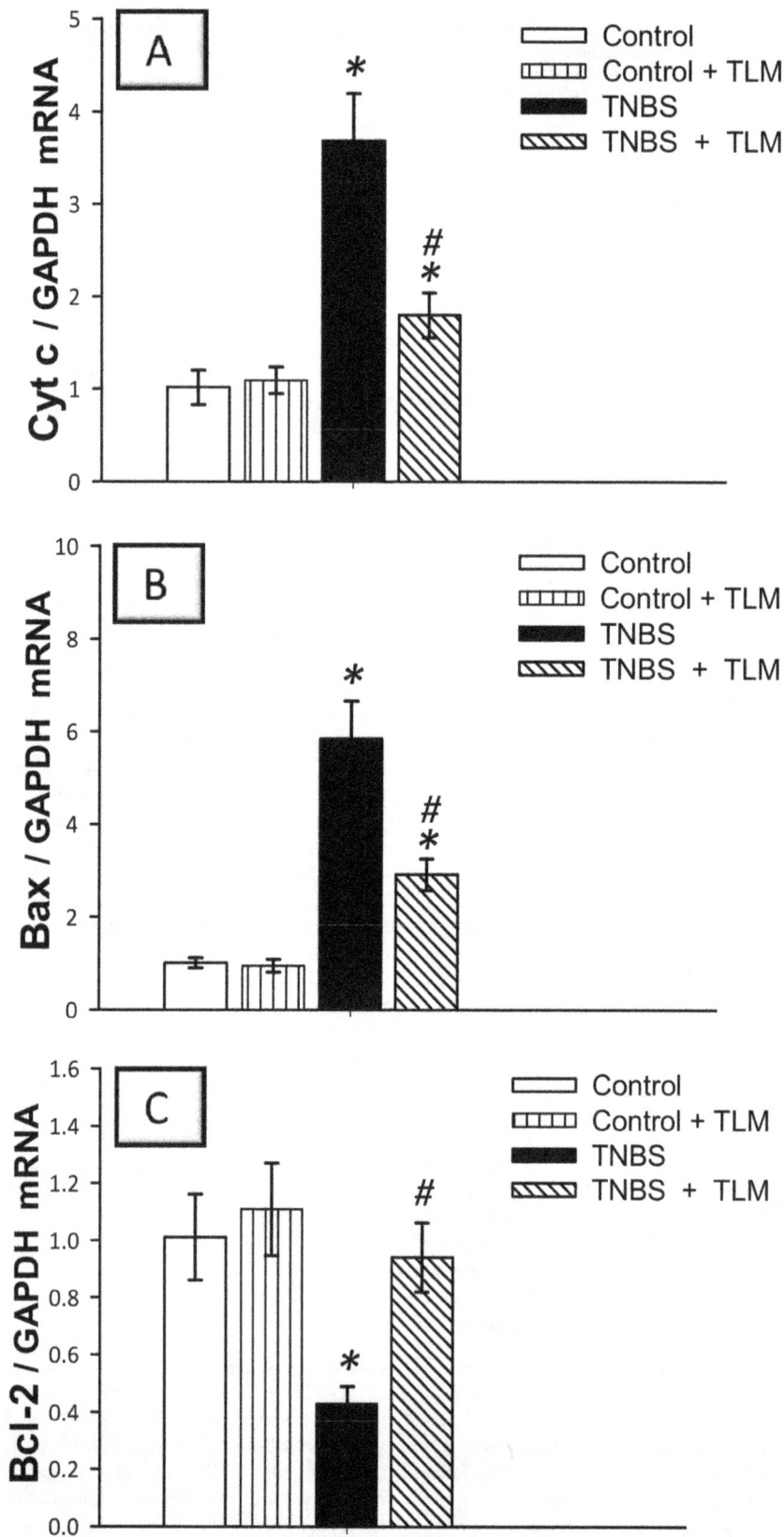

Figure 9. Effect of telmisartan on mRNA expression of Cyt c, Bax and Bcl-2 apoptotic genes in colon of rats with TNBS colitis. (A) Cytochrome c; Cyt c. (B) Bcl-2 associated x protein; Bax. (C) B cell lymphoma-2; Bcl-2. mRNA expression was detected by quantitative real-time RT-PCR. Measurements were performed 5 days post TNBS instillation and TLM was administered for 12 days starting 1 week before colitis induction. Data are expressed as mean ± SD (n= 6). *Significant difference from control gp at $p<0.05$, # Significant difference from TNBS colitis gp at $p<0.05$. TLM; telmisartan, TNBS; tri-nitrobenzene sulfonic acid.

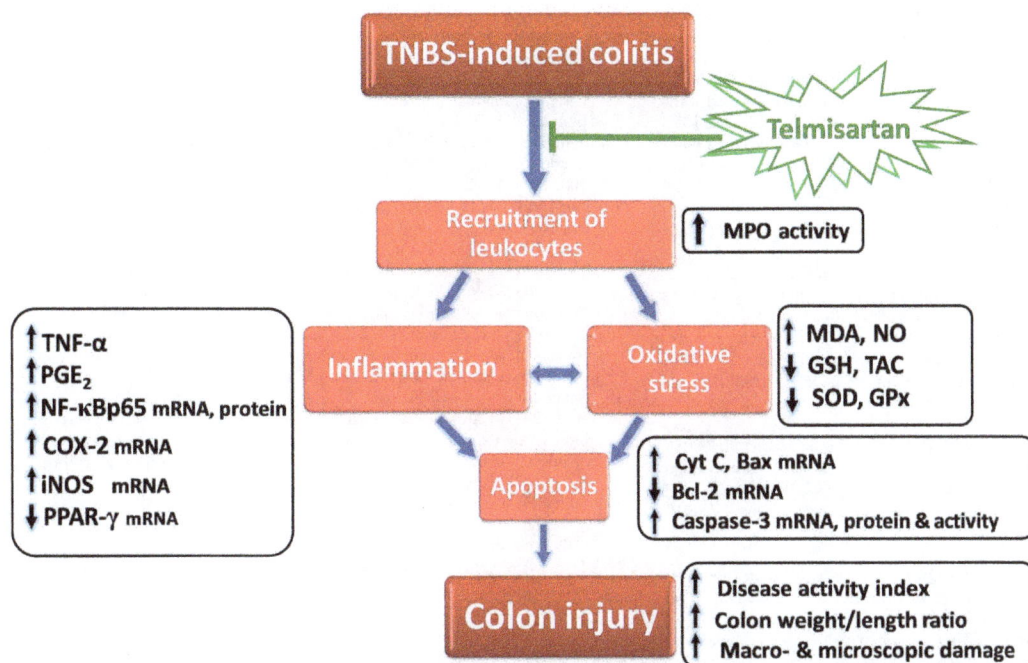

Figure 10. Diagram depicting the alleviating actions of telmisartan in TNBS-induced colitis.

TLM in the management of IBD following the manifestation of symptoms. Besides, the exact molecular mechanisms and signaling networks implicated in TLM actions need to be identified.

Acknowledgments

The authors are grateful to Prof. Adel Kholoussy, Department of Pathology, Faculty of Veterinary Medicine, Cairo University, Egypt for the kind help in histopathology and immunohistochemistry.

Author Contributions

Conceived and designed the experiments: HA MA DA NN. Performed the experiments: HA MA DA NN. Analyzed the data: HA MA DA NN. Contributed reagents/materials/analysis tools: HA MA DA NN. Wrote the paper: HA MA DA NN.

References

1. Fiocchi C (1998) Inflammatory bowel disease: etiology and pathogenesis. Gastroenterology 115: 182–205.

2. Sanchez-Munoz F, Dominguez-Lopez A, Yamamoto-Furusho JK (2008) Role of cytokines in inflammatory bowel disease. World J Gastroenterol 14: 4280–4288.

3. Kretzmann NA, Fillmann H, Mauriz JL, Marroni CA, Marroni N, et al. (2008) Effects of glutamine on proinflammatory gene expression and activation of nuclear factor kappa B and signal transducers and activators of transcription in TNBS-induced colitis. Inflamm Bowel Dis 14: 1504–1513.

4. Kucharzik T, Stoll R, Lugering N, Domschke W (1995) Circulating antiinflammatory cytokine IL-10 in patients with inflammatory bowel disease (IBD). Clin Exp Immunol 100: 452–456.

5. Barada KA, Mourad FH, Sawah SI, Khoury C, Safieh-Garabedian B, et al. (2007) Up-regulation of nerve growth factor and interleukin-10 in inflamed and non-inflamed intestinal segments in rats with experimental colitis. Cytokine 37: 236–245.

6. Tomoyose M, Mitsuyama K, Ishida H, Toyonaga A, Tanikawa K (1998) Role of interleukin-10 in a murine model of dextran sulfate sodium-induced colitis. Scand J Gastroenterol 33: 435–440.

7. Becker C, Watson AJ, Neurath MF (2013) Complex roles of caspases in the pathogenesis of inflammatory bowel disease. Gastroenterology 144: 283–293.

8. Hume GE, Radford-Smith GL (2008) ACE inhibitors and angiotensin II receptor antagonists in Crohn's disease management. Expert Rev Gastroenterol Hepatol 2: 645–651.

9. Bregonzio C, Armando I, Ando H, Jezova M, Baiardi G, et al. (2003) Anti-inflammatory effects of angiotensin II AT1 receptor antagonism prevent stress-induced gastric injury. Am J Physiol Gastrointest Liver Physiol 285: G414–423.

10. Nagib MM, Tadros MG, Elsayed MI, Khalifa AE (2013) Anti-inflammatory and anti-oxidant activities of olmesartan medoxomil ameliorate experimental colitis in rats. Toxicol Appl Pharmacol 271: 106–113.

11. Santiago OI, Rivera E, Ferder L, Appleyard CB (2008) An angiotensin II receptor antagonist reduces inflammatory parameters in two models of colitis. Regul Pept 146: 250–259.

12. Destro M, Cagnoni F, Dognini GP, Galimberti V, Taietti C, et al. (2011) Telmisartan: just an antihypertensive agent? A literature review. Expert Opin Pharmacother 12: 2719–2735.

13. Sanchez-Hidalgo M, Martin AR, Villegas I, de la Lastra CA (2007) Rosiglitazone, a PPARgamma ligand, modulates signal transduction pathways during the development of acute TNBS-induced colitis in rats. Eur J Pharmacol 562: 247–258.

14. Takaya T, Kawashima S, Shinohara M, Yamashita T, Toh R, et al. (2006) Angiotensin II type 1 receptor blocker telmisartan suppresses superoxide production and reduces atherosclerotic lesion formation in apolipoprotein E-deficient mice. Atherosclerosis 186: 402–410.

15. Goyal S, Arora S, Bhatt TK, Das P, Sharma A, et al. (2010) Modulation of PPAR-gamma by telmisartan protects the heart against myocardial infarction in experimental diabetes. Chem Biol Interact 185: 271–280.

16. Toba H, Tojo C, Wang J, Noda K, Kobara M, et al. (2012) Telmisartan inhibits vascular dysfunction and inflammation via activation of peroxisome proliferator-activated receptor-gamma in subtotal nephrectomized rat. Eur J Pharmacol 685: 91–98.

17. Yamagishi S, Nakamura K, Matsui T (2007) Potential utility of telmisartan, an angiotensin II type 1 receptor blocker with peroxisome proliferator-activated receptor-gamma (PPAR-gamma)-modulating activity for the treatment of cardiometabolic disorders. Curr Mol Med 7: 463–469.

18. Remuzzi A, Remuzzi G (2006) Potential protective effects of telmisartan on renal function deterioration. J Renin Angiotensin Aldosterone Syst 7: 185–191.

19. Attia YM, Elalkamy EF, Hammam OA, Mahmoud SS, El-Khatib AS (2013) Telmisartan, an AT1 receptor blocker and a PPAR gamma activator, alleviates liver fibrosis induced experimentally by Schistosoma mansoni infection. Parasit Vectors 6: 199.

20. Thoene-Reineke C, Rumschussel K, Schmerbach K, Krikov M, Wengenmayer C, et al. (2011) Prevention and intervention studies with telmisartan, ramipril and their combination in different rat stroke models. PLoS One 6: e23646.

21. Kushwaha S, Jena GB (2013) Telmisartan ameliorates germ cell toxicity in the STZ-induced diabetic rat: studies on possible molecular mechanisms. Mutat Res 755: 11–23.

22. Sukumaran V, Watanabe K, Veeraveedu PT, Ma M, Gurusamy N, et al. (2011) Telmisartan ameliorates experimental autoimmune myocarditis associated with inhibition of inflammation and oxidative stress. Eur J Pharmacol 652: 126–135.

23. Goyal SN, Bharti S, Bhatia J, Nag TC, Ray R, et al. (2011) Telmisartan, a dual ARB/partial PPAR-gamma agonist, protects myocardium from ischaemic reperfusion injury in experimental diabetes. Diabetes Obes Metab 13: 533–541.

24. Morris GP, Beck PL, Herridge MS, Depew WT, Szewczuk MR, et al. (1989) Hapten-induced model of chronic inflammation and ulceration in the rat colon. Gastroenterology 96: 795–803.

25. Qin HY, Xiao HT, Wu JC, Berman BM, Sung JJ, et al. (2012) Key factors in developing the trinitrobenzene sulfonic acid-induced post-inflammatory irritable bowel syndrome model in rats. World J Gastroenterol 18: 2481–2492.

26. Cooper HS, Murthy SN, Shah RS, Sedergran DJ (1993) Clinicopathologic study of dextran sulfate sodium experimental murine colitis. Lab Invest 69: 238–249.

27. Tsune I, Ikejima K, Hirose M, Yoshikawa M, Enomoto N, et al. (2003) Dietary glycine prevents chemical-induced experimental colitis in the rat. Gastroenterology 125: 775–785.

28. Bobin-Dubigeon C, Collin X, Grimaud N, Robert JM, Le Baut G, et al. (2001) Effects of tumour necrosis factor-alpha synthesis inhibitors on rat trinitrobenzene sulphonic acid-induced chronic colitis. Eur J Pharmacol 431: 103–110.

29. Galvez J, Coelho G, Crespo ME, Cruz T, Rodriguez-Cabezas ME, et al. (2001) Intestinal anti-inflammatory activity of morin on chronic experimental colitis in the rat. Aliment Pharmacol Ther 15: 2027–2039.

30. Krawisz JE, Sharon P, Stenson WF (1984) Quantitative assay for acute intestinal inflammation based on myeloperoxidase activity. Assessment of inflammation in rat and hamster models. Gastroenterology 87: 1344–1350.

31. Buege JA, Aust SD (1978) Microsomal lipid peroxidation. Methods Enzymol 52: 302–310.

32. Miranda KM, Espey MG, Wink DA (2001) A rapid, simple spectrophotometric method for simultaneous detection of nitrate and nitrite. Nitric Oxide 5: 62–71.

33. Beutler E, Duron O, Kelly BM (1963) Improved method for the determination of blood glutathione. J Lab Clin Med 61: 882–888.

34. Marklund S, Marklund G (1974) Involvement of the superoxide anion radical in the autoxidation of pyrogallol and a convenient assay for superoxide dismutase. Eur J Biochem 47: 469–474.

35. Lowry OH, Rosebrough NJ, Farr AL, Randall RJ (1951) Protein measurement with the Folin phenol reagent. J Biol Chem 193: 265–275.

36. Paglia DE, Valentine WN (1967) Studies on the quantitative and qualitative characterization of erythrocyte glutathione peroxidase. J Lab Clin Med 70: 158–169.

37. Livak KJ, Schmittgen TD (2001) Analysis of relative gene expression data using real-time quantitative PCR and the 2(-Delta Delta C(T)) Method. Methods 25: 402–408.

38. Neurath M, Fuss I, Strober W (2000) TNBS-colitis. Int Rev Immunol 19: 51–62.

39. Eiserich JP, Hristova M, Cross CE, Jones AD, Freeman BA, et al. (1998) Formation of nitric oxide-derived inflammatory oxidants by myeloperoxidase in neutrophils. Nature 391: 393–397.

40. Atreya I, Atreya R, Neurath MF (2008) NF-kappaB in inflammatory bowel disease. J Intern Med 263: 591–596.

41. Kruidenier L, Kuiper I, Lamers CB, Verspaget HW (2003) Intestinal oxidative damage in inflammatory bowel disease: semi-quantification, localization, and association with mucosal antioxidants. J Pathol 201: 28–36.

42. Mizushima T, Sasaki M, Ando T, Wada T, Tanaka M, et al. (2010) Blockage of angiotensin II type 1 receptor regulates TNF-alpha-induced MAdCAM-1 expression via inhibition of NF-kappaB translocation to the nucleus and ameliorates colitis. Am J Physiol Gastrointest Liver Physiol 298: G255–266.

43. Wang YH, Ge B, Yang XL, Zhai J, Yang LN, et al. (2011) Proanthocyanidins from grape seeds modulates the nuclear factor-kappa B signal transduction pathways in rats with TNBS-induced recurrent ulcerative colitis. Int Immunopharmacol 11: 1620–1627.

44. Witaicenis A, Luchini AC, Hiruma-Lima CA, Felisbino SL, Garrido-Mesa N, et al. (2012) Suppression of TNBS-induced colitis in rats by 4-methylesculetin, a natural coumarin: comparison with prednisolone and sulphasalazine. Chem Biol Interact 195: 76–85.

45. Schreiber S, Heinig T, Thiele HG, Raedler A (1995) Immunoregulatory role of interleukin 10 in patients with inflammatory bowel disease. Gastroenterology 108: 1434–1444.

46. Autschbach F, Braunstein J, Helmke B, Zuna I, Schurmann G, et al. (1998) In situ expression of interleukin-10 in noninflamed human gut and in inflammatory bowel disease. Am J Pathol 153: 121–130.

47. Liu X, Wang JM (2011) Iridoid glycosides fraction of Folium syringae leaves modulates NF-kappaB signal pathway and intestinal epithelial cells apoptosis in experimental colitis. PLoS One 6: e24740.

48. Talero E, Sanchez-Fidalgo S, Villegas I, de la Lastra CA, Illanes M, et al. (2011) Role of different inflammatory and tumor biomarkers in the development of ulcerative colitis-associated carcinogenesis. Inflamm Bowel Dis 17: 696–710.

49. Sukumaran V, Veeraveedu PT, Gurusamy N, Yamaguchi K, Lakshmanan AP, et al. (2011) Cardioprotective effects of telmisartan against heart failure in rats induced by experimental autoimmune myocarditis through the modulation of angiotensin-converting enzyme-2/angiotensin 1-7/mas receptor axis. Int J Biol Sci 7: 1077–1092.

50. Fujita H, Fujishima H, Morii T, Sakamoto T, Komatsu K, et al. (2012) Modulation of renal superoxide dismutase by telmisartan therapy in C57BL/6-Ins2(Akita) diabetic mice. Hypertens Res 35: 213–220.

51. Tuzun A, Erdil A, Inal V, Aydin A, Bagci S, et al. (2002) Oxidative stress and antioxidant capacity in patients with inflammatory bowel disease. Clin Biochem 35: 569–572.

52. Cai H, Griendling KK, Harrison DG (2003) The vascular NAD(P)H oxidases as therapeutic targets in cardiovascular diseases. Trends Pharmacol Sci 24: 471–478.

53. Cianchetti S, Del Fiorentino A, Colognato R, Di Stefano R, Franzoni F, et al. (2008) Anti-inflammatory and anti-oxidant properties of telmisartan in cultured human umbilical vein endothelial cells. Atherosclerosis 198: 22–28.

54. Crespo I, San-Miguel B, Prause C, Marroni N, Cuevas MJ, et al. (2012) Glutamine treatment attenuates endoplasmic reticulum stress and apoptosis in TNBS-induced colitis. PLoS One 7: e50407.

55. Wang R, Zagariya A, Ang E, Ibarra-Sunga O, Uhal BD (1999) Fas-induced apoptosis of alveolar epithelial cells requires ANG II generation and receptor interaction. Am J Physiol 277: L1245–1250.

56. Yue G, Lai PS, Yin K, Sun FF, Nagele RG, et al. (2001) Colon epithelial cell death in 2,4,6-trinitrobenzenesulfonic acid-induced colitis is associated with increased inducible nitric-oxide synthase expression and peroxynitrite production. J Pharmacol Exp Ther 297: 915–925.

57. Liu HR, Tao L, Gao E, Lopez BL, Christopher TA, et al. (2004) Anti-apoptotic effects of rosiglitazone in hypercholesterolemic rabbits subjected to myocardial ischemia and reperfusion. Cardiovasc Res 62: 135–144.

58. Dey I, Beck PL, Chadee K (2013) Lymphocytic colitis is associated with increased pro-inflammatory cytokine profile and up regulation of prostaglandin receptor EP4. PLoS One 8: e61891.

59. Zhang M, Deng C, Zheng J, Xia J, Sheng D (2006) Curcumin inhibits trinitrobenzene sulphonic acid-induced colitis in rats by activation of peroxisome proliferator-activated receptor gamma. Int Immunopharmacol 6: 1233–1242.

60. Gillberg L, Berg S, de Verdier PJ, Lindbom L, Werr J, et al. (2013) Effective treatment of mouse experimental colitis by alpha 2 integrin antibody: comparison with alpha 4 antibody and conventional therapy. Acta Physiol (Oxf) 207: 326–336.

61. Hassan A, Ibrahim A, Mbodji K, Coeffier M, Ziegler F, et al. (2010) An alpha-linolenic acid-rich formula reduces oxidative stress and inflammation by regulating NF-kappaB in rats with TNBS-induced colitis. J Nutr 140: 1714–1721.

19

The Stimulatory Adenosine Receptor ADORA2B Regulates Serotonin (5-HT) Synthesis and Release in Oxygen-Depleted EC Cells in Inflammatory Bowel Disease

Rikard Damen[1⑨], **Martin Haugen**[1⑨], **Bernhard Svejda**[1], **Daniele Alaimo**[1], **Oystein Brenna**[2], **Roswitha Pfragner**[3], **Bjorn I. Gustafsson**[2], **Mark Kidd**[1*]

1 Gastrointestinal Pathobiology Research Group, Yale University School of Medicine, New Haven, Connecticut, United States of America, **2** Department of Cancer Research and Molecular Medicine, Norwegian University of Science and Technology, Trondheim, Norway, **3** Institute of Pathophysiology and Immunology, Centre for Molecular Medicine, Graz, Austria

Abstract

Objective: We recently demonstrated that hypoxia, a key feature of IBD, increases enterochromaffin (EC) cell 5-HT secretion, which is also physiologically regulated by the ADORA2B mechanoreceptor. Since hypoxia is associated with increased extracellular adenosine, we wanted to examine whether this nucleotide amplifies HIF-1α-mediated 5-HT secretion.

Design: The effects of hypoxia were studied on IBD mucosa, isolated IBD-EC cells, isolated normal EC cells and the EC cell tumor derived cell line KRJ-1. Hypoxia (0.5% O_2) was compared to NECA (adenosine agonist), MRS1754 (ADORA2B receptor antagonist) and SCH442146 (ADORA2A antagonist) on HIF signaling and 5-HT secretion. Antisense approaches were used to mechanistically evaluate EC cells *in vitro*. PCR and western blot were used to analyze transcript and protein levels of HIF-1α signaling and neuroendocrine cell function. An animal model of colitis was evaluated to confirm hypoxia:adenosine signaling *in vivo*.

Results: HIF-1α is upregulated in IBD mucosa and IBD-EC cells, the majority (~90%) of which express an activated phenotype *in situ*. Hypoxia stimulated 5-HT release maximally at 30 mins, an effect amplified by NECA and selectively inhibited by MRS1754, through phosphorylation of TPH-1 and activation of VMAT-1. Transient transfection with *Renilla* luciferase under hypoxia transcriptional response element (HRE) control identified that ADORA2B activated HIF-1α signaling under hypoxic conditions. Additional signaling pathways associated with hypoxia:adenosine included MAP kinase and CREB. Antisense approaches mechanistically confirmed that ADORA2B signaling was linked to these pathways and 5-HT release under hypoxic conditions. Hypoxia:adenosine activation which could be reversed by 5'-ASA treatment was confirmed in a TNBS-model.

Conclusion: Hypoxia induced 5-HT synthesis and secretion is amplified by ADORA2B signaling via MAPK/CREB and TPH-1 activation. Targeting ADORA2s may decrease EC cell 5-HT production and secretion in IBD.

Editor: Jörn Karhausen, Duke University Medical Center, United States of America

Funding: These studies were funded by National Institutes of Health (NIH) R01DK080871 (Kidd) and Kontaktutvalget (Gustafsson) at St Olavs University Hospital and Faculty of Medicine, NTNU, Trondheim, Norway. The funders had no role in study design, data collection and analysis, decision to publish, or preparation of the manuscript.

Competing Interests: The authors have declared that no competing interests exist.

* E-mail: mark.kidd@yale.edu

⑨ These authors contributed equally to this work.

Introduction

Inflammatory Bowel Disease (IBD) is highly prevalent in Europe and North America and a recent systematic review demonstrated an increasing incidence (for UC: 6.3–24.3/100,000; for CD: 5–20.2) [1]. This coupled with the long duration of the illness make IBD one of the most common gastroenterological diseases with a prevalence per 100,000 of 505 and 249 for UC and 322 and 319 for CD in Europe and the US, respectively [1]. The etiology and pathogenesis of IBD, however, remains largely

unknown. While defects in local immune responses (both innate as well as adaptive) to commensal microflora and food antigens are assumed to play pathogenic roles in IBD [2,3], recent studies have also demonstrated a role for the enterochromaffin (EC) cell in the pathogenesis of this disease.

The EC cell is the most common neuroendocrine cell in the epithelia lining the lumen of the gut and plays a key regulatory role in gut secretion, motility, pain, and nausea [4]. The monoamine neurotransmitter serotonin (5-hydroxytryptamine: 5-HT) has proven central in EC cell regulatory function and these cells synthesize, store, and release the vast majority (95%) of the body's store of this amine [5]. EC cells function as "taste buds of the gut" and represent sensory transducers responding to mechanical events, luminal acidification, or nutrients such as glucose and short chain fatty acids, bile salt, tastants and olfactants [6–13]. In addition, EC cell secretion can be activated by neural, bacterial and immunological input [14,15]. Specifically, development of IBD is associated with altered EC cell serotonin release [15,16].

Serotonin is considered to play a role in IBD through activation of immune cell types which express receptors for this amine [15,17]. *TPH-1* knockout mice respond to chemically-induced colitic agents with a less severe phenotype and delayed onset of disease compared to wild-type mice treated in the same protocol [15]. A variety of other studies [18–20] support a role for serotonin in modulating immune signaling and the promotion of interactions between innate and adaptive immune responses within the context of gut inflammation.

Recently, rhythmic mechanical strain that mimics normal bowel movements (mediated by ADORA2B receptors) has been identified to induce EC cell secretion and transcription of EC cell secretory products – responses that are accentuated by neoplasia [21]. We have also demonstrated that gut EC cells are oxygen-responsive and alterations in O_2 levels differentially activate HIF-1α signaling and serotonin release [22]. This results in alterations in serotonin production and secretion, effects amplified by inflammation. In addition, to the latter, alterations in neuroendocrine signaling as well as activation of hypoxia-mediated responses are features recently identified in a TNBS animal model [23] and in IBD samples through transcriptome analyses [24].

Hypoxia is also strongly associated with an increase in extracellular/mucosal adenosine levels [25] and with stabilization of HIF-1α [26]. HIF-1α induces transcription and increases the activity of 5'ecto-nucleotidase (CD73), the enzyme that converts AMP to adenosine [27]. CD73 also regulates transcription of the ADORA2B receptor while suppressing transcription of the adenosine re-uptake transporters, equilibrative nucleoside transporters 1 and 2 (ENT1 and 2). Furthermore, CD73 decreases the intracellular metabolism of adenosine by suppressing the transcription of adenosine kinase [28]. In IBD, localized hypoxia occurs as a result of chronic inflammation increasing the metabolic needs of the tissue [29], and thus potentially up-regulates the adenosine-ADORA pathway. ADORA2B is the predominant ADORA receptor in colonic mucosa [30] and is also up-regulated by TNFα [31]. Activation of the receptor is thought to regulate cytokine production including IL-10 [32]; colitis is reduced in knockout mice [33,34] suggesting a protective role.

We hypothesized that the increase in 5-HT observed in IBD may, in part, be due to hypoxia increasing functional HIF-1α which triggers an increase in extracellular adenosine signaling, leading to increased production and secretion of 5-HT via ADORA2B receptor activation. Gut mucosal tissue from IBD patients, isolated EC cells and the well-characterized EC cell line KRJ-1 were studied. This cell line possesses similar properties (e.g. similar signaling pathways, enzyme activity and secretory products) and have similar responsiveness to stimuli, as normal EC cells and is therefore an appropriate model to study 5-HT regulation [13,21,35,36].

Materials and Methods

Materials

5'-(N-Ethylcarboxamido) adenosine (NECA) (Sigma-Aldrich, St. Louis, MO), a general adenosine receptor agonist that targets all subtypes (ADORA1, 2A, 2B and 3), curcumin (a HIF-1α inhibitor), SCH442146, a specific A2A receptor antagonist, and MRS1754 hydrate, a specific A2B receptor antagonist were used [37]. The following antibodies for western blot were obtained from Cell Signaling Technology: PKA C-alpha (5842S), MAPK (4695S), pMAPK (4370S), CREB (9197S), pCREB (9198S), Rb IgG (7074S), Mouse IgG (7076S), from Abcam: VMAT-1 (58170) and pTPH-1 (30574), from Alomone labs: A2B adenosine receptor (AAR-003), from Novis Biologicals: TPH-1 (110-57629), from BD Biosciences: HIF-1α (610958), from DAKO: Chromogranin A (CgA: MO869) and from Sigma-Aldrich, β-actin (011M4793).

Human Samples

Tissue was collected from twenty-one patients (M:F = 12:9; median age [range] = 53 yr [29–67]). CD tissue ($n = 12$) was obtained from patients who had undergone surgery for CD ileitis ($n = 3$) or colitis ($n = 9$). Only grossly affected tissue was studied. Macroscopically "normal" tissue was obtained from matched samples when available ($n = 6$). All tissue was collected between 2008 and 2013 at Yale University, Department of Surgery following written informed consent from patients *per protocol* (Yale University School of Medicine IRB approval, HIC#0805003870).

Animals

For the TNBS-colitis model, female Sprague Dawley rats (200–250 g; Taconic) ($n = 9$) were used including controls (vehicle [0.6 ml 50%, ethanol]: $n = 3$), TNBS (29.3 mg/ml, FLUKA; $n = 3$) or TNBS +5-aminosalicylic acid (5-ASA) (4 g/60 ml, volume 1.4 ml; $n = 3$). Volumes were rectally instilled and colitis was confirmed by endoscopy [23]. The study was terminated day 12 (after instillation) with blood and tissue collection. An additional 11 rats were used for EC cell isolation for the antisense studies.

ADORA2B Knockdown

A 19-mer oligonucleotide antisense corresponding to 461–480 of the rat ADORA2B receptor (NM_01716.1) was designed to induce a steric obstacle for protein translation (Yale Medical School Keck Oligonucleotide Synthesis Facility) [38]. Control nucleotides were prepared with randomized sequence of matching nucleotides per protocol. In these experiments, isolated EC cells [39] were exposed to oligonucleotides (antisensense: TCCCTCTTGCTCGTGTTCC, or control: CTGTTCCGTCCGTTCCCTT –150 pmol) for 12 hrs (FITC-uptake of oligonucleotides was noted as early as 2 hrs within cells, with peri-nuclear uptake complete by 14–16 hrs), and then assessed for mRNA, flow cytometry (receptor expression), secretion and by western blot. These experiments were conducted within 16 hrs following oligonucleotide uptake.

EC Cell Isolation

EC cells (>98% purity) were isolated from human or rat samples by mucosal stripping, enzymatic digestion, and a combination of Nycodenz gradient fractionation and fluorescence activated cell sorting (FACS) as described [13,16,35,39]. Approximately 1×10^6 cells were obtained per mucosal sample, a quantity sufficient for real-time PCR, short-term culture and western blots.

Cell Culture Studies

KRJ-I cells [40] were maintained as floating aggregates in Quantum 263 complete tumor growth medium (PAA) supplemented with penicillin (100 IU/ml) and streptomycin (100 ug/ml). EC cells (normal, IBD or isolated from rat) were maintained in short-term culture (<12 hrs after isolation) under the same conditions. All experiments were performed without antibiotics; the cell line was *mycoplasma* free.

Hypoxic conditions were induced using a modular incubator chamber (MIC-101, Billups-Rothenberg Inc, Del Mar, CA). Briefly, short-term cultured EC cells or cultured KRJ-I cells (48 hrs) were transferred to the humidified hypoxic chamber; the chamber was flushed with CO_2 for 4 min to maintain hypoxic conditions (0.5% O_2). KRJ-I cells (4×10^5 cells/ml, $n = 6$) were seeded in 6 well plates (Falcon, BD, Franklin Lakes, NJ) NECA, curcumin, SCH442146, MRS1754, and DMSO were added to the wells. DMSO was added to the controls to compensate for NECA and MRS1754 being solubilized in DMSO (<0.1% final concentration). Cells were then incubated for 15 minutes. They were then exposed to hypoxia for 0, 15, 30, 60, 120 and 240 mins.

After cells were harvested, whole-cell lysates were prepared by adding 200 µl of ice-cold cell lysis buffer ($10 \times$ RIPA lysis buffer [Millipore, Billerica, MA], complete protease inhibitor [Roche, Indianapolis, IN], phosphatase inhibitor set 1&2 [Calbiochem, Gibbstown, NJ], 100 mM PMSF [Roche], 200 mM Na_3VO_4 [Acros Organics], 12.5 mg/ml SDS [American Bioanalytical, Natick, MA]). Tubes were centrifuged at 12,000 g for 20 min and protein amount in the supernatant was quantified using the BCA protein assay kit (Thermo Fisher Scientific, Rockford, IL).

Serotonin Secretion

5-HT levels were analyzed using commercially available ELISA assays (5-HT: BA 10-0900; Rocky Mountain Diagnostics) as previously described [13] in supernatant according to the manufacturer's instructions.

RLU Studies

The Cignal HIF Pathway Reporter Assay Kit (LUC) (CCS-007L) was used to evaluate HIF signaling in EC cells (human, ADORA2B-antisense treated rat) and in KRJ-I cells. Briefly, the basis of this protocol is transient transfection with a HIF-responsive luciferase construct that encodes the firefly luciferase reporter gene under the control of a minimal (m)CMV promoter and tandem repeats of the hypoxia transcriptional response element (HRE). This is designed to monitor the activity of HIF-regulated signal transduction pathways in cultured cells. Each reporter is premixed with constitutively expressing *Renilla* luciferase, which serves as an internal control for normalizing transfection efficiencies and monitoring cell viability. Short-term cultured CD EC cells (10,000/well) or KRJ-I cells (10,000/well) were transfected per protocol. *Renilla* luciferase activation following ADORA2 activation was measured using the dual luciferase assay (Glomax). The average maximum response per kit is 4 RLU; in these experiments 2 RLU were identified.

Western Blot Analysis

Analyses were performed on 30 min hypoxia samples to evaluate total TPH, p-TPH, total CREB, p-CREB, total ERK, p-ERK, HIF-1α and PKA. Total protein lysates (20 µg) were denatured in SDS sample buffer, separated on a Tris-Glycine gel (10%) and transferred to an Immobilon P (PVDF) membrane (Milipore Corporation, Bedford, MA). After blocking (5% BSA for 60 min at room temperature) the membrane was incubated with primary antibodies (Cell Signaling Technology and BD Biosciences) in 5% BSA/PBS/Tween20 overnight at 4°C. The membranes were incubated with the horseradish peroxidase-conjugated secondary antibodies (Cell Signaling Technology) for 60 min at room temperature and immunodetection was performed using the Western Lightning™ Plus-ECL (PerkinElmer, MA). Blots were exposed on X-OMAT-AR films [40,41]. The optical density of the appropriately sized bands was measured using ImageJ software (NIH, USA).

RNA Isolation, Reverse Transcription and RT-PCR Analyses

RNA was extracted from mucosa (macroscopically normal human or rat – normal, TNBS and TNBS-treated with 5'ASA), isolated normal and CD EC cells (1×10^6), isolated normal and ADORA2B-deficient (antisense) rat EC cells, and KRJ-I cells (1×10^6, $n = 4$–7) using TRIZOL® (Invitrogen, Carlsbad, CA) then cleaned (Qiagen, RNeasy kit, Qiagen, Valencia, CA) and converted to cDNA (High Capacity cDNA Archive Kit, Applied Biosystems, Carlsbad, CA) [36,42]. RT-PCR analyses were performed using Assays-on Demand™ and the ABI 7900 Sequence Detection System [36,42]. Primer sets (*HIF-1α* (human and rat) and *ADORA2B* (rat)) were all obtained from Applied Biosystems and PCR mix on gels were performed to confirm presence of single bands for each primer set. PCR Data was normalized using the $\Delta\Delta C_T$ method; *ALG9* was used as a housekeeping gene[43] for human, *GAPDH* was used for rat [23].

Immunostaining

An established immunohistochemical protocol was used to identify target proteins [44,45]. Briefly, de-paraffinized sections were incubated with a combination of antibodies (mouse HIF-1α 1:50 and goat polyclonal Chromogranin A 1:50) overnight at 4°C and then with goat anti-mouse HRP conjugated (1:25) and donkey anti-goat Alexa Fluor 488 conjugated (1:25). A Cy-5 tyramide protocol was used to identify HIF-1α. 4',6-diamidino-2-phenylindole (1:100) was used for nuclear identification. Bound antibodies were visualized using immunofluorescent microscopy. A total of 10 clinical samples were examined, HIF-1α staining was identified and quantitated as a subset of chromogranin A-positive cells. Crohn's mucosa was compared to macroscopically normal mucosa.

Flow Cytometry

Rat EC cells (control or antisense at 12 hrs) were stained with ADORA2B (1:500) and flow cytometry was conducted on a BD FACS Aria Cell Sorter (BD Biosciences, Bedford MA). Positive cells were identified for unstained, and the two EC cell populations (antisense-treated and control).

Statistics

Results were expressed as mean±standard error (SEM). All statistical analyses were performed using Prism 4 (GraphPad Software, San Diego, CA). Results were compared between control and stimulated cells using the Mann-Whitney test. A $p < 0.05$ was considered significant.

Results

HIF-1α Expression in Normal and IBD Mucosa and EC Cells

HIF-1α transcripts were increased 3.5-fold in IBD mucosa compared to macroscopically normal CD mucosa (**Figure 1A**). A similar pattern was evident at the EC cell level, with CD EC cells demonstrating a ~2.5-fold increase of *HIF-1α* mRNA compared to normal EC cells. Assessment of protein expression confirmed HIF-1α activation both in mucosa as well as in EC cells isolated from Crohn's mucosa (**Figure 1B**). Immunofluorescent staining of CgA and HIF-1α (**Figure 1C**) identified double positive cells in the mucosa (yellow arrows), confirming that the HIF-1α-positive

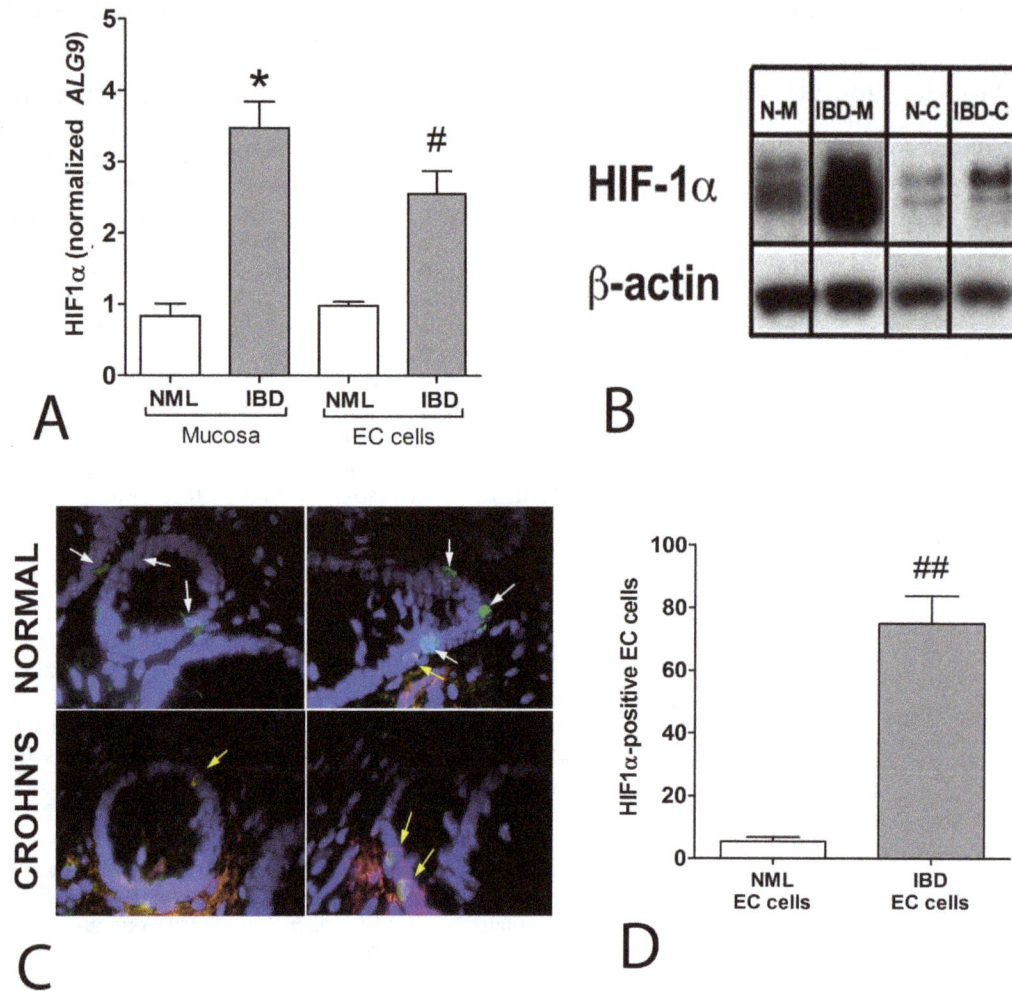

Figure 1. *HIF-1α* **transcripts and protein in normal mucosa, IBD mucosa, isolated normal and IBD-EC cells. 1A)** Transcript of HIF-1α was significantly elevated in IBD-associated conditions (mucosa: 3.4±0.63 fold, cells: 2.4±0.41). **1B)** Protein levels were significantly elevated in IBD-associated conditions (mucosa: 12.2±3.4, cells: 2.6±0.36). **1C)** Immunohistochemical staining of HIF-1α and Chromogranin A (white arrows) in normal mucosa and Crohn's mucosa identified co-staining (yellow arrows) predominantly in IBD mucosa. **1D)** Quantitation identified significantly more enteroendocrine cells to be HIF-1α positive in IBD mucosa. Mean±SEM, $n = 4–7$, *$p = 0.03$ vs. normal mucosa, #$p = 0.04$ vs. normal EC cells, ##$p < 0.001$ vs. normal EC cells. DAPI – nuclei (blue), FITC-CgA (green), Cy5-HIF-1α (red), co-localization (yellow). N–M = normal mucosa, IBD-M = IBD mucosa, N–C = normal EC cells, IBD-C = IBD EC cells.

cells were enteroendocrine. Significantly more EC cells (~90%, $p < 0.001$) were positive in Crohn's mucosa than in macroscopically normal mucosa (**Figure 1D**). These results suggest that EC cells are exposed to hypoxia during inflammation and predominantly exhibit an activated hypoxia-mediated signaling pathway (HIF-1α).

The 5-HT Secretory Pathway

To evaluate whether adenosine-mediated HIF1α activation increased 5-HT release from EC cells, we examined the effects of hypoxia with and without ADORA2 antagonists on KRJ-I cells over a 4 hr time period. Hypoxia significantly increased 5-HT between 15 and 120 mins with a maximal effect (2.2 fold, $p < 0.05$ versus no hypoxia, **Figure 2A**). Curcumin, a known HIF-1α inhibitor through transcriptional repression [46], reversed hypoxia-mediated secretion at all time points. NECA, increased 5-HT release (30–120 min), while MRS1754 but not SCH442146, decreased it (15–120 min). This suggests that 5-HT release by

hypoxia is driven, at least in part, by activation of ADORA2B receptors, and that adenosine can modulate 5-HT secretion.

We next evaluated expression of enzymes involved in 5-HT synthesis and vesicle uptake (TPH-1 and VMAT-1) and in secretion per se, chromogranin A (CgA). We focused on 30 mins as this identified the time point at which 5-HT was maximally secreted. Total protein levels of TPH-1 were unchanged by hypoxia at 30 min (**Figure 2B**) but the phosphorylated form of this enzyme, which identifies activated TPH-1, was increased. This was amplified by NECA and inhibited by MRS1754. Analysis of the ratio of activated to total TPH-1 protein identified that this was increased 1.6±0.16 by hypoxia ($p < 0.05$ vs. controls) and 2.4±0.2 (by NECA: $p < 0.05$ vs. hypoxia) and was reduced to 0.91±0.17 (by MRS, $p < 0.05$ vs. hypoxia). VMAT-1 functions to accumulate cytosolic monoamines, like 5-HT, into secretory vesicles [47]. No significant changes were noted for VMAT-1 by hypoxia, but levels were significantly elevated by NECA (2.83±0.07, $p < 0.05$) (**Figure 2C**), indicating that adenosine signaling activates 5-HT uptake into vesicles. CgA is important for granulogenesis and

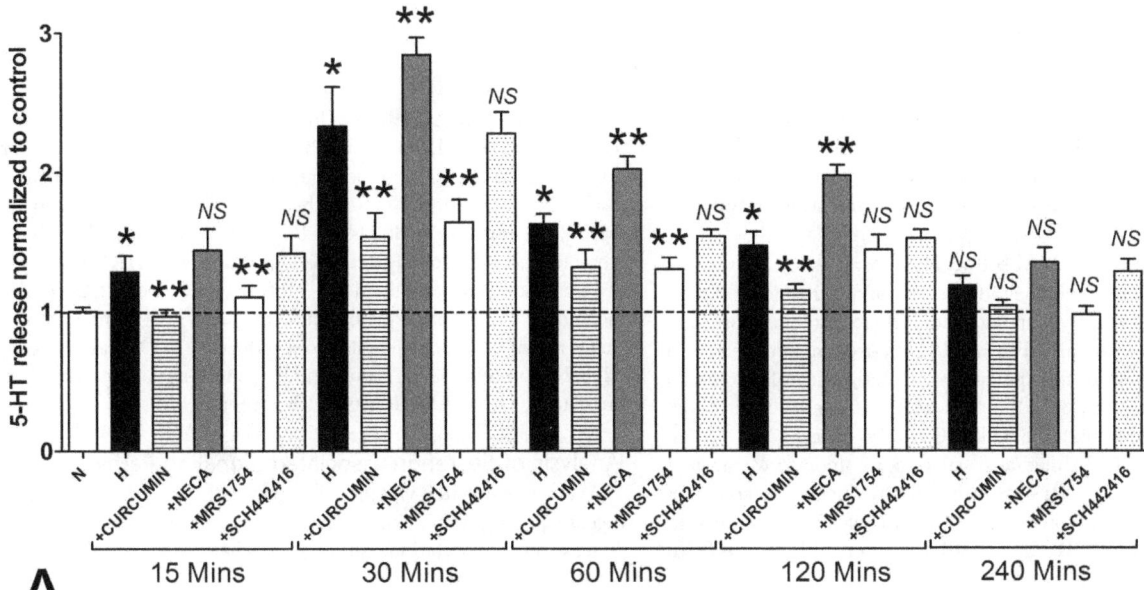

A

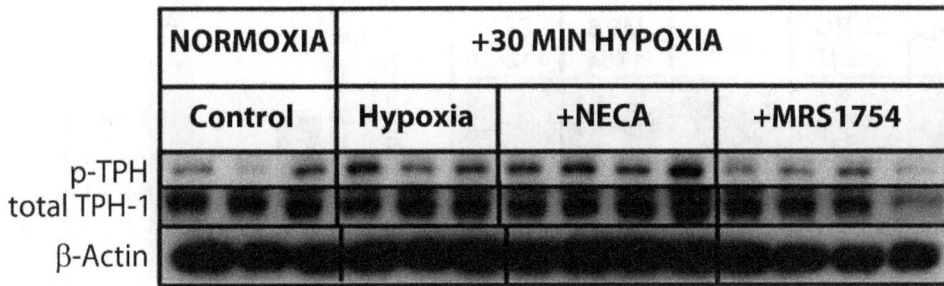

B

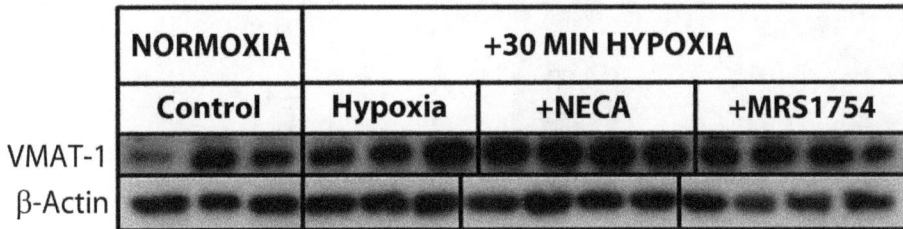

C

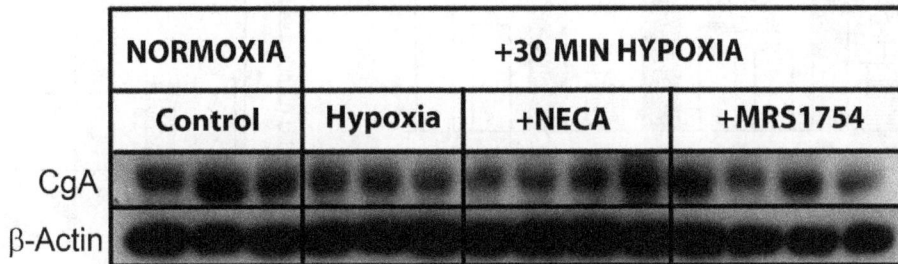

D

Figure 2. Effect of adenosine on the hypoxia-activated 5-HT pathway in KRJ-I cells. 2A) 5-HT was increased by hypoxia between 15–120 min, with a maximal effect at 30 min (2.28±0.12 fold). Curcumin and MRS1754 inhibited while NECA augmented secretion at all time points up to 120 mins. SCH442146 had no significant effect. **2B)** Total TPH-1 protein levels were unchanged after 30 min of hypoxia and after NECA or MRS1754 stimulation. Phosphorylated TPH-1 was significantly increased under hypoxia (1.80±0.26), was amplified by NECA (2.66±0.28) and reduced by MRS1754 to baseline. **2C)** VMAT-1 protein levels were significantly increased (2.83±0.31) by NECA during hypoxia and reduced by MRS1754

(2±0.1). **2D)** Chromogranin A protein levels did not change significantly after hypoxia or with the addition of NECA or MRS 1754. Mean±SEM, $n = 3$–8, *$p < 0.05$ vs. control, **$p < 0.05$ vs. hypoxia. NS = not significant.

secretion in neuroendocrine cells [48]. No alterations were identified (**Figure 2D**). We interpret this to indicate that hypoxia and adenosine directly activate pathways associated with the formation of components essential to neuroendocrine secretion.

Directly Linking ADORA2B and HIF-1α

We next evaluated whether adenosine could activate HIF-1α. In KRJ-I cells, 30 min hypoxia-induced HIF-1α protein expression was reversed by curcumin (**Figure 3A**). Pre-treatment of cells with NECA (15 mins prior to hypoxic challenge) significantly increased HIF-1α protein (~1.3-fold) while MRS1754 significantly decreased this (~0.8-fold). SCH442146 had no effect.

To evaluate HIF-1α mediated signaling we undertook transient transfection with a HIF-responsive firefly luciferase construct under HRE-transcription control (*Renilla* luciferase-constructs) in KRJ-I cells (**Figure 3B**) and in IBD-EC cells (**Figure 3C**). In

KRJ-I cells NECA activated luciferase (RLU) under normoxic conditions while MRS1754 inhibited this; no effect was noted for SCH442146. Under hypoxic conditions, NECA amplified luciferase activity (3-fold, $p < 0.05$ vs. hypoxia) which was inhibited by MRS1754 but not by SCH442146. In IBD-EC cells (which have an activated HIF-1α–**Figure 1A–C**), activation of HRE-mediated transcription was amplified by NECA (~1.5-fold RLU) under normoxic conditions and inhibited by MRS1754. These results suggest that adenosine, similar to a reduction in O_2, can increase HIF-1α protein levels and induce HRE-signaling which is mediated via the ADORA type 2B receptor.

Analysis of Secretion-associated Signaling Pathways

We next evaluated whether signaling pathways related to 5-HT release [21,49] were altered by hypoxia and adenosine. MAPK kinease phosphorylation, although unchanged by hypoxia, was

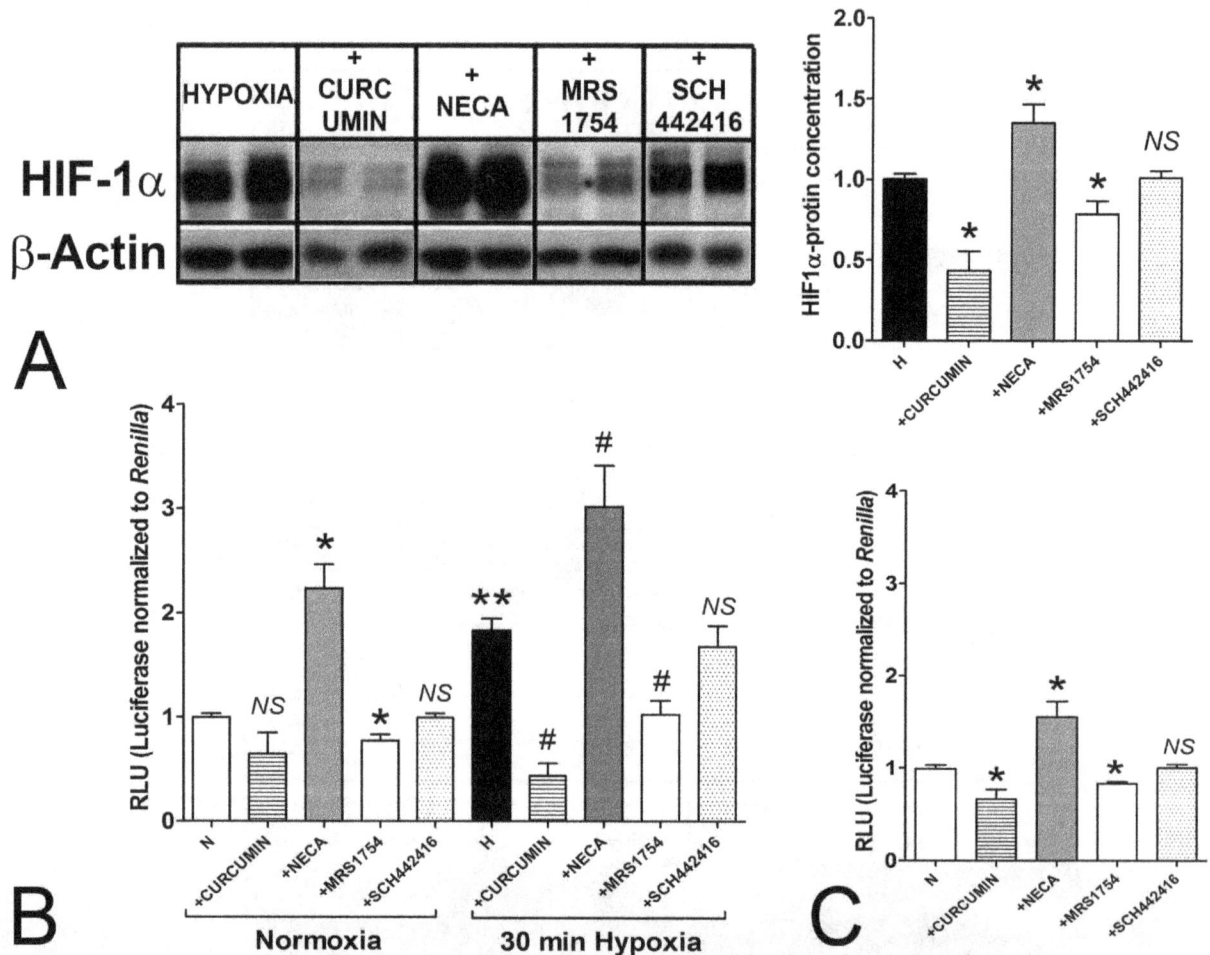

Figure 3. HIF-1α, adenosine signaling and HRE activation. 3A) Curcumin inhibited (022±0.04 fold) while NECA (1.24±0.06 fold) stimulated and MRS1754 (0.74±0.02) inhibited HIF-1α protein levels compared to 30 minutes hypoxia in KRJ-I cells. SCH442146 had no effect. **3B)** Transient transfection with *Renilla* luciferase-encoding constructs in KRJ-I cells. Under normoxic conditions, NECA amplified activation of luciferase (RLU) while MRS1754 inhibited this. Curcumin and SCH442416 had no effect. Hypoxic conditions activated RLU (1.81±0.12), which was inhibited by curcumin and MRS1754 and amplified by NECA. **3C)** In IBD-EC cells, RLU was elevated in normoxic conditions. This could be reduced by curcumin and MRS1754 and amplified by NECA. Mean±SEM, $n = 3$–7, *$p < 0.05$ vs. 30 min hypoxia or control, **$p < 0.05$ vs. normoxic cells, #$p < 0.05$ vs. 30 min hypoxia. NS = not significant.

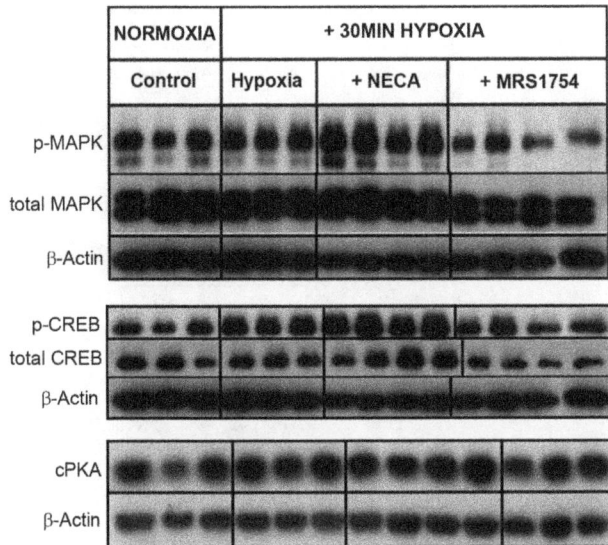

Figure 4. Effects of hypoxia and adenosine on signaling pathways. 4A) Phosphorylated MAPK was not significantly altered by hypoxia but was amplified by NECA (1.29±0.06)and reduced by MRS1754 (0.40±0.09); total MAPK protein amount was unchanged. **4B)** Neither total CREB nor phosphorylated CREB were altered after 30 min of hypoxia. NECA, however, stimulated p CREB compared (1.55±0.07; this was reduced by MRS1754 (0.7±0.12). **4C)** Free catalytically active PKA protein levels were unchanged after 30 min of hypoxia, as well as after NECA and MRS1754. Mean±SEM, $n = 5-8$.

amplified by NECA, and reduced by MRS-1754 (**Figure 4A**). This suggests that the ADORA2B receptor under hypoxic conditions regulates MAP kinase activity – a known regulator of 5-HT secretion and TPH-1 phosphorylation [13,35].

CREB is an important transcription factor for *TPH-1* transcription [50–52]. While not significantly increased by hypoxia, the phosphorylated form was significantly increased by NECA (**Figure 4B**), an effect that was reversed by MRS1754. This suggests a role for ADORA-mediated signaling in the regulation of hypoxia-mediated *TPH1* transcription.

PKA, which mediates the adenosine signal for 5-HT production and secretion under mechanical stress [21], was not significantly changed by hypoxia and was not altered by either NECA or MRS1754 (**Figure 4C**) suggesting that this pathway does not regulate 5-HT secretion under these conditions.

Mechanistic Analysis of Hypoxia-adenosine Signaling Pathways in EC Cells

We used an antisense approach to mechanistically dissect the pathways associated with hypoxia-adenosine signaling in isolated rat EC cells. ADORA2B antisense decreased transcription (~50%) and was associated with a significant and almost complete reduction in ADORA2B membrane protein expression (**Figure 5A**). These cells could respond to hypoxia with 5-HT release, but this was significantly lower than cells with normal ADORA2B expression (**Figure 5B**). The latter cells responded similar to human EC cells with adenosine-regulated hypoxia-mediated 5-HT release, while the antisense-treated cells had largely lost adenosine mediated effects. At a protein level, we identified reduced pMAPK, pCREB and pTPH-1 in antisense treated hypoxic cells (**Figure 5C**) identifying that these are the principle pathways involved in adenosine-mediated 5-HT secretion.

Hypoxia and ADORA2B in an Animal TNBS-induced Colitis Model

Finally, we evaluated expression of HIF-1α and ADORA2B in intestinal mucosa from a rat animal TNBS-induced colitis model and evaluated the effect of 5-ASA. A real-time PCR analysis confirmed significant upregulation of HIF-1α and ADORA2B mRNA by TNBS (**Figure 6A**). The expression levels were decreased by 5-ASA treatment. Protein levels followed a similar expression pattern (**Figure 6B**). We interpret these data to confirm activation of a hypoxia-adenosine pathway in a colitis model – similar to observations in clinical samples.

Discussion

IBD is associated with abnormalities in the pro-inflammatory 5-HT system. Previously, we have demonstrated that LPS and IL1β induce a significantly elevated 5-HT response in IBD mucosa [16]. This may partly explain the hypersecretion of 5-HT noted in the IBD disease process. As IBD mucosa is also exposed to significant hypoxic stress, we examined the effects of hypoxia on EC cell 5-HT secretion. We have identified that hypoxia induces 5-HT secretion from EC cells and that this can be reversed by targeting HIF-1α. HIF-1α is also associated with increased mucosal adenosine availability, a known regulator of 5-HT production and secretion [22]. Based on these observations, we investigated the relationship between hypoxia, the ADORA signaling system and 5-HT production/secretion in EC cells from CD and normal mucosa to evaluate whether these factors are involved in the amplified 5-HT production noted in IBD.

We demonstrated that HIF-1α was increased both at the mRNA and protein levels in IBD mucosa, in an animal model of colitis and in IBD-EC cells. The latter almost predominantly (~90%) expressed a hypoxia activated phenotype and active HRE signaling. These data confirm that the inflamed mucosa is under hypoxic stress [53,54], and that EC cells, in particular, are hypoxia-activated. We have previously identified increased ADORA2B receptors both at protein and transcript levels in EC cells isolated from IBD patients compared to controls [21]. In the current study, we identified that adenosine amplified HIF-1α expression and activity, which suggests that it can act as a positive feedback mechanism for 5-HT synthesis and release.

Activating ADORA signaling via NECA increased 5-HT release which could specifically be inhibited by MRS1754 identifying that, under low oxygen mucosal levels such as found with hypoxia, EC cell secretion is regulated by adenosine and specifically, via activation of ADORA2B receptors. The inhibitory effect of MRS1754 was complete for the time period 15–90 mins but at 120 mins, we could identify no inhibition by this agent. This suggests that the adenosine (ADORA2B):hypoxic signaling pathway occurs early (within 30 mins) and that other ADORA receptors may play a role later in hypoxia-mediated 5-HT release; it is unlikely that this is ADORA2A. A combination of HIF-1α signal activation and adenosine-mediated ADORA2 signaling appears to play important roles in EC cell 5-HT secretion in IBD.

HIF-1α itself may directly regulate transcription of the rate-limiting enzyme in 5-HT synthesis TPH-1. The promoter region of this gene encodes hypoxia responsive elements (HRE) [55]; hypoxia may therefore directly increase 5-HT production by increasing *TPH-1* expression. Transcriptional alterations in TPH-1 were not consistently identified in our current study (*data not shown*) suggesting the major route regulating 5-HT release occurred at the level of protein regulation and via pathways cross-activated by HIF-1α signaling.

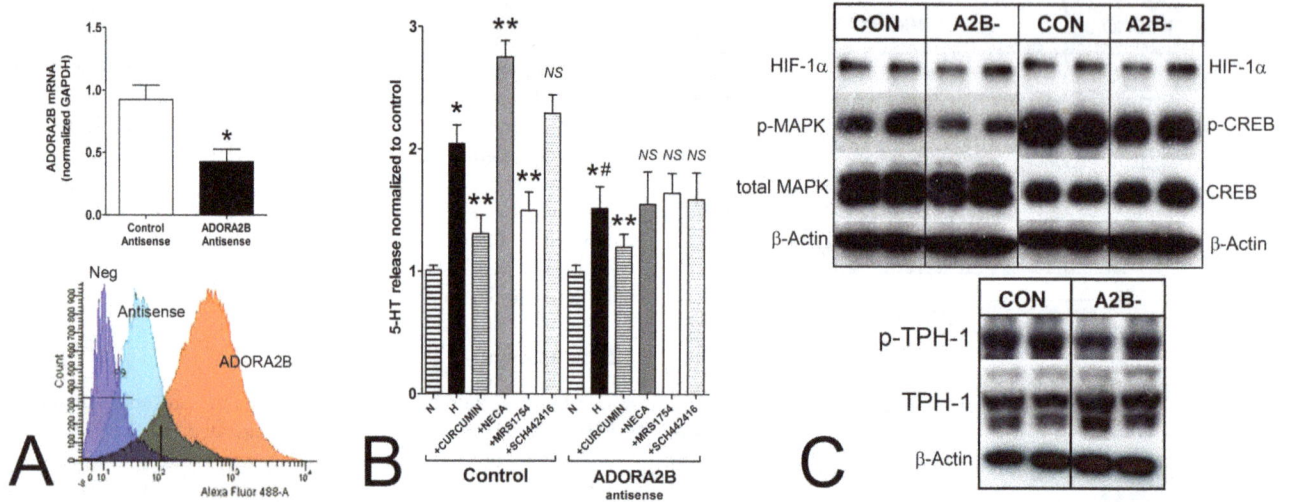

Figure 5. Analysis of 5-HT release and signaling pathways in ADORA2B-deficient rat EC cells. 5A) A 12 hr antisense approach inhibited ADORA2B transcript (real-time PCR) and protein expression (membrane-bound, flow cytometry) in isolated rat EC cells. Membrane expression was reduced to an estimated 5% of non-targeted cells. **5B)** In non-targeted cells, 5-HT release was elevated by hypoxia and inhibited by curcumin. Adenosine signaling responses were similar to human EC cells. Antisense reduced hypoxic-mediated responses (compared to controls) and ameliorated cell responses to NECA and MRS1754. **5C)** Western blot identified decreased pMAPK (0.56 ± 0.09), pCREB (0.75 ± 0.11) and pTPH-1 (0.63 ± 0.07) in antisense treated cells confirming down-regulation of these pathways with loss of ADORA2B expression under hypoxic conditions. Mean $\pm$ SEM, $n = 3$. *$p < 0.05$ vs. control, **$p < 0.05$ vs hypoxia, #$p < 0.05$ vs. hypoxia (in non-antisense treated cells). NS = not significant.

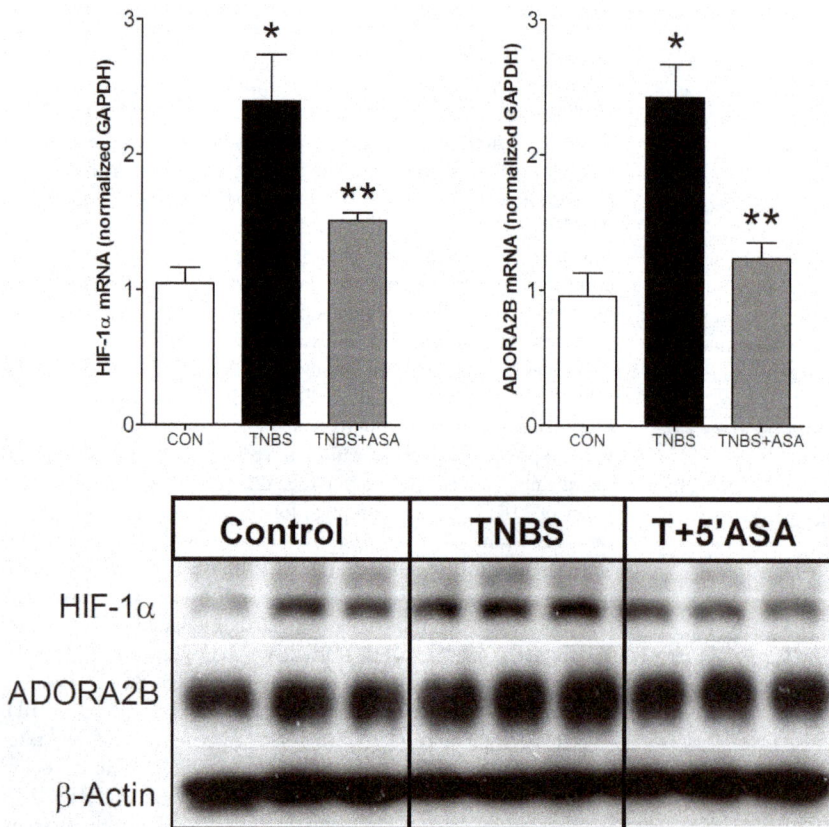

Figure 6. Analysis of HIF-1α and ADORA2B in mucosa from the animal TNBS-induced colitis model with or without 5-ASA-treatment. 6A) TNBS was associated with a significant elevation in HIF-1α and ADORA2B transcripts. Treatment with 5-ASA reversed these values to those similar to untreated rats. 6B) Protein expression was elevated by TNBS (HIF-1α: 1.68 ± 0.11; ADORA2B: 1.37 ± 0.09) and reversed by 5-ASA in mucosa. Mean $\pm$ SEM, $n = 3$. *$p < 0.05$ versus control, **$p < 0.05$ versus TNBS.

We have previously demonstrated that the adenosine/ ADORA2B/cAMP/PKA/CREB pathway plays a pivotal role in regulating 5-HT secretion from the EC cell when subject to mechanical stress [21]. In the current study, we demonstrated that the activation of the ADORA2B receptor was important for the increased levels of 5-HT noted during hypoxia. The intracellular signaling pathways involved in the hypoxic response, however, exhibit differences to that identified for EC cell mechanoresponsivity. We failed to detect differences in PKA suggesting that activation of cAMP-responsive pathways is not PKA-regulated under these conditions. In contrast, we identified ADORA2B mediated activation of MAPK signaling as well as increased phosphorylation (and thereby activation) of TPH-1. TPH-1 is a MAPK target and it is likely, under hypoxic conditions, that MAPK phosphorylates and thereby activates this enzyme, leading to an increase in 5-HT synthesis. Antisense approaches mechanistically confirmed roles for both MAPK as well as TPH-1 in EC cells under hypoxic conditions.

Other factors involved in 5-HT secretion were altered by adenosine-ADORA2B signaling. Specifically, protein levels of the rate-limiting enzyme involved in 5-HT vesicular accumulation, VMAT1, were increased. We postulate that the excess 5-HT produced by activated TPH-1, is actively transported into vesicles which then provides a large pool for release. We interpret this to demonstrate that vesicle maturation [47,48], is directly regulated by adenosine under hypoxic conditions.

Adenosine plays a complex role in IBD. Apart from activating EC cell 5-HT secretion, this nucleotide can also decrease SERT activity [56]; the combination resulting in a increased mucosal 5-HT signal. One prediction, given the pro-inflammatory activity of 5-HT, is an exacerbation of colitis under these conditions. Other studies have demonstrated an increased severity of colitis in ADORA2B−/− mice suggesting that targeting this receptor may be a potential therapeutic target. Currently, loss of ADORA2B is considered to result in down-regulation of IL10 production, with accentuation of colitis. Our studies indicate that loss of ADORA2B decreases 5-HT and, presumably, the mucosal aminergic signal.

Elevated mucosal adenosine, induced in hypoxic conditions or during abnormalities in peristalsis, may activate EC cell 5-HT synthesis and release, and reduce enterocyte-mediated SERT production with a resultant overall increase in 5-HT pro-inflammatory signaling. In the context of ADORA signaling, our studies and others, highlight both the complexity of the mucosal pathways involved in IBD as well as the importance of delineating individual cell signaling. This may help better direct targeted therapy.

Author Contributions

Conceived and designed the experiments: RD MH BS BIG MK. Performed the experiments: RD MH BS DA OB MK. Analyzed the data: RD MH BS DA OB BIG MK. Contributed reagents/materials/ analysis tools: RD MH BS RP BIG MK. Wrote the paper: RD MH BS RP BIG MK.

References

1. Molodecky NA, Soon IS, Rabi DM, Ghali WA, Ferris M, et al. (2012) Increasing incidence and prevalence of the inflammatory bowel diseases with time, based on systematic review. Gastroenterology 142: 46–54 e42.
2. Xavier RJ, Podolsky DK (2007) Unravelling the pathogenesis of inflammatory bowel disease. Nature 448: 427–434.
3. Strober W (2006) Immunology. Unraveling gut inflammation. Science 313: 1052–1054.
4. Gershon MD, Tack J (2007) The serotonin signaling system: from basic understanding to drug development for functional GI disorders. Gastroenterology 132: 397–414.
5. Bertaccini G (1960) Tissue 5-hydroxytryptamine and urinary 5-hydroxyindoleacetic acid after partial or total removal of the gastro-intestinal tract in the rat. J Physiol 153: 239–249.
6. Kalhan A, Vazquez M, Jasani B, Stott J, Neal J, et al. Adenosine Receptor Signal Pathways in Neuroendocrine Tumours 2008; London. Bioscientifica.
7. Kellum J, Albuerqueque F, Stoner M, Harris R (1999) Stroking human jejunal mucosa induces 5-HT release and Cl- secretion via afferent neurons and 5-HT4 receptors. Am J Physiol 277: G515–G520.
8. Kellum J, Jaffe B (1976) Validation and application of a radioimmunoassay for serotonin. Gastroenterolology 70: 516.
9. Bulbring E, Lin R (1958) The effect of intraluminal application of 5-hydroxytryptamine and 5-hydroxytryptophan on peristalsis: the local production of 5-HT and its release in relation to intraluminal pressure and propulsive activity. J Physiol 140: 381.
10. Zhu J, Wu X, Owyang C, Li Y (2001) Intestinal serotonin acts as a paracrine substance to mediate vagal signal transmission evoked by luminal factors in the rat. J Physiol 530: 431–442.
11. Raybould H, Glatzle J, Robin C, Meyer J, Phan T, et al. (2003) Expression of 5-HT3 receptors by extrinsic duodenal afferents contribute to intestinal inhibition of gastric emptying. Am J Physiol 284: G367–372.
12. Fukumoto S, Tatewaki M, Yamada T, Fujimiya M, Mantyh C, et al. (2003) Short-chain fatty acids stimulate colonic transit via intraluminal 5-HT release in rats. Am J Physiol 284: R1269–1276.
13. Kidd M, Modlin IM, Gustafsson BI, Drozdov I, Hauso O, et al. (2008) Luminal regulation of normal and neoplastic human EC cell serotonin release is mediated by bile salts, amines, tastants, and olfactants. Am J Physiol Gastrointest Liver Physiol 295: G260–272.
14. Cooke HJ (2000) Neurotransmitters in neuronal reflexes regulating intestinal secretion. Ann N Y Acad Sci 915: 77–80.
15. Ghia JE, Li N, Wang H, Collins M, Deng Y, et al. (2009) Serotonin has a key role in pathogenesis of experimental colitis. Gastroenterology 137: 1649–1660.
16. Kidd M, Gustafsson BI, Drozdov I, Modlin IM (2009) IL1beta- and LPS-induced serotonin secretion is increased in EC cells derived from Crohn's disease. Neurogastroenterol Motil 21: 439–450.
17. Leon-Ponte M, Ahern GP, O'Connell PJ (2007) Serotonin provides an accessory signal to enhance T-cell activation by signaling through the 5-HT7 receptor. Blood 109: 3139–3146.
18. Muller T, Durk T, Blumenthal B, Grimm M, Cicko S, et al. (2009) 5-hydroxytryptamine modulates migration, cytokine and chemokine release and T-cell priming capacity of dendritic cells in vitro and in vivo. PLoS One 4: e6453.
19. Idzko M, Panther E, Stratz C, Muller T, Bayer H, et al. (2004) The serotoninergic receptors of human dendritic cells: identification and coupling to cytokine release. J Immunol 172: 6011–6019.
20. Li N, Ghia JE, Wang H, McClemens J, Cote F, et al. (2011) Serotonin activates dendritic cell function in the context of gut inflammation. Am J Pathol 178: 662–671.
21. Chin A, Svejda B, Gustafsson BI, Granlund A, Sandvik AK, et al. (2011) The role of mechanical forces and adenosine in the regulation of intestinal enterochromaffin cell serotonin secretion. Am J Physiol Gastrointest Liver Physiol 28: 28.
22. Haugen M, Damen R, Svejda B, Gustafsson B, Pfragner R, et al. (2012) Differential signal pathway activation and 5-HT function: the role of gut enterochromaffin cells as oxygen sensors. Am J Physiol Gastrointest Liver Physiol 303: G1164–1173.
23. Brenna Ø, Furnes M, Drozdov I, Granlund A, Flatberg A, et al. (2013) Endoscopic, histological and transcriptomic characterization of TNBS-colitis in rats, a model for IBD. Plos One 8: e54543.
24. Van Beelen Granlund A, Flatberg A, Ostvik A, Drozdov I, Gustafsson B, et al. (2013) Whole Genome Gene Expression Meta-analysis of Inflammatory Bowel Disease Colon Mucosa demonstrates lack of major differences between Crohn's Disease and Ulcerative Colitis. Plos One 8: e56818.
25. Eltzschig HK (2009) Adenosine: an old drug newly discovered. Anesthesiology 111: 904–915.
26. Semenza GL (2001) HIF-1, O(2), and the 3 PHDs: how animal cells signal hypoxia to the nucleus. Cell 107: 1–3.
27. Synnestvedt K, Furuta GT, Comerford KM, Louis N, Karhausen J, et al. (2002) Ecto-5′-nucleotidase (CD73) regulation by hypoxia-inducible factor-1 mediates permeability changes in intestinal epithelia. J Clin Invest 110: 993–1002.
28. Sitkovsky MV (2008) Damage control by hypoxia-inhibited AK. Blood 111: 5424–5425.
29. Taylor CT, Colgan SP (2007) Hypoxia and gastrointestinal disease. J Mol Med 85: 1295–1300.
30. Strohmeier GR, Reppert SM, Lencer WI, Madara JL (1995) The A2b adenosine receptor mediates cAMP responses to adenosine receptor agonists in human intestinal epithelia. J Biol Chem 270: 2387–2394.
31. Kolachala V, Asamoah V, Wang L, Obertone TS, Ziegler TR, et al. (2005) TNF-alpha upregulates adenosine 2b (A2b) receptor expression and signaling in

intestinal epithelial cells: a basis for A2bR overexpression in colitis. Cell Mol Life Sci 62: 2647–2657.

32. Nemeth ZH, Lutz CS, Csoka B, Deitch EA, Leibovich SJ, et al. (2005) Adenosine augments IL-10 production by macrophages through an A2B receptor-mediated posttranscriptional mechanism. J Immunol 175: 8260–8270.

33. Frick JS, MacManus CF, Scully M, Glover LE, Eltzschig HK, et al. (2009) Contribution of adenosine A2B receptors to inflammatory parameters of experimental colitis. J Immunol 182: 4957–4964. doi: 4910.4049/jimmunol.0801324.

34. Kolachala VL, Vijay-Kumar M, Dalmasso G, Yang D, Linden J, et al. (2008) A2B adenosine receptor gene deletion attenuates murine colitis. Gastroenterology 135: 861–870. doi: 810.1053/j.gastro.2008.1005.1049. Epub 2008 May 1021.

35. Modlin IM, Kidd M, Pfragner R, Eick GN, Champaneria MC (2006) The functional characterization of normal and neoplastic human enterochromaffin cells. J Clin Endocrinol Metab 91: 2340–2348.

36. Kidd M, Eick GN, Modlin IM, Pfragner R, Champaneria MC, et al. (2007) Further delineation of the continuous human neoplastic enterochromaffin cell line, KRJ-I, and the inhibitory effects of lanreotide and rapamycin. J Mol Endocrinol 38: 181–192.

37. Kalhan A, Gharibi B, Vazquez M, Jasani B, Neal J, et al. (2011) Adenosine A(2A) and A (2B) receptor expression in neuroendocrine tumours: potential targets for therapy. Purinergic Signal 27: 27.

38. Lauffer JM, Tang LH, Zhang T, Hinoue T, Rahbar S, et al. (2001) PACAP mediates the neural proliferative pathway of Mastomys enterochromaffin-like cell transformation. Regul Pept 102: 157–164.

39. Kidd M, Modlin IM, Eick GN, Champaneria MC (2006) Isolation, functional characterization, and transcriptome of Mastomys ileal enterochromaffin cells. Am J Physiol Gastrointest Liver Physiol 291: G778–791. Epub 2006 Feb 2002.

40. Svejda B, Kidd M, Kazberouk A, Lawrence B, Pfragner R, et al. (2011) Limitations in small intestinal neuroendocrine tumor therapy by mTor kinase inhibition reflect growth factor-mediated PI3K feedback loop activation via ERK1/2 and AKT. Cancer.

41. Kidd M, Modlin IM, Pfragner R, Eick GN, Champaneria MC, et al. (2007) Small bowel carcinoid (enterochromaffin cell) neoplasia exhibits transforming growth factor-beta1-mediated regulatory abnormalities including up-regulation of C-Myc and MTA1. Cancer 109: 2420–2431.

42. Kidd M, Eick G, Shapiro MD, Camp RL, Mane SM, et al. (2005) Microsatellite instability and gene mutations in transforming growth factor-beta type II receptor are absent in small bowel carcinoid tumors. Cancer 103: 229–236.

43. Kidd M, Nadler B, Mane S, Eick G, Malfertheiner M, et al. (2007) GeneChip, geNorm, and gastrointestinal tumors: novel reference genes for real-time PCR. Physiol Genomics 30: 363–370.

44. Kidd M, Modlin IM, Eick GN, Camp RL, Mane SM (2007) Role of CCN2/CTGF in the proliferation of Mastomys enterochromaffin-like cells and gastric carcinoid development. Am J Physiol Gastrointest Liver Physiol 292: G191–200.

45. Kidd M, Modlin IM, Mane SM, Camp RL, Shapiro MD (2006) Q RT-PCR detection of chromogranin A: a new standard in the identification of neuroendocrine tumor disease. Annals of Surgery 243: 273–280.

46. Bae MK, Kim SH, Jeong JW, Lee YM, Kim HS, et al. (2006) Curcumin inhibits hypoxia-induced angiogenesis via down-regulation of HIF-1. Oncol Rep 15: 1557–1562.

47. Eiden LE, Schafer MK, Weihe E, Schutz B (2004) The vesicular amine transporter family (SLC18): amine/proton antiporters required for vesicular accumulation and regulated exocytotic secretion of monoamines and acetylcholine. Pflugers Arch 447: 636–640.

48. Modlin IM, Gustafsson BI, Moss SF, Pavel M, Tsolakis AV, et al. (2010) Chromogranin A–biological function and clinical utility in neuro endocrine tumor disease. Ann Surg Oncol 17: 2427–2443.

49. Damen R, Haugen M, Svejda B, Pfragner R, Modlin I, et al. (2013) The stimulatory adenosine receptor ADORA2B regulates serotonin (5-HT) synthesis and release in oxygen-depleted EC cells in IBD. Plos One (in press).

50. Zubenko GS, Jones ML, Estevez AO, Hughes HB 3rd, Estevez M (2009) Identification of a CREB-dependent serotonergic pathway and neuronal circuit regulating foraging behavior in Caenorhabditis elegans: a useful model for mental disorders and their treatments? Am J Med Genet B Neuropsychiatr Genet 150B: 12–23.

51. Garcia-Osta A, Del Rio J, Frechilla D (2004) Increased CRE-binding activity and tryptophan hydroxylase mRNA expression induced by 3,4-methylenedioxymethamphetamine (MDMA, "ecstasy") in the rat frontal cortex but not in the hippocampus. Brain Res Mol Brain Res 126: 181–187.

52. Drozdov I, Svejda B, Gustafsson B, Mane S, Pfragner R, et al. (2011) Gene Network Inference and Biochemical Assessment delineates GPCRPathways and CREB Targets in Small Intestinal Neuroendocrine Neoplasia Plos One 6: e22457.

53. Pierdomenico M, Stronati L, Costanzo M, Vitali R, Di Nardo G, et al. (2011) New insights into the pathogenesis of inflammatory bowel disease: transcription factors analysis in bioptic tissues from pediatric patients. J Pediatr Gastroenterol Nutr 52: 271–279.

54. Hirota SA, Beck PL, MacDonald JA (2009) Targeting hypoxia-inducible factor-1 (HIF-1) signaling in therapeutics: implications for the treatment of inflammatory bowel disease. Recent Pat Inflamm Allergy Drug Discov 3: 1–16.

55. Pocock R, Hobert O (2010) Hypoxia activates a latent circuit for processing gustatory information in C. elegans. Nat Neurosci 13: 610–614.

56. Matheus N, Mendoza C, Iceta R, Mesonero JE, Alcalde AI (2009) Regulation of serotonin transporter activity by adenosine in intestinal epithelial cells. Biochem Pharmacol 78: 1198–1204.

20

Pancreatitis-Associated Protein does not Predict Disease Relapse in Inflammatory Bowel Disease Patients

Tiago Nunes[1], Maria Josefina Etchevers[1], Maria Jose Sandi[2], Susana Pinó Donnay[1], Teddy Grandjean[3,4,5,6], Maria Pellisé[1], Julián Panés[1], Elena Ricart[1], Juan Lucio Iovanna[2], Jean-Charles Dagorn[2], Mathias Chamaillard[3,4,5,6], Miquel Sans[7]*

1 Department of Gastroenterology, Hospital Clinic of Barcelona (IDIBAPS/Centro de Investigació Bioméica en Red de Enfermedades Hepáicas y Digestivas [CIBEREHD]), Barcelona, Catalonia, Spain, **2** Centre de Recherche en Cancérologie de Marseille (CRCM), INSERM U1068, CNRS UMR 7258, Aix-Marseille Université and Institut Paoli-Calmettes, Parc Scientifique et Technologique de Luminy, Marseille, France, **3** University Lille Nord de France, F-59000, Lille, France, **4** Institut Pasteur de Lille, Center for Infection and Immunity of Lille, F-59019, Lille, France, **5** Centre National de la Recherche Scientifique, UMR8204, F-59021, Lille, France, **6** Institut National de la Santé et de la Recherche Médicale, U1019, Team 7, Equipe FRM, F-59019, Lille, France, **7** Department of Digestive Diseases, Centro Medico Teknon, Barcelona, Catalonia, Spain

Abstract

Background: The pancreatitis-associated protein (PAP) is increased in the serum of active inflammatory bowel disease (IBD) patients and its levels seem to be correlated with disease activity. Our aim was to evaluate the usefulness of serum and fecal PAP measurements to predict relapse in patients with inactive IBD.

Materials and Methods: We undertook a 12-month prospective study that included 66 Crohn's disease (CD) and 74 ulcerative colitis (UC) patients. At inclusion, patients were in clinical remission, defined by a Harvey-Bradshaw (HB) Index$\leq$4 (CD) or a partial Mayo Score (MS)$<$3 (UC), along with a normal serum C reactive protein (CRP) and fecal calprotectin. Patients were followed every 3 months. Blood and stool samples were collected and a clinical evaluation was performed at each visit. Serum PAP and CRP levels as well as fecal concentrations of PAP and calprotectin were assessed.

Results: Active CD patients had an increased mean serum PAP at the diagnosis of the flare (104.1 ng/ml) and 3 months prior to activity (22.68 ng/ml) compared with patients in remission (13.26 ng/ml), p$<$0.05. No significant change in serum PAP levels in UC and fecal PAP levels in CD and UC were detected during disease activity. In CD, serum PAP was a poor diagnostic predictor of disease activity, with an AUC of 0.69. In patients in remission, fecal PAP was barely detectable in UC compared with CD patients.

Conclusion: Serum PAP is increased only in active CD patients, but this marker does not predict disease activity. Inactive UC patients have marked low levels of PAP in fecal samples compared with CD patients.

Editor: Simon Patrick Hogan, Cincinnati Children's Hospital Medical Center, University of Cincinnati College of Medicine, United States of America

Funding: This work was supported by the Fondation pour la Recherche Médicale and by the Broad Medical Research Program on Inflammatory Bowel Disease, The Eli and Edythe Broad Foundation grant number IBD-0222R. The funders had no role in study design, data collection and analysis, decision to publish, or preparation of the manuscript.

Competing Interests: The authors have declared that no competing interests exist.

* E-mail: sans@dr.teknon.es

Introduction

The pancreatitis-associated protein (PAP), also known as regenerating islet-derived protein 3 β (Reg3β) in mice, is a soluble calcium-dependent carbohydrate-binding protein which is expressed by intestinal epithelial cells.[1] It has been shown that colonization of germ-free mice with pathogens increases the expression PAP/Reg3β in the murine ileum and that this protein is directly bactericidal for gram-positive bacteria.[1] PAP/Reg3β also plays a protective role against intestinal translocation of gram-negative bacteria probably through interference with virulence mechanisms or host responses to these pathogens.[1] PAP/Reg3β triggers bacterial aggregation and displays bactericidal activity through its ability to directly bind some carbohydrate components of peptidoglycan.[2,3] Recently, a protective role has been proposed for PAP/Reg3β in liver and pancreas, which is apparently independent of its bactericidal properties.[4,5] *In vitro* studies showed that this protein plays an essential role in the negative regulation of cytokine signaling.[6,7]

The gastrointestinal tract and the pancreas are major sources of PAP/Reg3β.[2,8] In the colon, PAP/Reg3β is primarily secreted in the lumen by goblet cells and metaplastic Paneth cells[9] and in the *lamina propria* by intraepithelial lymphocytes[10]. Colonic expression of PAP/Reg3β is higher during inflammation-induced colorectal cancer and in the course of acute and chronic chemically-induced colitis in mice, whereas no significant changes are observed during the recovery phase.[11–13] In human subjects, PAP/Reg3β is over-expressed in the intestinal mucosa of patients with inflammatory bowel disease (IBD).[9,11,14] Importantly, clinical and endoscopic disease severity seems to correlate with serum PAP/Reg3β in parallel with C reactive protein (CRP) levels and erythrocyte sedimentation rate.[9]

The natural history of IBD is unpredictable and characterized by a succession of relapses and remissions. Furthermore, an overall 25–30% of therapy-refractoriness is seen, regardless of the available therapies.[15,16] This usually results in a significant delay until the appropriate treatment is started and also in accumulation of adverse events. To help predicting clinical relapses in IBD, valuable non-invasive biomarkers are eagerly awaited. Previous preliminary data suggests that measurements of serum PAP/Reg3β have fine sensitivity and specificity in active ileal CD with positive and negative predictive values of 84% and 81%, respectively[14].

Collectively, our hypothesis is that an aberrant production of PAP/Reg3β takes place in IBD and that the measurement of PAP/Reg3β in humans could function as an inflammation marker with future clinical application. Our aim was to determine the clinical value of PAP/Reg3β testing in predicting clinical relapse in CD and UC patients.

Materials and Methods

Study design and definitions

This is a 12-month prospective study that included consecutive patients with inactive UC and CD recruited at the Hospital Clinic of Barcelona, in a 6-month period. All enrolled patients had an established diagnosis of IBD confirmed by standard radiological, endoscopic and histological features. Since endoscopy had not been performed before inclusion in most patients, the partial Mayo Clinic score (pMS) was used to establish remission in UC patients and the Harvey-Bradshaw (HB) Index was used for CD patients. Patients were considered in remission and suitable for study inclusion if they presented pMS<3 or HB≤4 and normal levels of CRP and calprotectin. Patients with previously known intestinal disorders or inflammatory diseases other than IBD, acute or chronic pancreatitis or chronic renal failure were excluded to avoid possible confounders in the PAP/Reg3β measurement.

During the follow-up, disease activity was evaluated by the same clinical scores used to define remission at inclusion (pMS or the HB index). At each visit, serum and fecal samples were collected to determine CRP and fecal calprotectin levels as standard biomarkers currently used in clinical practice. As the samples for CRP and calprotectin measurements were collected on the same day of the visit, they were not used to determine disease activity. For the PAP/Reg3ß measurements in sera and stool, blood and fecal samples were also collected at each visit and stored at −80 for posterior analysis.

After inclusion, patients were followed every 3 months until clinical disease activity was detected or the scheduled 12-month follow-up was completed. Data regarding demographics and disease description were collected from patient's charts. UC and CD characteristics were defined according to the Montreal Classification.

PAP, Calprotectin and CRP measurements

Serum and fecal PAP/Reg3β was measured using a commercially available ELISA kit (Dynabio SA, Marseille, France) at the Institut Pasteur de Lille and results were expressed as ng of PAP/Reg3β per ml of serum or ng of PAP/Reg3β per mg of fecal material. The quantitative measurement of fecal calprotectin was performed at the Institut Pasteur de Lille by ELISA and results are given as ng/mg of stool sample. The CRP measurement was performed at the Hospital Clinic of Barcelona, and an elevated CRP was defined as higher than 0.8 mg/dL according to the

hospitals standard normal range. The measurement of all biological samples was investigator-blinded.

Ethical issues

This Study was approved by the Ethics Committee of Hospital Clinic of Barcelona, Spain. All patients gave their written informed consent before enrolment. Data was anonymously analysed to preserve patient's confidentiality.

Statistical analysis

Qualitative variables were expressed using frequencies. Continuous variables were expressed using median and interquartile range for demographics and mean with standard error of the mean (SEM) for laboratory measurements. A Kolmogorov–Smirnov test was used to evaluate whether serum and fecal PAP/Reg3ß, CRP and calprotectin values followed a normal distribution. Student's t tests or the Wilcoxon–Mann–Whitney test were performed for these continuous variables. A P-value<0.05 was considered statistically significant. The global yield of the serum PAP/Reg3ß to predict IBD relapse was calculated using the area under the ROC (receiver operating characteristic) curve.

Results

Patients characteristics, follow-up and relapse rate

UC patients. 74 patients were enrolled. About 35% of the recruited UC patients had disease limited to the rectum, 42% extensive disease and 23% left-sided involvement. Additional data on patients characteristics are shown in **Table 1.** 67 patients completed the scheduled 12-month follow-up. 7 patients were excluded: 5 patients as a result of initiating treatment for disease activity on their own before stool and serum sample collection, 1 refused to continue in the study and 1 moved to a different city.

CD patients. 66 patients were enrolled in the longitudinal study and 62 completed the follow-up. 34 had ileal disease (52%), 10 colonic (15%), 21 Ileocolonic (32%) and 1 patient upper GI disease (1%). Regarding disease behavior, most patients had non-stricturing non-penetrating disease. Additional information on patients characteristics are also shown in **Table 1.** In addition to the 62 recruited patients who continued in the study, 4 patients were excluded: 1 as a result of not reporting a flare and auto-medication and 3 refused to continue in the study.

Relapse rates. Overall, 7 CD (11.2%) and 17 UC (25.3%) patients who completed the follow-up had disease activity during the 1-year follow-up period, **Figure 1.** Most patients with disease activity in the CD group had mild disease according to the HB index (5−7 points) and only 2 patients had moderate disease (8−16 points) with no patients with severe flare (>16 points). For UC patients, all patients had a moderate-severe flare with pMS always higher than 5 points.

Mean serum and fecal PAP/Reg3β, CRP and calprotectin in UC

Mean values for serum and fecal PAP/Reg3β, CRP and calprotectin in UC are shown in **Figure 2**. Mean serum (**Figure 2C**) and fecal (**Figure 2D**) PAP/Reg3β levels were similar in relapsing and inactive UC patients. In contrast, serum CRP and fecal calprotectin levels (**Figures 2A and 2B**) were higher at disease relapse compared with patients in remission (p<0.005). In addition, no differences were observed in serum and fecal PAP/Reg3β between active and relapsing UC patients at any time point, including the visit prior to flare diagnosis.

Table 1. Main characteristics of CD and UC patients.

Characteristics	CD patients	UC patients
Number of patients	66	74
Male	35 (53)	35 (47)
Age at diagnosis (years)	30 (25–44)	34 (27–45)
Disease duration (months)	90 (53–120)	90 (48–149)
Disease location		
Ileal/Proctitis	34 (52)	26 (35)
Colonic/Left-sided	10 (15)	17 (23)
Ileocolonic/Extensive	21 (32)	31 (42)
Upper GI	1 (1)	
Perianal disease	10 (15)	
Extraintestinal manifestations	17 (26)	19 (26)
Disease behavior		
Inflammatory	36 (55)	
Stricturing	19 (29)	
Penetrating	11 (17)	
Bowel resection	20 (30)	
Maintenance therapy		
5-ASA	1 (2)	47 (39)
Immunosuppressants	32 (48)	20 (15)
Anti-TNF	6 (9)	2 (2)
No treatment	29 (44)	7 (6)

Categorical variables are represented as frequencies (percentages) and continuous variables are represented as median and inter-quartile range.

Mean serum and fecal PAP/Reg3β, CRP and calprotectin in CD

Mean values for serum and fecal PAP/Reg3β, CRP and calprotectin in CD are shown in **Figure 3**. Serum CRP (**Figure 3A**) and PAP/Reg3β (**Figure 3C**) levels were higher at disease relapse compared with patients in remission (p<0.0005 and p<0.05 respectively). Likewise, serum CRP (**Figure 3A**) and PAP/Reg3β (**Figure 3C**) were also increased at the visit prior to disease relapse (p<0.05). In contrast, fecal calprotectin (**Figure 3B**) and fecal PAP/Reg3β (**Figure 3D**) levels were similar in relapsing and inactive CD patients.

Receiver operating characteristics (ROC) analysis

Given the differences regarding serum PAP/Reg3β levels between CD patients in flare and remission, the efficacy of serum PAP/Reg3β as a diagnostic marker for intestinal inflammation was evaluated. The area under the ROC curve to predict CD relapse using PAP/Reg3β was 0.69 (**Figure 4**). The best global cutoff point was 16.85 ng/ml (sensitivity 50%, specificity 73%). ROC curves for serum PAP/Reg3β in UC patients and in IBD patients in general are also shown (**Figure 4**).

Mean serum and fecal PAP/Reg3β during follow-up in patients in remission

During remission, serum PAP/Reg3β (**Figure 5A**), fecal PAP/Reg3β (**Figure 5B**) and calprotectin levels were stable over time. Surprisingly, fecal PAP/Reg3β (**Figure 5B**), but not systemic (**Figure 5A**), was barely detectable in inactive UC patients when compared with CD patients. In contrast, no differences in fecal calprotectin levels were observed between UC and CD patients during remission (**Figure 5C**).

Discussion

Growing evidence indicates that mucosal healing is a surrogate marker of sustained remission in CD and UC and should be the ultimate therapeutic goal in the management of IBD patients.[17] Endoscopic evaluation is still the gold standard for assessment of mucosal healing though the procedure is invasive and costly.[18] As alternative non-invasive inflammatory markers, increased fecal levels of calprotectin and lactoferrin indicate intestinal inflammation of any cause, showing good positive predictive values for endoscopically active disease in IBD.[18] As for serum CRP, however, these fecal parameters lack specificity for IBD-related mucosal inflammation, being also elevated in the infectious involvement of the gut.[19−21] In addition, many patients in clinical practice have endoscopically active inflammation and fecal protein and CRP levels within the normal range.[18] New and better non-invasive diagnostic tools, therefore, are urgently needed.

The notion that intestinal PAP/Reg3β production is increased in active IBD patients had already been suggested by studies measuring PAP/Reg3β mRNA in intestinal tissue.[11,22,23] In addition, PAP/Reg3β levels were previously shown to be elevated in sera of patients with IBD compared with controls.[9,14] In the most recent study, performed by Gironella et al, UC and CD patients had higher serum PAP/Reg3β levels than controls even in

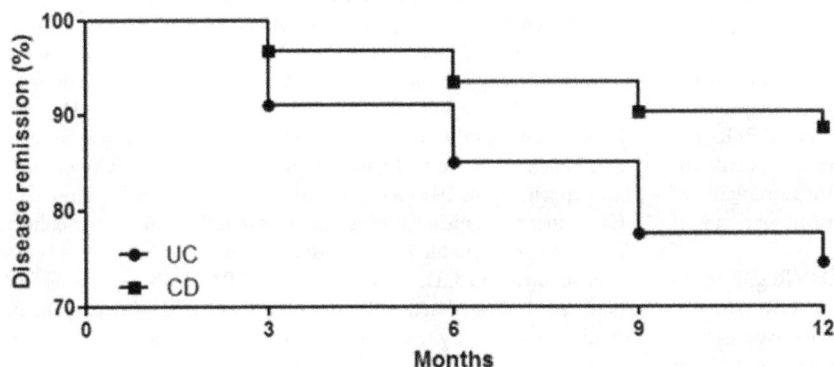

Figure 1. Remission rates in CD (n = 62) and UC (n = 67) patients over the 12-month period of follow-up. 17 out of the 67 UC patients (25%) who completed the follow-up had disease activity with a mean pMS score of 8. In the CD leg, 7 out of the 62 patients (11%) had clinical disease activity with a mean HB index of 6.

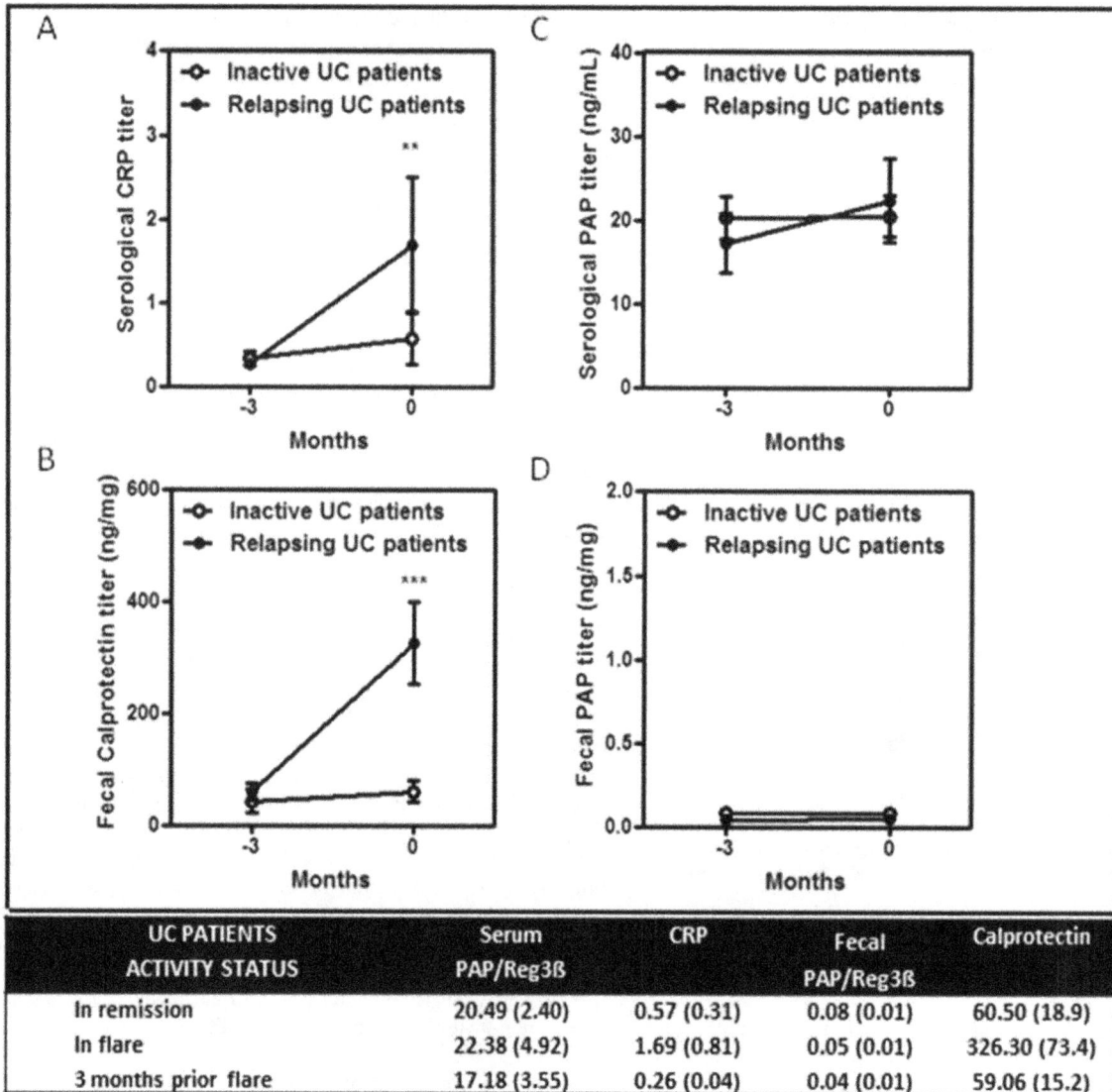

UC PATIENTS ACTIVITY STATUS	Serum PAP/Reg3ß	CRP	Fecal PAP/Reg3ß	Calprotectin
In remission	20.49 (2.40)	0.57 (0.31)	0.08 (0.01)	60.50 (18.9)
In flare	22.38 (4.92)	1.69 (0.81)	0.05 (0.01)	326.30 (73.4)
3 months prior flare	17.18 (3.55)	0.26 (0.04)	0.04 (0.01)	59.06 (15.2)

Figure 2. Graphics for mean serum and fecal PAP/Reg3β, CRP and calprotectin levels in UC patients at disease relapse and 3 months before the diagnosis of disease activity. In the table, mean values and standard error of the mean of serum and fecal PAP/Reg3β (ng/ml in serum and ng/mg in stool), CRP (mg/dL) and calprotectin (ng/mg) in UC patients in remission, flare and 3 months before the episode of disease activity.

disease remission. In contrast to current non-invasive diagnostic markers available in clinical practice, the authors showed that the increase in serum PAP/Reg3β followed in parallel with disease activity and it seemed to be specific for IBD as protein levels were not elevated in subjects with infectious diarrhea.[9] These previous findings led us to hypothesize that higher levels of PAP/Reg3β could function as a disease activity serological marker specific for IBD-related inflammation and that prospective measurements of this protein could predict future disease activity in patients in clinical remission.

In keeping with these previous data, serum PAP/Reg3β levels were higher at disease relapse than in inactive CD patients. Importantly, patients with active disease also had increased levels of PAP/Reg3β compared with subjects in remission at the visit prior to disease flare suggesting that this marker could help predict future clinical relapse. As serum PAP/Reg3β, serum CRP was also elevated at these two time points, at clinical recognizable disease

flare and 3 months before activity was diagnosed. Nevertheless, in the Receiver operating characteristics (ROC) analysis, serum PAP/Reg3β had poor predictive diagnostic accuracy to detect disease activity in patients with CD. We could not confirm, therefore, the findings of a previous study performed by Desjeux et al. which found that a serum PAP concentration above 50 ng/mL indicated active CD with a good accuracy (sensitivity of 60% and specificity of 94%).[14] In this regard, the small number of CD patients relapsing during the 1-year follow-up in our cohort might be accountable for these differences.

In contrast to CD, an increase in PAP/Reg3β levels was not detected in sera of active UC subjects compared with patients in remission. Contrary to the study by Gironella et al [9] which found higher levels of serum PAP/Reg3β in random UC samples compared with controls, the present study has the strength of being the first to follow patients prospectively with several PAP/Reg3β measurements during different time points. One can

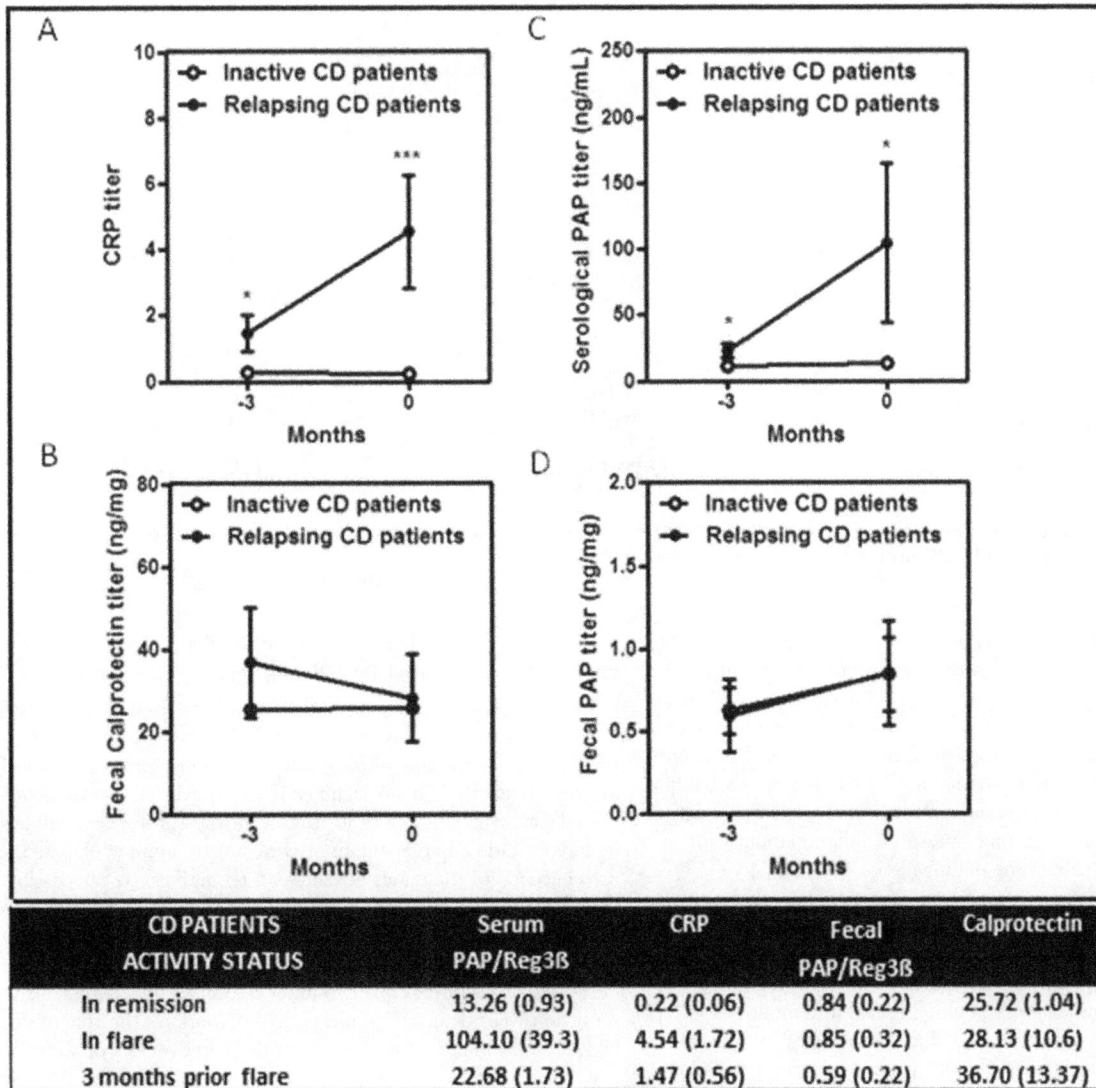

CD PATIENTS ACTIVITY STATUS	Serum PAP/Reg3ß	CRP	Fecal PAP/Reg3ß	Calprotectin
In remission	13.26 (0.93)	0.22 (0.06)	0.84 (0.22)	25.72 (1.04)
In flare	104.10 (39.3)	4.54 (1.72)	0.85 (0.32)	28.13 (10.6)
3 months prior flare	22.68 (1.73)	1.47 (0.56)	0.59 (0.22)	36.70 (13.37)

Figure 3. Graphics for mean serum and fecal PAP/Reg3β, CRP and calprotectin levels in CD patients at disease relapse and 3 months before the diagnosis of disease activity. In the table, mean values and standard error of the mean of serum and fecal PAP/Reg3β (ng/ml in serum and ng/mg in stool), CRP (mg/dL) and calprotectin (ng/mg) in CD patients in remission, flare and 3 months before the episode of disease activity.

hypothesize that, even though an elevated clinical score was measured, patients with UC in this series did not have actual intestinal inflammation. In our study, however, disease activity in UC patients was not only documented with elevation in the clinical activity score but this group also had significant elevations of serum CRP and fecal calprotectin compared with patients in remission. Our results support the notion that there is no role for the measurement of PAP/Reg3β in sera of UC patients. In keeping with this finding, Desjeux *et al.* found that an increase in serum PAP/Reg3β was specific for ileal inflammation as CD patients with active colonic disease had normal levels of PAP/Reg3β compared with controls.[14]

When it comes to the utility of PAP/Reg3β measurements in stool, results are more clearly negative. In this regard, there were no differences in fecal PAP/Reg3β levels in CD regardless of disease activity. Surprisingly, though active CD patients had a marked increase in CRP compared with subjects in remission, no differences with respect to fecal calprotectin were found at any

time point. The lower sensitivity of calprotectin to assess proximal gut inflammation [18] (most active patients presented ileal or upper GI inflammation) and the low number of CD patients who had clinical activity in our cohort could account for these results. The fact that there were also no differences in fecal PAP/Reg3β levels between active UC patients and subjects in remission further indicates that there is no role for fecal PAP/Reg3β in the assessment of IBD-related gut inflammation.

Overall, we do not recommend PAP/Reg3β testing in patients with UC. In contrast, in CD patients, the low relapse rate in our cohort makes it difficult to definitely exclude the potential utility of PAP/Reg3β, especially for serological measurements. Given that patients were in remission at inclusion, it is likely that CD patients with mild disease course were selected. Accordingly, most active CD patients had only mild disease activity and no patient with a severe flare was detected.

Our study is the first to report on the patterns of fecal and serum PAP/Reg3β levels over time in IBD in remission. In these patients,

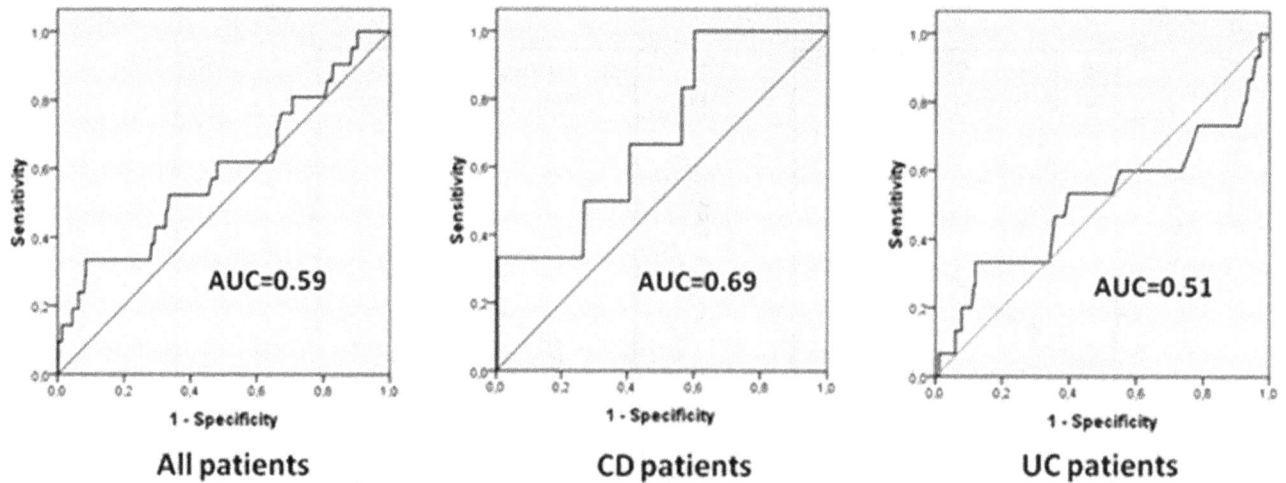

Figure 4. Area under the receiver operating characteristic (ROC) curve to predict inflammatory bowel disease relapse using serum PAP/Reg3β determination in CD, UC and in the combined group of IBD subjects.

serum and fecal PAP/Reg3β levels were very stable during the 12-month follow-up. Interestingly, a constant decreased intraluminal secretion of PAP/Reg3β in UC patients with no disease activity was observed. As mentioned before, this protein is believed to have an important role in the homeostasis of the intestine. It has been suggested that an increased production of PAP/Reg3β probably related to hyperplasia/metaplasia of Paneth cells might have anti-inflammatory effects in chronic intestinal inflammation with a potential protective role in the pathogenesis of IBD.[9]

Two mechanisms have been proposed to explain these anti-inflammatory properties, both through down-regulation of NFkB. First, NFkB-dependent secretion of pro-inflammatory cytokines in the intestine of IBD subjects was shown to be down-regulated by PAP/Reg3β in endothelial cells, epithelial cells and monocytes.[9] Second, it has been demonstrated that PAP/Reg3β can inhibit leukocyte recruitment into the bowel by monitoring up-regulation of E-selectin, ICAM-1, and VCAM-1.[9] Sustained low intraluminal levels of PAP/Reg3β, therefore, could impact the immunological balance of the intestinal mucosa in these patients, contributing to the pathogenesis of bowel chronic inflammation.

These interesting findings linking for the first time UC and low intraluminal secretion of PAP/Reg3β require further evaluation.

In conclusion, our study further confirms that serum PAP/Reg3β levels are increased in active CD patients and show that these serum levels are also elevated 3 months prior to clinical activity. Even though no significant predictive value was determined for serum PAP/Reg3β in CD, further prospective studies including endoscopic evaluation, with larger number of patients are needed to definitely exclude this marker as a possible diagnostic tool in this setting. On the contrary, fecal PAP/Reg3β concentrations are not associated with disease activity in both CD and UC patients and have no clinical utility. Constant marked decreased levels of PAP/Reg3β in fecal samples of UC patients in remission were detected requiring further work on the role of this alleged anti-inflammatory protein in the pathogenesis of IBD.

Author Contributions

Conceived and designed the experiments: MS MC. Performed the experiments: TN MJE MJS SPD TG MP JP ER JI JCD. Analyzed the

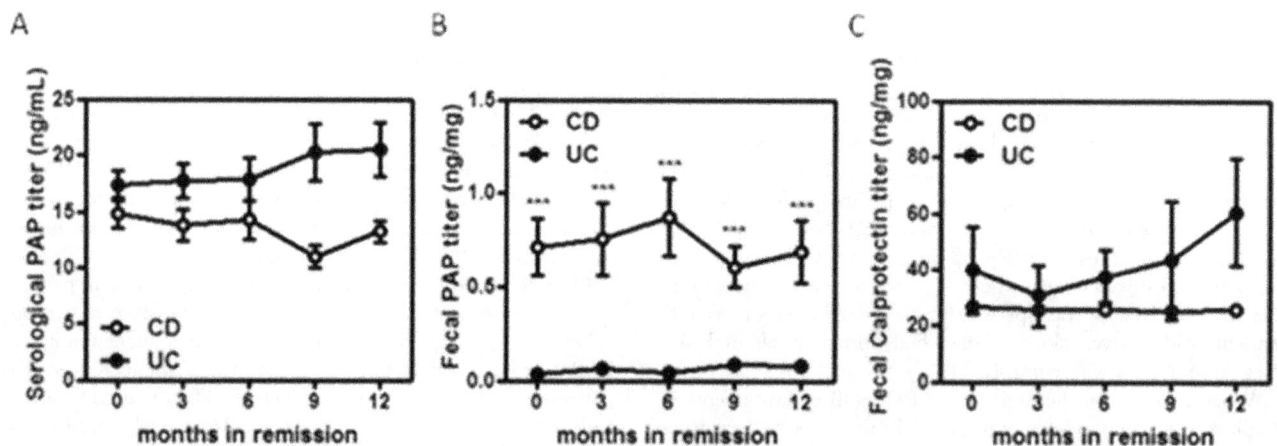

Figure 5. Graphics representing the mean serum and fecal PAP/Reg3β and calprotectin levels at different time points over time in UC and CD patients in remission.

data: TN MJE. Contributed reagents/materials/analysis tools: MJS SPD TG MP JP ER JI JCD. Wrote the paper: TN MJE.

References

1. van Ampting MT, Loonen LM, Schonewille AJ, Konings I, Vink C, et al. (2012) Intestinally secreted C-type lectin Reg3b attenuates salmonellosis but not listeriosis in mice. Infect Immun 80: 1115–1120.

2. Iovanna J, Orelle B, Keim V, Dagorn JC (1991) Messenger RNA sequence and expression of rat pancreatitis-associated protein, a lectin-related protein overexpressed during acute experimental pancreatitis. J Biol Chem 266: 24664–24669.

3. Cash HL, Whitham CV, Behrendt CL, Hooper LV (2006) Symbiotic bacteria direct expression of an intestinal bactericidal lectin. Science 313: 1126–1130.

4. Moniaux N, Song H, Darnaud M, Garbin K, Gigou M, et al. (2011) Human hepatocarcinoma-intestine-pancreas/pancreatitis-associated protein cures fas-induced acute liver failure in mice by attenuating free-radical damage in injured livers. Hepatology 53: 618–627.

5. Baeza N, Sanchez D, Christa L, Guy-Crotte O, Vialettes B, et al. (2001) Pancreatitis-associated protein (HIP/PAP) gene expression is upregulated in NOD mice pancreas and localized in exocrine tissue during diabetes. Digestion 64: 233–239.

6. Gironella M, Folch-Puy E, LeGoffic A, Garcia S, Christa L, et al. (2007) Experimental acute pancreatitis in PAP/HIP knock-out mice. Gut 56: 1091–1097.

7. Folch-Puy E, Granell S, Dagorn JC, Iovanna JL, Closa D (2006) Pancreatitis-associated protein I suppresses NF-kappa B activation through a JAK/STAT-mediated mechanism in epithelial cells. J Immunol 176: 3774–3779.

8. Iovanna JL, Keim V, Bosshard A, Orelle B, Frigerio JM, et al. (1993) PAP, a pancreatic secretory protein induced during acute pancreatitis, is expressed in rat intestine. Am J Physiol 265: G611–G618.

9. Gironella M, Iovanna JL, Sans M, Gil F, Penalva M, et al. (2005) Anti-inflammatory effects of pancreatitis associated protein in inflammatory bowel disease. Gut 54: 1244–1253.

10. Ismail AS, Behrendt CL, Hooper LV (2009) Reciprocal interactions between commensal bacteria and gamma delta intraepithelial lymphocytes during mucosal injury. J Immunol 182: 3047–3054.

11. Ogawa H, Fukushima K, Naito H, Funayama Y, Unno M, et al. (2003) Increased expression of HIP/PAP and regenerating gene III in human inflammatory bowel disease and a murine bacterial reconstitution model. Inflamm Bowel Dis 9: 162–170.

12. Rakoff-Nahoum S, Medzhitov R (2007) Regulation of spontaneous intestinal tumorigenesis through the adaptor protein MyD88. Science 317: 124–127.

13. Mizoguchi E, Xavier RJ, Reinecker HC, Uchino H, Bhan AK, et al. (2003) Colonic epithelial functional phenotype varies with type and phase of experimental colitis. Gastroenterology 125: 148–161.

14. Desjeux A, Barthet M, Barthellemy S, Dagorn JC, Hastier P, et al. (2002) Serum measurements of pancreatitis associated protein in active Crohn's disease with ileal location. Gastroenterol Clin Biol 26: 23–28.

15. Munkholm P, Langholz E, Davidsen M, Binder V (1995) Disease activity courses in a regional cohort of Crohn's disease patients. Scand J Gastroenterol 30: 699–706.

16. Cosnes J, Gower-Rousseau C, Seksik P, Cortot A (2011) Epidemiology and natural history of inflammatory bowel diseases. Gastroenterology 140: 1785–1794.

17. Papi C, Fasci-Spurio F, Rogai F, Settesoldi A, Margagnoni G, et al. (2013) Mucosal healing in inflammatory bowel disease: Treatment efficacy and predictive factors. Dig Liver Dis 45: 978–985.

18. Van AG, Dignass A, Panes J, Beaugerie L, Karagiannis J, et al. (2010) The second European evidence-based Consensus on the diagnosis and management of Crohn's disease: Definitions and diagnosis. J Crohns Colitis 4: 7–27.

19. Shastri YM, Bergis D, Povse N, Schafer V, Shastri S, et al. (2008) Prospective multicenter study evaluating fecal calprotectin in adult acute bacterial diarrhea. Am J Med 121: 1099–1106.

20. Chen CC, Huang JL, Chang CJ, Kong MS (2012) Fecal calprotectin as a correlative marker in clinical severity of infectious diarrhea and usefulness in evaluating bacterial or viral pathogens in children. J Pediatr Gastroenterol Nutr 55: 541–547.

21. Sykora J, Siala K, Huml M, Varvarovska J, Schwarz J, et al. (2010) Evaluation of faecal calprotectin as a valuable non-invasive marker in distinguishing gut pathogens in young children with acute gastroenteritis. Acta Paediatr 99: 1389–1395.

22. Dieckgraefe BK, Stenson WF, Korzenik JR, Swanson PE, Harrington CA (2000) Analysis of mucosal gene expression in inflammatory bowel disease by parallel oligonucleotide arrays. Physiol Genomics 4: 1–11.

23. Lawrance IC, Fiocchi C, Chakravarti S (2001) Ulcerative colitis and Crohn's disease: distinctive gene expression profiles and novel susceptibility candidate genes. Hum Mol Genet 10: 445–456.

21

Systemic and Mucosal Immune Reactivity upon *Mycobacterium avium* ssp. *paratuberculosis* Infection in Mice

Arzu Koc[1◑], **Imke Bargen**[2◑], **Abdulhadi Suwandi**[2], **Martin Roderfeld**[1], **Annette Tschuschner**[1], **Timo Rath**[1,3], **Gerald F. Gerlach**[4], **Mathias Hornef**[5], **Ralph Goethe**[6], **Siegfried Weiss**[2¶], **Elke Roeb**[1*¶]

1 Justus-Liebig-University Giessen, Department of Gastroenterology, Giessen, Germany, 2 Helmholtz Centre for Infection Research, Molecular Immunology, Braunschweig, Germany, 3 Medical Clinic 1, Friedrich-Alexander University Erlangen-Nuernberg, Erlangen, Germany, 4 IVD GmbH, Hannover, Germany, 5 Department of Microbiology, Hannover Medical School, Hannover, Germany, 6 Institute for Microbiology, Department of Infectious Diseases, University of Veterinary Medicine Hannover, Hannover, Germany

Abstract

Mycobacterium avium ssp. paratuberculosis (MAP) is the cause of Johne's disease, an inflammatory bowel disorder of ruminants. Due to the similar pathology, MAP was also suggested to cause Crohn's disease (CD). Despite of intensive research, this question is still not settled, possibly due to the lack of versatile mouse models. The aim of this study was to identify basic immunologic mechanisms in response to MAP infection. Immune compromised C57BL/6 $Rag2^{-/-}$ mice were infected with MAP intraperitoneally. Such chronically infected mice were then reconstituted with $CD4^+$ and $CD8^+$ T cells 28 days after infection. A systemic inflammatory response, detected as enlargement of the spleen and granuloma formation in the liver, was observed in mice infected and reconstituted with $CD4^+$ T cells. Whereby inflammation in infected and $CD4^+CD45RB^{hi}$ T cell reconstituted animals was always higher than in the other groups. Reconstitution of infected animals with $CD8^+$ T cells did not result in any inflammatory signs. Interestingly, various markers of inflammation were strongly up-regulated in the colon of infected mice reconstituted with $CD4^+CD45RB^{lo/int}$ T cells. We propose, the usual non-colitogenic $CD4^+CD45RB^{lo/int}$ T cells were converted into inflammatory T cells by the interaction with MAP. However, the power of such cells might be not sufficient for a fully established inflammatory response in the colon. Nevertheless, our model system appears to mirror aspects of an inflammatory bowel disease (IBD) like CD and Johne's diseases. Thus, it will provide an experimental platform on which further knowledge on IBD and the involvement of MAP in the induction of CD could be acquired.

Editor: Mathias Chamaillard, Inserm, France

Funding: This work was supported by the German Ministry for Science and Education (BMBF; ZooMAP 01KI1003E, ZooMAP 01KI0750, ZooMAPII 01KI1003A, 01KI1003B), by grants from the Deutsche Forschungsgemeinschaft (RO 957/8-1), the von-Behring-Roentgen Foundation and the University Medical Center Giessen and Marburg (10/2012 GI, UKGM). The funders had no role in study design, data collection and analysis, decision to publish, or preparation of the manuscript.

Competing Interests: One of the authors is employed by a commercial company IVD GmbH.

* E-mail: Elke.Roeb@innere.med.uni-giessen.de

◑ These authors contributed equally to this work.

¶ These authors also contributed equally to this work.

Introduction

Crohn's disease (CD) belongs to the family of human inflammatory bowel diseases and is believed to result from an excessive mucosal immune response towards the enteric microbiota in a genetically susceptible host [1]. Its histopathological characteristics are very similar to Johne's disease, a chronic granulomatous inflammation of the small intestine of ruminants that is caused by *Mycobacterium avium* ssp. *paratuberculosis* (MAP). Due to the histomorphological similarities MAP has already been suggested to be involved in the pathogenesis of CD in 1913 [2]. Indeed, a number of studies reported the detection of MAP in material obtained from CD patients [3–6]. However, other groups could not confirm these results and could detect MAP in a significant number of apparently healthy individuals as well [7]. A possible causative role of MAP for CD is therefore still under debate.

MAP is one of the mycobacteria that exhibits a very long generation time. Similar to other species of this genus, MAP is able to survive even under harsh environmental conditions for long periods of time [8,9]. Infections are mainly observed in ruminants although sporadic infections of primates and many other species have been described [10]. In most instances, transmission occurs during the neonatal/infant period via the oral-faecal route and M cells are believed to represent the main mechanism of mucosal translocation followed by phagocytosis in subepithelial macrophages [11,12].

Similar to other pathogenic mycobacterial species, MAP is able to survive and proliferate in the phagosome. Infected macrophages might further function as "trojan horse" and facilitate dissemination of MAP to other tissues [11,13,14]. Animals develop clinical signs of infection as recently as months to years after infection. Weight loss, reduced lactation and chronic diarrhea associated with wasting and shedding of large numbers of bacteria are observed [15]. Histopathological analysis reveals severe intestinal mucosal inflammation and granulomas in the small and large intestine as well as the liver [16].

The delayed onset of disease after an extended period of latency led us to hypothesize that MAP might initially be controlled by the host's immune system. After impairment of immune function by stress or additional infection, proliferation of MAP might cause clinically apparent infection and fatal outcome. The well-described reactivity of both the innate as well as the adaptive immune system towards mycobacteria might then drive the inflammatory symptoms observed during manifest disease.

In order to simulate such a situation, we selected immune compromised mice that lack the recombination activating genes ($Rag^{-/-}$). These genes are required for the rearrangement of the gene segments forming the T and B cell receptors. As consequence, such mice lack cells of the adaptive immune system and are severely immune compromised [17]. Infection by intraperitoneal injection was selected since no *in vivo* mouse model of mucosal translocation has been reported. Infected mice were subsequently reconstituted with various T cell subpopulations and liver and intestinal tissues were screened for signs of immune activation such as granuloma formation or up-regulation of matrix metalloproteinases (MMPs), tissue inhibitors of metalloproteinases (TIMPs), Toll like receptors (TLR), and pro-inflammatory cytokines. MMPs are the most potent proteases in the turnover of the extracellular matrix [18] but also known to either stimulate or maintain inflammation by proteolytic processing of inflammatory cytokines [19]. Importantly, MMPs are known to play a critical role in mucosal barrier function and inflammatory bowel disease (IBD) [20,21].

CD45RB is a member of protein tyrosine phosphatase family expressed on leukocytes and known as an essential regulator in T lymphocytes [22]. Adoptive transfer of CD4$^+$CD45RB^{hi} T cells (naive T cells) from healthy wild-type to lymphopenic mice leads to colitis and small bowel inflammation at 5–8 weeks following T cell transfer which represents an important model to study specific T cells involvement in dysregulation [23]. Coinjection of CD4$^+$CD45RB^{lo} cells (activated/memory T cells) could prevent the development of colitis. It was shown that the CD4$^+$CD45RB^{lo} population contains CD25$^+$Foxp3$^+$ regulatory T cells (Treg cells), which are responsible for the regulatory activity of this T cells subset [24].

By T-cell reconstitution of MAP-infected immune compromised $Rag2^{-/-}$ mice we now show for the first time that MAP-induced systemic inflammation is mainly driven by CD4$^+$CD45RB^{hi} T cells. Under the influence of MAP CD4$^+$CD45RB$^{lo/int}$ T cells convert into effector cells during enteric mucosal inflammation.

Materials and Methods

Bacterial culture

The MAP strain DSM 44135 was cultured and prepared for infection as previously described [25]. For infection experiments, bacteria were transferred to Dulbecco's Modified Eagle Medium and bacterial suspensions were vortexed in the presence of glass beads (3 mm diameter) for 15 min, centrifuged for 10 min at 2900 g and washed with PBS. Infection doses were calculated by determining the optical density measured at 600 nm of the supernatants containing single bacteria. An OD$_{600}$ of 0.1 corresponds to 10^7 MAP/ml [26].

Animals

C57BL/6 $Rag2^{-/-}$ mice were bred at the animal facility of the Helmholtz Centre for Infection Research (HZI) and maintained under specific pathogen-free conditions. Wild type (WT) C57BL/6 mice were purchased from Janvier (France). All animal experiments were done at HZI using adult mice between 8 and 12 weeks of age. Intraperitoneal (i.p.) infection was done with 10^8 MAP in 200 µl PBS. Control mice were always inoculated with the same amount of PBS, respectively. This study was carried out in strict accordance with the German Law for the Protection of Animals. The protocol was approved by the Lower Saxony authorities (anim. exp. no. 33.11.42502-04-090/08, Niedersächsisches Landesamt für Verbraucherschutz und Lebensmittelsicherheit).

Adoptive transfer experiments

Two groups of 4 mice each were inoculated i.p. with 10^8 CFU MAP in 200 µl PBS. Additionally, 2 groups of 4 mice each were inoculated i.p. with PBS as control. 28 days later one group of infected and one group of uninfected mice were reconstituted by adoptive transfer. Spleen cells from naive C57BL/6 wild type mice were used for reconstition of C57BL/6 $Rag2^{-/-}$ mice. In all groups recipient and donor mice were gender-matched. Murine spleens were flushed on ice with IMDM (Gibco BRL, Eggenstein, Germany) supplemented with 10% heat inactivated FCS and 0.25 mM β-mercaptoethanol. Red blood cells were lysed for 2 min in ACK lysis buffer (0.15 M NH$_4$Cl, 10 mM KHCO$_3$, 0.1 mM Na$_2$EDTA in ddH$_2$O) and B cells were removed using 25 µl/ml magnetic B cell removal beads (Invitrogen Dynabeads Mouse pan B (B220) 114.41D 4×10^8 beads/ml). Cells were then incubated for 7′ with 500 µl 1:500 diluted mouse serum (Biowest S2160-020) to block Fc receptors. The suspension was diluted to 14 ml with PBS and centrifuged 7′ at 1000 rpm (209×g). The pellet was resolved in 3 ml PBS and FcBlock (rat anti-mouse CD16/CD32 BD Pharmingen #5531422.4G2 0.01 µg/ml) and incubated for 7′ on ice. Cells were mixed with an equal volume of antibody solutions (1:1) and incubated for 15′ in the dark. Cells were then washed and incubated with PI (Sigma P4170, 0.5 µg/ml) or DAPI (Sigma 9564, 10 µg/ml) for live/dead discrimination. For sorting cells were gated on live cells leaving out doublets. Dependent on the set up the following cell populations were sorted using a FACSAriaII cell sorter (Becton Dickinson, NJ, USA. using FACSDiva software): CD3$^+$CD19$^-$CD11c$^-$CD4$^+$CD45RB$^{lo/int}$ (CD4$^+$CD45RB$^{lo/int}$ T cells), CD3$^+$CD19$^-$CD11c$^-$CD4$^+$CD45RB^{hi} (CD4$^+$CD45RB^{hi} T cells), CD3$^+$CD19$^-$CD11c$^-$CD8$^+$ (CD8$^+$ T cells). For staining the following antibodies were used: hamster anti mouse CD3e 145-2C11 PE (BD Pharmingen 20 µg/ml), rat anti mouse CD19 1D3 APC (BD Pharmingen 2 µg/ml), hamster anti mouse CD11c N418 PECy7 (eBioscience 6.7 µg/ml), rat anti mouse CD4 RM4-5 APCeFlour780 (eBioscience 10 µg/ml), rat anti mouse CD45RB 16A FITC (BD Pharmingen 1.7 µg/ml), rat anti mouse CD8a 53-6.7 PacificBlue (eBioscience 10 µg/ml). After sorting, the cells were counted and the cell number was adjusted to 2×10^6 cells in 150 µl PBS and injected i.v. Body weight of the mice was monitored regularly as read out for the general health of the animals. Four weeks after adoptive transfer the mice were sacrificed and organs were removed for further analysis.

Liver plating

Liver were homogenized with sterile PBS in the presence of sterile 3 mm glass beads 2 times for 20 seconds using the homogenizer FastPrep-24 (MP Biomedicals). The liver homogenates were plated on Middlebrook 7H10 agar (Difco TM) containing Mycobactin J (IDVet Innovative Technology). The plates were incubated at 37°C for up to 4 weeks. After this incubation time the plates were analyzed. Every single white dot was defined as one colony forming unit (CFU). The CFU of the whole plate were counted and the CFU/g liver was calculated according the dilution factor.

DNA preparation with Qiagen QIAmp DNA Stool kit

300 mg liver was homogenized with 1.4 ml buffer ASL and 0.1 mm, 1.4 mm and 3 mm glass beads 6 times 40″ with the MP FastPrep-24. After centrifugation for 1′ at 13000 rpm (16089×g), the solution was incubated 20′ at 95°C. For further steps Qiagen QIAmp DNA Stool kit was used due to manufacturers' instructions. The DNA was used for PCR as a 1:100 dilution in ddH_2O.

Polymerase chain reaction

Polymerase chain reaction (PCR) was done with Fermentas True Start Hot Start Taq DNA polymerase. Mastermix for one reaction was prepared as follows: 7.7 µl water (Ampuwa Fresenius Kabi), 1.6 µl $MgCl_2$, 2 µl buffer, 1 µl forward primer (5 pmol/µl), 1 µl reverse primer (5 pmol/µl), 1.6 µl dNTPs (10 mM dNTP mix Bioline), 0.1 µl Taq polymerase. 15 µl mastermix were mixed with 5 µl DNA. The PCR program was as follows: 3′ at 95°C 35 cycles of 30″ 95°C, 30″ 61°C and 30″ 72°C followed by 3′ 72°C and 5′ 8°C (peqLab Biotechnologie GmbH peqStar).

Primer: MAP-IS900-F 5′-AATGACGGTTACGGAGGTGGT-3′ and MAP-IS900-R 5′-GCTGCGCGTCGTCGTTAATA-3′

RNA extraction and mRNA expression

Shock-frozen tissue samples (10–20 mg) from the colon (middle part) and small intestine (end part) were homogenized with Precellys Ceramic Beads, 1.4 mm (Peqlab, Erlangen, Germany) and total cellular RNA was extracted using Qiagen RNeasy Mini Kit reagent (Qiagen, Hilden, Germany) according to the manufacturer's protocol. First strand cDNA synthesis was performed using iScript reverse transcriptase (Bio-Rad Laboratories CA), according to the manufacturer's instructions. qRT-PCR was performed in duplicates using a Mx3005P Cycler (Stratagene, La Jolla, CA). Primers were purchased from Qiagen, Hilden, Germany (Table S1). The specificity and sensitivity of the qPCR was confirmed by analysis of molecular weight and melting points of the products. The expression of the gene of interest was normalized against r18S mRNA. All data were analyzed by the $\Delta\Delta Ct$ model [27,28].

Immunohistological analysis

Immunohistological stainings of colon samples were performed as described [29].

Statistical analysis

Statistical analyses were performed with SPSS 19.0 software (SPSS Inc. Chicago, Illinois, USA). Considering not normally distributed parameters non-parametric tests were applied. The data were analysed using Mann-Whitney U-test. Results are presented as mean ± standard error of mean (SEM). A two-sided $p<0.05$ was considered significant.

Results

MAP Infection and T cell reconstitution of $Rag2^{-/-}$ mice

The experiments were outlined to simulate a situation in which MAP infected mice recover from cellular immune hyporesponsiveness. Immunocompromised $Rag2^{-/-}$ mice were left untreated or infected i.p. with 10^8 CFU MAP. After four weeks, animals

were reconstituted with purified total spleen cells (data not shown), CD4+ or CD8+ T cell subpopulations (Figure 1). The CD4+ T cells were further separated according the expression levels of CD45RB. Whereas CD45RB[hi] have previously been shown to promote mucosal inflammation in immune compromised mice, this phenotype is not observed after transfer of CD45RB[lo/int] cells [23].

Purity of the cell populations was verified prior to reconstitution by FACS re-analysis (Figure 1A). In addition, reconstituted mice were assessed for splenic CD4+ and CD8+ T cells. No CD8+ T cells were detected in 4 of 4 mice reconstituted with CD4+ T cells. Vice versa, in 4 of 4 mice reconstituted with CD8+ T-cells, no CD4+ T cells were found, thereby verifying the specificity of the reconstitutions (Figure 1B). Interestingly, the percentage of vital CD4+ T cells in reconstituted mice infected with MAP is higher compared with controls. Possibly MAP infection led to activation of such T cells. As a general indicator of health status, no changes in the body weight were observed after infection and/or reconstitution (Figure 2).

Signs of systemic inflammation in reconstituted MAP infected $Rag2^{-/-}$ mice

In addition, total organ weight of spleen tissue was assessed. Interestingly, spleens from 3 of 4 infected mice reconstituted with colitogenic CD4+CD45RB[hi] T cells exhibited markedly enhanced weight (Figure 3). In contrast, reconstitution of infected $Rag2^{-/-}$ mice with CD4+CD45RB[lo/int] or CD8+ T cells did not result in enhanced spleen weight in 2 of 4 mice (Figure 3).

MAP is known to induce liver granulomas in cattle. Similarly, granuloma formation has been observed in MAP infected wild type mice (data to be published). Therefore, liver tissues from all groups were formalin fixed and stained with haematoxylin/eosin. As expected no granulomas were observed in control $Rag2^{-/-}$ mice and non-reconstituted $Rag2^{-/-}$ mice infected with MAP (Figure S1). This finding is in accordance with the critical role of the adaptive immune system (and in particular the critical role of certain T cells) for the generation of granulomas. Also, no granulomas were observed in mice reconstituted with CD8+ T cells consistent with the previous finding that CD8+ T cells are not involved in granuloma formation [30,31].

Surprisingly, liver granulomas were found in 1 of 4 MAP infected mice reconstituted with CD4+CD45RB[lo/int] T lymphocytes but not in their uninfected counterparts (Figure 4 and Figure S1). In contrast, granulomas were observed in liver tissue of mice reconstituted with the colitogenic subpopulation of CD4+CD45RB[hi] T cells even in the absence of MAP infection. However, in MAP infected animals reconstituted with CD4+CD45RB[hi] T cells more and significantly larger granulomas were found in all 4 mice compared to mice that received CD4+CD45RB[hi] T cell reconstitution but no MAP infection (Figure 4 and Figure S1).

Thereby, it is apparent that MAP infection is either an absolute prerequisite for the development of T cell mediated granuloma formation (as seen for CD4+CD45RB[lo/int] T cells) or a strongly promoting factor in this process (as seen for CD4+CD45RB[hi] T cells). In addition, granulomas were only found in liver tissue in which MAP could be detected. Although MAP was only occasionally detected by Ziehl-Neelsen staining in liver sections of infected mice, the presence of low numbers of viable MAP was confirmed either by serial dilution and plating of liver homogenates (Figure 5) or alternatively by PCR (for results please refer to Table S2).

A

B

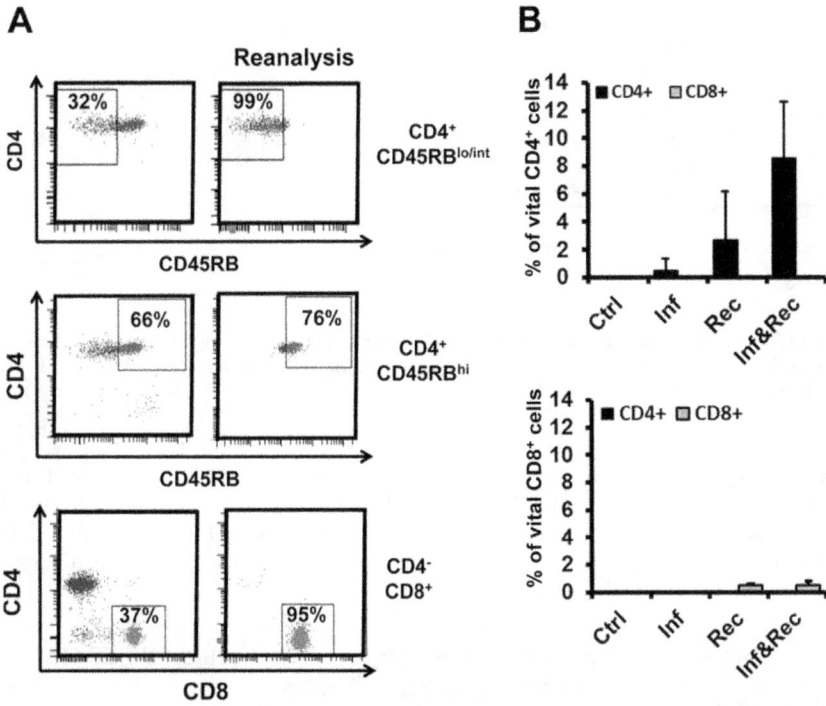

Figure 1. Adoptive transfer of T cell populations into MAP infected *Rag2*$^{-/-}$ mice. A. Sorting strategy and reanalysis of CD4$^+$CD45RB$^{lo/int}$, CD4$^+$CD45RB^{hi} and CD8$^+$ T cells from spleen of naïve mice. Gates were set to sort pure population of CD3$^+$CD19$^-$CD4$^+$CD45RB$^{lo/int}$, CD19$^-$CD3$^+$CD8$^-$CD4$^+$CD45RB^{hi}, CD3$^+$CD19$^-$CD4$^-$CD8$^+$ T cells. **B.** Analysis of reconstituted mice for CD4$^+$ and CD8$^+$ T cells four weeks after transfer i.e. day 56 of the experiment. Ctr – control; Inf – only infected with MAP at the beginning of the experiment, Rec – reconstituted with the T cell population indicated; Inf & Rec – infected at the beginning of the experiment and reconstituted after 4 weeks.

Colonic inflammatory response by CD4$^+$CD45RB$^{lo/int}$ T cells in MAP infected mice

CD4$^+$ T cells of the CD45RB^{hi} type are known to induce colitis in lymphopenic mice most likely due to the absence of regulatory T cells in this lymphocyte population. We therefore concentrated on the question whether CD4$^+$ T cells of the CD45RB$^{lo/int}$ type would be converted into inflammatory T cells by the interaction with MAP. We hypothesized that, in the presence of MAP, CD4$^+$CD45RB$^{lo/in}$ T cells could produce inflammatory factors by themselves or stimulate other cells to produce them, and thus be converted into a pro-inflammatory phenotype.

First, we analyzed tumor necrosis factor-α (*TNF*-α) and interleukin 1β (IL-1β). *TNF*-α is a potent pro-inflammatory cytokine with elevated levels found in several autoimmune diseases including rheumatoid arthritis and CD [32–34]. Consistent with our hypothesis, transcriptional levels of *TNF*-α were significantly increased (4.9-fold, p = 0.049) in the colon of mice with MAP infection and CD4$^+$CD45RB$^{lo/int}$ T-cell reconstitution, but not mice with MAP infection only (without concomitant T cell reconstitution) or those with CD4$^+$CD45RB$^{lo/int}$ reconstitution only. *IL-1β* expression was higher by trend in mice with MAP infection and CD4$^+$CD45RB$^{lo/int}$ T-cell reconstitution (Figure 6A).

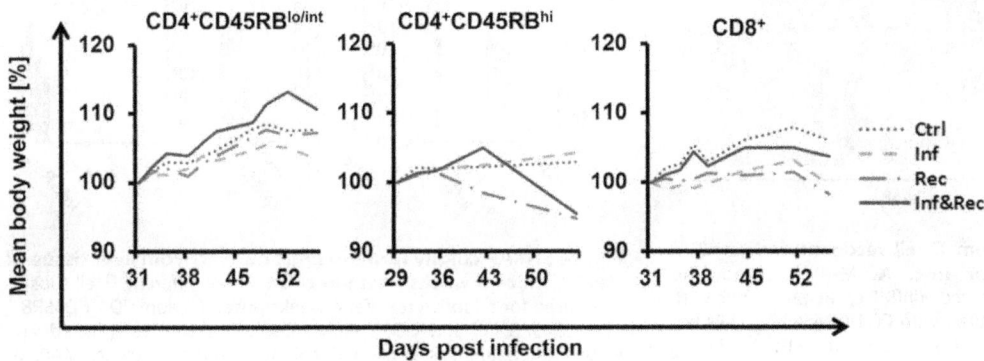

Figure 2. Body weight of *Rag2*$^{-/-}$ mice after MAP infection and/or T cell reconstitution. Infection with MAP led to hardly any decrease of body weight even not in the first week. Adoptive transfer of CD4$^+$CD45RB^{hi}, CD4$^+$CD45RB$^{lo/int}$ or CD8$^+$ T cells on day 28 had no influence on the body weight, neither of uninfected nor of infected mice. n = 4 mice in each group.

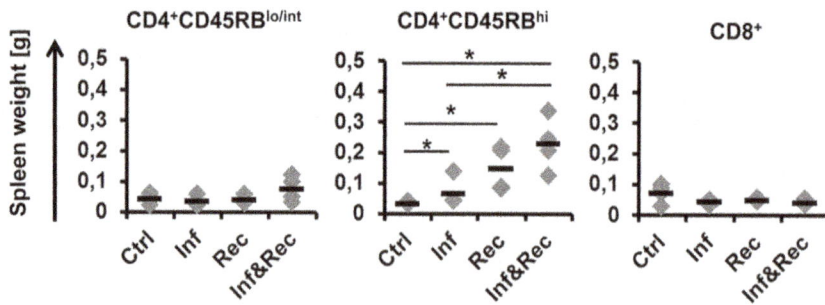

Figure 3. Increase of spleen weight in MAP infected and CD4⁺ T cell reconstituted *Rag2⁻/⁻* mice 8 weeks. Three different T cell subsets were used for adoptive transfer 4 weeks post infection: CD4⁺CD45RB^{hi}, CD4⁺CD45RB$^{lo/int}$ and CD8⁺. Each group with n = 4 mice. Mann-Whitney U-Test p = 0.05*, p = 0.01**. The experiment was carried out at least twice with similar results.

Having shown an increase of the pro-inflammatory cytokine *TNF-α* in the presence of MAP and CD4⁺CD45RB$^{lo/int}$ T cells, we turned our attention to factors responsible for maintaining inflammation and tissue destruction and therefore determined the expression levels of *MMPs* as well as their inhibitory regulators, the *TIMPs* [35,36].

As demonstrated in Figure 6B, a significant increased expression of *MMP-9* (4-fold, p = 0.043), *MMP-13* (4.5-fold, p = 0.021), *MMP-14* (2.6-fold, p = 0.043) and *TIMP-1* (3-fold, p = 0.021) was observed in MAP-infected *Rag2⁻/⁻* mice reconstituted with CD4⁺CD45RB$^{lo/int}$ T cells. Similarly to the results seen for *TNF-α*, these markers remained unaltered in their expression level in *Rag2⁻/⁻* mice infected with MAP only or those reconstituted with CD4⁺CD45RB$^{lo/int}$ T cells only. Thus, strengthening our hypothesis that both, MAP and CD4⁺CD45RB$^{lo/int}$ T cells, and possibly their interaction, are critical for the induction and maintenance of inflammation in the model used.

TLRs are critically involved in the recognition of microbe-associated molecular patterns and in the initiation of an innate immune response upon bacterial challenge. Therefore, we further quantified the expression of TLRs involved in the recognition of mycobacterial components. Consistent with its prominent role for the recognition of MAP [29,37,38], we found a significant upregulation of *TLR-6* (2.2-fold, p = 0.043) in mice that received both, MAP infection and concomitant CD4⁺CD45RB$^{lo/int}$ T-cell

reconstitution compared to mice with MAP infection or T cell reconstitution only. *TLR-2, -3,* and *-9* showed similar trends of expression in mice with MAP infection and CD4⁺CD45RB$^{lo/int}$ T-cell reconstitution, although did not reach statistical significance (Figure 6C).

Immunohistochemistry of MAP infected CD4⁺CD45RB$^{lo/int}$ reconstituted *Rag2⁻/⁻* mice

Despite the fact that the peritoneum was chosen as the site of MAP infection in the current study, MAP was occasionally detected in colonic tissue of all 4 MAP infected mice (reconstituted with CD4⁺CD45RB$^{lo/int}$) using a polyclonal antiserum against the protein MAP 1775 (Figure 7). In contrast, no staining was detected in non-infected animals, thereby confirming that these results were indeed due to the i.p. infection with MAP, but not due to an environmental presence of MAP. These results were further corroborated using a highly MAP-specific PCR, by which MAP transcripts were detected in the colon of all mice, that received MAP infections but not in non-infected controls. Interestingly, immunofluorescence staining demonstrated intracellular clusters of MAP associated with and surrounded by aggregates of CD45⁺ leukocytes (Figure 7A). Further, *MMP-9* expressing cells could be demonstrated in close proximity or directly adjacent to MAP clusters (Figure 7B).

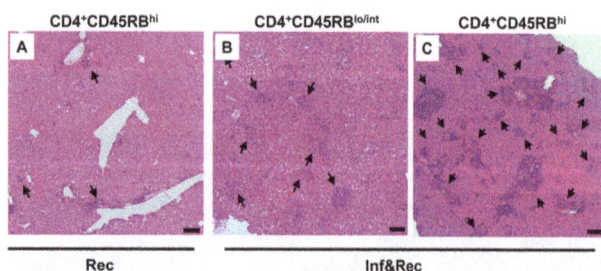

Figure 4. Histology of liver from T cell reconstituted *Rag2⁻/⁻* mice infected with MAP or not. A. MAP infected and CD4⁺CD45RB$^{lo/int}$ T cell reconstituted (Inf&Rec) *Rag2⁻/⁻* mice. **B.** Control of *Rag2⁻/⁻* mice reconstituted with CD4⁺CD45RB^{hi} T cells not infected with MAP. **C.** *Rag2⁻/⁻* mice infected with MAP and reconstituted with CD4⁺CD45RB^{hi} T cells. Controls are shown in Fig. S1. Arrow heads point at the granulomatous structures. Adoptive transfer of CD8⁺ T cells after MAP infection did not lead to formation of granulomatous structures. Bars depict 100 μm. The data are representative from 4 mice per group and the experiments were carried out at least twice with similar results.

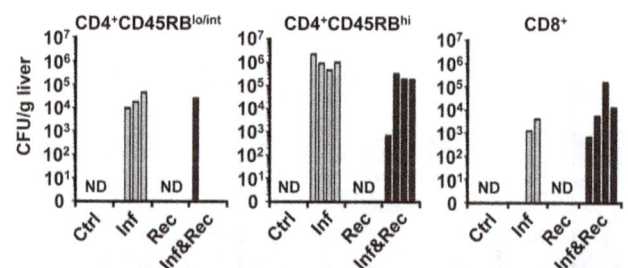

Figure 5. MAP colony forming units derived from liver tissue of *Rag2⁻/⁻* mice 8 weeks post infection. Three different T cell subsets were used for adoptive transfer 4 weeks post infection: CD4⁺CD45RB^{hi}, CD4⁺CD45RB$^{lo/int}$ and CD8⁺. Only infected as well as infected and reconstituted animals contained colony forming units i.e. MAP, as expected. Although all mice of a group were injected i.p. with 10⁸ MAP, plating 8 weeks later did not indicate a homogeneous infection. From some infected mice viable MAP could not be revealed from liver. Similar data were obtained using PCR. Each group n = 4 mice. The experiments were carried out twice with similar results.

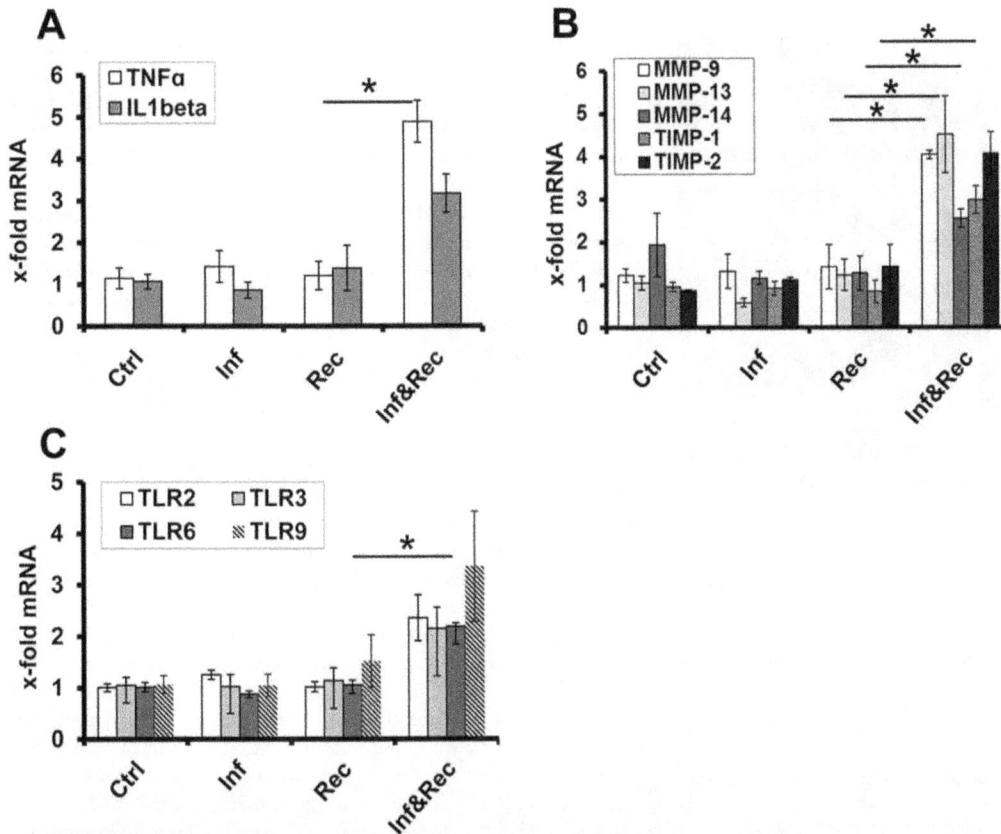

Figure 6. Colonic inflammatory response reconstitution of MAP infected $Rag2^{-/-}$ mice with CD4$^+$CD45RB$^{lo/int}$. A. Colonic expression of TNF-α and IL-1β. **B.** Colonic expression of MMP-9, MMP-13, MMP-14, TIMP-1 and TIMP-2. **C.** Colonic expression of TLRs. Mice had been infected i.p. with 10^8 CFU MAP and 4 weeks later reconstituted with CD4$^+$CD45RB$^{lo/int}$ T-cells. Reconstituted and MAP infected mice compared to mice with reconstitution only. No differences in expression of the indicated genes were found in samples without T-cell reconstitution (data not shown). The expression of the genes of interest was normalized against r18S RNA. Ctrl = $Rag2^{-/-}$ mice treated with PBS only; Inf = $Rag2^{-/-}$ mice infected with MAP; Rec = $Rag2^{-/-}$ mice reconstituted with CD4$^+$CD45RB$^{lo/int}$; Inf&Rec = $Rag2^{-/-}$ mice infected with MAP and reconstituted with CD4$^+$CD45RB$^{lo/int}$. n = 4. Bars depict median ± SEM. Statistical significance (p<0.05) is indicated by *.

Discussion

Based on pathological similarities between human CD and Johne's disease in ruminants MAP was suggested as causative agent of CD almost 100 year ago. However, epidemiological and clinical studies have since then failed to provide unambiguous evidence for a causative role of MAP in the pathogenesis of CD [15]. Geographical variation in MAP exposure, major technical difficulties to culture MAP from primary tissue samples and multiple variants of this complex disease entity might, however, have blurred the picture. In the past, the establishment of animal models and the use of defined, genetically homogenous groups of individuals facilitated deeper insights into fundamental questions of mucosal inflammation and provided clearly defined hypotheses to be subsequently investigated in humans. Unfortunately, no mouse or small animal model has been reported to date that would allow experimental approaches on the association of MAP with CD. One might argue that this, among other factors, might be one of the reasons why the potential role of MAP in the pathogenesis of CD still has remained unresolved.

In the present work we aimed to mimic the situation that might underlie the pathogenesis of CD and Johne's disease. We considered that MAP infection in ruminants takes place during the neonatal period, a transient period of immunosuppression, leading to manifest clinical disease in later years of life. Based on

these considerations, we injected MAP i.p. into immunocompromised $Rag2^{-/-}$ mice that lack B and T cells and by complementation with defined lymphocyte subpopulations subsequent to MAP infection. This approach allowed the identification of the cellular immune function responsible for MAP-induced inflammation. Although the way of infection utilized by us does not represent the physiological route of MAP infection, it consistently resulted in chronic infection within the current study. In this context the following is important to note: in contrast to i.p. injection, oral infection of adult mice with MAP does not allow reliable infection and thus is not suitable to study MAP host interaction [39]. Further, as shown within this study, i.p. infection leads to systemic spread of MAP, infection of liver tissue and significant infection-induced immunological alterations in the colon, thereby illustrating its potential value for the analysis of MAP-induced inflammation.

Using this approach, we are able to demonstrate that systemic inflammation, granuloma formation and intestinal expression of TNF-α was linked to CD4$^+$ T cell populations whereas, as expected, CD8$^+$ T cells did not induce MAP mediated pathology. To be more precise, granuloma formation mediated by CD4$^+$CD45RB$^{lo/int}$ T cells was exclusively detected in MAP infected mice whereas transfer of CD45RB^{hi} cells induced granuloma formation even in the absence of MAP infection, illustrating the potent inflammatory potential of this cell popula-

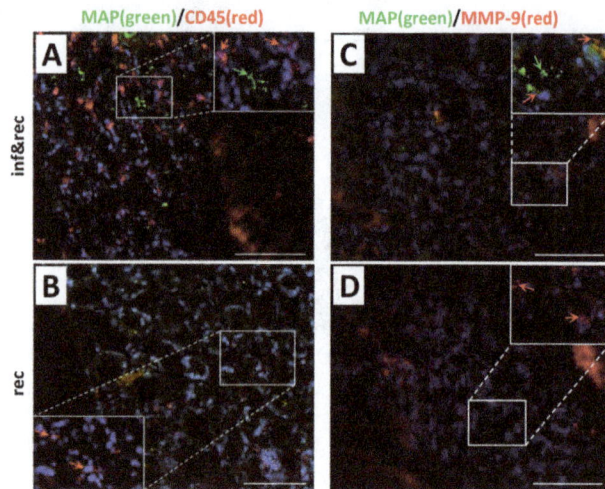

Figure 7. Immunofluorescence staining of murine colon from MAP infected *Rag2*$^{-/-}$ mice reconstituted with CD4$^+$CD45RB$^{lo/int}$ T-cells and in non-infected but reconstituted mice for control. A–B. Samples were stained for MAP (green) and leukocytes (CD45: red). Green arrows indicate colonies of MAP in the epithelium and red arrows indicate leukocytes most likely macrophages. **C–D.** Samples were stained for MAP (green) and MMP-9 (red). Green arrows indicate colonies of intracellular MAP. Red arrows indicate MMP-9 expressing leukocytes. In reconstituted and non-infected mice no MAP clusters could be detected and showed a normal histology of colon mucosa. Magnification 200x&1000x, bar = 100 µm. Blue staining in all samples: DAPI. The data are representative from 4 mice per group and the experiment was carried out at least twice with similar results.

tion, as reported before [16]. Nevertheless, granulomas were clearly increased in numbers and size in mice with both, MAP infection and reconstitution of CD4$^+$CD45RB^{hi} T cells, indicating that MAP infection significantly increases the potential of distinct T cell subpopulations to attract inflammatory cells like macrophages and neutrophils to the site of infection.

As CD4$^+$CD45RB^{hi} T cells apparently exhibited pro-inflammatory properties per se [40], we focused on the effect of CD4$^+$CD45RB$^{lo/int}$ T cells in subsequent analyses. Several markers of inflammation and tissue regeneration and MAP recognition were quantified.

We started off by analyzing expression levels of *TNF-α* and *IL-1β* as broad and potent pro-inflammatory cytokines and the utilized experimental strategy that allowed us to dissect the effects of combined MAP infection and CD4$^+$CD45RB$^{lo/int}$ T cell reconstitution, and of both components (MAP and CD4$^+$CD45RB$^{lo/int}$ T cells) alone on expression of these cytokines. Using this approach, we were able to show that MAP infection and subsequent reconstitution of the CD4$^+$CD45RB$^{lo/int}$ T cell population led to strong induction of *TNF-α* (results for *IL-1β* were not significant). Of note, this increase of *TNF-α* was not observed in mice with MAP infection alone or CD4$^+$CD45RB$^{lo/int}$ T cell reconstitution alone, we take this as evidence that MAP converts the reconstituted CD4$^+$CD45RB$^{lo/int}$ T cells into a pro-inflammatory phenotype. These findings are consistent with data in the literature: elevated *TNF-α* level have been found in several diseases with autoimmune components including rheumatoid arthritis and CD and importantly, in the context of MAP infection, *in vitro* studies demonstrated *TNF-α* secretion by mucosal organ cultures obtained from MAP positive CD patients [32,34].

Based on previous results from our group [41,42] we further chose to quantify *MMPs* and *TIMP-1* which are key enzymes in

the matrix turnover and tissue destruction in inflammatory bowel diseases and also indicate pathogenic relevance during mycobacterial infections [43]. In this regard, previous studies have identified *MMP-9* as a key enzyme during mycobacterial infections [44,45]. Consistent with these data, the observed enhanced expression of *MMP-9* in MAP infected and CD4$^+$CD45RB$^{lo/int}$ T cell reconstituted mice, but not in mice with MAP infection or T cell reconstitution alone, could represent a part of the host immune response towards MAP and might disclose an essential role in mediating mycobacterial pathogenicity [29,46]. Apart from *MMP-9*, we observed an induction of *MMP-13* and *MMP-14* in MAP infected and T cell reconstituted mice. Nevertheless, as we could not observe any tissue destruction by histological examination, the role of induced MMP-expression in the interplay with CD4$^+$CD45RB$^{lo/int}$ T cells is still incomprehensible.

As TLRs play a key role in the recognition of microbe associated molecular patterns and the initiation of an innate immune response towards infectious agents, we further quantified members of the TLR family. Especially *TLR-2* and *TLR-6* have been shown to play an important role in the innate immune response against mycobacterial infections [47–49]. Consistent with reported data on the role of *TLR-6* for the recognition of MAP, we observed a significantly increased expression of *TLR-6* after MAP infection in CD4$^+$CD45RB$^{lo/int}$ T cells reconstituted *Rag2*$^{-/-}$ mice.

In summary and consistent with our hypothesis that both, MAP and T cells are required for the induction of inflammation and tissue pathology, we herein describe the induction of *TNF-α* and tissue destructive proteases only in the presence of MAP and CD4$^+$CD45RB$^{lo/int}$ T cells, but not under conditions where only one of the later factors is present. This might led to the hypothesis that MAP is, upon its recognition by the host, capable to initiate a host response that induces a pro-inflammatory and tissue destructive environment that subsequently might lead to manifest inflammation.

However, within this study, microscopic inflammation was restricted to the colon and despite the presence of inflammatory cells and inflammatory effector molecules, neither macroscopic colonic inflammation was detected nor histologic alterations were observed. It might be argued that the observation period after T cell reconstitution was not long enough for the development of macroscopic inflammation. Also, it is conceivable that a further "hit" such as genetic predisposition is necessary for the manifestation of full macroscopic colitis and that MAP and induction of cytokines by MAP represent a potent trigger in this setting. Clearly, these issues have to be addressed in the future and the approach presented here may provide a suitable animal model.

Further, MAP was not always detected in colonic tissue by immunohistochemistry and PCR. Thus, even in the absence of high bacterial burden, MAP infection prompted transferred CD4$^+$ T cells particularly to inflammation and the formation of granulomas in liver tissue. This finding may be interesting in the context of the role of MAP in CD patients that show great variability in the detection rate of MAP in a number of recent studies.

In conclusion, we present an infection model that allows the analysis of the MAP induced stimulation and pro-inflammatory activity of CD4$^+$ T cells. Following systemic infection, we observed significant signs of systemic infection, granuloma formation within the liver and inflammatory reactions in the colon. In addition viable MAP was cultured from inflamed tissue and the MAP-induced inflammatory potential of T cell subpopulations was evaluated. All signs of inflammation such as increase in spleen weight and granuloma formation in the liver were linked to CD4$^+$ T cells. Our work reveals new mechanisms by which MAP induces inflammatory responses dependent on T-cell activity and might ultimately contribute to a better understanding of the role of MAP in chronic inflammatory disorders providing the basis for further investigations.

Supporting Information

Figure S1 Complete experiments of the panels shown in Figure 4 including all controls. MAP infected and CD4$^+$CD45RB$^{lo/int}$ T cell reconstituted (Inf&Rec) $Rag2^{-/-}$ mice. Control of $Rag2^{-/-}$ mice reconstituted with CD4$^+$CD45RB^{hi} T cells not infected with MAP. $Rag2^{-/-}$ mice infected with MAP and reconstituted with CD4$^+$CD45RB^{hi} T cells. All controls are shown. Arrow heads point at the granulomatous structures. Adoptive transfer of CD8$^+$ T cells after MAP infection did not lead to formation of granulomatous structures. Bars depict 100 μm. The data are representative from 4 mice per group and the experiments were carried out at least twice with similar results. (JPG)

Table S1 Primers for qRT-PCR. Table S1 presents ordering informations about the Quiagen primers used for qRT-PCR.

Table S2 Infection status at sacrifice. Analytical methods and MAP infection status at sacrifice for subgroups infected with MAP (IHC immunohistochemistry, n.a. not analysed, rec./inf. reconstituted and infected).

Author Contributions

Conceived and designed the experiments: ER RG MH SW. Performed the experiments: AK IB AS MR AT TR GG SW. Analyzed the data: AK IB AS MR AT TR GG SW. Contributed reagents/materials/analysis tools: GG RG. Wrote the paper: AK IB MH RG SW ER.

References

1. Abraham C, Cho JH (2009) Inflammatory bowel disease. N Engl J Med 361: 2066–2078.
2. El-Zaatari FA, Osato MS, Graham DY (2001) Etiology of Crohn's disease: the role of Mycobacterium avium paratuberculosis. Trends Mol Med 7: 247–252.
3. Abubakar I, Myhill D, Aliyu SH, Hunter PR (2008) Detection of Mycobacterium avium subspecies paratuberculosis from patients with Crohn's disease using nucleic acid-based techniques: a systematic review and meta-analysis. Inflamm Bowel Dis 14: 401–410.
4. Behr MA, Kapur V (2008) The evidence for Mycobacterium paratuberculosis in Crohn's disease. Curr Opin Gastroenterol 24: 17–21.
5. Feller M, Huwiler K, Stephan R, Altpeter E, Shang A, et al. (2007) Mycobacterium avium subspecies paratuberculosis and Crohn's disease: a systematic review and meta-analysis. Lancet Infect Dis 7: 607–613.
6. Kirkwood CD, Wagner J, Boniface K, Vaughan J, Michalski WP, et al. (2009) Mycobacterium avium subspecies paratuberculosis in children with early-onset Crohn's disease. Inflamm Bowel Dis 15: 1643–1655.
7. Rath T, Roderfeld M, Blocher S, Rhode A, Basler T, et al. (2011) Presence of intestinal Mycobacterium avium subspecies paratuberculosis (MAP) DNA is not associated with altered MMP expression in ulcerative colitis. BMC Gastroenterol 11: 34.
8. Grant IR (2005) Zoonotic potential of Mycobacterium avium ssp. paratuberculosis: the current position. J Appl Microbiol 98: 1282–1293.
9. Zurbrick BG, Czuprynski CJ (1987) Ingestion and intracellular growth of Mycobacterium paratuberculosis within bovine blood monocytes and monocyte-derived macrophages. Infect Immun 55: 1588–1593.
10. Waddell LA, Rajic A, Sargeant J, Harris J, Amezcua R, et al. (2008) The zoonotic potential of Mycobacterium avium spp. paratuberculosis: a systematic review. Can J Public Health 99: 145–155.
11. Momotani E, Whipple DL, Thiermann AB, Cheville NF (1988) Role of M cells and macrophages in the entrance of Mycobacterium paratuberculosis into domes of ileal Peyer's patches in calves. Vet Pathol 25: 131–137.
12. Ponnusamy D, Periasamy S, Tripathi BN, Pal A (2013) Mycobacterium avium subsp. paratuberculosis invades through M cells and enterocytes across ileal and jejunal mucosa of lambs. Res Vet Sci 94: 306–312.
13. Valentin-Weigand P, Goethe R (1999) Pathogenesis of Mycobacterium avium subspecies paratuberculosis infections in ruminants: still more questions than answers. Microbes Infect 1: 1121–1127.
14. Zhao BY, Czuprynski CJ, Collins MT (1999) Intracellular fate of Mycobacterium avium subspecies paratuberculosis in monocytes from normal and infected, interferon-responsive cows as determined by a radiometric method. Can J Vet Res 63: 56–61.
15. Over K, Crandall PG, O'Bryan CA, Ricke SC (2011) Current perspectives on Mycobacterium avium subsp. paratuberculosis, Johne's disease, and Crohn's disease: a review. Crit Rev Microbiol 37: 141–156.
16. Buergelt CD, Hall C, McEntee K, Duncan JR (1978) Pathological evaluation of paratuberculosis in naturally infected cattle. Vet Pathol 15: 196–207.
17. Oettinger MA, Schatz DG, Gorka C, Baltimore D (1990) RAG-1 and RAG-2, adjacent genes that synergistically activate V(D)J recombination. Science 248: 1517–1523.
18. Birkedal-Hansen H, Moore WG, Bodden MK, Windsor LJ, Birkedal-Hansen B, et al. (1993) Matrix metalloproteinases: a review. Crit Rev Oral Biol Med 4: 197–250.
19. McQuibban GA, Gong JH, Wong JP, Wallace JL, Clark-Lewis I, et al. (2002) Matrix metalloproteinase processing of monocyte chemoattractant proteins generates CC chemokine receptor antagonists with anti-inflammatory properties in vivo. Blood 100: 1160–1167.
20. Rath T, Roderfeld M, Graf J, Roeb E (2009) [Matrix metalloproteinases in inflammatory bowel disease - from basic research to clinical significance]. Z Gastroenterol 47: 758–769.
21. Woessner JF, Jr. (1994) The family of matrix metalloproteinases. Ann N Y Acad Sci 732: 11–21.
22. Trowbridge IS, Thomas ML (1994) CD45: an emerging role as a protein tyrosine phosphatase required for lymphocyte activation and development. Annu Rev Immunol 12: 85–116.
23. Powrie F, Leach MW, Mauze S, Caddle LB, Coffman RL (1993) Phenotypically distinct subsets of CD4+ T cells induce or protect from chronic intestinal inflammation in C. B-17 scid mice. Int Immunol 5: 1461–1471.
24. Asseman C, Read S, Powrie F (2003) Colitogenic Th1 cells are present in the antigen-experienced T cell pool in normal mice: control by CD4+ regulatory T cells and IL-10. J Immunol 171: 971–978.
25. Kuehnel MP, Goethe R, Habermann A, Mueller E, Rohde M, et al. (2001) Characterization of the intracellular survival of Mycobacterium avium ssp. paratuberculosis: phagosomal pH and fusogenicity in J774 macrophages compared with other mycobacteria. Cell Microbiol 3: 551–566.
26. Logar K, Kopinc R, Bandelj P, Staric J, Lapanje A, et al. (2012) Evaluation of combined high-efficiency DNA extraction and real-time PCR for detection of Mycobacterium avium subsp. paratuberculosis in subclinically infected dairy cattle: comparison with faecal culture, milk real-time PCR and milk ELISA. BMC Vet Res 8: 49.
27. Livak KJ, Schmittgen TD (2001) Analysis of relative gene expression data using real-time quantitative PCR and the 2(-Delta Delta C(T)) Method. Methods 25: 402–408.
28. Pfaffl MW (2001) A new mathematical model for relative quantification in real-time RT-PCR. Nucleic Acids Res 29: e45.
29. Roderfeld M, Koc A, Rath T, Blocher S, Tschuschner A, et al. (2012) Induction of matrix metalloproteinases and TLR2 and 6 in murine colon after oral exposure to Mycobacterium avium subsp. paratuberculosis. Microbes Infect 14: 545–553.
30. Ehlers S, Benini J, Held HD, Roeck C, Alber G, et al. (2001) Alphabeta T cell receptor-positive cells and interferon-gamma, but not inducible nitric oxide synthase, are critical for granuloma necrosis in a mouse model of mycobacteria-induced pulmonary immunopathology. J Exp Med 194: 1847–1859.
31. Hogan LH, Heninger E, Elsner RA, Vonderheid HA, Hulseberg P, et al. (2007) Requirements for CD4(+) T cell levels in acute Mycobacterium bovis strain bacille Calmette Guerin (BCG)-induced granulomas differ for optimal mycobacterial control versus granuloma formation. Int Immunol 19: 627–633.
32. Clancy R, Ren Z, Turton J, Pang G, Wettstein A (2007) Molecular evidence for Mycobacterium avium subspecies paratuberculosis (MAP) in Crohn's disease correlates with enhanced TNF-alpha secretion. Dig Liver Dis 39: 445–451.
33. Reimund JM, Wittersheim C, Dumont S, Muller CD, Kenney JS, et al. (1996) Increased production of tumour necrosis factor-alpha interleukin-1 beta, and interleukin-6 by morphologically normal intestinal biopsies from patients with Crohn's disease. Gut 39: 684–689.
34. Sibartie S, Scully P, Keohane J, O'Neill S, O'Mahony J, et al. (2010) Mycobacterium avium subsp. Paratuberculosis (MAP) as a modifying factor in Crohn's disease. Inflamm Bowel Dis 16: 296–304.
35. Brew K, Dinakarpandian D, Nagase H (2000) Tissue inhibitors of metalloproteinases: evolution, structure and function. Biochim Biophys Acta 1477: 267–283.
36. Gomez DE, Alonso DF, Yoshiji H, Thorgeirsson UP (1997) Tissue inhibitors of metalloproteinases: structure, regulation and biological functions. Eur J Cell Biol 74: 111–122.
37. Ferwerda G, Kullberg BJ, de Jong DJ, Girardin SE, Langenberg DM, et al. (2007) Mycobacterium paratuberculosis is recognized by Toll-like receptors and NOD2. J Leukoc Biol 87: 1011–1018.
38. Takeuchi O, Kawai T, Muhlradt PF, Morr M, Radolf JD, et al. (2001) Discrimination of bacterial lipoproteins by Toll-like receptor 6. Int Immunol 13: 933–940.

39. Mutwiri GK, Butler DG, Rosendal S, Yager J (1992) Experimental infection of severe combined immunodeficient beige mice with Mycobacterium paratuberculosis of bovine origin. Infect Immun 60: 4074–4079.

40. Mutwiri GK, Rosendal S, Kosecka U, Yager JA, Perdue M, et al. (2002) Adoptive transfer of BALb/c mouse splenocytes reduces lesion severity and induces intestinal pathophysiologic changes in the Mycobacterium avium Subspecies paratuberculosis beige/scid mouse model. Comp Med 52: 332–341.

41. Rath T, Roderfeld M, Graf J, Wagner S, Vehr AK, et al. (2006) Enhanced expression of MMP-7 and MMP-13 in inflammatory bowel disease: a precancerous potential? Inflamm Bowel Dis 12: 1025–1035.

42. Rath T, Roderfeld M, Halwe JM, Tschuschner A, Roeb E, et al. (2010) Cellular sources of MMP-7, MMP-13 and MMP-28 in ulcerative colitis. Scand J Gastroenterol 45: 1186–1196.

43. Quiding-Jarbrink M, Smith DA, Bancroft GJ (2001) Production of matrix metalloproteinases in response to mycobacterial infection. Infect Immun 69: 5661–5670.

44. Basu S, Pathak S, Pathak SK, Bhattacharyya A, Banerjee A, et al. (2007) Mycobacterium avium-induced matrix metalloproteinase-9 expression occurs in a cyclooxygenase-2-dependent manner and involves phosphorylation- and acetylation-dependent chromatin modification. Cell Microbiol 9: 2804–2816.

45. Dezzutti CS, Swords WE, Guenthner PC, Sasso DR, Wahl LM, et al. (1999) Involvement of matrix metalloproteinases in human immunodeficiency virus type 1-induced replication by clinical Mycobacterium avium isolates. J Infect Dis 180: 1142–1152.

46. Chang JC, Wysocki A, Tchou-Wong KM, Moskowitz N, Zhang Y, et al. (1996) Effect of Mycobacterium tuberculosis and its components on macrophages and the release of matrix metalloproteinases. Thorax 51: 306–311.

47. Bulut Y, Faure E, Thomas L, Equils O, Arditi M (2001) Cooperation of Toll-like receptor 2 and 6 for cellular activation by soluble tuberculosis factor and Borrelia burgdorferi outer surface protein A lipoprotein: role of Toll-interacting protein and IL-1 receptor signaling molecules in Toll-like receptor 2 signaling. J Immunol 167: 987–994.

48. Plain KM, Purdie AC, Begg DJ, de SK, Whittington RJ (2010) Toll-like receptor (TLR)6 and TLR1 differentiation in gene expression studies of Johne's disease. Vet Immunol Immunopathol 137: 142–148.

49. Ryffel B, Fremond C, Jacobs M, Parida S, Botha T, et al. (2005) Innate immunity to mycobacterial infection in mice: critical role for toll-like receptors. Tuberculosis (Edinb) 85: 395–405.

Permissions

List of Contributors

Florian Beigel, Matthias Deml, Fabian Schnitzler, Simone Breiteneicher, Burkhard Göke and Stephan Brand
Department of Medicine II, University Hospital Munich-Grosshadern, Ludwig-Maximilians-University, Munich, Germany

Thomas Ochsenkühn
Isarmedizin Zentrum, Munich, Germany

Zhi-Feng Zhang, Gang Zhao, Lei Zhu and Li-Xia Wang
Department of Gastroenterology, The First Affiliated Hospital of Dalian Medical University, Dalian, China

Ning Yang
Department of Nephrology, The First Affiliated Hospital of Dalian Medical University, Dalian, China

Anupa Kamat and Dana Gabuzda
Department of Cancer Immunology and AIDS, Dana Farber Cancer Institute, Harvard Medical School, Boston, Massachusetts, United States of America

Petronela Ancuta
Departement de Microbiologie et Immunologie, Centre de Recherche du Centre Hospitalier de l'Universite de Montreal (CRCHUM) Universite de Montreal and INSERM Unit 743, Montreal, Quebec, Canada

Richard S. Blumberg
Department of Medicine, Brigham and Women's Hospital, Harvard Medical School, Boston, Massachusetts, United States of America

Anne Phillips, Jason A. Hackney and Yan Ma
Department of Bioinformatics and Computational Biology, Genentech Inc, South San Francisco, California, United States of America

Svetlana Pidasheva and Hilary F. Clark
Department of Bioinformatics and Computational Biology, Genentech Inc, South San Francisco, California, United States of America
Department of Immunology, Genentech Inc, South San Francisco, California, United States of America

Sara Trifari, Sue J. Sohn and Hergen Spits
Department of Immunology, Genentech Inc, South San Francisco, California, United States of America

Timothy W. Behrens
ITGR Biomarker Discovery Group, Genentech Inc, South San Francisco, California, United States of America

Ashley Smith and Lee Honigberg
ITGR Early Development, Genentech Inc, South San Francisco, California, United States of America

Nico Ghilardi
Department of Immunology, Genentech Inc, South San Francisco, California, United States of America
Department of Molecular Biology, Genentech Inc, South San Francisco, California, United States of America

Randall D. Little
Genizon BioSciences, Inc., St. Laurent, Quebec, Canada

Xiangmin Jiao and Wei Zhu
Department of Applied Mathematics and Statistics, Stony Brook University, Stony Brook, New York, United States of America

Tianyi Zhang
Department of Applied Mathematics and Statistics, Stony Brook University, Stony Brook, New York, United States of America
Department of Medicine, Stony Brook University, Stony Brook, New York, United States of America

Robert A. DeSimone
Department of Medicine, Stony Brook University, Stony Brook, New York, United States of America

Ellen Li
Department of Medicine, Stony Brook University, Stony Brook, New York, United States of America
Department of Medicine, Washington University-St. Louis School of Medicine, Saint Louis, Missouri, United States of America

F. James Rohlf
Department of Ecology and Evolution, Stony Brook University, Stony Brook, New York, United States of America

Qing Qing Gong, Themistocles Dassopoulos and Rodney D. Newberry
Department of Medicine, Washington University-St. Louis School of Medicine, Saint Louis, Missouri, United States of America

Steven R. Hunt
Department of Surgery, Washington University-St. Louis School of Medicine, Saint Louis, Missouri, United States of America

Erica Sodergren and George Weinstock
The Genome Institute, Washington University-St. Louis School of Medicine, Saint Louis, Missouri, United States of America

Charles E. Robertson
Department of Molecular, Cellular and Developmental Biology, University of Colorado, Boulder, Colorado, United States of America

Daniel N. Frank
Department of Medicine, University of Colorado, Aurora, Colorado, United States of America

Hong Yang and Jiaming Qian
Department of Gastroenterology, Peking Union Medical College Hospital, Beijing, China

Yumei Li, Qingwen Sun, Hongbo Lv, Qing Xia and Haihua Li
Department of Gastroenterology, Daqing Longnan Hospital, Daqing, China

Wei Wu
Department of Gastroenterology, Daqing Oilfield General Hospital, Daqing, China

Yunzhong Zhang
Department of Gastroenterology, Daqing People Hospital, Daqing, China

Wei Zhao
Department of Gastroenterology, Daqing Fourth Hospital, Daqing, China

Pinjin Hu
Department of Gastroenterology, The First Affiliated Hospital of Sun Yat-sen University, Guangzhou, China

Zenaida P. Lopez-Dee, Bhumi Patel, Rebecca Stanton, Michelle Wakeley, Brittany Lippert, Anastasya Menaker, Bethany Eiche, Robert Terry and Linda S. Gutierrez
Department of Biology, Wilkes University, Wilkes-Barre, Pennsylvania, United States of America

Sridar V. Chittur
Center for Functional Genomics, University at Albany, State University of New York, Rensselaer, New York, United States of America

Christina M. Hamm
Department of Medicine, Stony Brook University, Stony Brook, New York, United States of America

Ellen Li
Department of Medicine, Stony Brook University, Stony Brook, New York, United States of America

Department of Microbiology and Molecular Genetics, Stony Brook University, Stony Brook, New York, United States of America
Department of Medicine, Washington University, St. Louis, Missouri, United States of America

Tianyi Zhang
Department of Medicine, Stony Brook University, Stony Brook, New York, United States of America
Department of Applied Mathematics and Statistics, Stony Brook University, Stony Brook, New York, United States of America

Hongyan Chen, Xiao Wu and Wei Zhu
Department of Applied Mathematics and Statistics, Stony Brook University, Stony Brook, New York, United States of America

F. James Rohlf
Department of Ecology and Evolution, Stony Brook University, Stony Brook, New York, United States of America

Charles E. Robertson and Norman R. Pace
Department of Molecular, Cellular and Developmental Biology, University of Colorado, Boulder, Colorado, United States of America

Ajay S. Gulati
Department of Pediatrics, University of North Carolina, Chapel Hill, North Carolina, United States of America,

R. Balfour Sartor
Departments of Medicine, Microbiology and Immunology, University of North Carolina, Chapel Hill, North Carolina, United States of America

Edgar C. Boedeker
Department of Medicine, University of New Mexico, Albuquerque, New Mexico, United States of America

Noam Harpaz
Department of Pathology, Mount Sinai School of Medicine, New York, New York, United States of America

Jeffrey Yuan
Department of Medicine, Washington University, St. Louis, Missouri, United States of America

George M. Weinstock and Erica Sodergren
Genome Institute, Washington University, St. Louis, Missouri, United States of America

Chi Gu
Division of Biostatistics, Washington University, St. Louis, Missouri, United States of America

Daniel N. Frank
Department of Medicine, University of Colorado Anschutz Medical Campus, Aurora, Colorado, United States of America

Yazan Ismail, Vikneswari Mahendran, Sophie Octavia, Ruiting Lan, Thi Anh Tuyet Tran and Li Zhang
The School of Biotechnology and Biomolecular Sciences, University of New South Wales, Sydney, Australia

Daniel Lemberg
Department of Gastroenterology, Sydney Children's Hospital, Sydney, Australia

Andrew S. Day
Department of Gastroenterology, Sydney Children's Hospital, Sydney, Australia
School of Women's and Children's Health, University of New South Wales, Sydney, Australia
Department of Paediatrics, University of Otago, Christchurch, New Zealand

Stephen M. Riordan
Gastrointestinal and Liver Unit, The Prince of Wales Hospital, Sydney, Australia
Faculty of Medicine, University of New South Wales, Sydney, Australia

Michael C. Grimm
St. George Clinical School, University of New South Wales, Sydney, Australia

Wei Yu, John P. Hegarty, Ashley A. Kelly, Yunhua Wang, Walter A. Koltun and Zhenwu Lin
Department of Surgery, Pennsylvania State University, Hershey, Pennsylvania, United States of America

Arthur Berg
Center for Statistical Genetics, Department of Public Health Sciences, Pennsylvania State University, Hershey, Pennsylvania, United States of America

Lisa S. Poritz
Department of Surgery, Pennsylvania State University, Hershey, Pennsylvania, United States of America
Department of Cellular & Molecular Physiology, Pennsylvania State University, Hershey, Pennsylvania, United States of America

Xi Chen
Department of Biostatistics, Vanderbilt University, Nashville, Tennessee, United States of America

Gail West
Department of Pathobiology, Lerner Research Institute, the Cleveland Clinic Foundation, Cleveland, Ohio, United States of America

Tina Zupancic and Apolonija Bedina-Zavec
National Institute of Chemistry, Ljubljana, Slovenia

Radovan Komel and Mirjana Liovic
National Institute of Chemistry, Ljubljana, Slovenia
Medical Centre for Molecular Biology, Faculty of Medicine, University of Ljubljana, Ljubljana, Slovenia

Jure Stojan
Medical Centre for Molecular Biology, Faculty of Medicine, University of Ljubljana, Ljubljana, Slovenia

Ellen Birgitte Lane
Institute of Medical Biology, Immunos, Singapore

Øystein Brenna, Arne K. Sandvik and Björn I. Gustafsson
Department of Gastroenterology and Hepatology, St. Olavs Hospital, Trondheim University Hospital, Trondheim, Norway
Department of Cancer Research and Molecular Medicine, Norwegian University of Science and Technology, Trondheim, Norway

Marianne W. Furnes, Atle van Beelen Granlund, Arnar Flatberg and Rosalie T. M. Zwiggelaar
Department of Cancer Research and MolecularMedicine, Norwegian University of Science and Technology, Trondheim, Norway

Ignat Drozdov
Bering Limited, Richmond, United Kingdom

Ronald Mårvik
Department of Cancer Research and MolecularMedicine, Norwegian University of Science and Technology, Trondheim, Norway
Department of Gastrointestinal Surgery, St. Olavs Hospital, Trondheim University Hospital, Trondheim, Norway

Ivar S. Nordrum
Department of Cancer Research and MolecularMedicine, Norwegian University of Science and Technology, Trondheim, Norway
Department of Pathology and Medical Genetics, St. Olavs Hospital, Trondheim University Hospital, Trondheim, Norway

Mark Kidd
Department of Surgery, Section of Gastroenterology,
Yale School of Medicine, New Haven, Connecticut,
United States of America

Pinyi Lu and Josep Bassaganya-Riera
Genetics, Bioinformatics, and Computational Biology
Program, Virginia Tech, Blacksburg, Virginia, United
States of America,
Nutritional Immunology and Molecular Medicine
Laboratory, Virginia Bioinformatics Institute, Blacksburg,
Virginia, United States of America
Center for Modeling Immunology to Enteric Pathogens,
Virginia Bioinformatics Institute, Blacksburg, Virginia,
United States of America

Raquel Hontecillas
Nutritional Immunology and Molecular Medicine
Laboratory, Virginia Bioinformatics Institute, Blacksburg,
Virginia, United States of America
Center for Modeling Immunology to Enteric Pathogens,
Virginia Bioinformatics Institute, Blacksburg, Virginia,
United States of America

David R. Bevan
Genetics, Bioinformatics, and Computational Biology
Program, Virginia Tech, Blacksburg, Virginia, United
States of America
Department of Biochemistry, Virginia Tech, Blacksburg,
Virginia, United States of America
Center for Modeling Immunology to Enteric Pathogens,
Virginia Bioinformatics Institute, Blacksburg, Virginia,
United States of America

Stephanie N. Lewis
Genetics, Bioinformatics, and Computational Biology
Program, Virginia Tech, Blacksburg, Virginia, United
States of America
Department of Biochemistry, Virginia Tech, Blacksburg,
Virginia, United States of America
Nutritional Immunology and Molecular Medicine
Laboratory, Virginia Bioinformatics Institute, Blacksburg,
Virginia, United States of America
Center for Modeling Immunology to Enteric Pathogens,
Virginia Bioinformatics Institute, Blacksburg, Virginia,
United States of America

Lera Brannan
Department of Biochemistry, Virginia Tech, Blacksburg,
Virginia, United States of America

Amir J. Guri
Nutritional Immunology and Molecular Medicine
Laboratory, Virginia Bioinformatics Institute, Blacksburg,
Virginia, United States of America

**Saroj K. Mohapatra, Amir J. Guri, Montse Climent,
Cristina Vives, Adria Carbo, William T. Horne, Raquel
Hontecillas and Josep Bassaganya-Riera**
Nutritional Immunology and Molecular Nutrition
Laboratory, Virginia Bioinformatics Institute, Virginia
Polytechnic Institute and State University, Blacksburg,
Virginia, United States of America

Ian Holmes
Department of Bioengineering, University of California,
Berkeley, California, United States of Americ

Keith Harris and Christopher Quince
School of Engineering, University of Glasgow, Glasgow,
United Kingdom

**Andreas Jenke, Gundula Wenzel, Jan Postberg,
Andreas Heusch and Stefan Wirth**
Department of Paediatrics, HELIOS Klinikum Wuppertal,
Germany

Matthias Zilbauer
Department of Paediatrics, HELIOS Klinikum
Wuppertal, Germany
Department of Paediatric Gastroenterology,
Addenbrooke's Hospital, Cambridge, United Kingdom

**Gabriele Noble-Jamieson, Franco Torrente, Camilla
Salvestrini and Robert Heuschkel**
Department of Paediatric Gastroenterology,
Addenbrooke's Hospital, Cambridge, United Kingdom

Alan D. Phillips
Centre for Paediatric Gastroenterology, Royal Free
Hospital, London, United Kingdom

**Luc Biedermann, Pascal Frei, Michael Scharl, Michael
Fried and Gerhard Rogler**
Division of Gastroenterology and Hepatology,
University Hospital Zurich, Zurich, Switzerland

Jonas Zeitz
Division of Internal Medicine, University Hospital
Zurich, Zurich,Switzerland

Jessica Mwinyi
Division of Gastroenterology and Hepatology,
University Hospital Zurich, Zurich, Switzerland
Division of Clinical Pharmacology and Toxicology,
University Hospital Zurich, Zurich, Switzerland

**Eveline Sutter-Minder, Markus Schuppler and
Martin J. Loessner**
Institute of Food, Nutrition and Health, ETH Zurich,
Zurich, Switzerland

Ateequr Rehman
Institute of Clinical Molecular Biology, Christian Albrechts University of Kiel, Kiel, Germany

Stephan J. Ott and Stefan Schreiber
Institute of Clinical Molecular Biology, Christian Albrechts University of Kiel, Kiel, Germany
Division of General Internal Medicine, University Hospital Schleswig-Holstein, Kiel, Germany

Claudia Steurer-Stey and Anja Frei
Institute of General Practice, University of Zurich, Zurich, Switzerland
Smoking Consulting Programme, University Hospital Zurich, Zurich, Switzerland

Stephan R. Vavricka
Division of Gastroenterology and Hepatology, University Hospital Zurich, Zurich, Switzerland
Division of Gastroenterology and Hepatology, Hospital Triemli, Zurich, Switzerland

Hany H. Arab
Department of Biochemistry, Faculty of Pharmacy, Cairo University, Cairo, Egypt

Muhammad Y. Al-Shorbagy, Dalaal M. Abdallah and Noha N. Nassar
Department of Pharmacology and Toxicology, Faculty of Pharmacy, Cairo University, Cairo, Egypt

Rikard Damen, Martin Haugen, Bernhard Svejda, Daniele Alaimo and Mark Kidd
Gastrointestinal Pathobiology Research Group, Yale University School of Medicine, New Haven, Connecticut, United States of America

Oystein Brenna and Bjorn I. Gustafsson
Department of Cancer Research and Molecular Medicine, Norwegian University of Science and Technology, Trondheim, Norway

Roswitha Pfragner
Institute of Pathophysiology and Immunology, Centre for Molecular Medicine, Graz, Austria

Tiago Nunes, Maria Josefina Etchevers, Susana Pinó Donnay, Maria Pellisé, Julián Panés and Elena Ricart
Department of Gastroenterology, Hospital Clinic of Barcelona (IDIBAPS/Centro de Investigació Bioméica en Red de Enfermedades Hepáicas y Digestivas [CIBEREHD]), Barcelona, Catalonia, Spain

Maria Jose Sandi, Juan Lucio Iovanna and Jean-Charles Dagorn
Centre de Recherche en Cancérologie de Marseille (CRCM), INSERM U1068, CNRS UMR 7258, Aix-Marseille Université and Institut Paoli- Calmettes, Parc Scientifique et Technologique de Luminy, Marseille, France

Teddy Grandjean and Mathias Chamaillard
University Lille Nord de France, F-59000, Lille, France
Institut Pasteur de Lille, Center for Infection and Immunity of Lille, F-59019, Lille, France
Centre National de la Recherche Scientifique, UMR8204, F-59021, Lille, France
Institut National de la Santéet de la Recherche Médicale, U1019, Team 7, Equipe FRM, F 59019, Lille, France

Miquel Sans
Department of Digestive Diseases, Centro Medico Teknon, Barcelona, Catalonia, Spain

Arzu Koc, Martin Roderfeld, Annette Tschuschner and Elke Roeb
Justus-Liebig-University Giessen, Department of Gastroenterology, Giessen, Germany

Imke Bargen, Abdulhadi Suwandi and Siegfried Weiss
Helmholtz Centre for Infection Research, Molecular Immunology, Braunschweig, Germany

Timo Rath
Justus-Liebig-University Giessen, Department of Gastroenterology, Giessen, Germany
Medical Clinic 1, Friedrich-Alexander University Erlangen-Nuernberg, Erlangen, Germany

Gerald F. Gerlach
IVD GmbH, Hannover, Germany

Mathias Hornef
Department of Microbiology, Hannover Medical School, Hannover, Germany

Ralph Goethe
Institute for Microbiology, Department of Infectious Diseases, University of Veterinary Medicine Hannover, Hannover, Germany

Index

www.ingramcontent.com/pod-product-compliance
Lightning Source LLC
Chambersburg PA
CBHW080534200326
41458CB00012B/4430